AF443153

MEDICINE MEETS VIRTUAL REALITY 15

Studies in Health Technology and Informatics

This book series was started in 1990 to promote research conducted under the auspices of the EC programmes' Advanced Informatics in Medicine (AIM) and Biomedical and Health Research (BHR) bioengineering branch. A driving aspect of international health informatics is that telecommunication technology, rehabilitative technology, intelligent home technology and many other components are moving together and form one integrated world of information and communication media. The complete series has been accepted in Medline. Volumes from 2005 onwards are available online.

Series Editors:
Dr. J.P. Christensen, Prof. G. de Moor, Prof. A. Famili, Prof. A. Hasman, Prof. L. Hunter,
Dr. I. Iakovidis, Dr. Z. Kolitsi, Mr. O. Le Dour, Dr. A. Lymberis, Prof. P.F. Niederer,
Prof. A. Pedotti, Prof. O. Rienhoff, Prof. F.H. Roger France, Dr. N. Rossing,
Prof. N. Saranummi, Dr. E.R. Siegel, Dr. P. Wilson, Prof. E.J.S. Hovenga,
Prof. M.A. Musen and Prof. J. Mantas

Volume 125

Recently published in this series

ISSN 0926-9630

Medicine Meets Virtual Reality 15

in vivo, in vitro, in silico: Designing the Next in Medicine

Edited by

James D. Westwood

Randy S. Haluck MD FACS

Helene M. Hoffman PhD

Greg T. Mogel MD

Roger Phillips PhD CEng FBCS CIPT

Richard A. Robb PhD

and

Kirby G. Vosburgh PhD

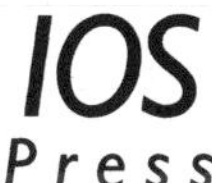

IOS
Press

Amsterdam • Berlin • Oxford • Tokyo • Washington, DC

ISBN 978-1-58603-713-0
Library of Congress Control Number: 2006939763

Publisher
IOS Press
Nieuwe Hemweg 6B
1013 BG Amsterdam
Netherlands
fax: +31 20 687 0019
e-mail: order@iospress.nl

Distributor in the UK and Ireland
Gazelle Books Services Ltd.
White Cross Mills
Hightown
Lancaster LA1 4XS
United Kingdom
fax: +44 1524 63232
e-mail: sales@gazellebooks.co.uk

Distributor in the USA and Canada
IOS Press, Inc.
4502 Rachael Manor Drive
Fairfax, VA 22032
USA
fax: +1 703 323 3668
e-mail: iosbooks@iospress.com

Medicine Meets Virtual Reality 15
J.D. Westwood et al. (Eds.)
IOS Press, 2007

v

Preface

in vivo, in vitro, in silico:
Designing the Next in Medicine

James D. WESTWOOD and Karen S. MORGAN
Aligned Management Associates, Inc.

Our culture is obsessed with design. Magazines, television, and websites publicize current trends in clothing, architecture, home furnishings, automobiles, and more. We design objects to convey ideas about wealth, status, age, gender, education, politics, religion, accomplishment, and aspiration. Design seems mysteriously vital to our well-being, like sleep and dreaming.

Sometimes designers can fuse utility and fantasy to make the mundane appear fresh—a cosmetic repackaging of the same old thing. Because of this, medicine—grounded in the unforgiving realities of the scientific method and peer review, and of flesh, blood, and pain—can sometimes confuse "design" with mere "prettifying."

Design solves real problems, however. It reshapes material, image, and data into something more useful than was previously available. It addresses challenges of increasing complexity and data overload. It simplifies tasks to reduce confusion and error. It accelerates adoption and training by making new tools more intuitive to use. It comforts clinicians as well as patients by giving engineering a friendly interface.

This year's theme acknowledges the importance of design—currently and as an opportunity—within the MMVR community.

in vivo. We design machines to explore our living bodies. Imaging devices, robots, and sensors move constantly inward, operating within smaller dimensions: system, organ, cell, DNA. Resolution and sensitivity are increasing. Our collaboration with these machines is burdened by vast quantities of input and output data. Physician to machine to patient to machine to physician and back again: it's a crowded information highway prone to bottlenecks, misinterpreted signals, and collisions. Out of necessity, we design ways to visualize, simplify, communicate, and understand complex biomedical data. These can be as basic as color-coding or as advanced as Internet2. In our measurement and manipulation of health, the design of information is critical.

in vitro. Using test tubes and Petri dishes, we isolate *in vivo* to better manipulate and measure biological conditions and reactions. The bold new field of tissue engineering, for example, relies on creating an imitation metabolic system for growing artificial body parts. Scientists carefully design the scaffolding to which cells will group themselves on their own. The artificial guides nature's path inside a glass container as we strive to improve what nature gives us.

in silico. We step out of the controlled *in vitro* environment and into a virtual reality. The silica mini-worlds of test tubes and Petri dishes are translated into mini-worlds contained within silicon chips. In the *in silico* lab, algorithms replace chemicals and proteins in the quest for new drugs. On a different scale, we design simulations of biological systems to serve as educational tools. A simulated human body improves learning by utilizing intuition, repetition, and objective assessment. In surgical training, we are replacing patients with computers, in part because the latter is less susceptible to pain and less likely to hire a lawyer.

The future of medicine remains within all three environments: *in vivo*, *in vitro*, and *in silico*. Design is what makes these pieces fit together—the biological, the informational, the physical/material—into something new and more useful.

And what is the next in medicine? We cannot say, but we hope it offers solutions to the very real challenges that are now upon us: an aging global population; disparities between rich and developing nations; epidemic, disaster, and warfare; and limited economic and natural resources. We are eager to see what new tools are designed to confront these old problems, each involving medicine in some way.

We are thankful to all who have made MMVR15 possible and that, after fifteen years, MMVR remains a place where so many talented, visionary, and hardworking individuals share their research to design the next in medicine.

MMVR15 Proceedings Editors

James D. Westwood
MMVR15 Program Coordinator
Aligned Management Associates, Inc.

Randy S. Haluck MD FACS
Associate Professor of Surgery
Chief, Minimally Invasive Surgery and Bariatrics
Penn State, Hershey Medical Center

Helene M. Hoffman PhD
Assistant Dean, Educational Computing
Adjunct Professor of Medicine
Division of Medical Education
School of Medicine
University of California, San Diego

Greg T. Mogel MD
Associate Professor of Radiology and Biomedical Engineering
Keck School of Medicine/Viterbi School of Engineering
University of Southern California

Roger Phillips PhD CEng FBCS CIPT
Research Professor, Simulation & Visualization Group
Director, Hull Immersive Visualization Environment (HIVE)
Department of Computer Science
University of Hull (UK)

Richard A. Robb PhD
Scheller Professor in Medical Research
Professor of Biophysics & Computer Science
Director, Mayo Biomedical Imaging Resource
Mayo Clinic College of Medicine

Kirby G. Vosburgh PhD
Associate Director, Center for Integration of Medicine and
Innovative Technology (CIMIT)
Brigham and Women's Hospital
Harvard Medical School

MMVR15 Organizing Committee

Michael J. Ackerman PhD
Office of High Performance Computing & Communications,
National Library of Medicine

Ian Alger MD
New York Presbyterian Hospital;
Weill Medical College of Cornell University

David C. Balch MA
DCB Consulting LLC

Steve Charles MD
MicroDexterity Systems;
University of Tennessee

Patrick C. Cregan FRACS
Nepean Hospital,
Wentworth Area Health Service

Henry Fuchs PhD
Dept of Computer Science,
University of North Carolina

Walter J. Greenleaf PhD
Greenleaf Medical Systems

Randy S. Haluck MD FACS
Dept of Surgery,
Penn State College of Medicine

David M. Hananel
Surgical Programs,
Medical Education Technologies Inc.

Wm. LeRoy Heinrichs MD PhD
Medical Media & Information Technologies/
Gynecology & Obstetrics,
Stanford University School of Medicine

Helene M. Hoffman PhD
School of Medicine,
University of California, San Diego

Heinz U. Lemke PhD
Institute for Technical Informatics,
Technical University Berlin

Alan Liu PhD
National Capital Area Medical Simulation Center,
Uniformed Services University

Greg T. Mogel MD
Keck School of Medicine/Viterbi School of Engineering,
University of Southern California

Kevin N. Montgomery PhD
National Biocomputation Center,
Stanford University

Makoto Nonaka MD PhD
Foundation for International Scientific Advancement

Roger Phillips PhD CEng FBCS CIPT
Dept of Computer Science,
University of Hull (UK)

Carla M. Pugh MD PhD
Center for Advanced Surgical Education,
Northwestern University

Richard A. Robb PhD
Mayo Biomedical Imaging Resource,
Mayo Clinic College of Medicine

Jannick P. Rolland PhD
College of Optics and Photonics,
University of Central Florida

Richard M. Satava MD FACS
Dept of Surgery,
University of Washington

Rainer M.M. Seibel MD
Inst of Diagnostic & Interventional Radiology,
University of Witten/Herdecke

Steven Senger PhD
Dept of Computer Science,
University of Wisconsin – La Crosse

Ramin Shahidi PhD
Image Guidance Laboratories,
Stanford University School of Medicine

Don Stredney
Interface Laboratory,
OSC

Julie A. Swain MD
Cardiovascular and Respiratory Devices,
U.S. Food and Drug Administration

Robert M. Sweet MD
Dept of Urology,
University of Minnesota

Kirby G. Vosburgh PhD
CIMIT/Brigham & Women's Hospital/
Harvard Medical School

Dave Warner MD PhD
Biodesign Institute/Decision Theater,
Arizona State University;
MindTel LLC; Inst for Interventional Informatics

Suzanne J. Weghorst MA MS
Human Interface Technology Lab,
University of Washington

Mark D. Wiederhold MD PhD FACP
The Virtual Reality Medical Center

Patricia Youngblood PhD
Medical Media & Information Technologies,
Stanford University School of Medicine

Contents

Medicine Meets Virtual Reality 15
J.D. Westwood et al. (Eds.)
IOS Press, 2007

1

Burrhole Simulation for an Intracranial Hematoma Simulator

Eric ACOSTA [a,1], Alan LIU [a], Rocco ARMONDA [b], Mike FIORILL [c],
Randy HALUCK [c], Carol LAKE [c], Gilbert MUNIZ [a], and Mark BOWYER [a]

[a] *The National Capital Area Medical Simulation Center, Uniformed Services University*
[b] *National Capital Neurosurgery Consortium, National Naval Medical Center*
[c] *Verefi Technologies, Inc.*

Abstract. Traumatic head injuries can cause internal bleeding within the brain. The resulting hematoma can elevate intracranial pressure, leading to complications and death if left untreated. A craniotomy may be required when conservative measures are ineffective. To augment conventional surgical training, a Virtual Reality-based intracranial hematoma simulator is being developed. A critical step in performing a craniotomy involves cutting burrholes in the skull. This paper describes volumetric-based haptic and visual algorithms developed to simulate burrhole creation for the simulator. The described algorithms make it possible to simulate several surgical tools typically used for a craniotomy.

Keywords. Surgical simulation, bone drilling, volume rendering, haptic feedback

Introduction

Head trauma commonly occurs on the battlefield. Resulting brain injuries and bleeding can elevate intracranial pressure, leading to complications and death if not treated. Training for head injury treatment is difficult to come by under battlefield conditions. Neurosurgery is a specialized skill that requires extensive training. Current training occurs on live patients. A surgical simulator can augment current training methods so trainees become proficient at the required surgical skills before working on the first patient. A craniotomy may be required for treatment when conservative measures are ineffective. This procedure involves removing a section of the skull in order to gain access to the brain. We are developing a Virtual Reality-based training simulator to practice this skill. A haptic workbench [9] is used to generate a virtual environment with 3D stereoscopic visual and haptic feedback. Surgical tools are controlled with a haptic device. The workbench allows the visual and haptic workspaces to be co-registered to preserve hand-eye coordination for surgical training. An important step of a craniotomy involves cutting burrholes in the skull using powered tools. This paper describes volumetric haptic, bone erosion, and visual algorithms developed to simulate bone cutting tools for the simulator.

The remainder of the paper is as follows. Section 1 describes the haptic rendering algorithm used in the simulator. Section 2 provides details of our method for computing

---

[1] Correspondence to: Eric Acosta, http://simcen.usuhs.mil; E-mail: eacosta@simcen.usuhs.mil.

bone erosion. Section 3 documents the visual rendering algorithms. Section 4 shows several surgical tools simulated with the described algorithms and the paper is concluded in Section 5.

1. Haptic rendering

A modified Voxmap point-shell algorithm [5,7] is created to simulate haptic interactions between bone cutting tools and bone. The original method used to compute force feedback in [5] and [7] can introduce considerable force discontinuities at voxel boundaries. We address the stability of the Voxmap point-shell haptic algorithm by modifying its surface boundary detection and force feedback calculation methods.

The haptic rendering algorithm represents a virtual environment using a spatial occupancy map called a voxmap. Bone is encoded within the voxmap using voxels. Each voxel encodes the bone density, density gradient vector, and color at its location. The tool bits are modeled as a set of haptic points that are spatially distributed to define the bits' shapes and sizes. The haptic points form a "point-shell" that approximates the surface of a tool bit. Each haptic point stores its position relative to the tool bit's center and an inward pointing tool normal that is used for calculating a collision force. The spatial positioning of the haptic points impacts force calculation [7]. To ensure even and symmetric point distributions, the positions and tool normals of haptic points are computed based on either a spherical or a cylindrical approximation of a tool bit. Several parameters, such as tool radius, height, and voxel size etc., help generate point-shells for bits of different shapes and sizes. Figure 1a shows the point-shell of a perforator and a round bit. The number of haptic points created for a tool bit is also controlled using the parameters.

Collisions between the haptic device and the virtual environment are checked by probing the voxmap with the haptic points. A collision occurs when a haptic point in-

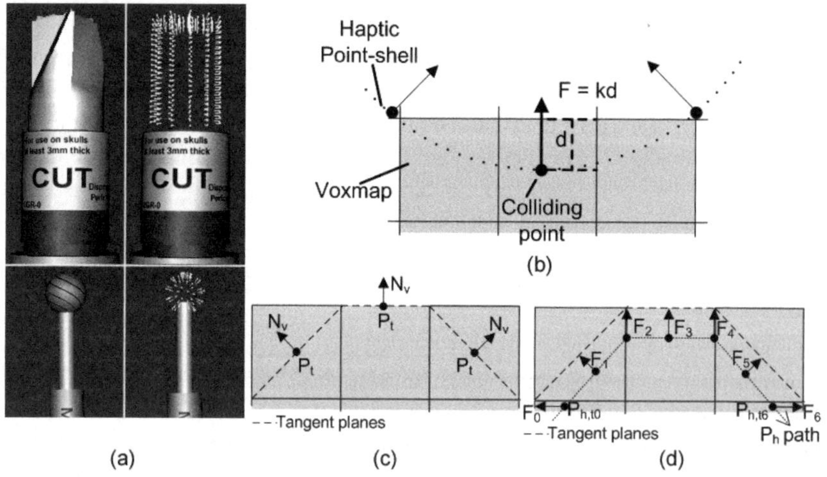

Figure 1. (a) Haptic point-shell approximations for a perforator bit (316 haptic points) and round bit (72 haptic points). (b) Point-shell interaction with a voxmap. (c) N_v and P_t used to construct "tangent planes" for force calculations. P_t placed on voxel boundary when exactly one facet exposed to surface, and at voxel center otherwise. (d) The force, F, for a haptic point, P_h, as it follows the bone's surface.

tersects a voxel with a density value greater than zero. A force is calculated for each colliding haptic point based on Hooke's law $F = kd$, where k is a stiffness constant and d is the point's penetration depth within the bone's surface. Figure 1b illustrates.

To help locate the surface for a haptic point, its tool normal is followed at voxel-sized intervals until a voxel with a non-zero gradient is encountered. The surface is then located by sampling along the gradient direction. Since bone material is stiff, little penetration is expected, and only a few samples are normally required. To avoid rendering artifacts, a threshold on the number of samples (e.g. 10 samples) is imposed. A haptic point is ignored if the bone's surface cannot be found within the set number of samples. In [5,7], voxels are labeled as interior, surface, or free. Since bone material is removed while drilling, a surface detection algorithm would be required in our case to dynamically update voxels' status. Instead, the currently sampled non-empty voxel is considered to be a surface voxel when the next voxel along the sampling vector has a zero density value.

Once a surface voxel is located, a "tangent plane" is constructed to compute d. With the original Voxmap point-shell algorithm, a force discontinuity can occur at every voxel for a haptic point whose tool normal is not perpendicular to the surface [5,7]. The discontinuities occur because the tangent plane's orientation and the computed force is based on the tool normal direction and not the surface's shape. We use the surface gradient to instead construct a plane perpendicular to the surface normal and to apply a force normal to the surface. A voxel returns a point, P_t, which lies on the tangent plane. P_t is placed on the voxel's surface boundary when exactly one facet is exposed. P_t is a voxel's center point in all other cases. Figure 1c is an example. Equation 1 is used to compute d as the distance from the haptic point (P_h) to the tangent plane. N_v is a voxel's unit gradient vector. The value of d is set to zero if the haptic point is above the plane. A haptic point's force is then computed in the direction of N_v with equation 2. The resultant force for the haptic device is the average of the colliding haptic points' forces.

$$d = (P_t - P_h) \cdot N_v \tag{1}$$

$$F = N_v kd \tag{2}$$

As shown in Figure 1d, force discontinuities are reduced by allowing a haptic point to transition across voxel boundaries. Additionally, voxels on curved surfaces or corners are smoothed out to reduce the "stair-step" feeling that is typical of voxel-based haptic interactions.

2. Bone drilling

Many existing bone drilling methods, such as [2] and [6], combine the voxel sampling methods required for haptics and bone erosion. This works well for spherical drill bits since all areas can cut bone. To model different types of tool bits, we separate the haptic and bone erosion sampling points.

A set of erosion points are generated to simulate the bone drilling capabilities of tools. Haptic points are only required along a tool bit's surface to compute a force response, as described in Section 1. However, it is necessary to generate interior and surface erosion points to prevent leaving residual bone material behind when the tool bit penetrates the bone's surface. Erosion points are generated by voxelizing either a sphere or cylinder. An erosion point is generated for each voxel whose center point falls within the boundaries of the chosen primitive shape, as shown in Figure 2. Parameters, such as tool radius, height, and voxel size etc., help control the size and shape of the tool bit. Erosion points store their position relative to the tool bit's center and an erosion factor that determines the amount of bone it can remove based on the rotational speed of the bit. An erosion point's position is based on the center point of its corresponding voxel during primitive voxelization. The erosion factor can be precomputed based on any erosion model. Different tool bits can be modeled by varying the erosion factor value, based on its position within a bit, to define areas that can/cannot remove bone and/or remove bone at different rates. For example, a perforator's cutting surface is restricted to its blades, whereas a ball bit has a spherical cutting surface. Interior points also erode bone faster than surface points to remove bone quicker as a surgeon applies more force with a tool.

A collision between the tool bit and bone material is detected when an erosion point intersects a voxel with a non-zero density value. The bone density at the colliding voxel (B_v) is reduced according to equation 3, where e is the point's erosion factor and s is the tool bit's rotational speed. The value of B_v is set to zero once it falls below a minimum threshold. A bounding box within the voxmap is tracked as bone density values are modified. The gradient values for the voxels within the bounding box are updated once all erosion points are processed. The bone material is also visually updated.

$$B_v' = B_v(1.0 - e \times s) \qquad\qquad (3)$$

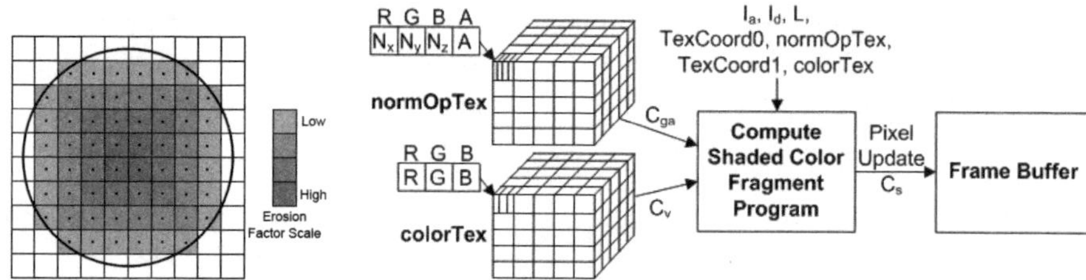

Figure 2. Erosion points generated by voxelizing tool bit shape. Voxels are color coded according to erosion factor.

Figure 3. RGBA normal/opacity map, RGB color texture, texture coordinates, and lighting parameters used by GPU fragment program to generate shaded color values.

3. Visual rendering

Three-dimensional texture-based volume rendering [3] is used for real-time visual display of bone. A fragment program [4] is created to compute volumetric shading on the video card's GPU as the volume is rendered. The program generates shaded color values that become pixels in the rendered frame buffer image, Figure 3. A fragment program can perform mathematical operations on the values stored within texture maps. Texture coordinates are used to access the color values within textures. This texture sampling capability makes it possible to compute the ambient and diffuse lighting to shade the volume. The following algorithm is implemented in the fragment program to shade voxels as they are rendered:

1. Get voxel color (C_v) by sampling colorTex.
2. Get voxel gradient and opacity (C_{ga}) from normOpTex and assign opacity to output color's (C_s) alpha component.
3. Compute shaded RGB components for C_s using the light model: $(I_a \times C_v) + (I_d \times C_v \times max(N \cdot L))$, where I_a is the ambient intensity, I_d the diffuse intensity, L the light vector, and N the surface normal acquired by expanding the gradient vector of C_{ga} with Equation 5.

The surface normal is estimated using the bone density gradient. The volume's gradient is stored in a special texture called normal map. Equation 4 is used to range compress normalized gradient vectors from a [-1.0, 1.0] range to an unsigned color value range of [0.0, 1.0] in order to encode the vectors into the normal map. The fragment program expands the range-compressed normals with Equation 5.

$$C = (0.5 \times N) + 0.5 \tag{4}$$

$$N = 2.0 \times (C - 0.5) \tag{5}$$

An opacity map is used to control the visibility of voxels. The voxels' opacity values are taken from the bone density values. Voxel opacity values are reduced while drilling until they become transparent due to bone erosion. The opacity and normal maps are updated when the volume is modified while drilling. To minimize texture updates, both maps are combined into a single RGBA three-dimensional texture, Figure 3. A sub-texture is used to only update values that fall within a modified bounding box region, which is tracked by the bone drilling algorithm. Color information for the bone is specified using a second RGB texture. The two textures and their texture coordinates are simultaneously specified to the fragment program using multi-texturing [8]. The lighting values are specified to the fragment program as input parameters.

4. Virtual tool simulation

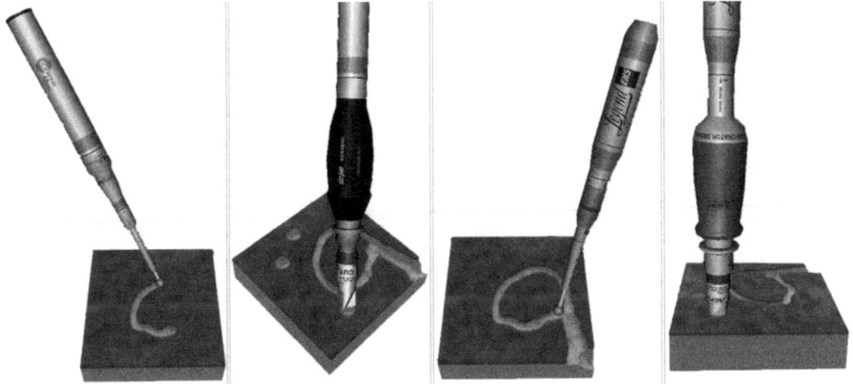

Figure 4. 3D models of tools typically used in clinical practice. (Left) Bone drill and perforator from Stryker. (Right) Bone drill and perforator from Medtronic.

The described algorithms make it possible to simulate several surgical tools, such as bone drills and perforators, typically used for a craniotomy. A haptic workbench [9] is used to generate a virtual environment with 3D stereoscopic visual and haptic feedback. Figure 4 shows realistic 3D models that are created from real surgical tools and controlled by a PHANTOM haptic device during their use.

5. Conclusion

A simulator can be a vital tool to help train for the difficulties and complications surrounding intracranial hematoma surgery. We have taken the first steps towards creating a simulator by developing the algorithms needed to simulate virtual tools for making burrholes. The generality of the methods used to model the tool bits and bit-bone interactions will make it possible for additional virtual tools to be simulated. The algorithms have been demonstrated for drilling on voxelized blocks. However, it will be possible to generate the voxmap directly from the voxel discretization of 3D CT and MR datasets to generate different virtual patients for a surgical simulator. Development of other surgical effects is also underway for the simulator.

Acknowledgments

We would like to thank Penny Christian from Medtronic and Jason Martin from Stryker for lending us the sets of surgical tools used to model the virtual tools.

This work is supported by the U.S. Army Medical Research and Materiel Command under Contract No. W81WH-05-C-0142. The views, opinions and/or findings contained in this report are those of the author(s) and should not be construed as an official Department of the Army position, policy or decision unless so designated by other documentation.

References

[1]　R.J. Adams and B. Hannaford. Stable haptic interaction with virtual environments. *IEEE Transactions on Robotics and Automation*, **15**(3), (1999), 465–474.

[2]　M. Agus, A. Giachetti, E. Gobbetti, G. Zanetti, and A. Zorcolo. Real-time haptic and visual simulation of bone dissection. *Presence*, **12**(1), (2003), 110–122.

[3]　K. Engel and M. Hadwiger and J. Kniss and et al. High-quality volume graphics on consumer PC hardware. *SIGGRAPH Course Notes*, (2002).

[4]　R. Fernando and M.J. Kilgard. *The Cg Tutorial*, Addison-Wesley, 2003.

[5]　W.A. McNeely, K. D. Puterbaugh, and J. J. Troy. Six degree-of-freedom haptic rendering using voxel sampling. *ACM SIGGRAPH*, (1999), 401–408.

[6]　D. Morris, C. Sewell, N. Blevins, F. Barbagli, and K. Salisbury. A collaborative virtual environment for the simulation of temporal bone surgery. *Medical Image Computing and Computer-Aided Intervention*, (2004).

[7]　M. Renz, C. Preusche, M. Potke, H.P. Kriegel, and G. Hirzinger. Stable Haptic interaction with virtual environments using an adapted voxmap-pointshell algorithm. *Eurohaptics*, (2001), 149–154.

[8]　D. Shreiner, M. Woo, J. Neider, and T. Davis. *OpenGL Programming Guide, Fourth Edition*, Addison-Wesley, 2004.

[9]　D. Stevenson, K. Smith, J. Mclaughlin, C. Gunn, and et al. Haptic workbench: A multisensory virtual environment. *PIE Stereoscopic Displays and Virtual Reality Systems VI*, **3639**, (1999), 356–366.

Medicine Meets Virtual Reality 15
J.D. Westwood et al. (Eds.)
IOS Press, 2007

Cranial Implant Design Using Augmented Reality Immersive System

Zhuming AI [a,1], Ray EVENHOUSE [a], Jason LEIGH [b], Fady CHARBEL [c], and Mary RASMUSSEN [a]

[a] *Virtual Reality in Medicine Lab*
Department of Biomedical and Health Information Sciences
University of Illinois at Chicago
1919 W. Taylor St, AHP, MC 530
Chicago, IL 60612
[b] *Electronic Visualization Lab*
University of Illinois at Chicago
851 S. Morgan St., MC 152, 1120 SEO
Chicago, IL 60607
[c] *Department of Neurosurgery*
University of Illinois at Chicago
912 South Wood Street (MC 799)
Chicago, IL 60612

Abstract. Software tools that utilize haptics for sculpting precise fitting cranial implants are utilized in an augmented reality immersive system to create a virtual working environment for the modelers. The virtual environment is designed to mimic the traditional working environment as closely as possible, providing more functionality for the users. The implant design process uses patient CT data of a defective area. This volumetric data is displayed in an implant modeling tele-immersive augmented reality system where the modeler can build a patient specific implant that precisely fits the defect. To mimic the traditional sculpting workspace, the implant modeling augmented reality system includes stereo vision, viewer centered perspective, sense of touch, and collaboration. To achieve optimized performance, this system includes a dual-processor PC, fast volume rendering with three-dimensional texture mapping, the fast haptic rendering algorithm, and a multi-threading architecture. The system replaces the expensive and time consuming traditional sculpting steps such as physical sculpting, mold making, and defect stereolithography. This augmented reality system is part of a comprehensive tele-immersive system that includes a conference-room-sized system for tele-immersive small group consultation and an inexpensive, easily deployable networked desktop virtual reality system for surgical consultation, evaluation and collaboration. This system has been used to design patient-specific cranial implants with precise fit.

Keywords. Implant Design, Virtual Reality, Augmented Reality, Haptic Rendering

---

[1]Corresponding Author: Zhuming Ai; E-mail: zai@uic.edu.

Introduction

Many different reasons, such as disease, accident, crime, and war, may cause large cranial defects. A technique for cranial implant design using patient CT data has been developed by Dujovny and Evenhouse et al., which builds patient-specific implants.[1] This method generates a computer polygonal model of the skull and defect from the patient's CT data, and a physical model of the skull with defect is built after the model is exported to a stereolithography machine. Using this model as a template, the implant is designed and fabricated using wax to sculpt the missing tissue. A mold is made to cast the implant. Although this method results in patient specific implants with near perfect fit, it is expansive and time-consuming.

Scharver and Evenhouse et al.[2] has developed a system to design cranial implant in a virtual environment. The system uses surface modeling, and the sculpting component was preliminary.

We have created software tools that utilize haptics for sculpting precise fitting cranial implants.[3] These tools use a haptic rendering algorithm[4] directly on patient CT data to provide a sense of touch, which is as crucial in virtual sculpting as in traditional physical sculpting. Our new approach replaced the expensive and time-consuming steps in the traditional sculpting methods.

In this paper, these tools are utilized in an augmented reality immersive system to create a virtual working environment for the modelers. The virtual environment is designed to mimic the traditional working environment as closely as possible, providing more functionality for the users.

1. Methods

To mimic the traditional sculpting workspace, the implant modeling augmented reality system includes stereo vision, viewer centered perspective, sense of touch, and collaboration. The Personal Augmented Reality Immersive System (PARIS^{TM})[5] developed at the Electronic Visualization Laboratory (EVL), University of Illinois at Chicago (UIC) has all these required features, and it is used in our study.

The implant design process uses patient CT data of a defective area. This volumetric data is displayed in an implant modeling tele-immersive augmented reality system where the modeler can build a patient specific implant that precisely fits the defect.

1.1. Augmented Reality Immersive System

Augmented Reality combines the real world with computer generated images. In our study, it allows the modeler to see his/her own hands immersed in the computer generated models and virtual sculpting tools.

The PARIS system used in this study (Fig. 1) is an augmented reality device with a $5' \times 4'$ screen that uses a DLP projector to display three-dimensional stereo images with a 1400×1050 pixel resolution. A half-silvered mirror mounted at an

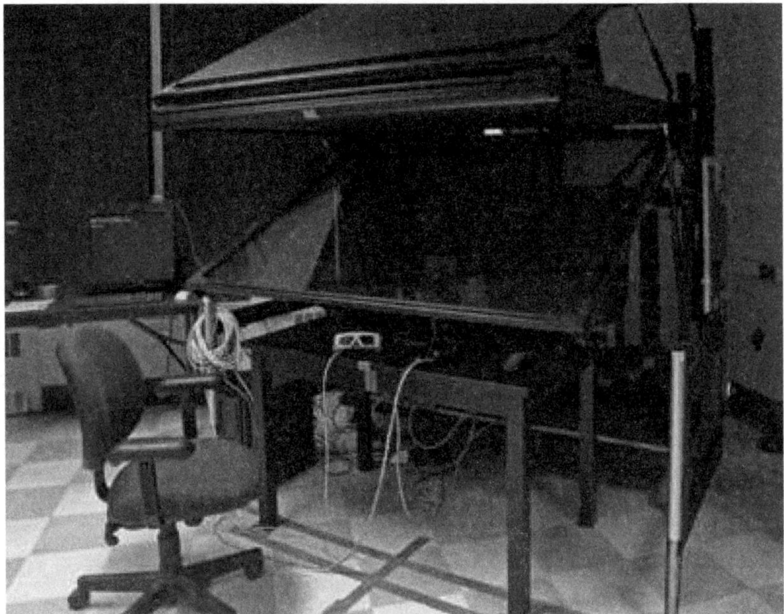

Figure 1. The Personal Augmented Reality Immersive System installed at the Virtual Reality in Medicine Lab (VRMedLab), UIC.

angle in front of the modeler prevents the computer generated image from being blocked by the user's hands. This not only provides augmented reality but also avoids an important stereo vision depth perception conflict.

The system uses trackers to follow the movement of the viewer's head and hand, so that it can generate stereo images from the viewer's perspective and let the user interact with the data directly in three-dimensions. A SensAble Technologies PHANTOM®desktop haptic device[6] is mounted on a desk in PARIS to provide sense of touch.

A Linux PC is used to drive the PARIS system. The PC controls two display devices at the same time; one is the projector on the PARIS, and the other is an ordinary monitor. With this dual-display configuration, we can separate the two-dimensional user interface, such as menus, buttons, dialogs, etc., from the three-dimensional working environment to avoid the complex, and often less effective, three-dimensional user interface programming.

1.2. Implant Design with PARIS

The sculpting software uses the haptic rendering algorithm we have developed[4] to provide the sense of touch. The algorithm is a proxy-based force feedback algorithm applied directly on volumetric data. It is accurate, and the force feedback from the volumetric data is calculated in real-time. The software tools we have developed[3] are used in the sculpting software to do the sculpting. CaveLib^{TM}[7] is used to interface with the tracking and the rendering system. The Visualization Toolkit (VTK)[8] is used for visualization, SensAble Technologies

OpenHaptics^{TM}Toolkit[9] is used for haptic rendering, and GTK[10] is used for user interface programming.

A hardware-assisted three-dimensional texture mapping based fast volume rendering algorithm has been implemented to render the patient CT data as well as the implant. The algorithm can render a CT data set of the scull at the speed of about 30 frames per second.

The speed of the volume rendering is a very important issue in this application. Latency between the visual feedback and the haptic feedback may make the user feel disconnected, so it is crucial to minimize it in virtual reality applications. Usually, 10 frames per second is considered real-time or interactive in computer graphics applications. In this application, 20 frames per second is necessary to make the latency between the visual feedback and the haptic feedback unnoticeable.

Both volume rendering and haptic rendering are processing intensive. To achieve optimized performance, this system includes a dual-processor PC, nVidia's high performance graphics card, fast volume rendering with three-dimensional texture mapping, the fast haptic rendering algorithm, and a multi-threading architecture. A rendering thread updates the stereo display of the volumetric data at nearly 30 frames/second. A haptic rendering thread calculates the force feedback at 1 kHz rate. And a much slower user interface thread handles the user commands. Patient CT data, implant data, and transformation matrices need to be shared among threads. A mutual exclusion algorithm (mutex) locking mechanism has been carefully designed to avoid data access conflicts. The result is an augmented reality system that has no noticeable latency between visual feedback and haptic feedback.

2. Results

The Augmented Reality Immersive System has been designed and built to design patient-specific cranial implants. The software application has been developed to provide medical modelers a working environment mimicking the traditional workspace. It includes viewer centered perspective, three-dimensional stereo vision, sense of touch, and augmented reality (the computer generated data lies in the same space as user's hands). The system replaces the expensive and time consuming traditional sculpting steps such as physical sculpting, mold making, and defect stereolithography.

Figure 2 shows that a researcher is designing a implant using the augmented reality immersive system.

3. Discussion and Conclusion

This augmented reality system is part of a comprehensive tele-immersive system that includes a conference-room-sized system for tele-immersive small group consultation and an inexpensive, easily deployable networked desktop virtual reality system for surgical consultation, evaluation and collaboration.

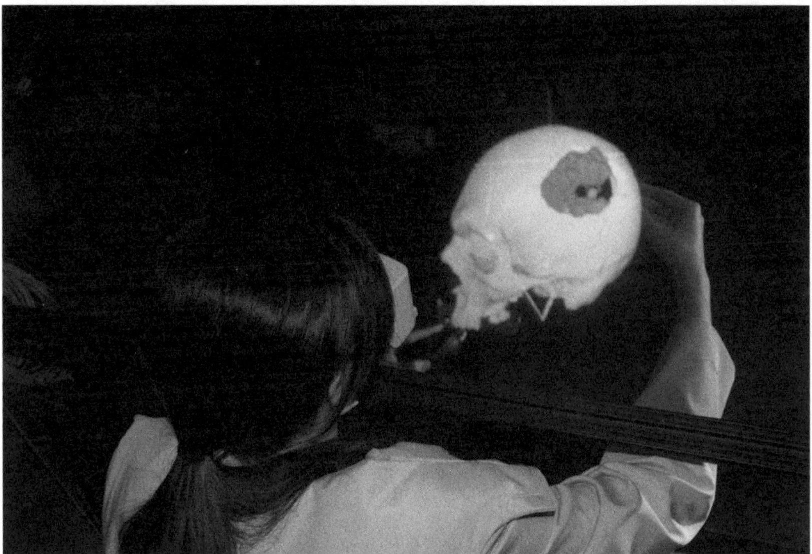

Figure 2. Cranial implant design using PARIS.

This system has been used to design patient-specific cranial implants with precise fit.

Acknowledgments

This publication was made possible by Grant Number N01-LM-3-3507 from the National Library of Medicine/National Institutes of Health.

References

[1] M. Dujovny, R. Evenhouse, C. Agner, F.T. Charbel, Sadler L., and D. McConathy. Preformed prosthesis from computed tomography data: Repair of large calvarial defects. In Benzel E.C. Rengachary SR, editor, *Calvarial and Dural Reconstructuion*, pages 77–88. American Association of Neurological Surgeons, Park Ridge, Ill, 1999.

[2] C. Scharver, R. Evenhouse, A. Johnson, and J. Leigh. Designing cranial implants in a haptic augment reality environment. *Communications of the ACM*, 27(8):32–38, August 2004.

[3] Zhuming Ai, R Evenhouse, J Leigh, F Charbel, and M Rasmussen. New tools for sculpting cranial implants in a shared haptic augmented reality environment. *Stud Health Technol Inform.*, 119:7–12, 2006.

[4] Zhuming Ai, Ray Evenhouse, and Mary Rasmussen. Haptic rendering of volumetric data for cranial implant modeling. In *The 27th Annual International Conference of the IEEE Engineering in Medicine and Biology Society*, Shanghai, China, Sept 2005.

[5] A. Johnson, D. Sandin, G. Dawe, Z. Qiu, S. Thongrong, and D. Plepys. Developing the paris: Using the cave to prototype a new vr display. In *CDROM Proceedings of IPT 2000: Immersive Projection Technology Workshop*, Ames, IA, Jun 2000.

[6] http://www.sensable.com/haptic-phantom-desktop.htm.

[7]   C. Cruz-Neira, D. J. Sandin, and T. A. DeFanti. Surround-screen projection-based virtual reality: The design and implementation of the CAVE. In *Proc. Siggraph 93*, pages 135–142, New York, 1993. ACM Press.

[8]   Will Schroeder, Ken Martin, and Bill Lorensen. *The Visualization Toolkit: An Object-Oriented Approach To 3D Graphics*. Prentice Hall PTR, 1996.

[9]   SensAble Technologies, Inc. *3D Touch SDK - OpenHaptics Toolkit Programmer's Guide*, 1999-2004.

[10] http://www.gtkmm.org.

Medicine Meets Virtual Reality 15
J.D. Westwood et al. (Eds.)
IOS Press, 2007

13

SOFA – an Open Source Framework for Medical Simulation

J. ALLARD [a] S. COTIN [a] F. FAURE [b] P.-J. BENSOUSSAN [b] F. POYER [b]
C. DURIEZ [b] H. DELINGETTE [b] and L. GRISONI [b]
[a] *CIMIT Sim Group - Harvard Medical School*
[b] *INRIA - Evasion, Alcove, and Asclepios teams*

Abstract. SOFA is a new open source framework primarily targeted at medical simulation research. Based on an advanced software architecture, it allows to (1) create complex and evolving simulations by combining new algorithms with algorithms already included in SOFA; (2) modify most parameters of the simulation – deformable behavior, surface representation, solver, constraints, collision algorithm, etc. – by simply editing an XML file; (3) build complex models from simpler ones using a scene-graph description; (4) efficiently simulate the dynamics of interacting objects using abstract equation solvers; and (5) reuse and easily compare a variety of available methods. In this paper we highlight the key concepts of the SOFA architecture and illustrate its potential through a series of examples.

1. Introduction

Computer-based training systems offer an elegant solution to the current need for better training in Medicine, since realistic and configurable training environments can be created. This can bridge the gap between basic training and performing the actual intervention on patients, without any restriction for repetitive training. However, in spite of the impressive developments in the field of medical simulation, some fundamental problems still hinder the acceptance of this valuable technology in daily clinical practice. In particular, the multi-disciplinary aspect of medical simulation requires the integration, within a single environment, of leading-edge solutions in areas as diverse as visualization, biomechanical modeling, haptics or contact modeling. This diversity of problems makes it challenging for researchers to make progress in specific areas, and leads rather often to duplication of efforts.

1.1. Objectives

For the past few years, there have been a few attempts at designing software toolkits for medical simulation. Examples include SPRING [7], GiPSi [3], VRASS [4], or SSTML [1]. These different solutions aim at the same goal: providing an open source answer to the various challenges of medical simulation research and development. Although our aim is identical, we propose a different approach, through a very modular and flexible software framework called SOFA. This open source framework allows independently developed algorithms to interact together within a common simulation while minimizing the development time required for integration.

The main objectives of the SOFA framework are:

- Provide a common software framework for the medical simulation community
- Enable component sharing / exchange and reduce development time
- Promote collaboration among research groups
- Enable validation and comparison of new algorithms
- Help standardize the description of anatomical and biomechanical datasets

Our main overall goal is to develop a flexible framework while minimizing the impact of this flexibility on the computation overhead. To achieve these objectives, we have developed a new architecture that implements a series of concepts described below.

2. The SOFA architecture

The SOFA architecture relies on several innovative concepts, in particular the notion of **multi-model representation**. In SOFA, most simulation components – deformable models, collision models, instruments, etc – can have several representations, connected together through a mechanism called mapping. Each representation can then be optimized for a particular task – e.g. collision detection, visualization – while at the same time improving interoperability by creating a clear separation between the functional aspects of the simulation components. As a consequence, it is possible to have models of very different nature interact together, for instance rigid bodies, deformable objects, and fluids. At a finer level of granularity, we also propose a **decomposition of physical models** – i.e. any model that behaves according to the laws of physics – **into a set of basic components**. This decomposition leads for instance to a representation of mechanical models as a set of degrees of freedom and force fields acting on these degrees of freedom. Another key aspect of SOFA is the **use of a scene-graph to organize and process the elements of a simulation** while clearly separating the computation tasks from their possibly parallel scheduling. These concepts not only characterize SOFA but also provide a mean to address the goals described in section 1.1.

2.1. High-Level Modularity

Any simulation involves, to some extent, the computation of visual feedback, haptic feedback, and interactions between medical devices and anatomical structures. This typically translates into a simulation loop where, at each time step, collisions between objects are detected, deformation and collision response are computed, and the resulting state can be visually and haptically rendered. To perform each of these actions, the various algorithms involved in the simulation rely implicitly on different data structures for the simulated objects. In SOFA we explicitly decompose an object into various representations, in such a way that each representation is more suited toward a particular task – rendering, deformation, or collision detection. Then, these representations are linked together so they can be coherently updated. We call the link between these representations a *mapping*. Various mapping functions can be defined, and each mapping will associate a set of primitives of a representation to a set of primitives in the other representation (see Figure 1). For instance, a mapping can connect degrees of freedom in a Behavior Model to vertices in a Visual Model.

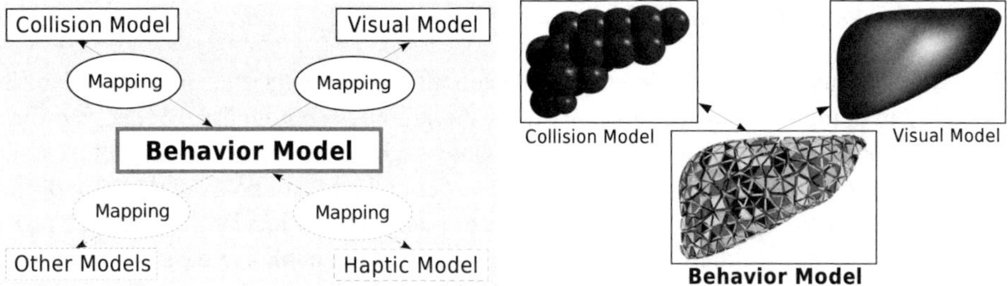

Figure 1. Illustration of the multi-model representation in SOFA. *Left*: possible representations for a simulated object, with the Behavior Model controlling the update of the other representations through a series of mappings. *Right*: examples of these representations for a liver model. Notice how the Visual Model is more detailed than the Behavior Model and how the Collision Model relies on a very different representation.

2.2. Fine Grain Modularity

One of the most challenging aspect of medical simulation is the computation, in real-time, of accurate biomechanical models of soft-tissues. Such models being computationally expensive, many strategies have been used to improve computation times or to reduce the complexity of the original model: linear elastic models have often been used instead of more complex non-linear representations, mass-spring methods as an alternative to finite element methods, etc. Each of these simplifications induces drawbacks, yet the importance of these drawbacks depends largely on the context in which they are applied. It becomes then very difficult to choose which particular method is most likely to provide the best results for a given simulation.

To address this issue in SOFA we have introduced, for the Behavior Model, a finer level of granularity than what is described in section 2.1. This permits for instance to switch from one solver to another in order to see the change in performance or robustness of the simulation, or to test different constitutive models. These changes can be done in a matter of seconds, without having to recompile any of the code, by simply editing an XML file. To achieve this level of flexibility, we have defined a series of generic primitives, or *components*, that are common to most physics-based simulations: `DoF`, `Mass`, `Force Field`, and `Solver`.

The `DoF` component describes the degrees of freedom, and their derivatives, of the object. This includes positions, velocities, accelerations, as well as other auxiliary vectors. The `Mass` component represents the mass of the object. Depending on the model, the mass can be represented by a single value – all the DoFs have the same mass, a vector – the DoFs have a different mass, or even a matrix as used in complex finite element models. The `Force Field` describes both internal forces associated with the constitutive equations of the model, and external forces that can be applied to this object. A variety of forces are currently derived from the abstract Force Field representation, including springs, linear and co-rotationnal FEM [5,6], Mass-Tensor, and Smoothed Particle Hydrodynamics (SPH). The `Solver` component handles the time step integration, i.e. advancing the state of the system from time t to time $t + \Delta t$. To this end, the solver sends requests to the other components to execute operations such as summation of forces, computation of accelerations, and vector operations on the DoFs such as $x = x + v \cdot \Delta t$. Currently SOFA integrates explicit Euler and Runge-Kutta 4 solvers, as well as implicit conjugate-gradient based Euler solver [2].

2.3. Scene Graph Representation

Building and maintaining the relations between all the elements of a simulation can become quite complex. Reusing concepts from the graphics community, we decided for a homogeneous scene-graph representation, where each component is attached to a node of a tree structure. While components are user-defined and can be extended at will, internal nodes are all the same. They only store pointers to their local components, as well as their parent and children nodes. This simple structure enables to easily visit all or a subset of the components in a scene, and dependencies between components are handled by retrieving sibling components attached to the same node. For instance, a `Force Field` component can access the `DoF` component by getting its pointer from the node. The scene-graph can also be dynamically reorganized, allowing for instance the creation of groups of interacting objects. Such groups can then be processed as a unique system of equations by the solver, thus permitting to efficiently handle stiff contact forces. Another advantage of using a scene-graph is that most computations performed in the simulation loop can be expressed as a traversal of the scene-graph. This traversal is called an *action* in SOFA. For instance, at each time step, the simulation state is updated by sending an `Animate` action to all `Solver` components. Each `Solver` then forwards requests to the appropriate components by recursively sending actions within its sub-tree.

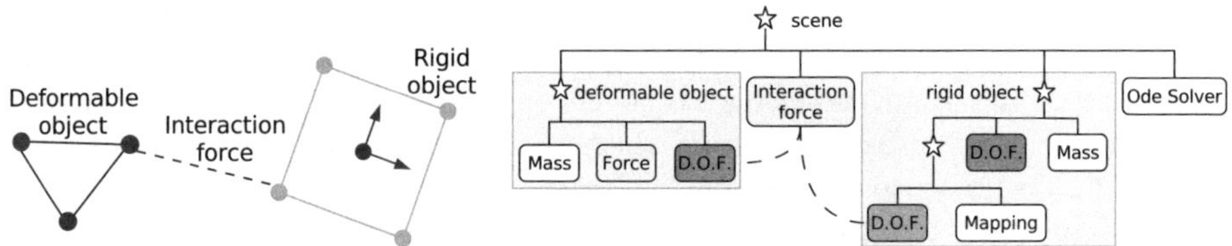

Figure 2. Left: two interacting bodies. The DoFs are shown as circles, and the forces as lines. A solid line describes an internal force, a dotted line an external force. Right: graph associated to the scene on the left. The nodes of the scene-graph, shown as stars, allow to model structured groups of components.

To illustrate the modularity in SOFA and the use of a scene-graph, we consider the example illustrated in Figure 2. In this example, two simulated objects – a rigid square and a simple Mass-Spring model – move through space and eventually collide. To compute the motion and deformation of the objects, we need to define for each of them a set of DoFs and a set of internal and external forces. The `DoF` component of the mass-spring model corresponds to the mass-points, while for the rigid object it corresponds to the position and orientation of the center of mass. This implies different data types for the DoFs of each object – a set of 3D vectors for the mass-spring and a 3D vector with a quaternion for the rigid object. Contacts between objects are possible through Collision Models associated with each object. The Collision Model for the mass-spring object consists of a set of vertices coincident with the DoFs of the object. The Collision Model for the rigid object – the square shape in Figure 2 – is rigidly attached to the body reference frame through a Mapping. The `Mapping` component is responsible for propagating the motion of the rigid body to the vertices of the Collision Model, and when collision occurs, the contact forces applied to the Collision Model are propagated back to the DoFs of the rigid body object. Since the vertices of the Collision Model do not coincide with the DoFs of the rigid object, we attach them to a different node of the scene-graph. However, as their motion is totally defined by the rigid body, they are not independent so this new node is created as a child of the rigid body node. The interaction force acts on the collision model vertices, independently of whether they are actual or mapped DoFs. At this point, actions can be propagated through the scene-graph to simulate both objects as a combined mechanical system.

3. Results

We present here several examples of simulations developed using SOFA. These examples illustrate the diversity and flexibility of the SOFA framework, in particular the ability to have objects with different behavior interact together. We also demonstrate some early results on the validation of algorithms used for simulating deformable structures.

Laparoscopic Simulation: the primary target for SOFA being Medical Simulation, we have developed an early prototype of a laparoscopic simulation system in which the liver and intestines are modeled as deformable models which can be manipulated using a laparoscopic instrument and can collide with the ribs, as illustrated in Figure 3. The modularity of the SOFA architecture allows us to easily experiment different constitutive models for the organs. In this example the liver is modeled as a co-rotational FEM and the intestines as a spring-based FFD grid. The separation between Visual, Collision, and Behavior models allows us to generate visually appealing simulations at interactive rates.

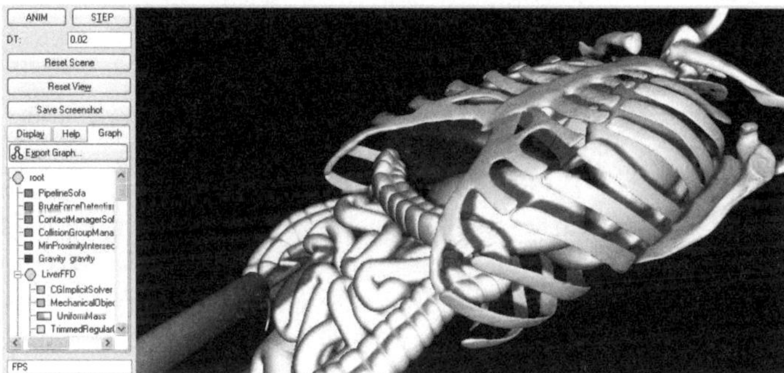

Figure 3. Simulation of laparoscopic surgery using SOFA at interactive rates (about 50Hz).

Quantitative validation and comparison of algorithms: comparing algorithms for soft-tissue deformation only makes sense if they are compared against reference models issued from the real world. To this end, we have built a cylinder using silicon gel of known material properties, and then applied controlled constraints to this object as it was being CT scanned. The resulting surface obtained after image processing is illustrated in Figure 4. This surface was used as a Visual Model to which various Behavior Models were assigned – mass-spring, co-rotational FEM, and linear FEM. It then becomes very easy to visually and quantitatively assess the accuracy of the various models.

Chain Links: handling interactions between heterogenous models is prone to stability issues. To test the robustness of different algorithms we experimented with falling chains where each link uses a different Behavior Model, as illustrated in Figure 5. No constraints between links were pre-defined, instead we relied on collision detection and stiff contact forces to handle the contacts. Using implicit integrator handling dynamically-created groups of interacting objects resulted in a stable simulation.

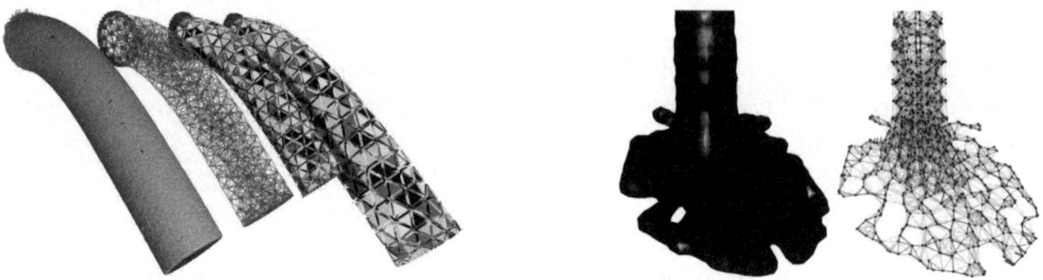

Figure 4. Left: surface of an actual soft cylindrical object compared to a mass-spring, co-rotational FEM, and linear FEM models, under the same constraints. Right: a fluid modeled in SOFA using a SPH method.

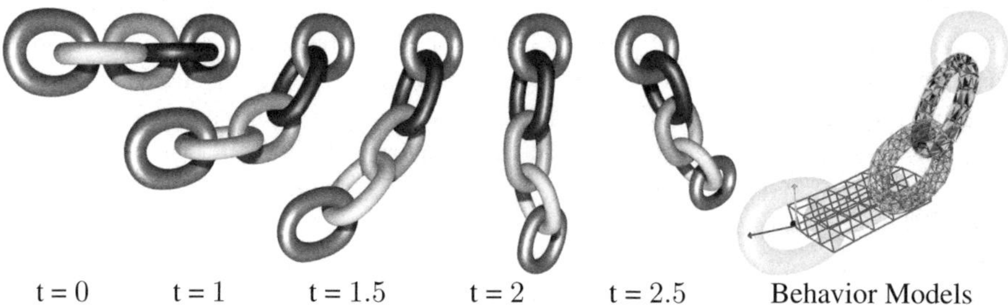

Figure 5. Animation of a chain combining a FEM model, a mass-spring model, a FFD grid, and a rigid body.

4. Conclusion and Future Work

The SOFA framework currently integrates, in the same environment, a variety of different algorithms, from springs and co-rotational FEM models to FFD deformation grids, as well as implicit and explicit solvers, and several collision detection methods, such as continuous or proximity-based algorithms. Our framework also supports hard constraints and stiff interaction forces, using implicit or multi-step explicit integrators that handle dynamically-created groups of interacting objects. Our future work includes the support for multi-processing, topological changes, and haptic feedback. The SOFA web site, *www.sofa-framework.org*, can be visited for more information on our most recent results.

Acknowledgments

We want to thank Sylvere Fonteneau, Damien Marchal, Xunlei Wu, Paul Neumann, Jeremie Dequidt, and Julien Lenoir for their contribution to the development of SOFA.

References

[1]   J. Bacon, N. Tardella, J. Pratt, and J. English. The Surgical Simulation and Training Markup Language: An XML-Based Language for Medical Simulation. In *Proceedings of MMVR*, pages 37–42, 2006.

[2]   D. Baraff and A. Witkin. Large steps in cloth simulation. In *Proceedings of SIGGRAPH*, 1998.

[3]   T. Goktekin, M. Cenk Cavusoglu, and F. Tendick. Gipsi: An open source software development framework for surgical simulation. In *International Symposium on Medical Simulation*, pages 240–248, 2004.

[4]   M. Kawasaki, M. Rissanen, N. Kume, Y. Kuroda, M. Nakao, T. Kuroda, and H. Yoshihara. VRASS (Virtual Reality Aided Simulation). In *www.kuhp.kyoto-u.ac.jp/ mi/research/vrass/index_en.shtml*.

[5]   M. Muller and M. Gross. Interactive virtual materials. In *Graphics Interface'04*, pages 239–246, 2004.

[6]   M. Nesme, Y. Payan, and F. Faure. Efficient, physically plausible finite elements. In *Eurographics*, 2005.

[7]   K. Montgomery *et. al.* Spring: A general framework for collaborative, real-time surgical simulation. In *Proceedings of MMVR*, pages 23–26, 2002.

Medicine Meets Virtual Reality 15
J.D. Westwood et al. (Eds.)
IOS Press, 2007

Integrated Lower Extremity Trauma Simulator

Bruce D. ANDERSON Ph.D.[1], Per NORDQUIST M.S.*, Eva SKARMAN Ph.D.*,
Mark T. BOIES M.S., Gina B. ANDERSON M.S. and David B. CARMACK MD**
*Simulution Inc., Melerit Medical AB*and Eastern Maine Medical Center***

Abstract. Severe limb trauma is prevalent in deployed U.S. Military forces since
the advent of body armor. To improve outcomes, improved pre-deployment
training is urgently needed. To meet this need, Simuluition Inc. and Melerit
Medical AB are expanding the capabilities of the TraumaVision™ Simulator,
originally designed for training surgeons in internal fixation procedures, to include
training in battlefield relevant trauma care for fractured femurs and compartment
syndrome. Simulations are being implemented for fractured femur reduction,
external fixation, measuring intercompartment pressure (ICP), and performing
fasciotomies. Preliminary validation work has begun to demonstrate content and
construct validity of the TraumaVision™ simulator. Future work will include
developing a SCORMs-compliant curriculum and completing the validation
studies.

Keywords. Fractured femur, compartment syndrome, virtual reality, simulation,
medical training.

1. Introduction

Lower extremity trauma can be life threatening, difficult to diagnose and complicated
to treat. With the advent of body armor, the US military has seen a substantial increase
in the number of traumatic limb injuries during recent deployments. To improve
outcomes, there is an urgent need to provide pre-deployment extremity trauma training
to military medical personnel. Improperly treated, severe femur fractures or acute
compartment syndrome can lead to massive hemorrhage, loss of limb or death.

The TraumaVision™ Simulator, a part task trainer for internal fixation of femur
and hip fractures, is being expanded to include training in triage and treatment of
combat relevant extremity trauma. Diagnosis and fracture reduction using the
TraumaVision™ Simulator is performed on a physical model while simulation of
surgical procedures including internal and external fixation, measuring
intercompartment pressure (ICP) and performing fasciotomies are done with Virtual
Reality. The VR simulation includes exterior and fluoroscopic views of the leg as well
as haptic feedback of inserting needles, making incisions and drilling into bone. When
complete, TraumaVision™ will be an integrated lower extremity trauma simulator
meeting military and civilian training needs.

---

[1] Correspondence to: Bruce D. Anderson, Simulution Inc., 16173 Main Ave., Prior Lake, MN 55372.
E-mail: banderson@simulution.com.

2. The Physical Model

The diagnosis and treatment of fractures and compartment syndrome require palpation and physical movement of the effected limb. Palpation is used to check pulses, locate positions to insert needles of pressure gauges and make incisions [1]. The leg is physically manipulated to reduce the fracture, which is checked with fluoroscopy. A physical model gives the trainee experience in palpating and manipulating a leg without cumbersome data gloves and head sets.

The physical model consists of a rigid plastic model of the leg bones encased in foam covered with an artificial skin. To simulate fractures, there are "pre-fractures" located at several places in the femur. At each fracture site there is a universal joint that allows two-axis angular movement as well as displacement of the bone fragments. This allows simulation of many different fractures at a given site. The miniBIRD 500/800 System from Ascension Technologies is used to determine the relative position of the two bone fragments. This information is used to update the VR views of the external leg as well as the VR fluoroscopic images. The bone model is surrounded with simulated soft tissues that include bladders for swelling and silicon tubes for simulating pulses. The miniBIRD system also includes a sensor that can be placed on the external portion of the physical model to identify points on the leg where external fixator pins are to be placed, needles are to be inserted, or incisions are to be made.

3. Virtual Reality Simulation of Internal Fixation: Techniques Developed

The TraumaVision™ Simulator was initially designed to train surgeons in internal fixation techniques for fractures of the femoral shaft and neck (i.e. hip fractures). Several techniques were developed that can be easily modified for the simulation of external fixation as well as many other orthopedic techniques. The TraumaVision™ Simulator includes VR images of both external and fluoroscopic views of the leg. The algorithms for simulating drilling provide variable resistance as the user drills through different layers of bone. The resistance encountered corresponds to the location of the drill in the simulated fluoroscopic image. Furthermore, the resistance encountered during drilling can be changed so the simulation can be modified to include healthy young soldiers as well as elderly patients with osteoporosis.

The internal fixation simulations include a suite of performance metrics that are use to generate a "medically-weighted" performance score. "Medically-weighted" means that an error's impact on the final score will vary according to its impact on the patient. Some metrics are important enough that their impact alone can lower the final score. Other metrics such as time and number of retries are not as medically critical and need to be summed together before the final score is affected. These metrics can be easily adapted to any fixation system.

To use the scoring system on diverse morphologies, a system was developed which reduces important anatomical features into a set of primitives. The primitives are simple geometrical shapes that can be used to model an anatomical feature. When a morphology is uploaded into the simulator, these primitives can be superimposed upon it and their coordinates uploaded into the simulation. Thus, the scoring system can be easily adapted to morphologies that can vary between patients of different age and sex. When the procedure is complete, the score is displayed and the user can scroll through the metrics and analyze appropriate views comparing the measured parameter to the acceptable range (Figure 1).

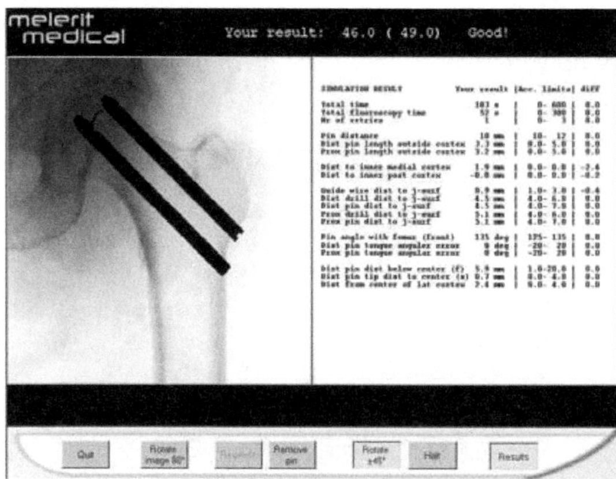

Figure 1. Display of the performance metrics after completion of a procedure.

4. Virtual Reality of External Fixation: Combat Relevant Simulations

4.1. Stab Incision and Bleeding Simulations

Recent development has focused on implementing simulations of external fixation. To place an external fixator, a small "stab" incision is made in the skin, and the fixator pin is inserted to the bone [1]. For a realistic simulation of external fixator placement, simulations of a stab incision and bleeding were developed. Making small incisions allows for a simplified simulation of an incision compared to longer incisions. In this scenario, the software detects the coordinates at which the scalpel encounters (collides) with the surface representing the skin and the incision begins at that point. The skin makes a small deformation until the scalpel "pops" through the skin when a threshold force is reached. The scalpel is then locked into a cutting direction and angle to simplify the algorithm. Once the cutting begins, the user controls only the depth and length of the incision along with the speed with which it was made. When the depth of the scalpel is outside the incision, the scalpel has made the incision and a gap in the skin is made and painted with a red texture.

To simulate the bleeding that occurs at a stab incision, as well as from wounds, a smoothed hydrodynamic particle system is used [2]. A particle system can be difficult to implement, but provides versatility in the scenarios that can be simulated. To realistically simulate bleeding, many blood particles need to be generated and they need to be "joined" to create a convincing fluid effect and add realism. Several methods to create this effect and add realism to the simulation have been employed.

First, the system has been optimized for speed by using shaders. Shaders are controlled by a low-level language and have a GPU (Graphics Processor Unit) which allows programs to be sent directly to the graphics card and makes graphics programs up to 100 times faster.

Secondly, the simulation of bleeding has been divided into several special cases, including "trickling" or "flowing", "spurting", and "pooling". The largest effort has been to simulate blood trickling or flowing down the leg after a small incision has been made (Fig. 2). When it is detected that the scalpel has punctured the skin, the particle system begins simulating a trickle of blood leaving the incision and flowing under the influence of gravity down the leg.

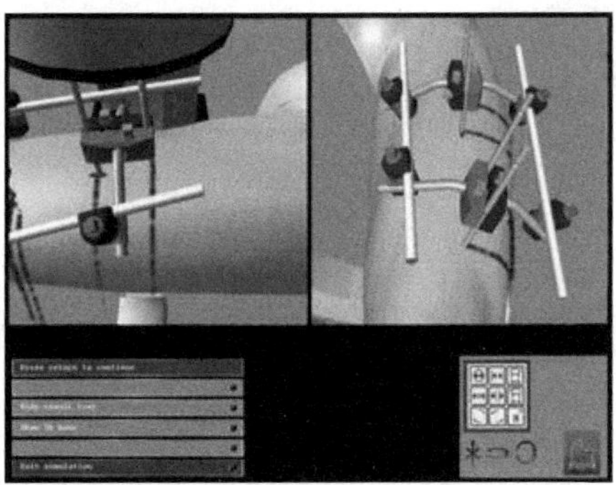

Figure 2. Stab incisions with blood trickling from them and the completed simulation of the Hoffmann II External Fixator System.

To prevent the simulation from becoming over-demanding of CPU time, steps have been taken to limit the number of particles. First, after particles flow to the bottom of the leg they disappear and new particles are generated at the incision site. Having the particles disappear keeps the total number of particles relatively constant and prevents the computational demands from becoming too great. Furthermore, after a trickle of blood runs down the leg, it leaves a static stain of the trail. Therefore, rather than the particle system continuously creating particles leaving the incision and running down the same path on the leg, after a short period of time, the trickle of blood is replaced with a series of red triangles that highlight the blood path. In these ways, the number of particles is decreased, so more bleedings can be simulated.

4.2. Hoffmann II External Fixator System Simulation

Our external fixator simulation is of the Stryker Hoffmann II External Fixator System used for long bone fractures . A field-kit version of this system is operational deployed by all branches of the U.S. military. The first step in placing an external fixator is to locate the sites where the pins are to be placed. This is done by observing the injury and palpating the leg. In our simulation, locating the pin positions is done by palpating the physical model. When the user locates the desired position, a stylus containing a PC MiniBird sensor is held at the desired spot which puts a "dot" at the corresponding location on the VR model of the leg.

After locating the desired placement position of the pins, the user turns to the VR Simulator to continue the simulation. The VR simulation allows the user to palpate the bone with the pins to determine the proper angle of placement, drill the pin into the bone, attach a clamp, and place and drill in subsequent pins and clamps. The user can choose a fluoroscopic view to evaluate their positioning of the pin relative to the bone. The fluoroscopic views can be used in the initial stages of training, but turned off when training for a field hospital environment and for evaluation. After all clamps are in place, the simulation automatically attaches the clamp connectors and rods, showing the external fixation configuration facilitated by the location of the pins and clamps chosen by the user (Fig. 2).

Metrics for evaluating the performance of a user applying an external fixator have been defined. These variables include basics such as fluoroscopy and total surgical time. They also include the new metrics for this procedure including the number of incisions made, the position of the external fixator pins in the bone, and in the future will include an evaluation of the structural stability of the external fixation construction. When complete, a medically-weighted score for external fixation will be provided.

5. Compartment Syndrome Simulations

TraumaVision™ includes a volumetric model of the lower leg for diagnosing and treating compartment syndrome as well as for treating tibia fractures. This model includes bones, muscles, fascia, nerves, blood vessels and skin. A model of the Stryker Pressure Gauge has also been completed (Figure 3A). The user can simulate inserting the needle of the gauge into all four anatomical compartments of the leg using the haptic feedback arm. The user feels a distinct "pop" as the needle passes though a layer of fascia. A pressure reading is displayed for each compartment, and the program tracks which compartments were entered and if any neurovascular structures were compromised. In this way, the instructor can determine if the student accessed all four compartments and if any major errors were made.

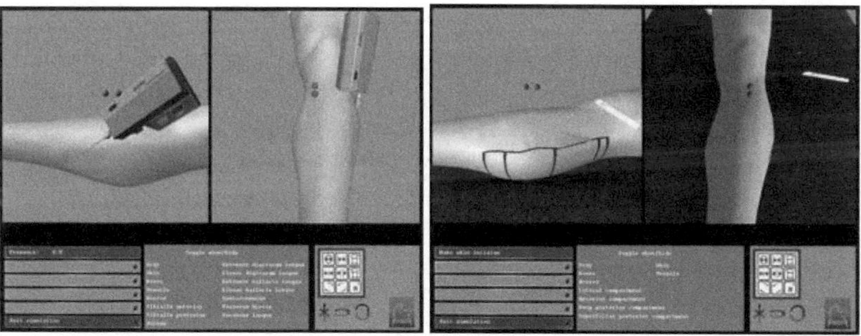

Figure 3. 3A. Measuring ICP with the Stryker Pressure Gauge. 3B. Making a fasciotomy incision.

If the pressure readings indicate that fasciotomy is necessary, the student can complete a simulated procedure. A novel graphical and haptic simulation of a long incision is used to incise the skin and fascia. As the incision is made, the particle system generates simulated blood trickles at intervals along the incision, as described above. The incision site is filled with a red surface simulating a pool of blood (Figure 3B). The system tracks which compartments have had their fascia incised as well as the length of the incision, to determine if the student has adequately relieved the pressure from the appropriate compartments.

6. Preliminary Validation Results

Content validity of the TraumaVision™ was done with a group of four orthopedic surgeons who rated various features on a seven-point Likert scale. The surgeons generally liked the look and feel of the physical model's skin and pulses (average score 4.6), but were not so positive on the ability to manipulate fractures (average score 3.15). The surgeons were very positive on a number of parameters related to the feel of drilling into bone (average score 4.9). In general the surgeons liked the simulator and felt that it provided an accurate assessment of a surgeons skill (average score 4.7).

A preliminary context validity study of the TraumaVision™ Simulator has been completed [3]. This study evaluated the performance differences between experienced orthopedic surgeons and medical students for simulation of the distal femoral nailing procedure. Surgeons had shorter total surgery times and fluoroscopy times than students did. Furthermore, the surgeons were able to stop the drill faster than students after drilling the medial cortex during femoral nailing of the distal femur. It was also demonstrated that students improved their performance on the simulator with repeated practice. Thus, TraumaVision™ has demonstrated construct validity for internal fixation procedures.

7. Conclusions and Future Work

TraumaVision™ is an expandable training system that can train various medical personnel in orthopedic trauma procedures including internal and external fixation as well as the care and dignosis of compartment syndrome. Future work on TraumaVision™ will include expanding procedural steps for combat relevant trauma treatments and completing a SCORMs compliant curriculum for management of orthopedic trauma. Validation studies will also be completed to demonstrate concurrent validity. When completed, TraumaVision™ will be a training system of value to civilian and military care providers.

8. Acknowledgements

This work is supported by the US Army Medical Research and Materiel Command under Contract Nos. W81XWH-04-C-0106 and W81XWH-06-C-0032.

9. References

[1] Crenshaw, A.H. *Campbell's Operative Orthopedics*. C.V. Mosby Company, 1987.
[2] Muller, M., Schrin, S., Teschner, M. Interactive Blood Simulation for Virtual Surgery based on Smoothed Particle Hydrodynamics. In Preparation. (2006).
[3] Tillander, B., Ledin, T., Nordqvist, P., Skarman, E., & Wahlstrom, O., A Virtual Reality Trauma Simulator, *Medical Teacher*, submitted, (2006).

Medicine Meets Virtual Reality 15
J.D. Westwood et al. (Eds.)
IOS Press, 2007

Data Acquisition and Development of a Trocar Insertion Simulator Using Synthetic Tissue Models

Veluppillai Arulesan, Govindarajan Srimathveeravalli, Thenkurussi Kesavadas,
Prashant Nagathan, Robert E. Baier {arulesan, gks2, kesh}@eng.buffalo.edu
Virtual Reality Lab, Dept. of Mechanical and Aerospace Engineering
State University of New York at Buffalo, Buffalo, NY 14260

Abstract: Realistic trocar insertion simulator requires reliable and reproducible tissue data. This paper looks at using synthetic surrogate tissue to facilitate creation of data covering a wide range of pathological cases. Furthermore, we propose to map the synthetic puncture force data to the puncture force data obtained on animal/human tissue to create a simulation model of the procedure. We have developed an experimental setup to collect data from surrogate synthetic tissue using a bladeless trocar.

1. Introduction

According to studies conducted by Food and Drug Administration, complications related to trocar insertion is the most commonly cited malpractice claim involving laparoscopic surgery [1]. A majority of these injuries are attributed to the use of excessive force by the surgeon [2]. In spite of a number of laparoscopic surgical simulators being developed [3], currently there exists no dedicated simulator which allows surgeons to practice the trocar insertion procedure in the abdomen covered by the rectus sheath. In our previous work [4], we utilized existing in-vitro porcine tissue data to construct a spring-mass model based simulator for trocar insertion. However, the range of force data and abdominal tissue models was not available to develop a reliable simulation. Hence in the present work we have first developed a methodology to ascertain tissue properties using synthetic materials and used this data to enhance our virtual trocar simulator.

2. Goal of Current Work

To simulate accurately the process of piercing, it is first necessary to obtain reliable and reproducible tissue data. Due to the nature of the procedure and instrumentation required, in-vivo determination of human tissue properties is both expensive and difficult. To facilitate creation of data covering various pathological cases in terms of tissue thickness and morbidity, we developed a methodology using synthetic surrogate material displaying similar properties.

We have used polyethylene to simulate the skin and fat layer and reinforcing nylon tape to simulate the tough muscle layer. The tissue was tested in both wetted conditions using physiologic saline solution and in dry conditions. Similar materials have been used in prior research by Baier et al [5] and have been validated against human tissue properties as an excellent yet cheap alternative for human skin tissues.

Multiple plies with different combination of thickness of these materials (Table 1) were formed and tested until puncture occurred to get a matrix of material properties. Using this data we mapped puncture force values of surrogate tissue and porcine test data. This allowed us to create a mapping between the thicknesses of surrogate tissue and those of actual tissue for similar puncture force values. For example, we had reported [4] puncture values between the range of 9-18 pound force for porcine data for different test conditions and trocars. Corresponding force values were obtained in our experiment for a set up of 1 polyethylene layer of 0.05 mm and 1 nylon tape of 0.14 mm thickness (Fig. 4). Similarly, a breaking strength of 0.6-7 pound force has been reported for rabbit abdominal walls [6]. We have obtained a similar puncture force range for a synthetic specimen consisting of 1 layer of polyethylene of 0.05mm (Fig. 3).We plan to carry out similar mapping of puncture forces for human abdominal tissue conditions in the future. This mapping, once established, can also then be used to predict surrogate tissue complements of actual tissue and subsequently the puncture force required. The determination of this force is important to the development of the simulator.

3. Experimental setup

A bladeless trocar with a diameter of 0.229' was used for the experimental procedure. The base of the trocar was cut and was fitted with a shaft of 0.25' diameter and 8' length (Fig 1). The other end of the shaft was fitted with a stud designed to fit in the Mechano-Chemical Tester (Fig. 2) (manufactured by Columbia Laboratories).

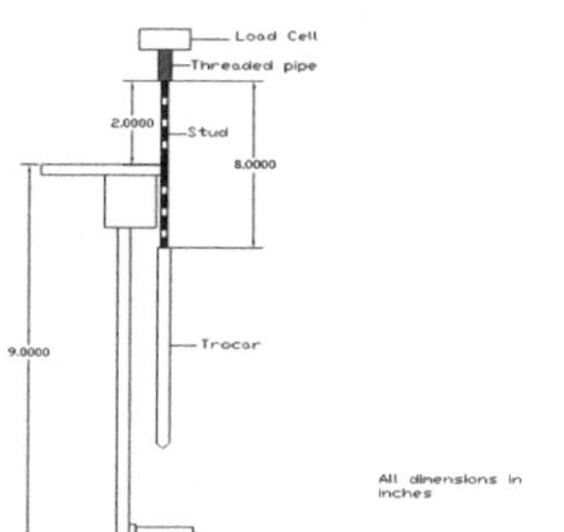

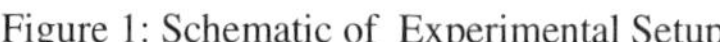

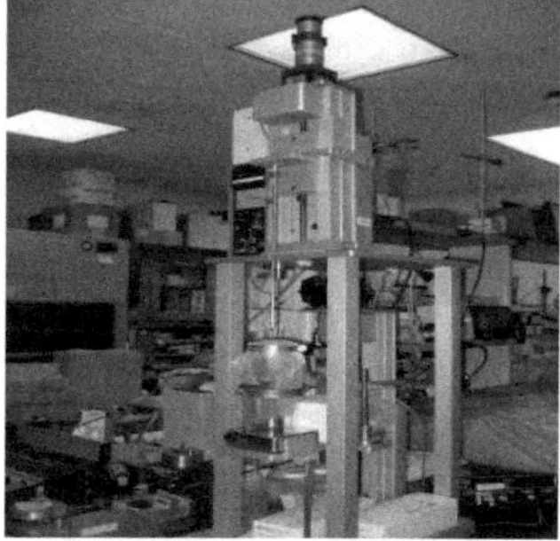

Figure 1: Schematic of Experimental Setup   Figure 2: Experimental Setup

The surrogate tissue was stretched and clamped over a cylinder using a metal clamp. The trocar was then advanced at constant velocities and the force and displacement of the trocar was recorded on a recording chart that was attached to the load cell on the testing device. This test was repeated for different velocities.

4. Results

We obtained force, time and displacement data for various configurations of tissue layers and thicknesses (Table 1). This data was used to create a base reference set of data for tissue properties.

Table 1 Experimental Values

Layers- Polyethylene (0.05mm each)	Layers-Reinforcing Nylon Tape (0.14mm each)	Velocity (cm/min)	Puncture Force (lb)
1	0	1.0583	0.88
1	1	3.6	18.99
1	2	3.6	25.43

A parametric force model was proposed previously to model the insertion process [4]. We will use these material properties and trocar-material coefficients of friction to determine a mathematical model to segregate the various components of the force.

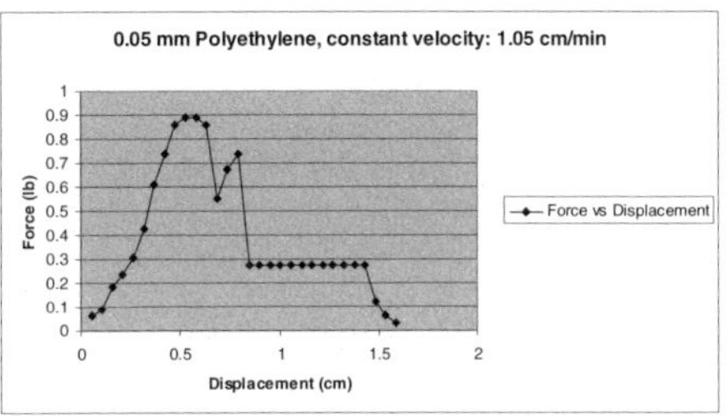

Figure 3: Polyethylene   Figure 4: Polyethylene with Nylon Tape

We are currently working on validating this force simulation obtained using a haptic device. We plan to present this simulation to a group of surgeons with expertise in trocar insertion procedure to obtain their initial feedback. Our long term goal is to develop a comprehensive simulator that can not only be used by surgeons to improve and hone their trocar insertion skills but also to determine whether new designs of trocars can help improve patient and procedural safety.

5. Reference:

1.   Fuller, J., Ashar, B.S and Carey-Corrado, J., *Trocar-associated injuries and fatalities: An analysis of 1399 reports to the FDA*. Journal of Minimally Invasive Gynecology, 2005. **12**(4): p. 302.
2.   Bhoyrul, S., et al., *Trocar injuries in laparoscopic surgery*. Journal of the American College of Surgeons, 2001. **192**(6): p. 677.
3.   Sutton, C., et al., *MIST VR. A laparoscopic surgery procedures trainer and evaluator*. Stud Health Technol Inform, 1997. **39**: p. 598-607.
4.   Kesavadas, T., Srimathveeravalli, G. and Arulesan, V., *Parametric modeling and simulation of trocar insertion*. Stud Health Technol Inform, 2006. **119**: p. 252-4.
5.   Baier, R.E., *Cutting Effectiveness of Heel Incision Devices*. 2006, Internal UB Technical Report.
6.   Nilsson, T., *Biomechanical studies of rabbit abdominal wall. Part I.--The mechanical properties of specimens from different anatomical positions*. J Biomech, 1982. **15**(2): p. 123-9.

Medicine Meets Virtual Reality 15
J.D. Westwood et al. (Eds.)
IOS Press, 2007

Centralized Data Recording for a Distributed Surgical Skills Trainer to Facilitate Automated Proficiency Evaluation

Christoph ASCHWANDEN[1,2], Craig CORNELIUS[3], Lawrence BURGESS[2]
Kevin MONTGOMERY[3], Aneesh SHARMA[3]
[1]*caschwan@hawaii.edu*
[2]*Telehealth Research Institute (TRI)*
[3]*Stanford-NASA National Biocomputation Center*

Abstract. Virtual reality simulators have the capability to automatically record user performance data in an unbiased, cost effective manner that is also less error prone than manual methods. Centralized data recording simplifies proficiency evaluation even more; however is not commonly available to date for surgical skills trainers. We will detail our approach in implementing a framework for distributed score recording over the Internet using a database for persistent storage.

Keywords. Surgery, Trainer, Simulator, Virtual Reality, Haptics, Force-Feedback, Touch, Fine-Motor Skills, Simulation, Laparoscope, Metrics, Benchmark, Recording, Proficiency, Evaluation, Distributed, Internet, TCP/IP, Database, Remote, HTTP, 3D, VR, Human-Computer Interaction, SPRING, VRMSS

1. Introduction

Minimal invasive surgery has been shown to have advantages over conventional open methods. Laparoscopic procedures now represent the 'gold standard' for various surgical procedures. However, lack of 3-D depth perception as well as the fulcrum effect of the body wall on instrument handling pose major obstacles that make effective training imperative. Surgeons are currently trained using conventional box trainers as well as virtual reality simulators.

Physical box trainers benefit from lower cost and much greater availability compared to VR simulators. However, their data recording and score taking capabilities are limited, and detailed performance assessment on inanimate box trainers requires subjective human-monitored evaluation, which is not only costly but also error-prone [7].

2. VRMSS and Distributed Score Taking

To broaden access to such training, a Virtual Reality Motor-Skills Simulator (VRMSS) was implemented [1]. VRMSS features distributed surgical 3D motor-skills training using Haptics for touch and feel feedback, and is designed as a low-cost alternative to current state-of-the-art practices in place. VRMSS is built using SPRING, a real-time soft-tissue modeling engine [5].

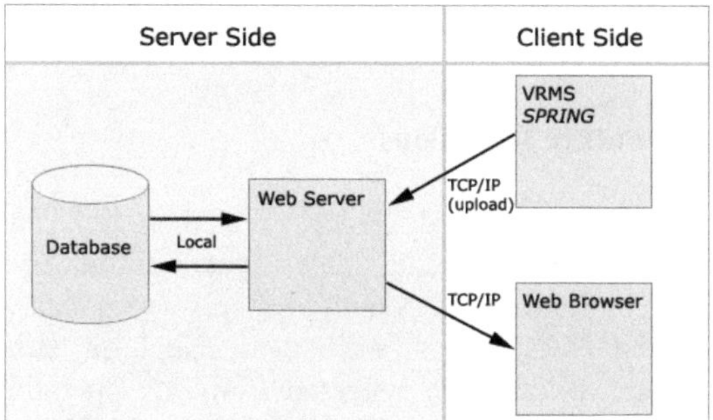

Figure 1 - System Setup

VRMSS has been equipped with automated logging capability which allows for data recording over TCP/IP, i.e., a local network or the Internet. See **Figure 1** for details. The system provides functionality for upload and download of training data on the client side, with the server offering persistent storage as well as basic data analysis/visualization capabilities for a single or multiple users.

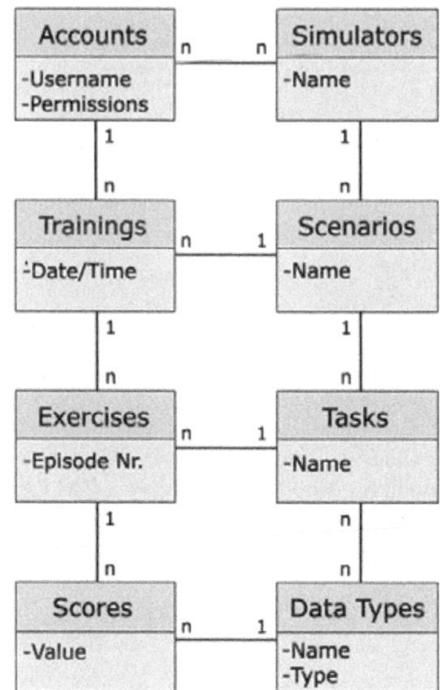

Figure 2 - Database Schema

A web-based prototype system to allow data recording for various types of simulators was constructed [2]. The database schema is depicted in **Figure 2**. The tables on the right-hand side hold the metadata defining the simulators, scenarios, tasks and data types to record. The tables on the left-hand side contain the actual data recorded including trainings, exercises and scores.

Current types of data elements recorded include task duration, collisions, distance, rotation, errors, hand jitter and steadiness. Preliminary pilot tests were completed successfully. Data was successfully recorded over the Internet and persistently stored in the database.

3. Contributions and Future Directions

A framework for remote data recording was created, tested and made available to interested 3rd parties [2]. The metadata tables in the framework allow for custom scenario creation, i.e., configuring the system to specify what data will be collected. To date, scenarios for the VRMSS as well as a Nephron simulation have been implemented. The framework can be accessed from any operating system including Windows, Macintosh, Linux and UNIX. A custom HTTP request allows data uploading/downloading to/from the framework. The HTTP protocol supports tunneling through Firewalls and Proxy servers, thus removing limitations of other available solutions. A MySQL database server in the background is responsible for persistent data storage, and the database is backed up regularly.

The ultimate goal is to provide wider access to surgical training, be it in the lab, at home, or in remote areas. Students can learn on their own time, being monitored through the automated data recording framework. Proficiency levels are determined automatically, and score-taking is unbiased.

References

[1]   Aschwanden C, Sherstyuk A, Burgess L, Montgomery K. A Surgical and Fine-Motor Skills Trainer for Everyone? Touch and Force-Feedback in a Virtual Reality Environment for Surgical Training. Medicine Meets Virtual Reality 14, 2006.

[2]   Data Recording Framework. http://www.tri.jabsom.hawaii.edu/surgicalsimweb

[3]   Dev P, Montgomery K, Senger S, et al. Simulated medical learning environments over the Internet. J Am Med Inform Assoc.

[4]   Heinrichs, W. L., Srivastava, S., Montgomery, K., and Dev, P. (2004).   The Fundamental Manipulations of Surgery: A Structured Vocabulary for Designing Surgical Curricula and Simulators, J Am Assoc Gynecol Laparasoc, 11(4), 450-456.

[5]   Montgomery, K., Bruyns, C., Brown, J., Sorkin, S., Mazzella, F., Thonier, G., Tellier, A., Lerman, B., Menon, A. (2002). Spring: A General Framework for Collaborative, Real-time Surgical Simulation, In: Westwood, J., et. al. (eds.): Medicine Meets Virtual Reality, IOS Press, Amsterdam, 2002.

[6]   Seymour, N. E., Gallagher, A. G., Roman, S. A., O'Brien, M. K., Bansal, V. K., Andersen, D. K. and Satava, R. M.(2002). Virtual reality training improves operating room performance: results of a randomized, double-blinded study, Ann. Surgery, 236(4), 458-464.

[7]   Woodrum DT, Andreatta PB, Yellamanchilli RK, Feryus L, Gauger PG, Minter RM. Construct validity of the LapSim laparoscopic surgical simulator. Am J Surg. 2006 Jan; 191(1):28-32.

Medicine Meets Virtual Reality 15
J.D. Westwood et al. (Eds.)
IOS Press, 2007

Precise Determination of Regions of Interest for Hepatic RFA Planning

Claire BAEGERT [a,1], Caroline VILLARD [b], Pascal SCHRECK [b] and Luc SOLER [a]

[a] *Institut de Recherche contre les Cancer de l'Appareil Digestif, France*
[b] *Laboratoire des Sciences de l'Image, de l'Informatique et de la Télédétection, France*

Abstract. Percutaneous radiofrequency ablation is a minimally invasive therapy for the treatment of liver tumors that consists in a destruction of tumors by heat. A correct insertion and placement of the needle inside the tumor is critical and conditions the success of the operation. We are developing a software that uses patients data to help the physician plan the operation. In this context, we propose a method that computes automatically, quickly and accurately the areas on the skin that provide a safe access to the tumor. The borders of the 3D mesh representing insertion areas are refined for a higher precision. Resulting zones are then used to restrict the research domain of the optimization process, and are visualized on the reconstructed patient as an indication for the physician.

Keywords. minimally invasive surgery, preoperative planning

Introduction

At present, open surgery is still the main curative treatment for liver cancer. However liver resection is a painful operation that is not always possible due to the patient's condition, multiple tumor location or insufficient hepatic reserve. Several minimal invasive procedures has been recently developed in order to treat patients that are not good candidates for surgery. These techniques are based on the local destruction of tumors either by temperature (radiofrequency ablation, cryoablation, focused ultrasound) or by the effects of chemical agents (ethanol injection). In this work we focus on percutaneous radiofrequency ablation (RFA) that offers a low rate of local recurrence (*i.e.* no tumor is found at the original site during the follow-up) and complications [3].

RFA consists in inserting through the patient's skin a RF-needle that heats tissues until destruction. The radiologist places his needle in the tumor in order to kill cancerous cells and a surrounding 1cm safe margin. Because of the limited visibility during this kind of operation (needle placement is generally guided by CT or US images), preoperative planning takes an important place in the success of the therapy. The physician has to choose a needle path that allows a safe access to the tumor and a secure ablation relying on 2D-slices of the patient obtained by CT-scan. Planning from 2D slices is not really intuitive and requires a long learning process. As advances in medical image processing

---

[1] Corresponding Author: Claire Baegert, IRCAD, 1 place de l'Hôpital, 67091 Strasbourg Cedex, France;
E-mail: Claire.Baegert@ircad.u-strasbg.fr

allow to rapidly reconstruct a virtual 3D model of the patient from CT-scan slices [8], we are developing a planning software based on the visualization of such 3D-reconstructed patients that would assist the physician in his decision. Our work is organized in 3 axis:

- Integration of constraints and rules governing RFA planning: strategies may vary from a specialist to another, however we have extracted recurrent information from their expertise and from medical literature [5,6] to define constraints included in the software.
- Resolution of the geometric problem corresponding to the previously specified constraints.
- Display facilities to browse the solution space: the physician may need to have access to various information concerning the different possible strategies.

We focus here on the second axis that is divided in two parts: firstly the determination of all solutions and secondly the choice of the optimal one. In this paper, we detail the method we developed for a fast computation of all needle trajectories that are technically feasible for each operation. The determination of an optimal trajectory among them is presented in [9]. Firstly, we briefly expose the approaches proposed in other studies concerning computer-aided planning of minimal invasive interventions. Then, we explain on which criteria we define a needle trajectory as being valid and we detail our method that computes with precision possible insertion zones on the skin, providing a safe access to the tumor. Finally we present and comment our results on several virtual patients.

1. Previous works

Various works have been recently published on computer assisted planning of different minimally invasive techniques, aiming at guiding the physician's decision. The problem of optimizing surgical tool placement has being addressed in a few studies. Optimizations have been performed regarding different criteria according to the therapy. In the case of thermal ablation, the different studies focus on minimizing damages to healthy tissues while killing the whole tumor [2,4]. Concerning robotically assisted heart intervention, the important criteria mainly concern distance between tools and angle between tools and patient [1,7]. In both cases, some trajectories could be immediately rejected for different reasons independent of the optimization criteria. For example the tools cannot cross bones in any case, the tools must be long enough to reach the surgical site or in case of the insertion of an endoscope, the surgical site must belong to the field of vision. These cases have to be taken into account otherwise there is no guarantee that the proposed optimized solution will be valid. In most of the studies this problem is avoided by the physician's intervention. The optimization is restricted within a limited number of solutions or an authorized access window that are provided by the surgeon and considered as valid. In one study [1], the set of insertion points proposed by the physician is controlled and insertion points that correspond to an intersection with an organ are eliminated.

While some studies propose an exhaustive examination of a limited number of possibilities preselected by the physician, our approach consist in an automatic selection of pertinent trajectories among the whole solution space. In a previous article [10] we presented a first approach that consisted in integrating the elimination of trajectories crossing vital organs in the optimization process. The optimization function was artificially modified by adding a huge penalty to these trajectories that were naturally avoided by the optimization process. However this method introduced artificial local minima in the optimization function, therefore we developed another approach consisting in computing an authorized insertion zone before the optimization step.

2. Objective

This study aims at designing and implementing a method that automatically computes possible trajectories for each operation. We must then define what we consider as a possible trajectory. A trajectory can be regarded as a possible choice if it satisfies all the required conditions for an operation. At this time, several constraints governing RFA planning have been identified thanks to bibliography and interviews with specialists. Among these constraints, some are strict constraints that define the validity of a trajectory, others are soft constraints that have to be optimized and combined with an appropriate weighting. In this paper, we focus on the processing of stricts constraints, that are directly involved in the determination of the feasible trajectories, as soft constraints only provide information on their quality. Among these strict constraints, we selected the two most obvious ones. Firstly the insertion depth has to be below the needle size. Secondly a valid trajectory cannot cross neither bones, large vessels nor surrounding vital organs. Nevertheless, our method could easily be adapted to additional strict constraints. For example, the physician could consider that a trajectory approaching a vital organ with less than 1 cm is not a possibility.

In order to precisely define the possible trajectories, we chose to determine what are the possible insertion points on the skin. Then the possible strategies are materialized by a simple area on the skin's mesh that is easily visualized. To each trajectory corresponds one insertion point, if it belongs to the possible insertion zone then the trajectory is valid. To each insertion point corresponds a set of trajectories and among them a few are pertinent. A trajectory can be viewed as pertinent if the target point belongs the tumor for example. Then an insertion point is accepted in the possible insertion zone if all the corresponding pertinent trajectories verify the constraints.

3. Method

We want then to determine precisely all the points of the skin that correspond to valid trajectories. A needle trajectory is considered as a valid solution if the needle passes through the skin and does not cross any organ. The initial possible trajectories are materialized by the surface mesh of the patient's skin. Triangles are progressively eliminated as the corresponding trajectories are declared not satisfactory regarding the previously specified conditions. Our algorithm could be summarized in:

Input :
$L = list\ of\ skin's\ triangles,$
$O = center\ of\ the\ tumor's\ bounding\ box,$
$E = set\ of\ organs\ to\ avoid$
Output :
$L = list\ of\ eligible\ triangles$

// Elimination of insertion points that are too far from the tumor
For *each triangle t in L*
   If *distAboveNeedleLength(O, t)*
     eraseFrom(L, t)
   Else if *distPartlyAboveNeedleLength(O, t)*
     eraseFrom(L, t) and subdivide(t, L)

// Elimination of insertion points that don't provide an access to the tumor
For *each voxel v in tumor's border*
   s = renderScene(v, E)
   For *each triangle t in L*
     If *hiddenFrom(s, t)*
       eraseFrom(L, t)
     Else if *partlyHiddenFrom(s, t)*
       eraseFrom(L, t) and subdivide(t, L)

The two parts of the algorithm resolve respectively our two constraints and follow the same principle: a triangle that does not respect the constraint is definitely eliminated. A triangle that partly fulfills a constraint is subdivided in four subtriangles that replace it and will be evaluated separately. Other triangles are kept in the possible insertion zone and will be evaluated regarding the other constraints. Finally the possible insertion zone only contains triangles that satisfy all the constraints. Other constraints could be added easily in this algorithm, assuming that it is possible to determine quickly if a needle insertion in a triangle fulfill the constraint in all the cases, in some cases or in no case.

Concerning our first constraint, the validity of an insertion triangle is determined by computing the distance between the center of the tumor's bounding box and the three corners of the triangle. The determination of the validity according to the second constraint requires a more complete verification. We chose to check the constraint not only for trajectories targeting the tumor's center but for an access to the whole tumor. It is important for this constraint that a light displacement from the trajectory does not compromise the validity of the trajectory. The test is then executed while targeting each voxel of the tumor's border. Our accessibility problem can be considered as a visibility problem. If a triangle is completely visible from the target point that means that no obstacle is on the way between any point of the triangle and the target. From a position, the visibility (partial visibility, total visibility or invisibility) of all candidate triangles can be determined by observing six renderings of the scene, each corresponding to a face of a virtual cube placed around the target position. More details can be found in [9] where we presented a first version of our computation of insertion zones.

The subdivision of border triangles results in the loss of neighbourhood information. However, in our context this kind of information is not necessary as we use the mesh of the insertion zone only to test if trajectories cross it. The subdivision of the triangles allows to compute precisely the insertion zone independently of the precision of the initial mesh of the skin. The maximum authorized subdivision level determines the precision of the borders of the insertion zone. Above this maximum subdivision level or below a significant size limit, triangles that do not completely fulfill a constraint are dismissed without subdivision. A reduced number of subdivisions enables to compute the insertion zone with a satisfying precision. We will detail our results in the next section.

4. Results

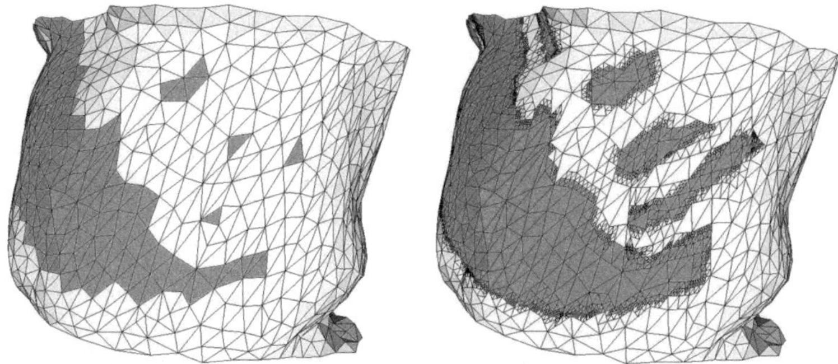

Figure 1. Insertion zones with 0 and 3 subdivision levels

Insertion zones have been computed for 15 tumors in 7 virtually reconstructed patients (represented in tab.1). The surfaces of zones are variable (10-300 cm^2) since tumors are more or less accessible. Although computing zones without triangles subdivisions provides a good idea of possible strategies, it discards many possible insertion points. The average surface loss between computations with 3 and no subdivision is 45% and often more important when the insertion zone is small. By observing fig. 1 we notice that the biggest zone is well represented in both cases while thin zones representing an insertion between ribs are almost occulted in the case of a computation without subdivisions. Computation with 3 subdivision levels provides insertion zones with a good precision in 4 seconds to 2 minutes (average: 30s) that represents 230% of the computation time without sudivision. With more subdivision levels, the resulting surface does not differ significantly from the zone computed with only 3 levels while taking much more time (140% of the time with 3 subdivisions). At a same subdivision level, the computation time can vary between tumors, that mainly depends on the number of tumor's voxels (150-13000) since it determines the number of time the visibility tests have to be done.

5. Conclusion

In this paper, we presented a method for computing automatically possible insertion zones on the skin for the planning of a radiofrequency ablation. Any needle insertion in this zone respects two constraints : it does not cross any vital organs, bone or large vessel and the needle can reach the tumor from the corresponding insertion point on the skin. Our method based on elimination and subdivision of triangles of the skin that do not respect the constraints quickly produces possible insertion zones on the skin with high precision. These zones are used in our patient-specific preoperative planning software to reduce the research domain for the optimization stage and provide valuable information to the physician who can easily see all possibilities for each operation.

Table 1. Surface of insertion zones and computation time for 15 tumors in 7 patients

case	surf. of insert. zones (cm^2)			computation time (s)		
	no subd.	3 subd.	4 subd.	no subd.	3 subd.	4 subd.
1	3	18	18	50	115	150
2	174	219	219	13	41	54
3	97	122	122	12	27	31
4	51	87	87	8	20	25
5	79	126	126	9	27	35
6	39	106	106	5	22	32
7	224	301	301	31	75	119
8	43	85	85	25	55	88
9	74	148	148	9	21	36
10	238	258	258	4	7	10
11	156	205	205	16	15	20
12	71	154	155	3	8	17
13	47	129	129	3	6	12
14	266	360	360	3	6	7
15	0	11	11	2	4	7

Acknowledgments

We would like to thank Region Alsace for its financial support.

References

[1] L. Adhami, E. Coste-Manière and J-D. Boissonnat, Planning and simulation of robotically assisted minimal invasive surgery, *Proceedings of Medical Image Computing and Computer Assisted Intervention (MICCAI'2000), LNCS* **1935**, 624–633, 2000.

[2] T. Butz, S.K. Warfield, K. Tuncali, S.G. Silverman, E. van Sonnenberg, F.A. Jolesz and R. Kikinis, Pre- and intra-operative planning and simulation of percutaneous tumor ablation, *Proceedings of Medical Image Computing and Computer Assisted Intervention (MICCAI'2000), LNCS* **1935**, 317–326, 2000.

[3] M. Kudo, Local ablation therapy for hepatocellular carcinoma: current status and future perspectives, *Journal of Gastroenterology* **39** (3), 205–214, 2004.

[4] D.C. Lung, T.F. Stahovitch and Y. Rabin, Local ablation therapy for hepatocellular carcinoma: current status and future perspectives, *Computer methods in Biomechanics and Biomedical Engineering* **7** (2), 101–110, 2004.

[5] Y. Ni, S. Mulier, Y. Miao, L. Michel and G. Marchal, A review of the general aspects of radiofrequency ablation, *Abdominal Imaging* **30**, 381–400, 2005.

[6] H. Rhim, S. Goldberg, G. Dodd, L. Solbiati, H.K. Lim, M. Tonolini and O.K. Cho, Essential techniques for successful radiofrequency thermal ablation of malignant hepatic tumors *Radiographics* **21**, S17–S35, 2001.

[7] S. Selha, P. Dupont, R. Howe and D. Torchiana, Dexterity optimization by port placement in robot-assisted minimally invasive surgery, *Proceedings of th SPIE* **4570**, 97–104, 2001.

[8] L. Soler, H. Delingette and G. Malandin, Fully automatic anatomical, pathological and functional segmentation from CT scans for hepatic surgery, *Computer Aided Surgery* **6** (3), 131–142, 2001.

[9] C. Villard, C. Baegert, P. Schreck, L. Soler and A. Gangi, Optimal trajectories computation within regions of interest for hepatic RFA planning, *Proceedings of Medical Image Computing and Computer Assisted Intervention (MICCAI'2005), LNCS* **3750**, 49–56, 2005.

[10] C. Villard, L.Soler and A. Gangi, Radiofrequenncy ablation of hepatic tumors: simulation, planning and contribution of virtual reality and haptics, *Journal of Computer Methods in Biomechanics and Biomedical Engineering* **8** (4), 215–227, 2005.

Medicine Meets Virtual Reality 15
J.D. Westwood et al. (Eds.)
IOS Press, 2007

Virtual Reality and Haptic Interface for Cellular Injection Simulation

P. Pat BANERJEE[1], Silvio RIZZI and Cristian LUCIANO
Department of Mechanical and Industrial Engineering
University of Illinois at Chicago

Abstract. This paper presents the application of virtual reality and haptics to the simulation of cellular micromanipulation for research, training and automation purposes. A collocated graphic/haptic working volume provides a realistic visual and force feedback to guide the user in performing a cell injection procedure. A preliminary experiment shows promising results.

Keywords. Virtual Reality, Haptics, Simulation, Cell Injection, ImmersiveTouch.

Introduction

Intracellular microinjection is a typical manipulation operation in a cell culture. Micromanipulation techniques for single cells have important role in applications such as in-vitro toxicology, cancer and HIV research [1].

ImmersiveTouch[™], the latest generation of augmented Virtual Reality (VR) technology [2], is the first system that integrates a haptic device with a head and hand tracking system, and a high resolution and high pixel density stereoscopic display (Figure 1). The haptic device collocated with the 3D graphics is a key factor to delivering extremely realistic simulations. The ImmersiveTouch has been successfully applied to the simulation of neurosurgical procedures and training of resident neurosurgeons [3].

This work presents the initial results of our research towards applying the ImmersiveTouch technology to the simulation of cellular micromanipulation for research, training, and automation purposes.

1. Background

A common setup in contact micromanipulation consists of an end-effector moved in a three-dimensional space by a micromanipulator [1]. Ammi and Ferreira [4] developed a 3-D micromanipulation system based on VR. Their system captures images from a microscope, extracts the shape of the cell using computer vision techniques, and displays a 3-D reconstruction of the cell on a head-mounted display. A haptic device is

---

[1] Corresponding Author: P. Pat Banerjee, Department of Mechanical & Industrial Engineering (M/C 251), University of Illinois at Chicago, 3029 Engineering Research Facility, 842 W. Taylor Street, Chicago, Illinois 60607. Email: banerjee@uic.edu

used to guide the injection pipette. The force feedback applied to the operator is modeled after a biomembrane point-load model. The system provides augmented visual and haptic guide to assist the operator during the process of cell injection. However, the lack of graphics/haptics collocation causes deficient hand-eye coordination during the procedure.

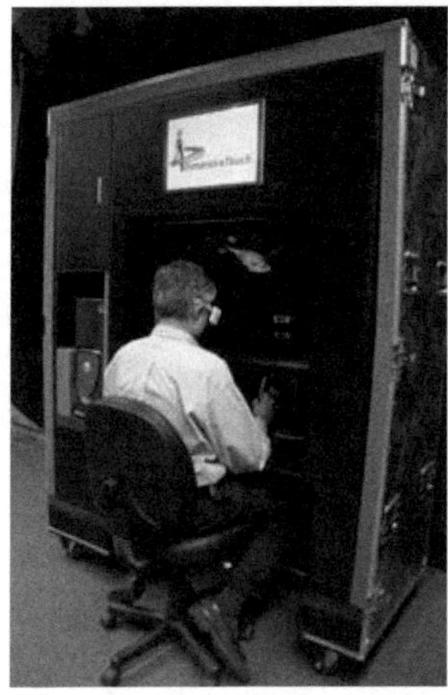

Figure 1. The ImmersiveTouch

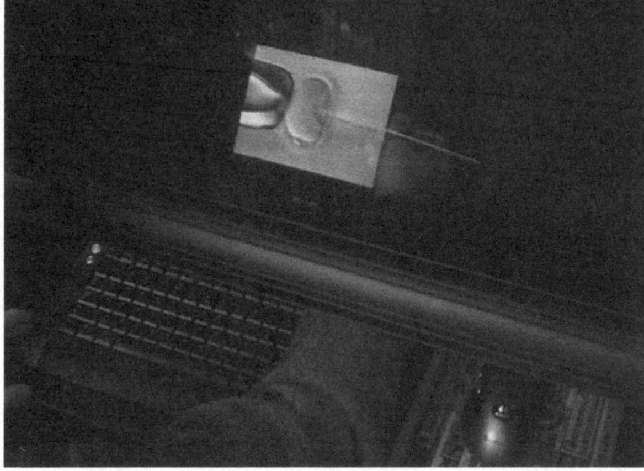

Figure 2. Cell Injection simulator on ImmersiveTouch

2. Implementation

The cellular injection simulator is implemented using the ImmersiveTouch platform. The graphics/haptics collocation (Figure 2) offers a significant improvement over the system described in [4]. In this preliminary version, images extracted from video frames of an actual procedure [5] are used. The haptic volume is defined as a sphere with its third dimension compressed by an adjustable factor. The image and haptic volume are collocated in the working volume of ImmersiveTouch while the radius of the haptic sphere is adjusted to match the cell boundary in the image.

Initially, an image is presented showing an intact cell attached to the holding pipette and the injection pipette in its initial position. The operator must pick the haptic stylus and guide the injection pipette to the cell along a straight line on the image plane. Once contact is made with the outer membrane of the cell, the simulator computes the penetration depth and presents the image that most closely represents this condition. In addition, haptic force is computed and fed back to the user. In this way, the user is immersed into a highly realistic simulation, visualizing actual images from the microscope, and interacting with the cell in a collocated working volume (Figure 2).

3. Preliminary experiments

An initial sample of six individuals were selected to test the prototype. A video from an actual experiment [5] was presented to each of them. Afterwards, each participant was invited to operate the simulator and try to reproduce the experiment previously shown in the video. A lapse of five minutes using the simulator was allotted to each participant. Finally, a questionnaire (see Table 1) consisting of six qualitative questions was handed out. The answer to each question consists of an integer number between 1 and 5, where 1 means "Strongly Disagree", and 5 means "Strongly Agree". The results are summarized in Table 1, showing the average answer for each question.

Table 1.

Question	Avg.
The simulator was easy to use	5.00
The simulator was responsive to your actions	4.33
You naturally interacted with the simulator	4.50
You adjusted quickly to the virtual environment experience	4.00
Considering the tactile aspect, the simulation was realistic	4.33
Considering the visual aspect, the simulation was realistic	4.17

4. Summary and Future Work

In this paper we have presented a promising new application for our ImmersiveTouch technology. We are actively developing and refining the application with the main goal of providing a high-fidelity simulator for complex and error-prone cellular injection tasks. A logical next step is interfacing the simulator to a microscope and microactuator to perform the injection procedures in real cells. In addition, the simulator could be extended to assist in other procedures, such as patch-clamp placement and other applications in cellular mechanotransduction.

Further validation experiments will be conducted by professionals of the field in future.

Acknowledgement: This work was supported in part by a grant from the Office of Naval Research under a NCSA TRECC Accelerator program.

References

[1] Kallio, P. & Kuncova, J. "Manipulation of Living Biological Cells: Challenges in Automation". The International Conference on Intelligent Robots and Systems, IROS'03, Las Vegas, September, 2003.

[2] Luciano, C.; Banerjee, P.; Florea, L.; Dawe, G., "Design of the ImmersiveTouch™: A High-Performance Haptic Augmented VR System," Proc. of Human-Computer Interaction (HCI) International Conf. Las Vegas, 2005.

[3] Luciano, C.; Banerjee, P.; Lemole, G.M.; Charbel,F., "Second Generation Haptic Ventriculostomy Simulator Using the ImmersiveTouch™ System," Proceedings of 14th Medicine Meets Virtual Reality, J.D. Westwood et al. (Eds.), IOSPress, pp. 343-348, 2006.

[4] Ammi, M.; Ferreira, A., "Biological cell injection visual and haptic interface", Advanced Robotics, Vol 20, No. 3, pp. 283-304, 2006.

[5] Intra-cytoplasmic sperm injection video. The Infertility Center of Saint Louis. St. Luke's Hospital, Saint Louis, Missouri. Retrieved 7/11/2006 from http://www.infertile.com/media_pages/technical/icsi.htm

Medicine Meets Virtual Reality 15
J.D. Westwood et al. (Eds.)
IOS Press, 2007

The Structure of the Radial Pulse - A Novel Noninvasive Ambulatory Blood Pressure Device

Martin BARUCH[a], Katherine Westin KWON[b], Emaad ABDEL-RAHMAN[b],
and Ross ISAACS[b]
[a] Empirical Technologies Corporation, [b] University of Virginia, Division of Nephrology

Abstract. A non-invasive wrist sensor, BPGuardian (Empirical Technologies C., Charlottesville, VA) has been developed that provides continuous pressure readings by de-convolving the radial arterial pulse waveform into its constituent component pulses (Pulse Decomposition Analysis). Results agree with the predictions of the model regarding the temporal and amplitudinal behavior of the component pulses as a function of changing diastolic and systolic blood pressure.

Keywords. Blood Pressure, Pulse Wave Analysis, Pulse Reflections, Pulse Wave Velocity

Introduction

A non-invasive wrist sensor, BPGuardian (Empirical Technologies C)) has been developed that provides a continuous pressure reading which requires minimal arterial compression. The device analyzes the radial arterial pulse waveform and de-convolves it into its constituent component pulses (Pulse Decomposition Analysis, PDA®).

Two small-scale studies, one involving patients undergoing dialysis, the other involving normo-tensive volunteers, were performed to establish correlations between readings obtained with the new device and accepted conventional monitors.

1. Methods

1.1 Study Protocols

Radial arterial pulse data were collected from nine patients undergoing regular dialysis sessions at the Kidney Center of the Department of Nephrology at the University of Virginia Medical Center. Blood pressures were collected with an automated cuff every 15 minutes, with the BPGuardian device on the wrist distal to the cuff. All of the patients were hypertensive and three were also diabetic.

To compare arterial pulse parameter results obtained from a group of patients with generally challenged vascular health with those of normo-tensives, a group of ten volunteers was recruited for purposes of inducing blood pressure variations by means of cold-pressor stimulation to the forehead, a well-established technique for raising vascular resistance [1]. The radial blood pressure of members of this group was monitored over the course of a 20 minute session with the volunteer in a supine position using the BPGuardian system, a continuous tonometric blood pressure monitor (Colin) on contralateral arms as well as an automatic cuff for verification (SunTech Medical).

1.2 Sensor Hardware

The BPGuardian physiological sensing system is a self-contained device controlled by a microprocessor that monitors and controls the coupling pressure in a sensing pad that pneumatically telemeters the radial arterial pulsations, digitizes the sensor signal at 512 Hz, and wirelessly transmits it to a PC computer using the Bluetooth protocol. The transmitted data stream is analyzed and parameterized by the Pulse De-Composition Analysis (PDA) algorithm using validated filtering and derivative techniques [2].

1.3 Pulse De-Composition Analysis (PDA)

The radial arterial pulse is a superposition of several component pulses. At the temporal front of the radial pulse envelope is the primary pressure pulse that results from the contraction of the left ventricle. This arterial pressure pulse travels away from the heart through the arterial tree and is reflected at two major reflection sites, one in the region of the renal arteries where the aorta's diameter decreases on the order of 17%, the other beyond the bifurcation of the iliac arteries [3].

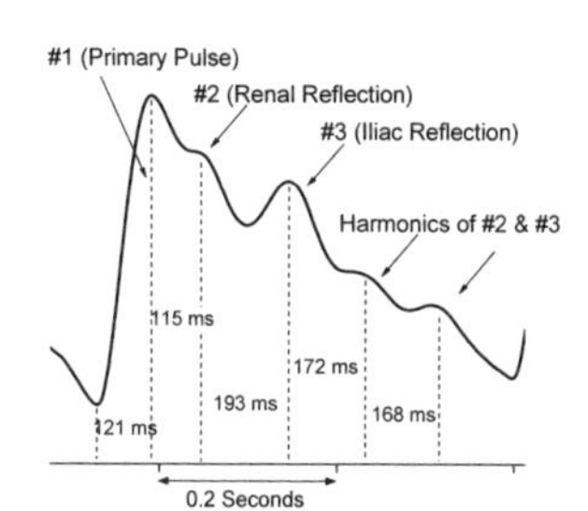

Figure 1: Distinct component pulse structure in the radial arterial pulse of a 44 y. male. Relative time intervals are given in milliseconds.

Figure 1 presents an example of the radial pulse of a 44 year old male and its various component pulses.

The PDA approach detects trends in blood pressure by tracking the relative time and amplitude evolutions of the three primary component pulses of the radial arterial pulsation. Trends in systolic blood pressure are monitored by tracking the ratio of the amplitudes of the #2 pulse to that of the #1 pulse (P2/P1). Due to the difference in arterial path lengths that the two pulses traverse, the ratio is proportional to the differential arterial compliance between the arteries of the arm complex and the thoracic aorta, which is very sensitive to variations in peak pulse pressure. The pulse pressure is tracked by monitoring the time delay between the #1 and the #3 (iliac reflection) pulses (T13). Both pulses travel at different velocities and sample different arterial path lengths. The different velocities are due to the fact that the pulses travel at different peak pressures. Furthermore, since the functional relation between arterial pressure and pulse propagation velocity is non-linear [4], particularly at systolic pressures, the T13 interval samples the differential slope that the two pulses are subject to as the pulse pressure changes.

2. Results

In the subjects who exhibited appreciable blood pressure changes the data displayed the predicted correlations. Figure 2 presents representative data correlating T13 delay times to pulse pressure and P2/P1 ratios to systolic blood pressure for normo-tensive volunteer #4. The correlation coefficients based on linear regression analysis were generally higher for relating P2/P1 to systolic pressure correlations than for relating T13 to pulse pressure. This is to be expected since the determination of pulse pressure requires the determination of diastolic pressure, which in the gold standards used here has been shown to be significantly more prone to errors and biases [5].

Correlations between the slope as well as offset parameters of the linear regression analysis of the patient and volunteer data and physiological parameters, specifically age, height, and vascular health were examined. These results are very preliminary due to the limited number of subjects observed. No correlations were found with age or height. Instead the only variable that correlated significantly was vascular health as quantified by heart rate variability (Figure 3), a well established link.

Preliminary results agree with predictions of the model regarding the temporal and amplitudinal behavior of the component pulses of the radial pulse as a function of changing diastolic and systolic blood pressure, taking into account the distensibilities of the central arteries. The device shows promise as a novel, non-occlusive method of monitoring blood pressure and assessing vascular health.

This research was supported by grants from the Office of Naval Research (ONR) and the Office of Technology Transfer and Commercialization (OTTC).

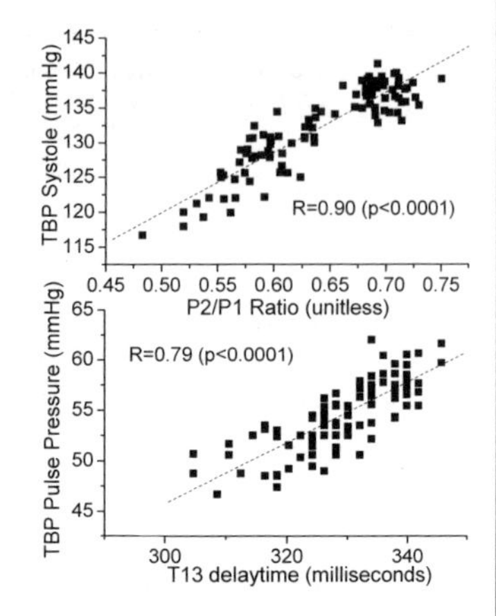

Figure 2: Sample correlations for normo-tensive volunteer #4.

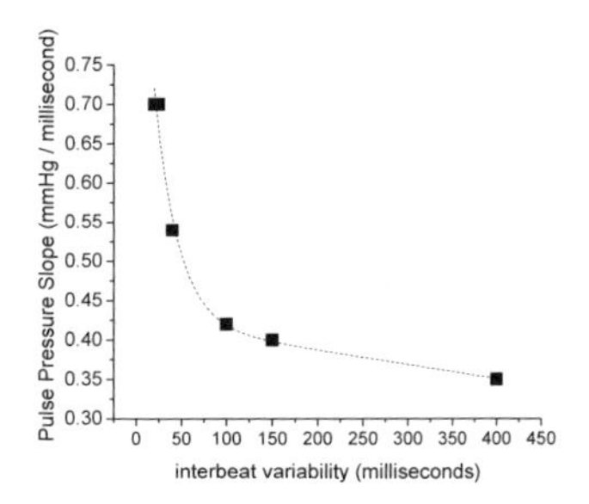

Figure 3: Slope of linear regression analysis correlating pulse pressure with P2/P1 ratio decrease with increasing heart rate variability.

References

[1]   Andrew Sherwood; Alan L. Hinderliter; Kathleen C. Light, Physiological Determinants of Hyperreactivity to Stress in Borderline Hypertension, *Hypertension.* 1995;25:384-390.

[2]   Thomas C. O'Haver, *et.al.* Derivative spectroscopy and its applications in analysis, ***Anal. Proc.***, 1982, **19**, 22 – 46.

[3]   Latham, RD *et.al*, Regional wave travel and reflections along the human aorta: a study with six simultaneous micromanometric pressures. *Circulation* 72, 1985, 1257-69.

[4]   Anliker M et.al, Transmission characteristics of axial waves in blood vessels, *J Biomech*, 1, p235-46, 1968.

[5]   Davies, JI, *et.al*, Peripheral blood pressure measurement is as good as applanation tonometry at predicting ascending aortic blood pressure, *J Hypertens* 2003, **21**:571-576.

Medicine Meets Virtual Reality 15
J.D. Westwood et al. (Eds.)
IOS Press, 2007

A 6DOF Gravity Compensation Scheme for a Phantom Premium Using a Neural Network

Matthew BIRTWISLE, Andy BULPITT
School of Computing, University of Leeds, UK
E-mail: matthewb@comp.leeds.ac.uk

Abstract. Current uses of haptic hardware such as the Phantom Premium 6DOF for surgical simulators lack the desired interface transparency and could cause artefacts in the training regime of a student training on a simulator. This problem is addressed and two neural networks are used to find a mapping between handle coordinates and orientation and force output required to counteract gravitational forces. A close fit to the data is achieved for both networks (errors of 0.00149 and 0.0157 between training and predicted forces) and 3DOF gravity compensation is achieved. A 6DOF simulator is created but requires further work to improve it accuracy.

1. Motivation

Using hardware such as a SensAble Phantom® [1] for the haptic feedback interface in a virtual surgery simulator comes at the cost of the weight of the device being present in the simulation. It may be a lightweight device, like the desktop Phantom Omni™, or partially counterweighted like the Phantom Premium, but there is still a lack of transparency that can detract from the perceived fidelity of a simulation. The problem is exacerbated in our research, that of developing a 6 degrees of freedom (DOF) suturing simulator, as the Phantom Premium 6DOF contains an additional three motors in the handle to produce handle torque. Our research builds on that of [2] and it was in the evaluation stage of this work that hardware was highlighted as an area requiring attention.

Not only is there a qualitative dislike of the use of a Phantom for some, but further to this the presence of undesired forces in a simulation could cause artefacts in the training regime of a student.

It is for these reasons that a gravity compensation system is developed; software will sample the coordinate and orientation information of the Phantom, calculate the necessary force to counteract gravitational forces, and send force and torque vectors back to the Phantom to control it. The scheme will run invisibly on-top of any other application using the Phantom so that non-gravitational forces can still be felt by the user. By doing so, the device is effectively removed from the simulation and the desired interface transparency is achieved.

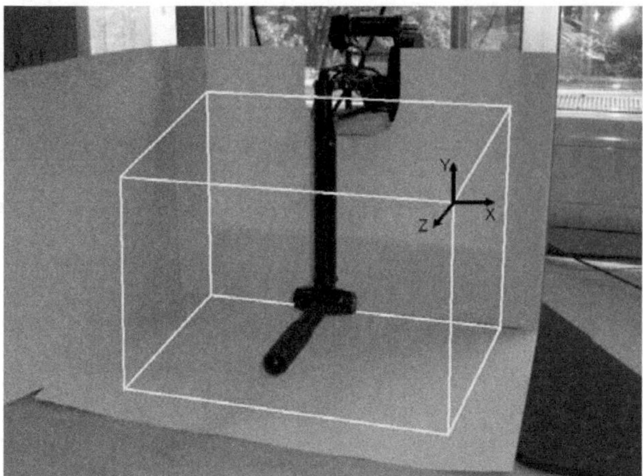

Figure 1. Workspace and coordinate system of the Phantom

2. Approaches

The kinematics of multi-component systems is not a new area and as such a forward kinematics approach was initially taken in an attempt to solve the problem [3,4]. For the 3DOF Phantom in [4] a gravity compensation system was proposed. However, for the Phantom Premium 6DOF, obtaining values for the additional unknown parameters such as the mass of the handle, the additional motors, and their centre of masses was insurmountable without physically deconstructing the device and as such, a new approach was sought.

As the overall function we require (that takes the coordinates and orientation of the device and returns a force and torque vector) should form a smooth continuous surface over of the problem space of all possible coordinates and orientations, a neural network is well suited to finding the mapping. Given a training set of coordinates and orientation inputs and the empirically found force and torque outputs, the network should be able to extrapolate for all coordinate and orientations in the workspace.

3. Methods

The *gravity compensation scheme* is split into two separate systems. The torque, required to prevent handle rotation as a result of gravity, and the force, to prevent any positional movement.

Torque Calculation

As direct control of individual motors is not possible, other than by using raw encoder values (where no consistent and reliable mapping between them and Newtons exists), the Phantom is sent a torque vector, split into components of torque about the global X-axis, Y-axis, and Z-axis. The motors then effect this torque.

The two components of handle orientation required for torque calculation are retrieved from the Phantom's Jacobian matrix, which maps device rotation to Cartesian space. These two components, J_X and J_Z, give the proportion of the handle currently present along the X-axis and Z-axis respectively, when projected onto an X-Z plane. To illustrate, a full alignment of the handle along the Z-axis whilst parallel to the plane (as shown in Figure 1), would yield a values of $J_X = 0$ and $J_Z = 1$; whereas if the handle pointed directly down, $J_X = J_Z = 0$.

The mass of the handle is estimated empirically by resting the device on a virtual surface with the top counterweight fixed so that only vertical movement is possible. The force required to hold the Phantom in position is then taken as the weight of the handle. This makes the assumption that second counterweight on the Phantom counters the weight of the two intermediate arms. The handle's torque-vector (τ) is given by:

$$\tau_X = -LgmJ_Z$$
$$\tau_Y = 0$$
$$\tau_Z = LgmJ_X$$

where $L = 75$mm and is half the length of the handle; $g = 9.80665$ ms^{-2}; $m = 0.12$N and is the combined mass of the handle components.

Force Calculation

Two forces are required, the upwards push along the Y-axis, and a second, push-pull force, to prevent movement in the X-Z plane. The latter of these forces is split into its X-axis and Z-axis components before it can be sent to the Phantom.

During training, to reduce complexity, the X-component remains zero so that all positional movement is limited to the Y Z plane. Once trained, the push-pull force can be split into its X-axis and Z-axis components depending on the current rotation of the device, by taking its sine and cosine components.

In an attempt to further reduce the complexity of the problem, the problem space is divided again. In the initial data capture stage, the handle remains parallel to the X-Z plane, and in line with the Z-axis as shown in Figure 1. This data set holds pairings of coordinate inputs to force outputs (for full details of data capture see below). A separate data set is also captured for a second network; where the coordinates of the handle remain constant but its orientation is varied. For this, it is the torque components to force pairings that are recorded.

These two networks are trained separately and then used in combination to form a system that produces an appropriate force. In use, the torque-force network is used twice, to produce a force vector for the current orientation, and a force vector for if it were oriented in the default position. The difference between the two is taken and then added to the output of the coordinate-force network, to give a force for the current position, corrected for the current orientation.

Neural Network Setup

During development a number of parameters were varied in an attempt to find a suitable network. Where possible, these were tailored to the data to ensure full use of the possible solution space. In other cases, such as number of hidden neurons, a range of values were tested, to find the most appropriate value.

The most successful network uses standard back-propagation and takes two inputs, representing the Y and Z coordinates (converted to be rotationally invariant), both of which are normalised [-1:1]. The output of the network is two forces, the upwards force and the push-pull force, which is subsequently broken into its X-axis and Z-axis components. There are 32 hidden neurons, in a single layer and all neurons use a standard bipolar sigmoid activation function (limits [-1:2], sigma = 0.5). The learning rate is initially set to 0.00002 and interactively varied depending on the current rate of change in error; where error is the difference between the training data and the predicted output forces. The network is trained continually, intermittently running the gravity compensation scheme on the Phantom using the network, and moving the Phantom around to see if it holds.

The neural network used for learning the torque-force mapping uses the same architecture as above, except it contains ten hidden neurons instead of 32 due to it being a more simple mapping to model. Input is the torque (normalised to [-1:1]) and testing is carried by varying only the orientation and seeing if the Phantom holds.

Training Data

To automate data capture for the first network, two virtual planes are created, one vertical in the X-Y plane to hold the Phantom at the desired Z-distance, and one horizontal X-Z plane, that slowly moves up 6mm, waits for equilibrium, takes a measure of the force required to hold the handle in position and repeats. This is done at eight Z-distances over the workspace [-60, -30, -15, 0, 40, 70, 110, 150], over the full available height of the workspace to give a total of 300 coordinate-force training pairs, satisfying the suggested ratio of [5] for an error of 10%. During this phase, the handle remains inline with the Z-axis and parallel to the X-Z plane; this requires manual adjustment as the handle rises.

To capture data for the second network, two virtual planes hold the handle in position in the middle of the workspace and the handle orientation is altered by hand, stopping in a variety of possible configurations for force measurements to be taken. In total 50 handle orientations were captured. To allow further analysis, this was repeated for a second point in the workspace.

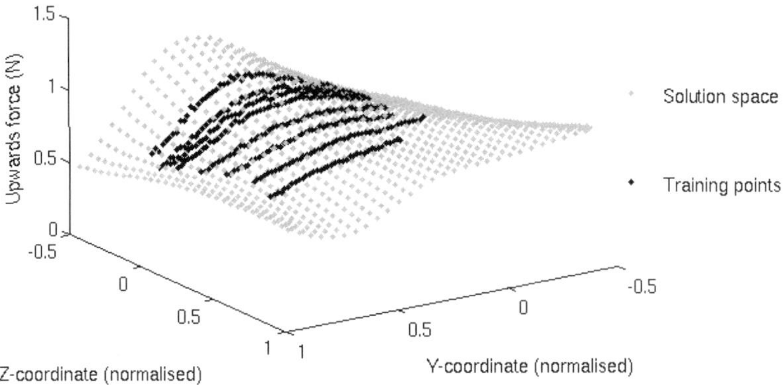

Figure 2. Upwards force surface and training data

4. Results

After approximately 4.5 million iterations the error in the coordinate-force network between the training set and the predicted values drops to 0.0149 (4 d.p.) and is able to provide gravity compensation reliably within approximately 80% of the physical workspace capable by the Phantom, this is approximated by the highlighted box in Figure 1. This is when the handle remains parallel to the X-Z plane and inline with the rest of the Phantom.

After around 2 million iterations, the error for the handle torque-force network drops to and levels off at 0.0157 (4 d.p.) and works for a variety of configurations, but does fail in several orientations even when the position is the same as the training position. Unfortunately, despite an apparent good fit to the data and low error rate, due to the need for a high level of accuracy, even minor errors can cause graceful failure.

The surfaces generated by the coordinate-force network along with the training data points are shown in Figure 2 and Figure 3 and show an excellent fit to the data. Figure 4 shows both surfaces generated for the torque-force.

The temperature of the six motors used in the Phantom were recorded whilst the Phantom was in use for twenty minutes. During this time, the hottest motor had yet to reach a third of its safety threshold, aptly demonstrating the capabilities of the hardware to run a gravity compensation scheme.

5. Discussion

Early qualitative evaluation of the presented gravity compensation scheme has been very positive and with a clear avenue of development to achieve a full 6DOF gravity compensated surgical simulator laid out, we look forward to its inclusion in our future work.

A neural network has been able to learn the required forces to hold a Phantom in place for the majority of the workspace, when the handle orientation matches that of training. This is equivalent to a 3DOF gravity compensation scheme, found by a method that could be used for other SensAble Phantom products.

In the development stage, data was captured with the top counterweight removed. The handle orientation was maintained and the coordinate-force network was trained.

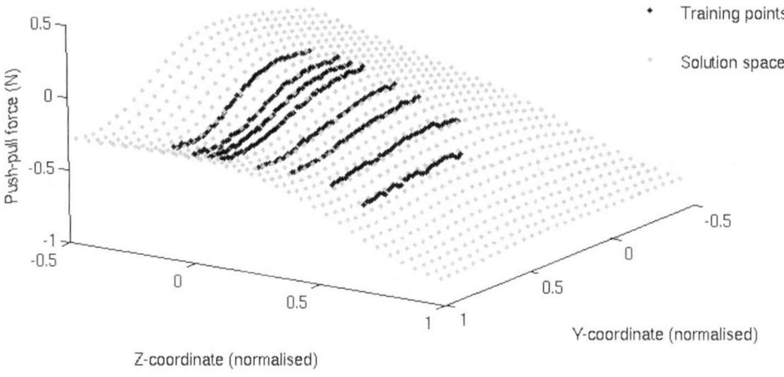

Figure 3. Push-pull force surface and training data

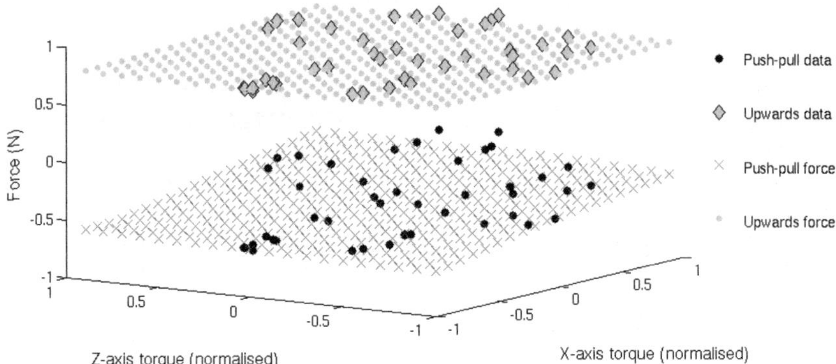

Figure 4. Both torque-force surfaces and training sets

But when tested the whole system worked, 6DOF as well. It would seem that by introducing the additional force required due to removal of one of the counterweights, the system seemed to lock up the handle to a point where it seemed a little stiff, but still very useable. This may be useful for those not interested in force accuracy, perhaps designers or such like, but it is not appropriate for our uses.

Initial evaluation suggests the 6DOF component of the system requires a richer data set in order to be successful, with various handle orientations being unsupported in the final model. The torque-force relationship is highly linear however, with a differing gradient over the workspace. As such coordinates and torques are required together to provide an accurate mapping and this will be the next step in its improvement.

In the slow surgical procedures such a scheme is aimed at, inertial effects are considered negligible.

The issues raised with a gravity compensation scheme used in a surgical simulator, such as the accuracy of the scheme and its affect on a highly accurate finite element model, along with a more qualitative evaluation of it will be important future work.

References

[1]   SensAble Technologies, Inc.®, http://www.SensAble.com – Last accessed 30/10/06
[2]   Holbrey, R., 2005, 'Virtual Suturing for Training in Vascular Surgery', PhD thesis, University of Leeds.
[3]   Horn, B. K. P., Hirokawa, K., and Vazirani, V., 1977, 'Dynamics of a Three Degree of Freedom Kinematic Chain', A.I. Memo 478.
[4]   Cavusoglu, M. C., Feygin, D., and Tendick, F., 2002, 'A Critical Study of the Mechanical and Electrical Properties of the Phantom Haptic Interface and Improvements for High Performance Control', Presence, 11(6) 555-568.
[5]   Baum, E. B., and Haussler, D., 1989, 'What Size Net Gives Valid Generalization?', Neural Computation, 1(1) 151-160.

Medicine Meets Virtual Reality 15
J.D. Westwood et al. (Eds.)
IOS Press, 2007

Endotracheal Intubation Training using Virtual Images: Learning with the Mobile Telementoring Intubating Video Laryngoscope

Ben H. Boedeker [€], MD, Scott Hoffman [F], MD, W Bosseau Murray [£] [1] , MD
[€] *University NE Medical Center, Omaha, NE; Omaha VAMC,TATRC, Ft Detrick, MD*
[F] *University NE Medical Center, Omaha, NE*
[£] *Simulation Development Lab, Pennsylvania State University College of Medicine,
Hershey, PA*

Abstract: Airway management and intubation skills are essential for in-hospital as well as out-of-hospital health care. However, these skills are difficult to learn and maintain. We tested the hypothesis that novice endoscopists (medical students) could rapidly learn intubation skills, and achieve success in routine as well as difficult intubations using an indirect video laryngoscope. Following the success of the students, we believe that indirect laryngoscopy could become a valuable technique in disaster medicine and personnel hampered by chem.-bio suits.

Keywords: Intubation, endotracheal tube, virtual reality, teaching, disaster medicine

Introduction

Airway management is a basic skill that must be acquired by many medical providers for routine use as well as during emergencies and disasters. With more operations being performed out of the operating room, including the use of conscious sedation, airway management and intubation skills are becoming even more necessary.

When an intubation is required during airway management, the standard method of direct visualization consists of aligning the oral, pharyngeal and laryngeal axes, to achieve direct visualization of the glottic opening. This is often technically challenging (especially with the obesity epidemic), difficult to teach, and even more difficult to maintain proficiency for the occasional endoscopist. We postulated that indirect methods of visualizing the glottic opening and vocal cords are easier to learn and

---

[1] **Corresponding Author**:
W Bosseau Murray,
Department of Anesthesiology H-187, 500 University Ave, Hershey, PA 17033,
tel 717 531 4265,   fax 717 531 5449   E-mail: Bosseau@Gmail.com

require less regular practice to maintain proficiency. The indirect laryngoscope used in this study was the Storz Medi Pack Mobile Imaging System™. This Medi Pack System consists of a light source and video camera head which is built into a modified Macintosh blade (3 or 4). A fiberoptic bundle interfaces with the camera head and runs to the distal end of the Macintosh blade[1]. The image seen at the distal blade tip is transmitted via this fiberoptic bundle to the camera head and projected onto a video monitor. This system allows the laryngoscopist to view an indirect image of a patient's glottic opening on the video monitor and introduce the endotracheal tube which has been shaped into a curve resembling the shape of the Macintosh blade. This curved shape in the endotracheal tube permits the laryngoscopist to maneuver it beyond the direct field of vision into the indirect field projected by the distal fiberoptic bundle; in effect "seeing around the corner" with the video laryngoscope. When using the indirect view, the image projected from the distal tip of the laryngoscope blade permits observation of the glottic structures without the need to align the basic airway axes to permit a direct line of sight. The resulting indirect glottic view is expected by the authors of this paper to be "better" than the direct view offered by conventional laryngoscopy.

The video laryngoscope may also offer advantages for training students in intubation techniques[2]. Projection of the laryngeal anatomy upon the viewing screen will permit both the student and instructor to visualize and discuss the anatomy. The image can be seen by multiple students who may watch the intubation process. When the video laryngoscope is used for training students in intubation, the device can be used in one of two modes: **a.)**   Indirect method – Where both the student and instructor are watching the video monitor. This will allow the instructor to explain the anatomy, mentor the intubation and perform laryngeal manipulations to improve the student's view if necessary.   **b.)**   Direct method – For more advanced students, the viewing monitor can be turned out of the student's view so a direct vision laryngoscopy must be performed. This achieves a training experience identical to the student using a standard laryngoscope blade. However, the instructor can still watch the video monitor during the student's intubation attempt to monitor the airway structures as the student attempts the intubation. This capability could significantly increase safety during intubation training by allowing the instructor to view a patient's airway during the entire intubation attempt. Moreover, if the airway appeared too challenging for the student, the more experienced laryngoscopist could intervene early in the intubation attempt, perform laryngeal maneuvers to enhance the student's view and prevent the student from unsafe intubation practices (e.g., use of excessive force to guide the tube through the glottic opening.) The indirect view from the video monitor also allows an instructor to more rapidly detect an esophageal intubation.

The purpose of this study was to determine whether use of the video laryngoscope in learning to intubate on an Laerdal Difficult Airway Mannequin™ improved three training factors: a) a student's view during laryngoscopy, b) the time to intubate; and c) the intubation success rate. The study also captured students' beliefs regarding whether the video laryngoscope would be useful in clinical practice, and whether they preferred the indirect viewing device compared to a standard intubating blade.

Methods

After Institutional Review Board approval, a convenience sample of students learning basic airway management and intubation skills were recruited from the University of Nebraska Medical Center. They voluntarily participated in this study and no further demographic indicators were recorded. The study consisted of 4 sections: a pre study web based learning program, a pre study questionnaire, a monitored simulation intubation exercise, and a post study questionnaire.

The pre study web based learning program consisting of a tutorial explaining basic intubation techniques. The pre-study questionnaire measured their confidence in being able to successfully intubate a normal airway patient on the first attempt, and if they had experience with a laryngoscope, whether they preferred, or usually used, a Macintosh or Miller intubating blade. Immediately prior to attempting to intubate the mannequin, subjects were again instructed in basic intubation technique by a senior anesthesiologist. After the simulation training a post-study questionnaire assessed their confidence in being able to successfully perform an intubation.

During the intubation simulation training four intubation exercises were conducted in succession using a Laerdal Difficult Intubation Mannequin[TM] by each study participant. These were:
1) intubation on a standard airway with <u>direct</u> visualization of the glottis (i.e., without using the video laryngoscope);
2) intubation of a standard airway with an <u>indirect</u> view (i.e., using the video monitor);
3) intubation on a difficult airway with direct view (i.e., without using the video laryngoscope monitor);
4) intubation on a difficult airway with <u>indirect</u> view. (i.e. using the video monitor).

Students were not restricted on intubation time, however, they were instructed to treat the mannequin as a real patient. The correct position of the 7.0 mm endotracheal tube used was monitored by the investigator by viewing the video monitor during both the direct and indirect view intubation attempts.

After placing the laryngoscopy device in the final position during the intubation attempt, and just before the students began to insert the endotracheal tube through the vocal cords, they recorded the laryngeal view on a modified 4 point Cormack and Lehane scoring system[3]. The mannequin was set at a consistent standard airway setting for standard intubations and set at a consistent difficult airway setting by inflating the tongue for the difficult intubation tests.

For each of the four intubation attempts, the following points were noted: The view of the vocal cords was noted on a 4 point Cormack and Lehane scoring system[3] (1 = good view, 4 = poor view). The success of the intubation was noted as well as the time required for the trainees to successfully intubate the trachea of the mannequin, or acknowledge failure. The instructors rated their ability to see and what the trainee was seeing, as well as their ability to advise the trainees.

Non-parametric data (e.g. ordinal data such as the classification of the view of the vocal cords and glottic opening) was analyzed with a two tailed Fisher Exact Probability test. Welche's modification (due to unequal variances) of Student's t-test was used for parametric data (duration of intubation attempts). A value of $p<0.05$ was considered significant.

Results

There were 45 participants in the study including 35 medical students, 3 residents, 1 respiratory technician, 1 internal medicine resident, and 1 fellow. The background and training was not recorded for the other 4 participants.

The students had a significantly better view of the vocal cords (Class I and II versus Class III and IV) with the video-laryngoscope, both in the normal airway mode ($p<0.001$, Fisher Exact Probability Test), as well as in the difficult airway mode ($p<0.0001$, Fisher Exact Probability Test). (see Table 1). The students also had a significantly greater success rate for intubation in the both in the normal airway mode ($p<0.05$), as well as in the difficult airway mode ($p<0.001$). (see Table 2). Most students, when attempting to intubate the mannequin in the difficult airway mode, almost immediately recognized that they would not succeed without excessive force, while others continued to try, and would not give up. This led to a short attempt time in most instances, but with excessively long times in other cases, resulting in a large variance in the duration of intubation with the direct mode (Macintosh blade). The students all realized that they would be able to intubate the difficult airway mannequin with the indirect mode, and therefore the durations of these attempts (with the indirect device) tended to be longer. (see Table 3)

Table 1: Number of trainees obtaining each view of the glottic opening as per Cormack and Lehane scoring system[3].

	View of Vocal Cords			
	Class I	**Class II**	**Class III**	**Class IV**
"Easy Mannequin" - airway set to standard mode				
Direct (Mac)	5	18	15	6
Indirect (VL)	37	5	0	0
"Difficult Mannequin" - airway set to difficult mode				
Direct (Mac)	0	1	6	32
Indirect (VL)	9	24	4	0

Where:
Indirect VL = is an indirect view using the video-laryngoscope,
Direct Mac = direct view of the vocal cords using the Macintosh intubating blade.

Table 2: Number of trainees who were successful and unsuccessful with each intubating device in each setting of the airway mannequin.

	Successful	Unsuccessful	Significance
"Easy Mannequin" - airway set to standard mode			
Direct	32	13	
Indirect	43	0	$p < 0.05$
"Difficult Mannequin" - airway set to difficult mode			
Direct	2	37	
Indirect	37	0	$p < 0.001$

For legend: see Table 1

Table 3: Intubation time required for trainees to complete the intubation, or acknowledge that they would not be successful.

Intubation Time in minutes					
	Avg	STD	Min	Max	Significance
"Easy Mannequin" - airway set to standard mode					
Direct	0.85	0.84	0.1	3.8	
Indirect	0.28	0.15	0.04	0.67	$p < 0.01$
"Difficult Mannequin" - airway set to difficult mode					
Direct	0.73	0.42	0.32	2.05	
Indirect	1.01	1.20	0.08	6.0	NS

Where: NS = not significant. For legend, see Table 1

Discussion

This study, comparing the video-laryngoscope with the standard Macintosh laryngoscope blade for early learning, has demonstrated that

a.) trainees had a statistically significantly better view of the larynx, as well as a greater success rate for intubation, especially in the difficult airway mode. They believed they had a better grasp of the anatomy due to the ability of the instructor to advise them, and therefore, they believed they could learn faster

b.) instructors indicated that they knew precisely what the trainees were seeing, therefore, they could better advise them, as well as better demonstrate the anatomy c.) it took less time to intubate the standard mannequin with the video laryngoscope compared to the standard Macintosh blade.

Future studies are needed to :

a. determine if these results (using virtual images, rather than direct visualization) are generally applicable to the training of other health care workers.

b. determine if the increased success rate of intubation carries through to the clinical environment, (for instance in patients with expected difficult airways such as subjects with Class 3 and 4 Mallampati scores[4].) Such an increased success rate would help to improve the safety of intubation.

Conclusions

The standard intubation technique has been direct laryngoscopy which requires alignment of the oral, pharyngeal and laryngeal axes to achieve a direct view of the glottic opening. With the introduction of video laryngoscopy, acquiring an indirect view of the glottic opening can be more easily achieved, even by novice endoscopists. We believe that it is likely that video laryngoscopy will become the gold standard for intubation in the future. It allows intubation to be performed faster, with less cervical strain to the patient, while achieving a better view of the glottic opening. The improved view will be of particular benefit to non-anesthesia personnel or first responders who do not frequently perform intubation. This technique may be the method of choice under special circumstances such as during intubation when wearing chemical protective gear.

References:

1. Kaplan M, Ward D, Berci G. A new video laryngoscope – an aid to intubation and teaching. J Clin Anest 14:620-626,2003.

2. Boedeker BH, Murray WB, et al. Basic review of endotracheal intubation for providers at a mass casualty event. . Journal of Clinical Anesthesia. Submitted for Publication 2006.

3. Cormack RS, Lehane J: Difficult tracheal intubation in obstetrics. *Anaesthesia* 39:1105, 1984

4. Mallampati SR, Gatti SP, Gugino LD: A clinical sign to predict difficult intubation: a prospective study. *Can Anaesth Soc J* 32:429-434, 1985

Disclaimer:

These views represent those of the authors and are not necessarily intended to represent the views of the United States Air Force and/or Veteran's Administration.

Acknowledgments:

We would like to acknowledge Dr. Allison Astorino-Courtois, Senior Policy Analyst at GISC-STRATCOM for statistical assistance, Dr George Berci of Cedars Sinai Medical Center Los Angeles for valuable insight provided for investigation and Georgia Purviance, RN for assistance with data collection.

Medicine Meets Virtual Reality 15
J.D. Westwood et al. (Eds.)
IOS Press, 2007

Efficient Modelling of Soft Tissue using Particle Systems

Oliver Buckley and Nigel W. John
University of Wales Bangor

Abstract. The ever improving price-performance ratio of personal computers is making a significant contribution to widening the accessibility of training simulators for a wide variety of medical procedures. High fidelity solutions are becoming more and more sought after. However, the problem of providing realistic soft tissue deformation in real time remains, particularly if haptic interaction is also required. This paper presents a new approach for efficient soft tissue deformation using particle systems to model both structure and haptic properties of anatomy. We are applying this technique to a simulator for interventional radiology procedures, but it can easily be adapted for other medical domains.

Keywords. Soft tissue deformation; particle systems

Introduction

The traditional apprenticeship model for medical training has been supplemented in recent years with the availability of virtual environments (VEs), as these offer the opportunity for unlimited practice for specific situations (see [1] for a comprehensive review). We are currently investigating the effective use of VEs for training interventional radiology (IR) procedures. Fixed anatomy models have been used to good effect for this purpose – see Fig 1, however, there are several drawbacks For example, such models do not allow for a diverse and varied challenge, and they can degenerate over time losing some of their effectiveness. Also, the deformation and reaction of a plastic tube is different from that of soft tissues and so the feel of the catheter and guidewire as they are inserted will be far from reality.

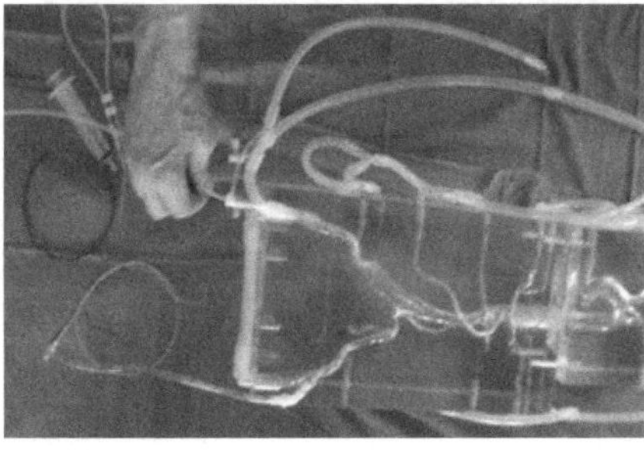

Figure 1. Fixed Model for IR. Good for understanding catheter manipulation but lacks realism. Image courtesy of Royal Liverpool Hospitals, UK

The motivation behind our work is to provide a viable and improved alternative to a fixed model. A substantial part of this work is to accurately simulate the haptic properties of various soft tissues and a new method to achieve this is described in this paper. When integrated within the IR simulator currently being developed at Bangor [2], we aim to provide a training option that is dynamic, varied, and fully customisable as well as being infinitely reusable, with no degradation or loss of accuracy over time.

1. Methods

Many of the current approaches to soft tissue modelling are physically based, relying on either a mass-spring system or finite element modelling – see [1, 3] for an overview of these and other commonly used techniques. We have found these models to be too slow or not realistic enough for our requirement to support soft tissue deformation and needle puncture, whilst also providing haptic feedback that is both visually and haptically realistic but will also run in real time on a standard desktop PC. Most of the current approaches focus on the surface of the object to be deformed, and offer little or no consideration to the internal structure of the object. When considering an application such a training simulator for IR, then the internal structure of the object in question becomes very important. It would be extremely useful to be able to model not only the surface of an organ, like the liver, but also to be able to model what is internal to the liver. Our approach explores a new use of particle systems [2] to support not only surface deformation but also needle puncture and the internal structure of an object.

Particle systems are used in computer graphics to model fuzzy phenomena such as fire or clouds using a large collection of independent objects, often represented as single points. Each particle has its own motion and property parameters, typically drawn from a random distribution. Particles may also be connected in some way to form objects with structure. For example, an object can be modelled inside a regular grid of particles. Associated with each particle are a number of attributes, which include: state, position, index number, nearest neighbours, displacement from origin, and presence.

To create anatomical objects we shape the grid structure by altering those particles that are present. Anything that has a zero value for presence will not be drawn. A particle in our structure is notionally linked to its six nearest neighbours. The structure as a whole has a value associated with it to determine the maximum allowable distance between a particle cell and its nearest neighbours. If this condition is broken then the neighbouring particles will be displaced to maintain the connectivity rules – see Fig. 2. This displacement is then propagated throughout the entire structure. By varying these maximum distance constraints we can model a variety of materials, a soft and malleable object by increasing the maximum allowable distance and conversely a rigid object by shortening the maximum allowable displacement. Once a particle becomes sufficiently displaced from its point of origin it will be destroyed and removed from the structure entirely. This removal of particles allows holes and pathways to be created within a structure, and so allows the simulation of needle puncture, and other tool interaction.

To achieve haptic feedback in a particle system, where a particle traditionally has no dimensions or mass, we have modelled each particle in the system as a gravity well.

By varying the sphere of influence of the gravity well, and the force required to leave the well, we can model materials with different properties.

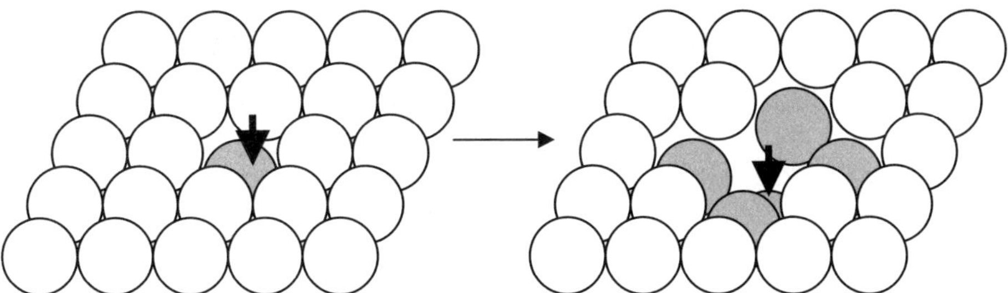

Figure 2. As the highlighted particle is displaced its nearest neighbours are further apart than the allowable distance. Therefore the neighbouring particles will be displaced to maintain displacement rules

2. Results and Conclusions

Irregular shapes such, such as human organs (liver, kidney, etc.) can be segmented from patient specific medical data scans. There are many published segmentation algorithms. We are now able to model these organs using a particle system approach and deform their shape in real time on a standard desktop PC, currently somewhere between 10 and 20 frames per second, depending on the size of structure modeled. Our method has been implemented using OpenGL, the OpenHaptics toolkit and a Phantom Omni Haptic Device. We are currently modelling realistic shapes, such as a liver, taken directly from CT/ultrasound data. The algorithm is being integrated into a simulator for image guided needle puncture that has been developed at Bangor and validated at teaching hospitals in the UK [2].

References

[1]   F.P. Vidal, et al, Principles and Applications of Computer Graphics in Medicine. Computer Graphics Forum, Vol. 25 Issue 1, 2006, pp113-137
[2]   F.P. Vidal, et al, Developing a Needle Guidance Virtual Environment with Patient Specific Data and Force Feedback. In Proc. of 19th International Congress of CARS - Computer Assisted Radiology and Surgery, Berlin, Germany, pp 418-423, 2005.
[3]   S.D. Laycock and A.M. Day, A Survey of Haptic Rendering Techniques, Computer Graphics Forum, Vol. 26, Issue 2, 2007. To appear.
[4] W. T. Reeves, Particle Systems - a Technique for Modeling a Class of Fuzzy Objects. ACM Transactions on Graphics (TOG), Vol. 2 Issue 2, 1983, pp91-108

Medicine Meets Virtual Reality 15
J.D. Westwood et al. (Eds.)
IOS Press, 2007

Requirement Specification for Surgical Simulation Systems with Surgical Workflows

Oliver BURGERT [a,1], Thomas NEUMUTH [a], Michel AUDETTE [a], Antje PÖSSNECK [a],
Rafael MAYORAL [a], Andreas DIETZ [a,b], Jürgen MEIXENSBERGER [a,c],
Christos TRANTAKIS [a,c]

[a] *Innovation Center Computer Assisted Surgery ICCAS, Universität Leipzig, Germany*
[b] *Department of ENT/Plastic Surgery, University Hospital Leipzig, Germany*
[c] *Department of Neurosurgery, University Hospital Leipzig, Germany*

Abstract. Surgical simulations are normally developed in a cycle of continuous refinement. This leads to high costs in simulator design and as a result to a very limited number of simulators which are used in clinical training scenarios. We propose using Surgical Workflow Analysis for a goal-oriented specification of surgical simulators. Based on Surgical Workflows, the needed interaction scenarios and properties of a simulator can be derived easily. It is also possible to compare an existing simulator with the real workflow to distinguish whether it behaves realistically. We are currently using this method for the design of a new simulator for transnasal neurosurgery with good success.

Keywords. Surgical Simulation, Requirements Specification, Design, Surgical Workflow

Introduction

Many medical simulation and training systems addressing different types of surgery and surgical skills have been developed [1]. The design of such systems generally follows a step-by-step approach to make the simulation as realistic as possible. However, the scene design depends heavily on the opinion of very few surgeons and is often done by intuition. This results in an increased number of iterations in the development cycle and, therefore, higher development costs.

The aim of this paper is to describe a novel goal-oriented method for the design of surgical simulation systems: we propose using "Surgical Workflows" (S-WF) [2] as basis for the definition of the surgical scene and the surgical skills which shall be trained. Surgical Workflows are an abstraction of many individual interventions and describe individual and average intervention courses.

---

[1] Corresponding Author: Oliver Burgert, Innovation Center Computer Assisted Surgery (ICCAS), Universität Leipzig, Philipp-Rosenthal-Str. 55, 04103 Leipzig, Germany; E-Mail: oliver.burgert@iccas.de

1. Tools and Methods

We employ the tools developed at our Centre for the analysis of surgical procedures, e.g. a "Surgical Workflow Editor" [3] which is used to record intervention courses. While recording, the surgeons can indicate important decisions, and structures or abnormalities. The number of recorded interventions needed for valid representation of the procedure depends on the complexity and variability of the intervention. The Surgical Workflows can be visualized either in a time-oriented or logically-oriented structure [4]. Using special techniques for the aggregation of Surgical Workflows, it is always possible to look at descriptions of single surgical processes, or at a union of all interventions for any specific type of procedure.

Intraoperative videos covering the situs are recorded either from the OR microscope or endoscope. In addition, it may be useful to document the whole scene and cover the motions of the surgeons for further analysis. Intraoperative photos are used to document situations indicated as of high importance by the surgeons.

The recorded workflows are enhanced by the intraoperative pictures and videos to represent the Surgical Workflow (see Figure 1). Now, both the logical and visual representations can be used to identify the relevant steps of the intervention. The surgeons together with the surgical scene designer and the simulator programmers can discuss the importance of each step for a specific training goal. In this way the necessary anatomical structures and their biomechanical behavior, instruments, and actions can be determined. This, in turn, results in a requirement specification for the surgical simulator.

Workflows allow great flexibility in the recording of the interventions regarding both the level of detail and the used concepts. It is also possible to consider online and offline recording. Therefore, workflows naturally support an iterative development process. Once specific critical portions of the initial workflow have been identified by the developing team, a second round of workflow recording is possible.

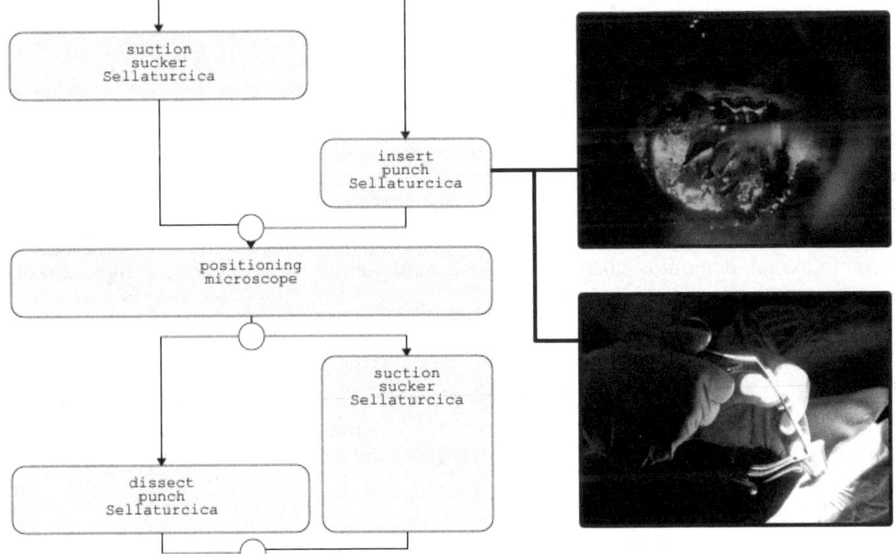

Figure 1. Excerpt from S-WF-graph with corresponding surgical action.

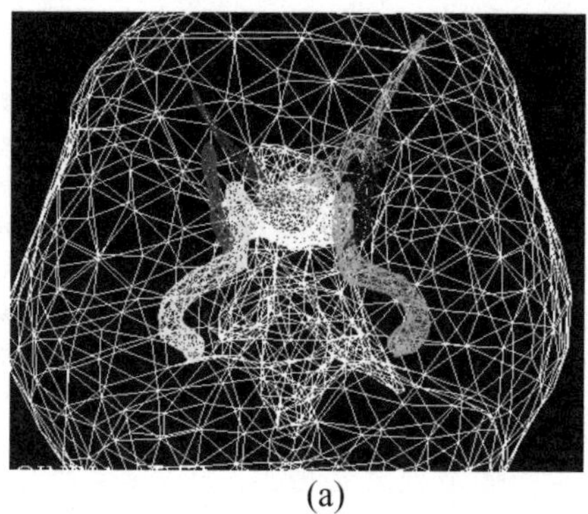
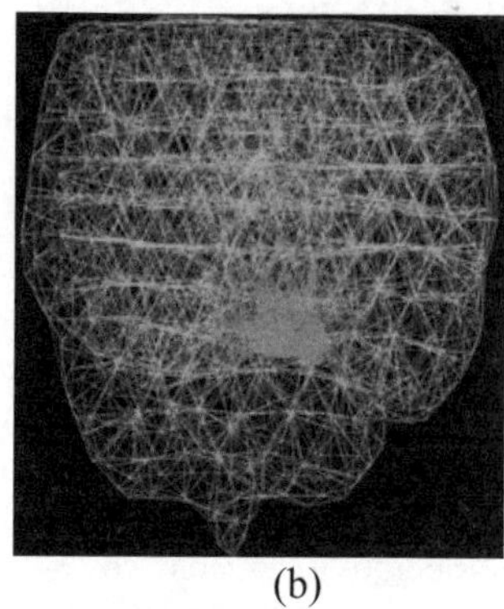

(a)   (b)

Figure 2. Topologically faithful, spatially varying meshing for endoscopic pituitary surgery simulation. (a) Brain surface mesh, bottom view with critical tissues; (b) tetrahedral mesh.

A viable scenario is to use intraoperative videos covering the situs and the critical sections to perform a more specific offline workflow recording. The same logical structure for the workflow recording is used, but the anatomical structures, instruments, and actions of interest will correspond to the more restricted situation. This possibility is in line with the goal-oriented approach to simulator development which is thus supported by the ability of recording highly specific workflows.

A characteristic example of workflow recruitment in surgery simulation can be seen in the elaboration of patient-specific anatomical meshing currently underway. We demonstrated the consideration of endoscopic surgery requirements in anatomical meshing of the pituitary gland and surrounding tissues [5], as shown in Figure 2. This method featured spatially varying mesh density [6] in order to reconcile the dense shapes required for endoscopic views and it focused haptic interaction for simulating transnasal pituitary surgery (Figure 3).

Additionally, we benefit from our experience in developing a virtual reality FESS (functional endoscopic sinus surgery) simulator (Figure 4). The simulator was developed without support of any precedent workflow analysis. The FESS simulator provides a force feedback via the PHANToM, a haptic device [7]. A study with the experienced and inexperienced surgeons was conducted to evaluate the simulator concerning criteria like anatomy, force feedback, and reality. The literature review (e.g. [8]-[14]) showed that the use of Surgical Workflows is a new specification method to define requirements of surgical simulators. We now use Surgical Workflows to get in-depth knowledge about the design flaws we made in our initial system design, and also in order to improve the simulator.

2. Results

Currently, we are using the proposed method for the design of a simulator for pituitary gland surgeries. Until Oct. 2006, we recorded 7 hypophysisadenoma for the first specification phase.

Because of the transnasal approach, two surgeons (ENT and Neurosurgery) are involved, each of them responsible for the specific anatomical region. The intervention requires highly-developed surgical skills because of the surrounding risk structures.

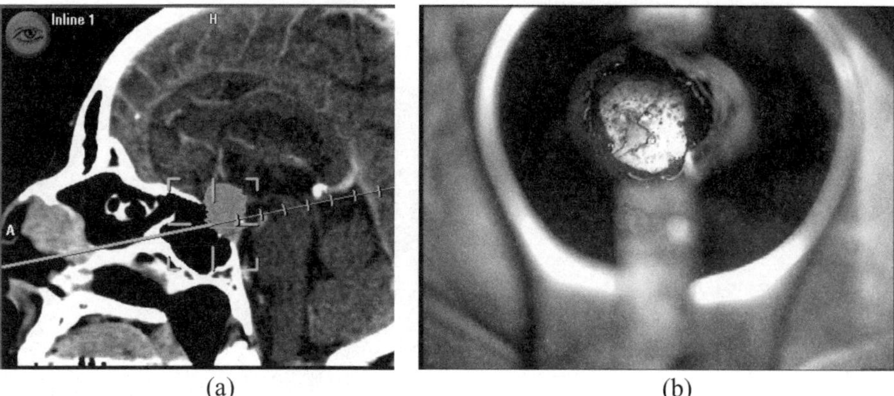

Figure 3. Illustration of trans-nasal pituitary surgery: (a) navigation view; (b) intraoperative situs.

The employment of enriched Surgical Workflows allows the cooperation of researchers coming from various scientific disciplines. Working together, they generate the necessary requirement specification. Consequently, the aims of the simulator can be determined more easily, and for each intervention step it is possible to define sub-goals which can be modeled and trained separately.

The implication is that anatomical meshing should also account for the separability of tissues around the relevant sulcus, e.g. the Sylvian fissure, by using semi-automatic procedures to detect them [16], as well as by enforcing this separability on the surface mesh by performing the required cut to the simplex mesh by topological operatoι [6][17], and ultimately on the volumetric meshing bounded by the surface mesh. Without a formal workflow analysis, it is unlikely that the anatomical meshing would be sufficiently expressive for the simulation.

Regarding the results of the evaluation study of our FESS simulator, we state that it is inalienable to record a workflow of the intervention that should be simulated and to do an offline analysis of the workflow using additional endoscopic video material. Anatomical particularities, their treatment, and the adjustment of the force feedback need an objective analysis, definition, and discussion in advance. Also, the accurate definition of surgical actions performed at anatomical or pathological structures is crucial. For example, the surgeon performs ripping motions with a Blakesley to remove ethmoid air cells. In the first version of the simulator the same task could be accomplished by a much simpler clipping motion. This reduced the level of realism achievable by the simulator. The analysis of important simulation steps can only be realized in cooperation with the surgeons who can define critical tasks of an intervention that need training, the needed force feedback, and tissue behavior during surgery.

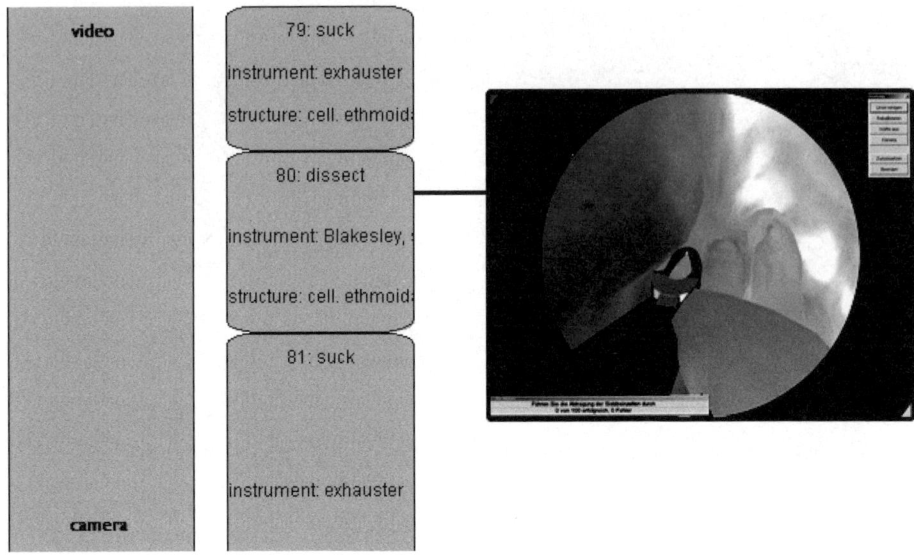

Figure 4. Surgical Workflow with a corresponding image of the simulated scene in the FESS training simulator.

3. Conclusion and Discussion

The method for requirement specification proposed in this paper helps in the goal-oriented requirement specification of surgical simulators. Workflows allow anticipating and identifying the pitfalls of real surgery. Visualized workflows including photographs and movie clips are an excellent communication tool enabling interdisciplinary discussions between surgeons and computer scientists. Not only the relevant scenarios for training can be derived from them, but also different surgical schools can be supported by one system. As a refinement step, we propose employing techniques like in [18] to analyze and model the single skills needed at specific steps, thus increasing the learning effect.

Acknowledgements

The Innovation Center Computer Assisted Surgery (ICCAS) at the Faculty of Medicine at the University of Leipzig is funded by the German Federal Ministry for Education and Research (BMBF) and the Saxon Ministry of Science and the Fine Arts (SMWK) in the scope of the initiative "Unternehmen Region" with the grant numbers 03 ZIK 031 and 03 ZIK 032.

References

[1]   P. Leskovsky, M. Harders, G. Székely: *A Web-Based Repository of Surgical Simulator Projects*, Medicine Meets Virtual Reality (MMVR) 14, p. 311-315, 2006.

[2]   O. Burgert, T. Neumuth, M. Fischer, V. Falk, G. Strauß, C. Trantakis, S. Jacobs, A. Dietz, J. Meixensberger, F.W. Mohr, W. Korb, H.U. Lemke: *Surgical Workflow Modeling*, Medicine Meets Virtual Reality (MMVR) 14, pp. 267, 2006.

[3]   T. Neumuth, N. Durstewitz, M. Fischer, G. Strauß, A. Dietz, J. Meixensberger, P. Jannin, K. Cleary, H.U. Lemke, O. Burgert: *Structured Recording of Intraoperative Surgical Workflows*, in S.C. Horii, O.M. Ratib (Eds.): SPIE Medical Imaging 2006 – PACS and Imaging Informatics, vol. 7(31), CID61450A, San Diego.

[4]   T. Neumuth, G. Strauß, J. Meixensberger, H.U. Lemke, O. Burgert: *Acquisition of Process Descriptions from Surgical Interventions*, in S. Bressan, J. Kueng, R. Wagner (Eds.): Database and Expert Systems Applications, Lecture Notes in Computer Science 4080, p. 602-611, Springer Berlin/Heidelberg.

[5]   P. Cappabianca et al.: *Atlas of Endoscopic Anatomy for Endonasal Intracranial Surgery*, Springer 2001.

[6]   M.A. Audette, H. Delingette, A. Fuchs, O. Astley and K. Chinzei: *A Topologically Faithful, Tissue-guided, Spatially Varying Meshing Strategy for Computing Patient-specific Head Models for Endoscopic Pituitary Surgery Simulation*, Computer Vision for Biomedical Image Applications International Conference on Computer Vision (ICCV) Workshop, Beijing, LNCS 3765, pp. 178-188, 2005. Accepted for publication in Journal of Computer Aided Surgery (2006).

[7]   A. Pößneck, E. Nowatius, C. Trantakis, H. Cakmak, H. Maaß, U. Kühnapfel, A. Dietz, G. Strauß: *A virtual training system in endoscopic sinus surgery*. Proceedings of the 19thCongress and Exhibition CARS 2005, Elsevier International Congress Series 1281 526-30.

[8]   M. Hilbert, W. Müller, J. Strutz: *Developement of a surgical simulator for interventions of the paranasal sinuses. Techniquel principles and initial prototype*, Laryngorhinootologie, 1998 Mar; 77(3) 153-6. Germany.

[9]   C.V. Edmond jr, D. Heskamp, D. Sluis et al.: *ENT Endoscopic Surgical Training Simulator*, Stud Health Technol Inform 1997;39 518-28.

[10] C.Trantakis, J.Meixensberger, G.Strauß et al.: *IO-Master 7D – a new device for virtual neuroendoscopy*, Proceedings of the 18thCongress and Exhibition CARS 2004, Elsevier International Congress Series 1268 707-7.

[11] S. Weghorst, C. Airola, P. Oppenheimer et al.: *Validation of the Madigan ESS Simulator*, Stud HealthTechnol Inform 1998;50 399-405.

[12] T. Rudman, Stredney, D., Sessanna, D., et al.: *Functional Endoscopic Sinus Surgery Training Simulator*, Laryngoscope 1998;108 1643-1647.

[13] U. Ecke, L. Klimek, W. Müller et al.: *Virtual Reality: Preparation and execution of sinus surgery*, Comput Aided Surg 1998; 3 45-50.

[14] M. Caversaccio, A. Eichenberger, R. Häusler,: *Virtual Simulator as a Training Tool for Endonasal Surgery*, Am J Rhinol 2003; 17 283-90.

[15] L.N. Sekhar, E. de Oliveira: *Cranial Microsurgery – Approaches and Techniques*, Thieme, 1999.

[16] G. Le Goualher, E. Procyk, L. Collins, R. Venegopal, C. Barillot, and A. Evans: *Automated extraction and variability analysis of sulcal neuroanatomy*, IEEE Transactions on Medical Imaging, TMI, 18(3):206--217, 1999.

[17] H. Delingette: *General Object Reconstruction Based on Simplex Meshes*, Int. J. Computer Vision, Vol. 32, No. 2, pp. 111-146, 1999.

[18] S. Sinigaglia, G. Megali, O. Tonet, P. Dario: *A machine learning approach to understand surgical performance*, Computer Assisted Radiology and Surgery (CARS) 2006, Osaka, Japan.

Medicine Meets Virtual Reality 15
J.D. Westwood et al. (Eds.)
IOS Press, 2007

3D Visualization and Open Planning Platform in Virtual Fluoroscopy

G. CHAMI [1,b], R. PHILLIPS [a], J.W. WARD [a], M.S. BIELBY [a], A.M.M.A. MOHSEN [b]
[a] *Department of Computer Science, University of Hull, Hull, UK, HU6 7RX*
[b] *Hull and East Yorkshire Hospitals NHS Trust, UK*

Abstract. Typically virtual fluoroscopy systems display the tracked instruments as a projected shadow on a number of 2D x-ray images completely missing the depth information of the third dimension. This paper describes an extra tool for 3D reconstruction in virtual fluoroscopy which is useful to clarify the position of instruments or anatomy and can be used in planning and assessing surgical procedure without further x-ray images. Two examples are given: displaced subtrochanteric fracture and slipped upper femoral epiphysis is presented.

Keywords. Surgical navigation, virtual fluoroscopy, CAOS.

1. Introduction

Virtual fluoroscopy (VF) systems display tracked instruments as a projected shadow on a number of 2D fluoroscopic images, enabling interactive guidance. Surgeons must infer 3D position and structure from these 2D projections. Visualization in 3D is currently achieved either by pre-operative CT scan [1] or intraoperative Iso-C3D (Siemens); both involving significant x-ray exposure. However, such detailed 3D images are not always needed; for long bone fracture reduction the use of numerous x-ray exposures to obtain a precise 3D shape can not be justified. Our aim is to provide 3D reconstructions of anatomy, implants or virtual operative plan, without additional x-ray exposure using an ordinary C-arm. The detail of the reconstructions must be of sufficient quality to perform most tasks during surgery and be easy to comprehend. A further aim is to provide a generic 3D planning platform based on in VF.

2. Methods and results

The VF equipment comprises a computer workstation and an optical tracking system for tracking surgical instruments, anatomy and a registration phantom [2]. A minimum of two sets of images from the C-arm are acquired while the registration phantom is placed in the fluoroscopic imaging space which permits determination of the position of the x-ray source and the image plane [2]. From this an additional 3D visualization is produced showing the images, the x-ray cone beam and the tracked instruments in their correct 3D positions. In this view, a 3D reconstruction of the anatomy is created and displayed as a shaded surface model. This is achieved by outlining one or many areas

---

[1] Email: george.chami@doctors.org.uk

of interest in the fluoroscopic images which could be bone, pathological lesion or implant. Our VF system then automatically projects the outlined areas outwards from the x-ray source for each image. The intersections of these areas are used to compute a 3D bounded colour coded volume which encloses areas of interest (Figure 1). The tracked instruments are visualized in real-time on the same 3D view for navigation and implementation of a plan. Planning could be achieved by outlining the optimal position of an implant which is verified visually in the same 3D view. Additional fluoroscopic images can be taken if needed, to improve the detail of the 3D reconstruction.

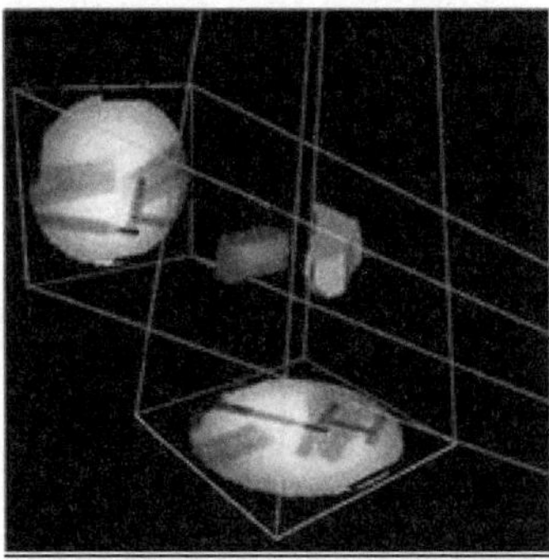

Figure 1: Reconstruction of the subtrochanteric fracture.

For displaced subtrochanteric femoral fracture a 3D-model is reconstructed from two 2D fluoroscopic images. This reconstruction shows the degree of displacement and angulation of the fracture in 3D. It also clearly includes a reconstruction of the fracture line, the position and the alignment of the medullary canal and the piriformis fossa position in 3D. This provides sufficient information to establish the direction of the manocuvre needed for fracture reduction, insertion of guide wire in the direction of the medullary canal and nail insertion for fracture fixation. This information is displayed in 3D space, instead of projective 2D images, to ease comprehension.

In order to assess flexibility in planning a reconstruction of the slipped upper femoral epiphysis was performed. For the measurement of the head-shaft angle, the epiphysis was reconstructed, a perpendicular column to the epiphyseal reconstruction was extended toward the shaft of femur, a further column which is aligned with the anatomical axis of femoral shaft was reconstructed by outlining the medullary canal, intersection of the two columns forms the head-shaft angle (Figure 2). Furthermore, to assess the degree and the direction of displacement, the femoral neck was reconstructed along with the femoral epiphysis. The result showed the degree and the direction of displacement (Figure 3). To verify the position of a guide wire in the femur; the femoral epiphysis, the femoral neck and the guide wire was outlined and reconstructed, the position of the guide wire can be visualized either in the two separate views (Figure 4) or as a combined view. To assess the distance between the wire-tip and the subchondral bone a further x-ray image was needed. For this new x-ray image the fluoroscope was positioned so that its x-ray cone beam was perpendicular to the long axis of the guide wire and centered over the wire-tip.

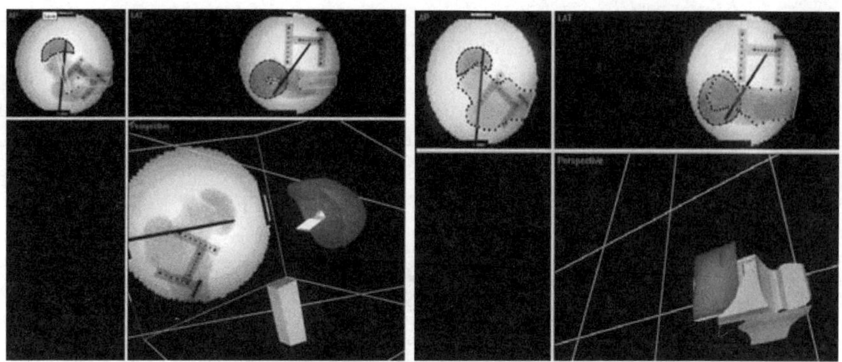

Figure 2: Head-shaft angle.   Figure 3: Degree of displacement.

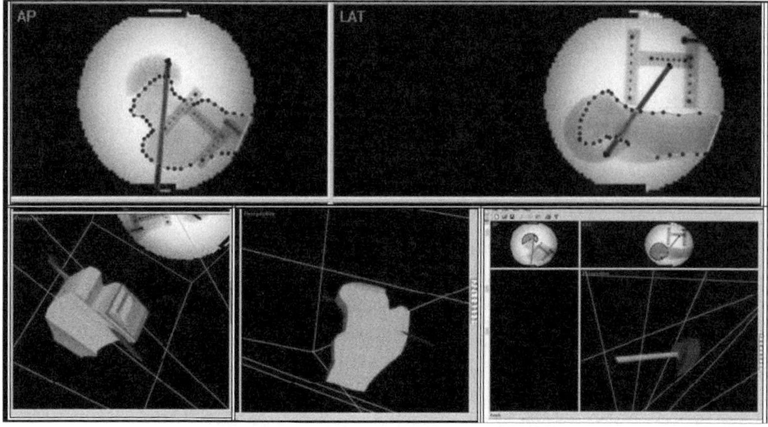

Figure 4: Reconstruction of slipped femoral epiphysis with wire insitu.

3. Discussion

Current VF systems provide planar projections of 3D reality, thus missing the depth information of the third dimension [3]. However, it is often important to verify the correct anatomy in all three dimensions. The system presented builds on the existing Hull's CAOSS [4], bridges the gap between 2D image visualization and precise 3D reconstruction allowing the surgeon to rationalise the radiation exposure and tailor it to the needs of different operations. It also provides a generic 3D planning platform and provides a clear demonstration of the potential benefits of virtual fluoroscopy.

References

[1]   Joskowicz, L., et al., *FRACAS: a system for computer-aided image-guided long bone fracture surgery.* Comput Aided Surg, 1998.3(6): 271-88.
[2]   Phillips R, et al, *A phantom based approach to fluoroscopic navigation for orthopaedic surgery.* Medical Image Computing & Computer Assisted Intervention, MICCAI 2004, 2004. Part 2, 621-628.
[3]   Langlotz F, *Potential pitfalls of computer aided orthopedic surgery.* Injury 2004. 35 Suppl 1: S-A17-23.
[4]   Phillips R, et al, *Hip Trauma.* In Computer and Robotic Assisted knee and Hip Surgery, eds. A.M. DiGioia, et al. 2004, Oxford: Oxford University Press. 283-296.

Medicine Meets Virtual Reality 15
J.D. Westwood et al. (Eds.)
IOS Press, 2007

Intra-operative Registration for Image Enhanced Endoscopic Sinus Surgery using Photo-consistency

Min Si CHEN [a], Gerardo GONZALEZ [a] and Rudy LAPEER [a,1]

[a] *School of Computing Sciences, University of East Anglia, Norwich, UK*

Abstract. The purpose of this paper is to present an intensity based algorithm for aligning 2D endoscopic images with virtual images generated from pre-operative 3D data. The proposed algorithm uses photo-consistency as the measurement of similarity between images, provided the illumination is independent from the viewing direction.

Keywords. endoscopy, augmented reality, registration, photo-consistency

1. Introduction

Anatomical images are vital parts of a large number of clinical applications, such as diagonsis, surgical guidances, and surgical evaluation. Medical imaging modalities include CT (computed tomography), MRI (magnetic resonance imaging) and video from endoscopes. Each modality is designed to capture specific types of anatomical information, e.g. X-ray based CT can distinctively respond to bones, whereas MRI works more effectively on soft tissues. Due to the nature of different sensors, it is often desireable to fuse images from different modalities in order to "complete" the anatomical picture. The process of fusing two images is often referred to as *registration*.

Registration is also an important procedure for augmented reality applications, in which computer generated imagery needs to be correctly aligned with its real counterpart. In order to solve the alignment problem, the pose of a virtual entity used for generating the virtual image must be correctly estimated from a sequence of video images. In this paper, we present an intensity based registration method using the *Photo-consistency* metric [2]. We demonstrate the use of this method for aligning volumetric voxel data with video images of the corresponding subject.

2. Previous Work

Intensity based registration techniques have been well studied in the field of computer vision and medical imaging processing. The essence of this type of algorithm is to establish

---

[1]Corresponding Author: School of Computing Sciences, University of East Anglia, Norwich, UK; E-mail: rjal@cmp.uea.ac.uk

a cost function that has a desired characteristic in colour/intensity when two images are considered to be accurately aligned. One well-known cost function is based on *mutual information* [7,9], which has been extensively studied and used in multi-modal registration. Recently, Clarkson *et al* [2] proposed a cost function based on *photo-consistency*. They demonstrate that it is feasible to use photo-consistency as a cost function to estimate the pose of a polygonal surface model from a sequence of images, provided the assumed illumination model obeys the Lambertian rule. A further development of a photo-consistency based algorithm was presented by Janko and Chetveriko [4,5]. They eliminate the prerequisite for camera calibration. Camera parameters and a rigid transformation representing the pose of the object are solved together using a genetic algorithm. However, the execution time of their method is lengthy due to the dimensionality of the cost function. This is mainly caused by the inclusion of camera parameters to the cost function.

3. Methodology

3.1. Photo-consistency

We assume that the illumination of an object is independent from the viewing direction, i.e. with a Lambertian model, the image of a visible surface point should exhibit similar intensity across different images when the lighting remains static. With our texture based direct volumetric renderer, the image formation process of a voxel can be expressed using Equation 1; where $\mathbf{v}'_{n,i}$ is the projection of the ith visible voxel in the nth image; $\mathbf{P}$ is the projection matrix that is constant for all images; $\mathbf{M}_n$ is the pose of the camera for the nth image.[2]

$$\mathbf{v}'_{n,i} = \mathbf{P}\mathbf{M}_n\mathbf{v}_i \tag{1}$$

The photo-consistency metric between two images is the defined by Equation 2:

$$C_{photo} = \frac{1}{L}\sum_{i=1}^{L}\left\|I_1(\mathbf{v}'_{n,i}) - I_2(\mathbf{v}'_{n,i})\right\|^2 \tag{2}$$

The corresponding pixel intensity of voxel $\mathbf{v}_i$ in each image is given by $I_1(\mathbf{v}'_{n,i})$ and $I_2(\mathbf{v}'_{n,i})$; L is the total number of visible voxel pairs in both images. Therefore, photo-consistency measures the intensity difference between the images of a voxel which appears in two or more endoscopic video images. The images are said to be consistent when the difference is small. If a model is correctly aligned with two or more images, the photo-consistency value should be minimal or ideally zero.

3.2. Registration of Volumetric Voxel Data and Video Images

In order to perform registration using photo-consistency, two images are captured by moving the endoscope around a visible anatomy. A pair of virtual views are generated

---

[2]In our experiment the total number of image used is 2, hence, $n \leq 2$.

using the tracked endoscope information together with the calibrated camera parameters. The objective of registration is to find an optimal rigid transformation $\widehat{\mathbf{M}}_1$ and $\widehat{\mathbf{M}}_2$ for each image to minimise Equation 2.

In general, the number of parameters involved in the cost function is twelve for two image cases. Because the movement of the endoscope is recorded by a tracking device, we can then relate $\widehat{\mathbf{M}}_1$ and $\widehat{\mathbf{M}}_2$ by Equation 3; where $\mathbf{M}_c$ denotes the relative camera motion between two images.

$$\widehat{\mathbf{M}}_2 = \widehat{\mathbf{M}}_1 \mathbf{M}_c \tag{3}$$

With this information only six parameters for $\widehat{\mathbf{M}}_1$ need to be included in the evaluation of cost function.

The complete registration process involves the following steps:

1. Perform camera calibration to obtain intrinsic and extrinsic parameters of the endoscope.
2. An initial estimation of the registration parameters is obtained using the ICP algorithm [1]. This is used as the starting point of the optimisation process.
3. Render the visible surface of the voxel data from two different view points using a modified direct volume rendering method.
4. Search corresponding visible voxels from both rendered images.
5. Evaluate the photo-consistency based cost function.

For the purpose of optimising the cost function, we chose Powell's method [8] as it does not require the derivative of the cost function. Step 3 and 4 are embedded within the optimisation routine, therefore every time a new set of parameters are computed the virtual images are re-rendered and correspondences are re-established.

To simplify the correspondences search, the volumetric data is preprocessed by assigning a unique RGB value for each voxel and store the intensity value of a voxel in the alpha channel. In this way, the volumetric data can be rendered as an iso-surface by using alpha testing in the fragment processing pipeline, e.g. a voxel whose intensity falls below the user defined threshold will not be rendered in the final image. This allows only the designated visible layer of the volume to be rendered. The choice of the threshold is completely manual and the chosen value should generate a virtual voxel surface which is similar to the region observed by the endoscope.

4. Result

The registration method was first used on simulated data. The simulated video images consist of two skull images acquired using surface rendering with Lambertian model. In our first experiment, we aim to study the behaviour of the cost function within a defined range of the parametric domain. The cost function is defined over six independent parameters, thus it is impractical to plot the function in six dimensions. We chose to study the effect of each parameter individually by performing a manual registration, and then each parameter is adjusted within a chosen range while keeping other parameters unchanged to trace the shape of the cost function. By fixing the value of the remaining parameters, this effectively reduces the dimensionality of the cost function to one dimension. Figure 1 shows the shape of the photo-consistency based cost function, when each parameter deviates from its optimal value. The vertical line in each graph denotes the value of the parameter at which the optimal alignment is reached. We can notice in most cases, the optimal parameter value is close to the global minimum of the cost function. This confirms that the photo-consistency based cost function can be used as a method for similarity measurement.

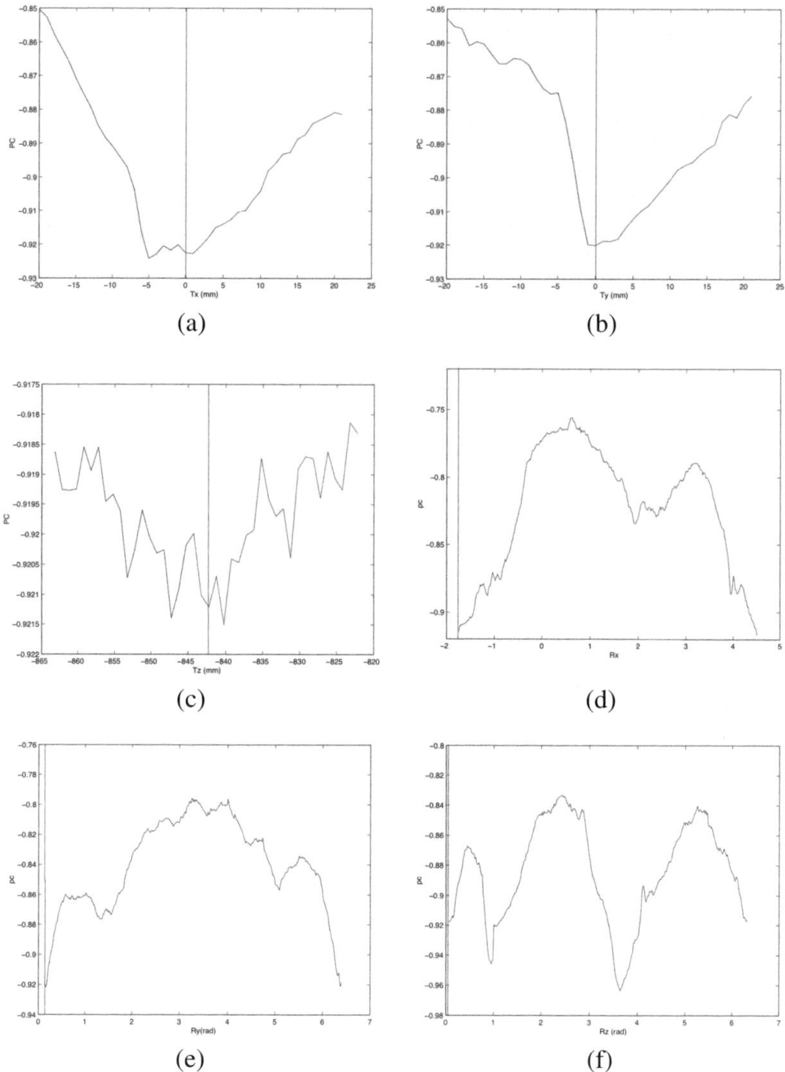

Figure 1. Plots of the photo-consistency cost function against each transformation parameter: (a) t_x, (b)t_y, (c)t_z, (d)r_x, (e)r_y, (f)r_z.

In our second experiment, we performed the registration routine on both simulated and real image data. Figure 2 shows the result of registering a CT scanned skull with a pair of simulated video images of the corresponding skull.

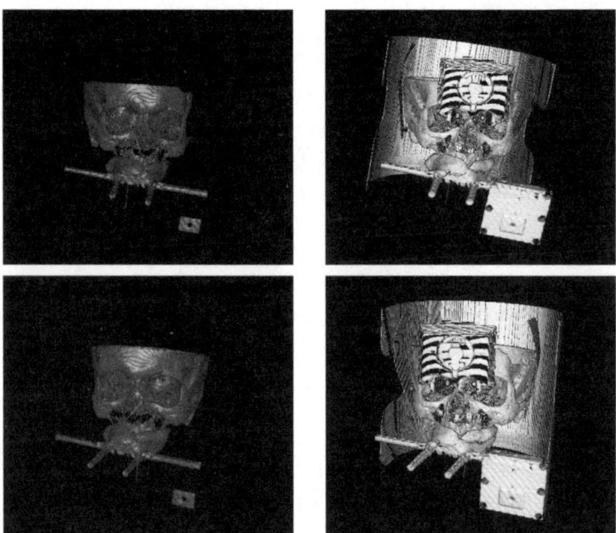

Figure 2. Registration of video images and CT volume using a pair of simulated images: left column shows the simulated video images; right column shows their corresponding reconstructed images after registration.

The experiment on real endoscopic images is performed using our augmented reality based surgical navigation software with real-time modeling of radial distortion [3,6].

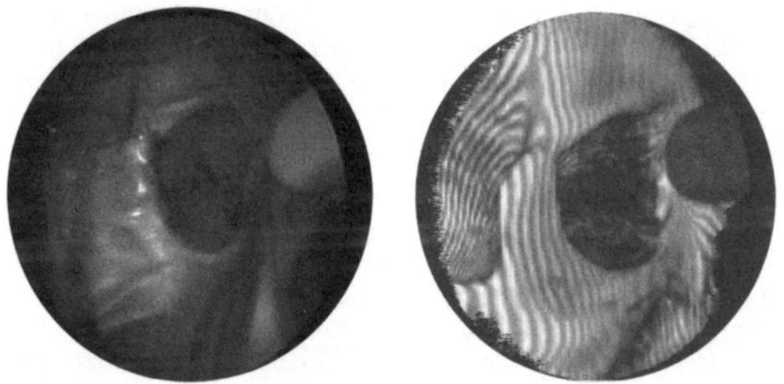

Figure 3. Registration of video images and CT volume using real endoscopic images: left image shows the video image of the orbit; right shows their corresponding reconstructed images after registration.

In both experiments, an average registration error in the range of 1-2mm was found. It is also important to estimate an initial transformation to place the volume close to the optimal alignment. This will improve the chance that the cost function will converge towards its global minimum. A good initial transformation estimate will also reduce the execution time for the algorithm, which currently takes between 120 to 200 seconds for a pair of 768x576 RGB images on a Pentium D 3.0GHz CPU.

5. Conclusion and Future Work

We have demonstrated the use of the photo-consistency metric for registering endoscopic images with anatomical volumetric data. This technique can be used to improve the initial registration obtained from the ICP algorithm and also provide an intra-operative registration update. In the current implementation, we take full advantage of graphics hardware to render the volumetric data at an interactive rate. Since our method also incorporates information from the tracking sensor, it could also be used as an additional tool for motion estimation. However, due to the iterative nature of the chosen optimisation method, it is difficult to achieve motion estimation at an interactive rate.

Acknowledgements

This work is conducted as part of the CASSPAR project which is funded by EP-SRC(6R/R86027). We would also like to thank Gus Alusi (St. Bartholomew Hospital, London UK) and Karl Storz UK Ltd. for providing necessary endoscopy equipment and test models.

References

[1]   P.J. Besl and N.D. McKay, A Method for Registration of 3D Shapes, *IEEE Trans. Pattern Analysis and Machine Intelligences* **14**(2):239-256, 1992.

[2]   M.J. Clarkson, D. Rueckert, D.L.G Hill, D.J. Hawkes, Using Photoconsistency to register 2D optical images of the human face to a 3D surface model, *IEEE Trans. Pattern Analysis and Machine Intelligences*, **23**(11):1266-1280, 2001.

[3]   M.S. Chen, R.J. Lapeer and R. Rowland, Real-time Rendering of Radially Distorted Virtual Scenes for Endoscopic Image Augmentation, *Medicine Meets Virtual Reality 13*, 87-79, 2005.

[4]   Z. Janko and D. Chetveriko, Photo-Consistency Based Registration of an Uncalibrated Image Pair to a 3D Surface Model Using Genetic Algorithm, *Proceedings of 3DPVT*, 616–622, 2004.

[5]   Z. Janko and D. Chetveriko, Registration of an Uncalibrated Image pair to a 3D Surface Model, *Proceedings of ICPR*, 208–211, 2004.

[6]   R.J. Lapeer, R. Rowland and M.S. Chen, PC-based Volume Rendering for Medical Visualisation and Augmented Reality based Surgical Navigation. *Proceedings of MediViz/IV04 conference*, 62–72, 2004.

[7]   M.E. Leventon, W.M. Wells, III and W.E.L. Grimson, Multiple View 2D-3D Mutual Information Registration, *Proceedings of IUW97*, 625-629,1997.

[8]   W.H. Press, B.P. Flannery, S.A. Teukolsky and W.T. Vetterling, *Numerical Recipes in C: The Art of Scientific Computing*, Cambridge University Press, 1992.

[9]   P.A Viola and W.M. Wells, III, Alignment by Maximization of Mutual Information, *International Journal of Computer Vision*, **24**(2), 137-154,1997.

Medicine Meets Virtual Reality 15
J.D. Westwood et al. (Eds.)
IOS Press, 2007

73

Evaluating Enhanced Volume Rendering Visualization of Cerebral Aneurysms

Marcelo Cohen[a], Ken Brodlie [b,1] and Nick Phillips[c]
[a]PUCRS - Brazil
[b] School of Computing, University of Leeds, UK
[c] Leeds General Infirmary, Leeds, UK

Abstract. The effective visualization of aneurysms is a very important issue in neurosurgery. However it is difficult to display both the aneurysm with sufficient detail, and the vessel network of the brain at the same time. This work offers a solution to both of these problems, applying the concept of focus and context to texture-based volume rendering. A flexible application has been developed, allowing different focus and context techniques to be used. This paper concentrates on the evaluation of the system by a group of neurosurgeons.

Keywords. Volume rendering, focus+context, volume distortion, aneurysms.

1. Introduction

The motivation for this work was the need to provide an easy-to-use, flexible system to aid in the visualization of 3D medical datasets. The driving application was neurosurgery where we were helping surgeons to identify the nature of a cerebral aneurysm. Such aneurysms can present themselves in a number of different configurations, and treatment needs to take into account the type of the aneurysm and its relation to the surrounding vascular network. Hence there is a need to view the aneurysm in detail, yet still have a full view of the cerebral vasculature of the patient. This is the classic 'Focus+Context' problem – much studied in Information Visualization [1], yet quite rarely considered in Scientific and Medical Visualization.

2. Approach

Our focus and context approach is to enlarge the region of interest around the aneurysm, while correspondingly shrinking the surrounding areas. We are interested in whether this volumetric distortion will be a help to surgeons, or whether it will prove confusing and therefore a handicap.

---

[1] Corresponding Author: Ken Brodlie, School of Computing, University of Leeds, Leeds, LS2 9JT, UK. E-mail: k.w.brodlie@leeds.ac.uk

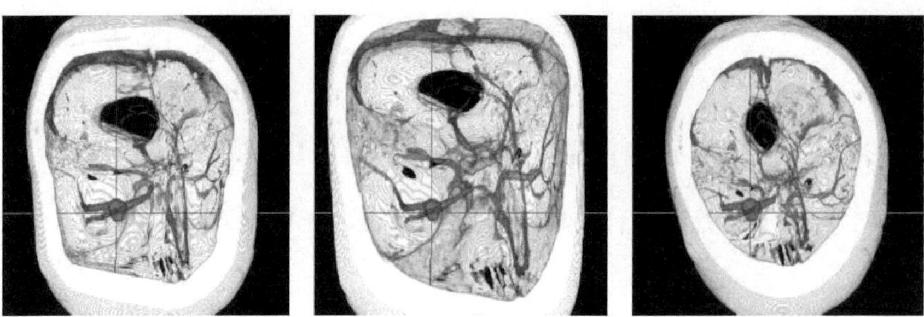

Figure 1. Bifocal, fisheye and volume lens distortion effects

We experimented with three different distortion techniques, illustrated in Figure 1. First, a bifocal distortion, similar to a bifocal display, but in 3D: it creates a focus region of uniform magnification, compressing everything outside, again uniformly. Note the clear separation between focus and context regions. Second, a fisheye distortion, again based on a 2D counterpart [1]: here there is no focus region, just a focal point and a distortion factor, producing a continuous distortion effect. Finally, a volume lens, similar to a real lens, in which the region under the lens is magnified and the region outside is unaffected – of course in order to fit within the original display region, there needs to be a transition region around the lens where the volume is highly compressed.

We have developed a volume rendering system (*VolFocus*) that provides each of these mapping effects, so that surgeons can experiment with the different techniques. In addition to the mapping effects, two other features are included: a *highlighting* effect (which uses colour to draw attention to the focus region); and an *attenuation* effect (which selectively changes the opacity of voxels, allowing one to see inner structures).

A key feature of our work is the exploitation of modern graphics hardware. The system uses texture mapping hardware present in modern graphics processors (GPUs), with the special effects being achieved through programming of a fragment shader. This allows the surgeon to navigate through the volume and apply the different effects, all at interactive speeds - a 512x512x146 dataset is rendered at 18 fps in 640x480 window, using a P4 3.6 GHz machine with a Quadro FX 4400. Details of the implementation are however outwith the scope of this paper and the reader is referred to the PhD thesis of one of the authors [2].

3. Evaluation

The focus of this paper is the evaluation of the system by members of the neurosurgery team at Leeds General Infirmary, including four consultant neurosurgeons, two registrars, a senior house officer – plus an interventional radiologist specializing in the treatment of aneurysms. Only the briefest training was given before the evaluation, since those involved were senior and busy clinicians – the training consisted of a presentation of the system plus a short hands-on coaching session.

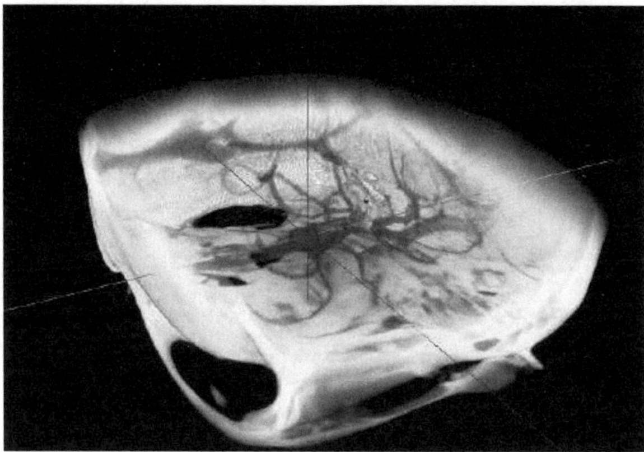

Figure 2. Fisheye distortion, highlighting and attenuation

The surgeons all found the ability to enlarge the aneurysm useful – with the fisheye technique most preferred because of the smoother transition between enlarged and compressed regions. The spatial distortion introduced by the mapping effects did not appear to confuse the surgeons. The radiologist was less enthusiastic. He made the observation that the interventional radiology approach of working from *inside* the arterial structure was quite different from the surgical approach of working from outside-to-in. This was felt to explain the differing level of acceptance. All subjects found the other two effects useful, with particular support for the effectiveness of attenuation in removing outer skull bone. An unexpected bonus was comment from a number of the subjects that the system had much wider potential in medicine – as a means of visualizing tumours, and as a general anatomy teaching tool where the ability to highlight features in an interactive demonstration would be extremely powerful.

The participants all found the system particularly easy to use. Our aim is for the system to be usable in the operating theatre and therefore the interface has been kept deliberately simple, with no requirement for a keyboard. At present a mouse is required, although it is recognized that even a mouse may not be ideal for an operating environment. Again a full description of the user interface is outside the scope of this paper; the reader is referred to the thesis [2]. Figure 2 shows output from the system, in which all effects are applied: to enlarge the aneurysm using fisheye, to colour the focus and to attenuate along the view direction so the bone does not obscure inner structures.

4. Conclusions

VolFocus provides a novel tool for the visualization of cerebral aneurysms, allowing a focus on an aneurysm while preserving the context of the surrounding cerebral vasculature. It runs at interactive speeds on conventional PC hardware, and its evaluation by the neurosurgical team demonstrates its potential for use in education, pre-operative planning and within the operating theatre itself.

References

[1]   R. Spence. *Information Visualization*. Addison Wesley. 2001
[2]   M. Cohen. *Focus and Context for Volume Visualization*. PhD Thesis, University of Leeds, 2006.

Medicine Meets Virtual Reality 15
J.D. Westwood et al. (Eds.)
IOS Press, 2007

Skills Acquired on Virtual Reality Laparoscopic Simulators Transfer into the Operating Room in a Blinded, Randomised, Controlled Trial

COSMAN, PH[a,b,c]; Hugh, TJ[b]; Shearer, CJ[c]; Merrett, ND[c]; Biankin, AV[c]; Cartmill, JA[a]
[a]University of Sydney, [b]Northern Clinical Skills Centre, and [c]South-Western Sydney Upper Gastrointestinal Surgical Service

Abstract: Virtual reality surgical simulators have proven value in the acquisition and assessment of laparoscopic skills. In this study, we investigated skill transfer from a virtual reality laparoscopic simulator into the operating room, using a blinded, randomised, controlled trial design. Surgical trainees using the LapSim System performed significantly better at their first real-world attempt at a laparoscopic task than their colleagues who had not received similar training, as measured independently by a number of expert surgical observers using four criteria.

1. Background

Simulation for the acquisition and assessment of surgical skills is not a novel concept; it has been advocated since ancient times, and live animal models, human cadaver models, animal tissue models, and synthetic inanimate bench-top models have been used to teach surgical skills for several decades, but critical examination of the literature reveals that none of these models has been examined with the same level of scrutiny as the virtual reality model. The feasibility of the virtual reality model has been repeatedly demonstrated in the context of laparoscopic skills and fibre-optic endoscopy. Virtual reality simulators have been shown to be a robust and reliable means of assessing surgical skills at all levels of experience. More recently, a single prospective, randomised study using the MIST-VR simulator has gone beyond construct validity and quasi-transfer to demonstrate transfer of training from a virtual reality simulator to the operating room[1].

To complement the results of a skill transfer trial using the MIST-VR simulator, we opted to replicate the study using the LapSim System laparoscopic surgery simulator[2] (Surgical Science Ltd; Haraldsgatan 5, SE 413 14 Gothenburg, SWEDEN). Transferability of training ought to be part of a core evaluation of any training modality. Unfortunately, few modalities other than virtual reality simulators have been evaluated for this critical property. We used the LapSim System to determine whether laparoscopic skills acquired on a virtual reality simulator would transfer into the operating suite.

2. Methods

We used version 1.5 of the Basic Skills package of the LapSim System, which comprises eight core modules of fundamental laparoscopic tasks, one of which involves the application of clips to, and division of, a blood vessel. In this exercise, a clip must be placed across the vessel in each of two delineated zones, and the vessel must be transected in another demarcated zone between them. Both jaws of the clip applicator must be seen around the vessel prior to clipping, otherwise the clip will not be placed correctly. Dropped clips must be retrieved prior to the end of the task. The vessel changes colour to indicate the degree of tension on it; too much tension will cause rupture of the vessel with accompanying haemorrhage, which must be controlled with clips. Once the task is completed, it is repeated with the instruments alternating between hands. The degree of difficulty can be determined by the instructor; we used a moderate level of difficulty. Haptic feedback was not yet featured in the LapSim System at the time the study was performed.

The performance parameters measured by the simulator include time to task completion, path length, angular path, number of incomplete targets, number of misplaced clips, number of dropped clips, maximum stretch damage (as a proportion of the amount of force required to rupture the vessel), and the amount of blood loss. The amount of blood loss recorded is a function of the blood flow rate, which is set by the instructor, and the amount of time required to completely control bleeding.

To ensure that the participants in the experiment achieved a sufficiently high standard of performance, we established a performance baseline by recruiting ten consultant laparoscopists to perform the clipping task on the simulator and recording their performance. We took the mean of their scores on each of the performance variables as the minimum standard required of the participants.

Once the performance baseline was established, volunteer basic surgical trainees were randomised to either the control group or the experimental group. The control group was tested on the simulator at enrolment into the study and again prior to performing the assessment task. They did not receive any simulator-based training in the interim, but may have received verbal instruction during the normal course of their employment, and were not otherwise prevented from learning laparoscopic clipping of structures. The experimental group was similarly tested on the simulator at enrolment and again prior to performing the assessment task. In the interim, they were required to practice the clipping task on the LapSim simulator, following a distributed training protocol, under which they were permitted access to the simulator for a maximum of one hour each day until they satisfied the performance criteria on two successive repetitions of the task. Once again, participants in this group may have received verbal or other instruction during the normal course of their employment.

All participants were then required to perform an assessment task which was video taped for subsequent analysis. Under consultant supervision, they were instructed to apply clips to and divide either the cystic duct or the cystic artery during laparoscopic cholecystectomy on a live human patient. The video recordings were then analysed independently by five laparoscopic surgeons who were unaware of the nature of training received by each participant. Each assessing surgeon was required to complete an error assessment scale for each participant; this was based on a similar instrument designed and validated by others[3] for assessment of performance during laparoscopic cholecystectomy. The scale comprised six parts: application of the grasper to

Hartmann's pouch; retraction of Hartmann's pouch; application of the patient-side clip; application of the specimen-side clip; transection; and miscellaneous.

Questions in each section identified significant departures from acceptable performance. In addition, reviewers were asked to assess the bimanual coordination of each participant using a 5-point Likert scale. Reviewers were also asked to provide a global assessment of the participants, again using a 5-point Likert scale. In addition, the time to task completion was recorded for each participant.

The data were interrogated using the Mann-Whitney U-Test to determine whether there were any differences between the performance of the experimental group and that of the control group for the pre-test, post-test, and assessment task, or whether there were differences between them in level of training or extent of laparoscopic experience. Finally, inter-rater reliability for assessment scales was calculated using the intra-class correlation (ICC) method[4, 5].

3. Results

The performance baseline was established by taking the mean performance of ten expert laparoscopic surgeons in each of the performance parameters. Their performance is summarised in *Table 1*, along with the baseline value that candidates had to achieve for each parameter, which appear in the final column of the table.

Table 1. Baseline Performance Values

	Mean	SD	Median	IQR	Baseline
Time (s)	102.06	69.14	83.13	84.33	120
PL (m)	0.96	0.59	0.76	0.62	1.0
AP (°)	182.49	125.42	138.90	138.22	200
Incomplete Targets (n)	0.79	0.89	0.00	2.00	0
Misplaced Clips (n)	0.97	1.49	0.00	1.00	1
Dropped Clips (n)	0.58	0.92	0.00	1.00	0
Max Stretch (%)	64.59	38.22	76.52	68.83	70
Blood Loss (L)	0.05	0.10	0.00	0.06	0.05

SD = Standard Deviation, IQR = Interquartile Range

A total of ten trainees were enrolled into the study; five were randomly allocated to the control group, and five to the experimental group. Based on the outcome of the Mann-Whitney U-Test for all variables, there were no measured differences between the two groups on the pre-test, and only time to task completion reached a statistically significant difference in the post-test ($U = 1$; $p = 0.04$), with those in the experimental group (median = 47.5 s) taking almost half the time to complete the task as those in the control group (median = 87.1 s). No statistically significant differences were recorded between the two groups in terms of level of training (mean $\pm$ SD = 1.3 $\pm$ 0.5 years) or number of laparoscopic cases performed (mean $\pm$ SD = 7.7 $\pm$12.8).

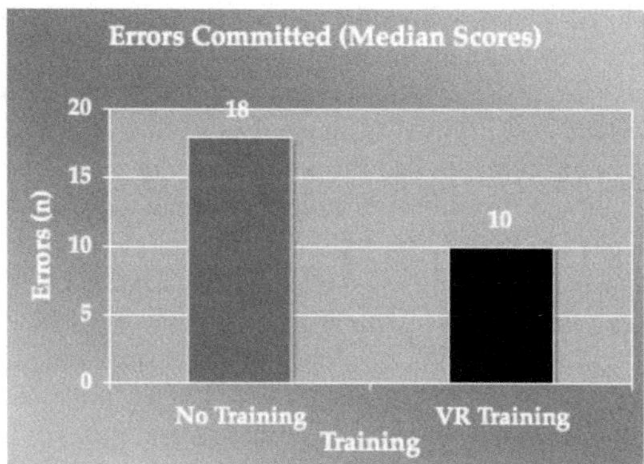

Figure 1. Median Value of Errors Committed (Fewer errors equates to superior performance)

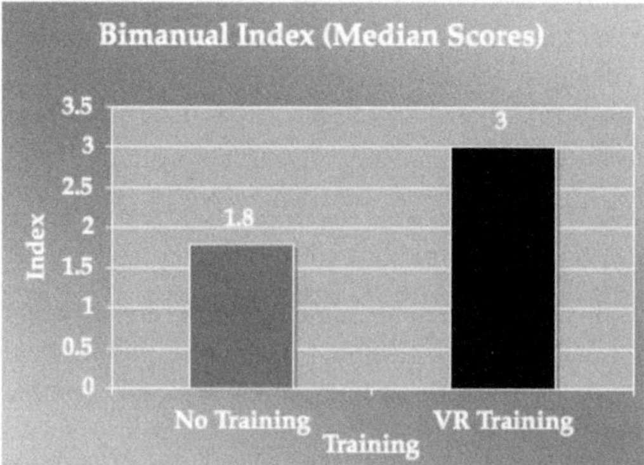

Figure 2. Median Value for Bimanual Index (A higher score is equivalent to superior performance)

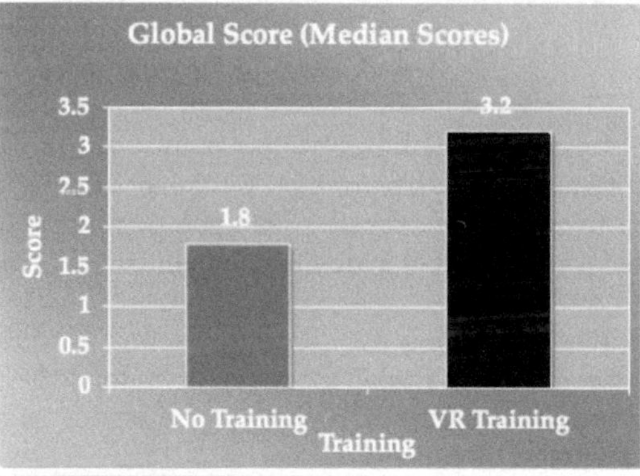

Figure 3. Median Values of Global Score (A higher value indicates better performance)

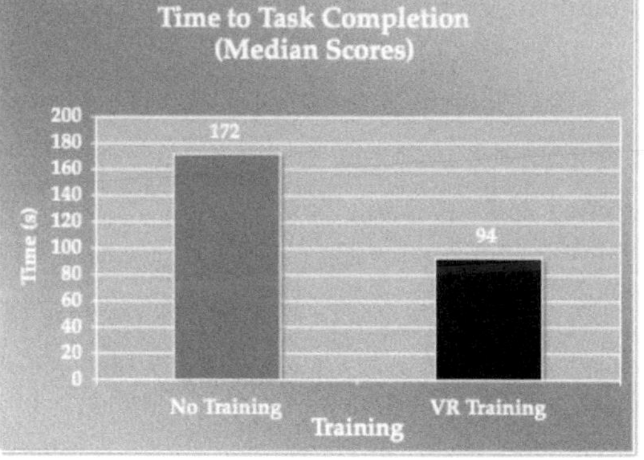

Figure 4. Median Value of Time to Task Completion (Less time taken equates to superior performance)

Significant differences were found, however, when the video recordings of their assessment tasks were analysed. Those who had trained on the simulator committed fewer than two-thirds as many errors (median = 10) as were committed by those who had not trained on the simulator (median = 18); this difference was significant (*Figure 1*; $U = 3.5$; $p = 0.05$). They also had better bimanual coordination (median = 3.0) when compared to those who had received no simulator training (median = 1.8); this difference was also significant (*Figure 2*; $U = 3$; $p = 0.05$). They also received a significantly higher global score *(Figure 3*; $U = 2.5$; $p = 0.04$). Those who had trained on the simulator took less time to complete the assessment task (median = 94 s) than those who had no training (median = 172 s), but this was only of borderline statistical significance (*Figure 4*; $U = 4$; $p = 0.075$).

The intra-class correlation (ICC) score for the error scale was calculated as 0.96, indicating 96% agreement between the five assessing surgeons for the error scale. The bimanual index and global rating each had an ICC score of 0.87, indicating 87% agreement between raters for these components of the assessment. Generally, scores above 0.7 are accepted as being indicative of significant correlation between independent reviewers.

4. Discussion

Unfortunately, from the time this study was planned in January 2001, it was beset by several delays. It did not actually commence until August 2002; the data-collection was completed in December 2002, but the performance analysis was not completed until April 2006. This delay reflects the difficulty encountered in finding surgeons willing to spend time performing the assessment analysis, although this generally took little over half an hour to complete. This should be borne in mind whenever criticism is raised about the expense of virtual reality based assessment of surgical skills when compared to assessment by experienced surgeons.

There are four important points to note from the results of this study.

Firstly, training conducted on a virtual reality laparoscopic simulator is definitely transferable to laparoscopic tasks on live human patients in the operating room; only one other study of this type using virtual reality laparoscopic simulators has been published to date, with similar results.

Secondly, by removing basic skill training from the operating room, this kind of training can significantly decrease the amount of time required for training in that expensive, mission-critical environment. Training efficacy is a measure of the effectiveness of simulation-based training. It quantifies the time saved by using simulators for training, and the Training Efficacy Ratio (TER) is given by the formula:

$$TER = A - \frac{A_S}{S} \qquad\qquad \textbf{Equation 1}$$

where: A = Duration of training without simulation;
            A_s = Duration of training with simulation; and
            S = Training time on simulator.

For simulator-based training in aviation, the Training Efficacy Ratio is 0.48[6], while in military applications, it is about 0.4[7]. The current study suggests that surgical simulation will also manifest a TER within a similar range of values. In this study, trainees required half the time to perform a procedure if they had previously trained on a virtual reality simulator than if they had received no such training. This cost saving in theatre time may help to amortise the acquisition and maintenance costs of virtual reality simulators.

Thirdly, virtual reality training can help minimise errors from the very first encounter with a patient. In the current climate of professional accountability, this result cannot be ignored.

Finally, there is no question that the paradoxical movement of the novice is eliminated by "training it out" on the simulator before approaching the patient; superior bimanual index and global rating scores were ascribed in this study to participants who had trained on the simulator, suggesting that paradoxical movement did not impede this group of trainees.

No other form of training in laparoscopic surgery has demonstrated these capabilities as conclusively as virtual reality simulation. The surgical community can no longer afford to ignore the potential impact of this training modality on the acquisition and assessment of laparoscopic skills.

References

[1]　Seymour, NE; AG Gallagher; SA Roman; MK O'Brien; VK Bansal; DK Andersen and RM Satava (2002). Virtual reality training improves operating room performance: results of a randomized, double-blinded study. *Annals of Surgery* **236(4)**: 458-63; discussion 63-4.

[2]　Larsson, A (2001). An open and flexible framework for computer aided surgical training. *Studies in Health Technology and Informatics* **81**: 263-5.

[3]　Eubanks, TR; RH Clements; D Pohl; N Williams; DC Schaad; S Horgan and C Pellegrini (1999). An objective scoring system for laparoscopic cholecystectomy. *Journal of the American College of Surgeons* **189(6)**: 566-74.

[4]　Ebel, RL (1951). Estimation of the reliability of ratings. *Psychometrika* **16**: 407-24.

[5]　Fleiss, JL and J Cohen (1973). The equivalence of weighted kappa and the intraclass correlation coefficient as measures of reliability. *Educational and Psychological Measurement* **33**: 613-9.

[6]　Higgins, GA and HR Champion. *The Military Simulation Experience: Charting the Vision for Simulation Training in Combat Trauma.* 2000, US Army Medical Research and Materiel Command: Fort Detrick, Maryland.

[7]　Farmer, E; Jv Rooij; J Riemersma; P Jorna and J Moraal. *Handbook of Simulator-Based Training.* Ashgate: Aldershot [Eng.]; Brookfield, VT, 1999.

Medicine Meets Virtual Reality 15
J.D. Westwood et al. (Eds.)
IOS Press, 2007

Implementing Virtual Worlds for Systematic Training of prehospital CPR in Medical School

J. CREUTZFELDT, MD[a,c,1], L. HEDMAN, PhD[c,f], C. MEDIN, MSc[c], C.J. WALLIN, MD, PhD[a,c], A. HENDRICK[e], P. YOUNGBLOOD, PhD[d], Wm. L. HEINRICHS, MD, PhD[d] and L. FELLÄNDER-TSAI, MD, PhD[a,c]

[a] *CLINTEC, division of anesthesiology,* [b] *CLINTEC, division of orthopedics,* [c] *Center for Advanced Medical Simulation all at Karolinska Institutet and Karolinska University Hospital Huddinge, 141 86 Stockholm, Sweden, Phone +46 8 585 82102, Fax + 46 8 585 8222,* [d] *SUMMIT, Stanford University, California, USA,* [e] *Forterra, California, USA,* [f] *Department of Psychology, Umeå University, Umeå, Sweden*

Abstract. We report on a study that investigates the relationship between repeated training of teams managing medical emergencies in the Virtual World and affective learning outcomes in a group of 12 medical students. The focus of the training was on individual actions, but also on interaction and behaviour in the team. Current CPR training seems to lack important team training aspects which this type of training is addressing. We found an increase in flow experience and in self efficacy. This type of training could probably be expanded to other groups for a similar purpose because of its easiness to use, adaptability and interactivity.

Keywords: CPR training, flow, medical students, MMOS, self-efficacy, serious games, simulation, virtual worlds

1. Introduction

Two major studies have demonstrated the ineffectiveness of standard CPR training of healthcare professionals [1,2]. One educational challenge of this project was to create and evaluate new and innovative methods of training students to perform CPR (cardio-pulmonary-resuscitation) because of the documented lack of retention of the resuscitation actions taught in traditional CPR training courses, even with the use of mannequins. McGaghie and collaborators [3] have emphasized the importance of simulation-based medical education by using clearly defined and objectively measured learning outcomes which document learner progress and are related to educational

---

[1] Corresponding author and reprint request: Johan Creutzfeldt at the above address and E-mail address: johan.creutzfeldt@karolinska.se

goals. The model of Flow experience has previously been used for assessment of affective learning outcomes [4]. Another individual variable and a powerful predictor of performance is self-efficacy; the belief that one can perform specific tasks and behaviours [5].

In this report, we explored if there was an association between the repetitive practice in our developed Virtual World prehospital CPR training program and affective learning outcomes. In particular, we analyzed if the practice improved flow and self-efficacy.

2. Material and Methods

A previously developed Virtual World prehospital CPR training program was implemented and evaluated in 12, 6 male and 6 female, Swedish medical students (year 1) at Karolinska Institutet (Forterra Systems, Inc.'s, OLIVE, game development platform) after approval in the local ethics committee. In Massively, Multi-player, Online Simulation (MMOS), virtual worlds, medical students played the role of a character, avatar, in a total of 4 scenarios. After a standardized CPR lecture, the students interacted with other avatars in the virtual world by using the keyboard and mouse to control movements and actions, and headsets to communicate in real time with the other players. After each virtual world role play, scenario, trainees participated in an instructor-led debriefing. Three students interacted with each other to practice the appropriate steps to rescue the victim, suffering from a cardiac arrest in a prehospital setting. Each group of subjects trained in all four scenarios.

Total flow was evaluated after scenario 1, 2 and 4, by using the Karolinska Flow Instrument (0-100 VAS). Medical students' perception of self efficacy was assessed before and after the training by using a subscale (five items on a 7 point Likert-type scale) constructed by Pintrich and collaborators [6]. Non-parametric methods, Mann-Whitney, were used for statistical analysis. A p-value less than .05 was considered statistically significant. Values below are presented as mean ± SD.

3. Results

The mean rating of the flow experience was 54 (scenario 1) to 63 (scenario 4). This increase in flow was highly statistically significant (P=.0053) (Table 1).

The mean value for the self-efficacy rating before the training was 5.83± .56 (median 5.90). After the training it was 6.40± .58 (median 6.50). This increase was statistically significant (p=.012).

Table 1. Measurements of total Flow experience by the Karolinska Flow Instrument (0-100 VAS). P-values were calculated comparing scenario 4 and 1, 4 and 2 and 2 and 1 respectively.

Scenario	Mean	Median	Std dev	Lower q	Upper q	Min	Max	P-value
1	52.21	54.13	13.72	43.00	64.94	31.88	76.33	.0053 (4:1)
2	58.66	60.44	15.79	51.88	66.06	29.88	88.63	.1200 (4:2)
4	63.10	61.75	13.59	55.00	73.63	37.13	83.50	.1027 (2:1)

4. Discussion

In this report, we explored if there was an association between the repetitive practice in our developed Virtual World prehospital CPR training program and affective outcomes. In particular, we analyzed if the practice improved values for flow and self-efficacy. Our findings clearly indicate that students practice was associated with positive experiences of total flow with scores being on the positive side – and above 50 - of the Karolinska Flow instrument. The second index for affective learning outcome used in this study - self-efficacy - was high already before the training. This could partly be explained by the fact that the subjects self enrolled and before the study had gone through a traditional CPR training program. However, a significant increase in self-efficacy after training was revealed. It is believed that simulation in general, as a training method, improves the student's confidence in related, real world tasks.

In the strive for improved teaching and learning the data that we have obtained could be considered promising. This study demonstrates the added value of MMOS for situated learning of CPR in which medical students are able to systematically practice the actions and behaviours necessary to respond appropriately.

5. Acknowledgments

This study was supported by research grants from the Wallenberg Global Learning Network, Karolinska Institutet, Karolinska University Hospital and Umeå University.

References

1. Wik L, Kramer-Johansen J, Myklebust H, et al. Quality of cardiopulmonary resuscitation during out-of-hospital cardiac arrest. *JAMA.* 2005; 293: 299-304.
2. Abella BS, Alvarado JP, Myklebust H, et al. Quality of cardiopulmonary resuscitation during in-hospital cardiac arrest. *JAMA.* 2005; 293: 305-31.
3. McGaghie W,Issenberg SB,Petrusa ER, Scalese RJ. Effect of practice on standardized learning outcomes in simulated-based medical education. *Medical Education* 2006; 40: 792-797.
4. Hedman L, Sharafi P. Early use of Internet-based educational resources: effects on students' engagement modes and flow experience. *Behaviour & Information Techn..* *2004*; 23(2): 137-146.
5. Bandura A. Self-Efficacy: The Exercise of Control, 1997, New York: Freeman.
6. Pintrich PR et al. Reliability and predictive validity of the motivated strategies for Learning Questionnaire (MSLQ), *Educational and Psychological Measurement. 1993*; 53: 801-813.

Medicine Meets Virtual Reality 15
J.D. Westwood et al. (Eds.)
IOS Press, 2007

Feasibility of Using Intraoperatively-Acquired Quantitative Kinematic Measures to Monitor Development of Laparoscopic Skill

Sayra M. CRISTANCHO[a,d,1], Antony J. HODGSON[a], Neely PANTON[b], Adam MENEGHETTI[b,c], Karim QAYUMI[b,c]

[a]*Dept. of Mechanical Engineering, The University of British Columbia, Canada*
[b]*Division of General Surgery, The University of British Columbia, Canada*
[c]*Centre of Excellence for Surgical Education & Innovation, Vancouver, Canada*
[d]*Facultad de Ingeniería Electrónica, Universidad Pontificia Bolivariana Bucaramanga, Colombia*

Abstract. The objective of this paper is to present the initial results of a study aimed at showing the feasibility of using kinematic measures to distinguish skill levels in manipulating surgical tools. Through a simulated surgical task (dissection of a mandarin orange), we acquired motor performance data from three sets of subjects representing different stages of surgical training. We computed the average lateral, axial and vertical tooltip velocities for each of the two main subtasks ('Peel Skin' and 'Detach Segment'). For each subject, we defined a 6-element vector to describe the kinematic measures extracted from the two tasks and used Principal Components Analysis (PCA) to extract the two dominant contributors to overall variability to simplify the presentation of the data to the trainer. We found that the first two principal components accounted for approximately 90% of the variance across all subjects and tasks. Moreover, the PCA plot showed good intrasubject repeatability, consistency within subjects with similar levels of training, and good separation between the subject groups. The results of this pilot study will allow us to design a future intraoperative study.

Keywords. Surgical training, Performance assessment, Minimally Invasive Surgery

Introduction

Surgical competence involves elements such as knowledge, judgement, communication, and technical dexterity. Due to the increasing technical difficulties involved in performing more advanced minimally invasive surgical procedures, there is widespread interest in designing objective methods for monitoring skill development in surgeons-in-training which incorporate performance measures such as time, tool kinematics and interaction forces [1-3]. Such quantitative measures are expected to be useful for several purposes [4]:

---

[1] Corresponding Author: Department of Mechanical Engineering, The University of British Columbia, 2054-6250 Applied Science Lane, Vancouver, BC, V6T 1Z4

a) <u>Self-monitoring of training</u> – to compare one's relative performance with respect to one's peer group to identify particular difficulties and strengths
b) <u>Comparison of different training programs</u> – to assess effectiveness and quality of training in different programs
c) <u>Selection of candidates</u> – to determine the feasibility of using motor skill measurements to screen candidates for special training programs

However, quantitatively assessing the motor skills of surgeons remains problematic and has become an important research topic, since current formal structured evaluation methodologies are time consuming and somewhat subjective. The current approaches rely on comments from the trainees' attending surgeons, which have been shown to be subject to bias [4]. Therefore, in order to better monitor the progress of trainees, quantitative and time-efficient methods are required to evaluate the trainees' developing motor skills in the live operative setting [5]. Furthermore, variability from one procedure to another represents a significant challenge that needs to be addressed while developing these methods.

Because of this interprocedure variability, most research on technical skill assessment in laparoscopic surgery has been performed on simulators [6] and has focussed on analyzing generic motor skills [7-9]. However, a complete surgical assessment process should assess not only a surgeon's technical skills, but their knowledge base and decision-making skills as well. Our group has developed a hierarchical motor/cognitive modelling approach that should enable us to represent live surgical tasks 'in context' and thereby facilitate making comparisons across real procedures and incorporating performance measures such as time and tool kinematics [10]. Ideally, we would use intraoperative data to evaluate this approach, but since it is comparatively expensive to run intraoperative tests, we have decided to first evaluate the feasibility of our proposed method with data from a physical surgical simulator in order to determine if it is able to distinguish between groups of subjects. More specifically, we wish to evaluate if (1) intrasubject repeatability is good, (2) scores for trainees with similar skill levels are similar, and (3) scores for trainees at different stages are significantly different. If these conditions are met, the technique will be worth testing in the live operative setting. Since there are many kinematic measures used, we also tested a dimension-reduction technique intended to present the differences between surgeons on a 2D plot that is more easily interpreted by trainers.

1. Protocol

We simulated a surgical dissection task by asking participants to peel and separate the segments of 2-3 mandarin oranges. The movements of the laparoscopic tools were tracked using a Polhemus Fastrak magnetic sensor attached to the tool's handle which continuously recorded position and orientation data at 120 Hz while the task was being executed. Following initial instruction in the task and demonstration by the investigator, subjects performed the task at their own pace. The acquired data was processed afterwards to calculate the kinematic features of the tool movements.

<u>Subjects:</u> We recruited three sets of subjects to represent different stages of training: novices (represented by three graduate students with no specific surgical training), novices with training (represented by three graduate students who received a half-hour of training from an expert surgeon), and experts (represented by three attending surgeons).

Experiment setup: We mounted the mandarin oranges in a laparoscopic training box and asked subjects to peel the skin off and release individual segments while attempting to avoid damaging the segments. The standard laparoscopic camera and tools were used, and the tasks were videotaped so that the investigator could later correlate the movement patterns with discrete phases of the task execution. A Polhemus Fastrak magnetic sensing system was used to acquire 3D position data by means of electromagnetic sensors attached to the handles of the laparoscopic tools.

Analytical methods: We computed the average tooltip velocities in each of the three cardinal directions for each of the two main subtasks of the simulated surgical task (Peel Skin and Detach Segment; the duration of each subtask was identified through a video analysis and the times records). For each subject and subtask, we defined a 6-element vector consisting of the three velocities for each of the two main subtasks. We then normalized the data by dividing each element by its own standard deviation, and used Principal Components Analysis (PCA) to extract the two dominant contributors to overall variability to simplify the presentation of the data to the trainer. The normalization ensures that the weights derived from the PCA are insensitive to the scaling of the measures used.

To test our three hypotheses, we computed the contributions to total variability from intrasubject, intragroup (ie, equivalent stages of training) and between group variations and report these numbers as percentages of total variation from the global data mean. In addition, as a measure of repeatability for specific subjects and groups, we report the ratio of mean square distance (MSD) in the weight space from the mean position of all trials executed by a specific subject or group to the MSD from the global mean position.

We hypothesize that plots of the extracted principal components and the derived variation measures will show consistency in individual performance, similarity amongst individuals at similar levels of training and distinctions between the different groups of subjects.

2. Results

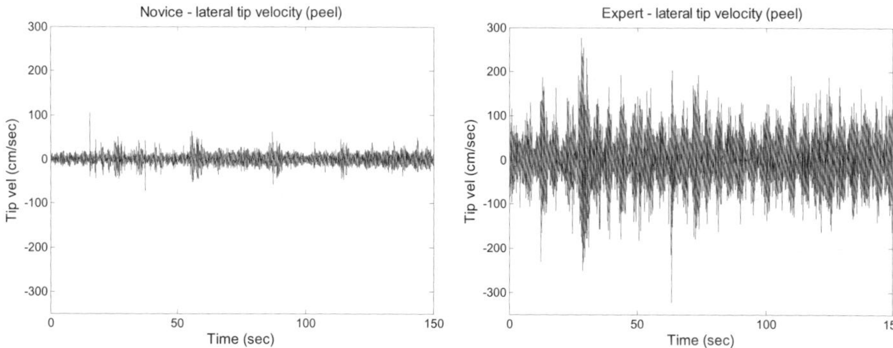

Figure 1A. Lateral tip velocity executed by a novice during a "peel" subtask

Figure 1B. Lateral tip velocity executed by an expert during a "peel" subtask

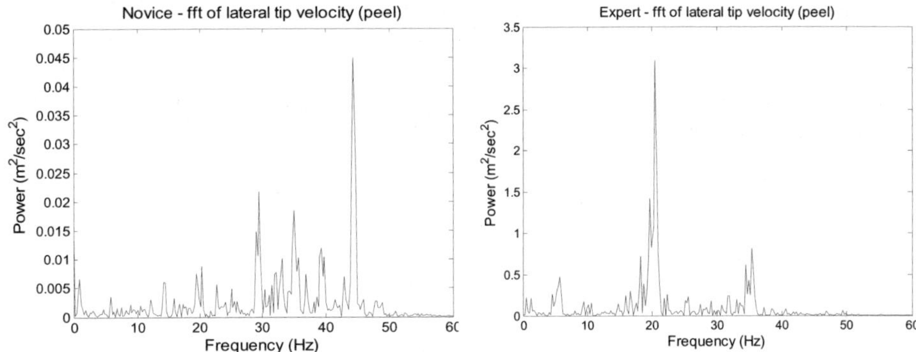

Figure 1C. Fast Fourier Transform for novice's
lateral tip velocity

Figure 1D. Fast Fourier Transform for expert's
lateral tip velocity

Figures 1A and 1B show samples of the lateral tip velocity data from a novice subject and an expert respectively. An expert executes faster movements than a novice possibly due to his/her familiarity with the use of the surgical tools, while novice needs to adjust him/herself to a new working setting for which there is no depth perception nor direct eye contact and therefore, caution is expressed in the form of slow motion. Figures 1C and 1D show the Fast Fourier Transform (FFT) for the novice's and expert's lateral tip velocities. The power spectrums indicate differences in the frequency components for which the stronger peaks occur (Highest for novice: 44Hz; Highest for expert: 20Hz) and in the magnitude of the power content (Novice in the range of $0.05\text{m}^2/\text{sec}^2$; and expert in the range of $3.5\text{m}^2/\text{sec}^2$).

With regard to the Principal Component Analysis, we found that the first two principal components accounted for approximately 90% of the variance across all subjects and tasks. This suggests that it is possible to describe the data in a two-dimensional space and still retain most of the information (Figure 2). Analysis of the coefficients of the first two principal components showed contrast between movements in the lateral and vertical directions, which indicates that the main source of variation is between subjects applying larger or smaller lateral velocities compared to vertical velocities. This effect was more prevalent in the 'detach' subtask.

The position of each trial in PCA-weight space is shown in Figure 2. It appears that intrasubject repeatability is generally high, that the data from subjects of comparable training level is in relatively close proximity to one another, and that there are significant variations between groups. The contributions to total variability are shown in Figure 3 (pieplot). The low values of intrasubject and intragroup variability support the qualitative observations that the greatest contributor to overall variability is difference in degree of training.

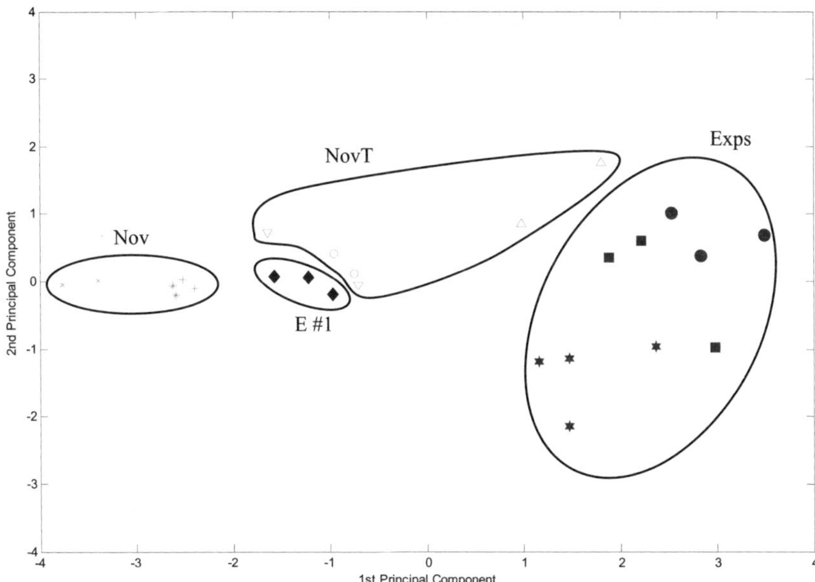

Figure 2. Cross-plot of the first 2 principal components for the three subject groups tested. [x,+,*]: novices (Nov); [▽,O,△]: novices with training (NovT); [(●◆)■✳]: experts (Exps); [◆]: expert #1 (E#1) measured while instructing novice group; [●]: expert #1 working alone at normal operating pace.

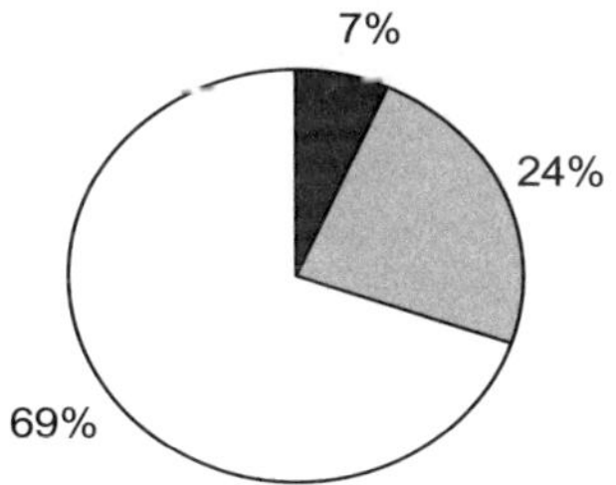

Figure 3. Contributions to total variability. [■]: intrasubject variability; [■]: intragroup variability; [ ]: intergroup variability

Our measure of repeatability shows that:

1. There is good intrasubject repeatability (e.g. Typical expert: 9%; Typical novice with training: 7%; Typical novice: 1%).
2. The intersubject repeatability for each group (Experts: 22%; Novices with training: 31%; Novices: 5%) seems larger after training which might suggest that training could enable operators to try more flexible strategies
3. The root-mean square (RMS) distances between different groups (Experts vs Novices: 5.43; Experts vs Novices with training: 2.65; Novices with training vs Novices: 3.30) are considerably larger than the RMS distances within groups

(Experts: 1.08; Novices with training: 1.29; Novices: 0.54); this is consistent with the idea that training changes motor patterns

The data for expert 1 suggests that instructing while working can significantly affect motor performance; in Figure 2, we see that expert #1's performance while instructing was more similar to that of the trainee group than to the expert group or to his own typical performance. The RMS distance of these instructional trials was 1.62 to the centre of the "Novices with training" group and 3.63 to the centre of the "Experts" group.

3. Conclusions

We have successfully shown that quantitative kinematic data obtained from real surgical tools used in a reasonable physical simulation of a dissection task can be used to distinguish between groups of trainees at different skill levels. Moreover, in the 2D space derived from a principal component analysis, the parameters derived from individuals performing the same task multiple times show good repeatability, and the separation between groups is readily apparent, which would make interpretation easier for the surgical trainer.   These results therefore provide sufficient justification to support us moving forward to a live intraoperative study involving experts and resident surgeons as they perform real surgical tasks such as laparoscopic cholecystectomies.

REFERENCES

[1]   Seymour N.E., et. al. (2004). Analysis of errors in laparoscopic surgical procedures. Surgical Endoscopy, 18, 4, p.592-5
[2]   Smith S.G. , et. al. (2001). Motion analysis. Surgical Endoscopy, 16,4, p.640-5
[3]   Rosen J., Hannaford B., Richards C., Sinanan M., (2001). Markov modeling of MIS based on force/torque signatures for evaluating surgical skills. IEEE Trans. Biom. Eng., 48, 5, p.579-591
[4]   Khan M., Snelling A., Tiernan E. (2005). The need for technical skills assessment in surgery. International Journal of Surgery, 3, p.83-86
[5]   Moorthy K, Muntz Y, Sarker SK, et al. Objective assessment of technical skills in surgery. Br Med J 2003;327:1032-7
[6]   Aggarwal R, Moorthy K, Darzi A. Laparoscopic skills training and assessment. Br J Surg 2004;91: 1549 –58
[7]   Sarker S., Chang A., Vincent C., Darzi A., 2006. Development of assessing generic and specific technical skills in laparoscopic surgery. The American Journal of Surgery, 191, p.238-244
[8]   Taffinder N, Sutton C, Fishwick RJ, et al. Validation of virtual reality to teach and assess psychomotor skills in laparoscopic surgery: results from randomised controlled studies using the MIST VR laparoscopic simulator. Stud Health Technol Inform 1998;50:124 –30
[9]   Martin JA, Regehr G, Reznick R, et al. Objective structured assessment of technical skill (OSATS) for surgical residents. Br J Surg 1997;84:273– 8
[10] Cristancho S., Hodgson A., Panton N., Meneghetti A., Qayumi K., (2006). Assessing Cognitive & Motor Performance in MIS for Training & Tool Design. MMVR14, p.108-113

Medicine Meets Virtual Reality 15
J.D. Westwood et al. (Eds.)
IOS Press, 2007

Parametric Eye Models

Jessica R. Crouch and Andrew Cherry
Department of Computer Science, Old Dominion University, Norfolk, Virginia

Abstract.
The shape of anatomic objects often depends in complex ways on the shapes and locations of neighboring objects. Shape parameter networks provide an approach for representing shape dependencies and producing multi-object models that share consistent boundary definitions. This paper provides an overview of the modeling framework provided by shape parameter networks, and demonstrates their use through the development of a detailed multi-object eye model. The eye model presented contains analytically defined shape equations that produce models matching user-specified physical measurements such as cornea width, cornea thickness, anterior chamber angle, and eye axial length.

Keywords. surgery simulation, shape model, eye model, cornea

1. Introduction

Three dimensional models of patient anatomy are an integral part of numerous medical computing applications, including surgery simulation [1], model-guided image segmentation, and planning for sophisticated interventions such as intensity modulated radiation therapy. For such applications the medical imaging and medical simulation communities have developed a wide variety of algorithms that construct models for parts of the human anatomy, many of which focus on the task of building one or more shape models for structures that are visible in medical image data. The construction of detailed eye models from clinical images is not feasible because important structures in the eye have thicknesses measured in microns while voxel dimensions for CT, MR, and other clinical imaging modalities are measured in millimeters. However, since the eye is accessible for direct observation, a rich set of metrics characterizing the size, thickness, curvature, relative orientations, or relative positions of structures can be measured or estimated to describe a patient's eye.

Because the eye is composed of many distinct structures that share boundary surfaces, boundary consistency between adjacent model objects must be ensured. Multi-object modeling methods that represent each object's shape independently generally only approximate consistent boundaries. Typically, such methods address the problem of boundary consistency by explicitly testing for and correcting unwanted gaps or overlaps between objects. This corrective approach to the boundary consistency problem involves a computationally intensive optimization, where each model's representation of its boundary is iteratively refined until the overlap or gap "error" between two adjacent models is sufficiently small. Shape parameter networks were developed to provide a method for producing anatomic shape models that does not require image input and guarantees boundary consistency without an expensive optimization step.

2. Shape Parameter Network

A shape parameter network is a directed acyclic graph whose nodes are shape parameters. Each node can be queried and will return a scalar, vector, or tensor that characterizes some aspect of an object's shape. Edges in the graph represent dependencies between parameters; data flows through the graph along edge paths. Parameters can be categorized according to whether they are *input* or *derived*, *local* or *global*, and *mapping* or *geometric*. These categorizations are defined below.

Input vs. Derived Parameters: When queried, an input parameter simply returns a value that has been assigned by a user. A derived parameter computes its value by evaluating a function that accepts other parameters' values as input.

Local vs. Global Parameters: Global parameters produce shape information that pertains to an entire object, whereas local parameters produce information that pertains to a particular point on an object. For example, in the eye model network the shape of the cornea is modeled as a patch on the surface of an ellipsoid. Since this ellipsoid is constant for a given instance of a model, the ellipsoid widths are computed by global parameters. Local shape parameters produce location specific information such as the world space coordinates of an object boundary point. Since there are an infinite number of points on a boundary surface, the world space coordinates computed will vary depending on the particular boundary location queried.

To provide local shape parameters with a means of uniquely identifying the points in a model, each object is defined with an object coordinate system. The shape of the eye's structures and their approximate symmetry about the anterior/posterior axis makes a spherical or cylindrical coordinate system a natural choice for use as the object coordinate system. Each eye object's coordinate space is defined for (θ, h, r), where θ is in the range $[0, 2\pi)$, and h and r are in the range $[0, 1]$. θ denotes an angle about the anterior/posterior axis, h varies along the anterior/posterior axis, and r represents a fraction an object's radius or thickness.

Mapping vs. Geometric Parameters: A mapping parameter transforms a point from its representation in one object's coordinate system to its representation in another object's coordinate system. For example the cornea and sclera meet at a shared boundary, and the `CorneaToScleraMapping` parameter maps (θ_C, h_C, r_C) cornea object coordinates to corresponding (θ_S, h_S, r_S) sclera object coordinates for points that lie on their shared boundary. In contrast, geometric parameters compute shape properties that pertain to an object's world space representation such as object boundary locations, intersection curves, and fiber orientation vectors.

When two objects share a patch of boundary surface, the position parameter for one of the objects computes point coordinates by evaluating a set of shape equations that could include functions for cubic splines, ellipsoids, and Gaussian blending, among others. The adjacent object computes boundary positions by using a mapping parameter to find the point's representation in its neighbor's coordinate system, and then requesting world coordinates from its neighbor's position parameter.

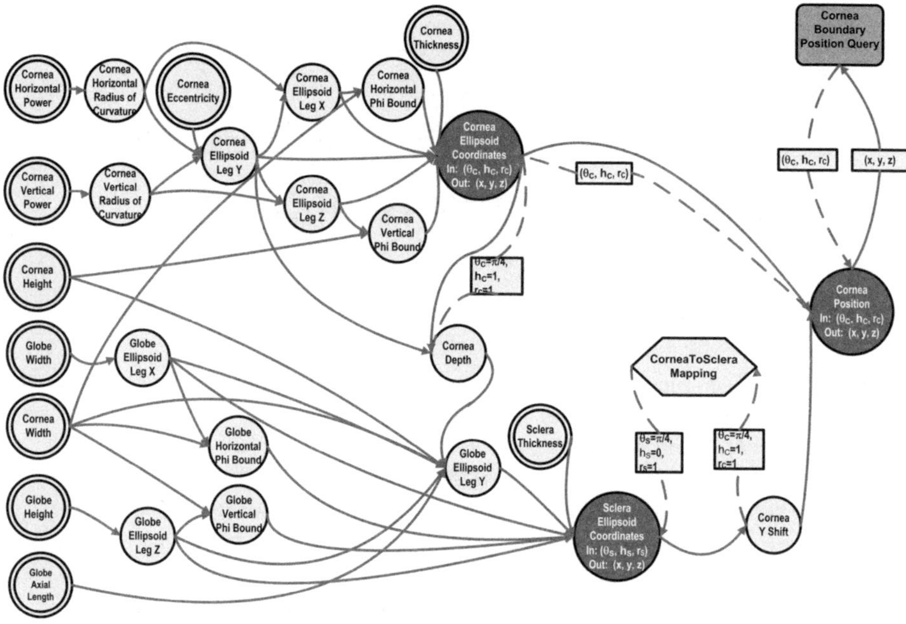

Figure 1. The cornea's parameter network shows input parameters with double borders, derived parameters with single borders, local parameters with dark backgrounds, and global parameters with light backgrounds. Solid edges indicate parameter values passing through the network, and dashed edges indicate object point coordinates traveling in the opposite direction. A mapping parameter is shown as a block with angled sides.

3. Eye Model

The portion of the eye shape parameter network that generates cornea geometry is shown in Fig. 1. Only three local parameters appear in this portion of the network, and only these three must be re-evaluated each time the position of a point on the cornea surface is computed. The entire shape parameter network for the eye contains 100 geometric parameters, a third of which are input parameters. The eye shape parameter network can generate a population of models by varying input parameter values. A single eye model instance is shown in Fig. 2. Generation of both 3D finite element meshes and surface meshes is supported [2].

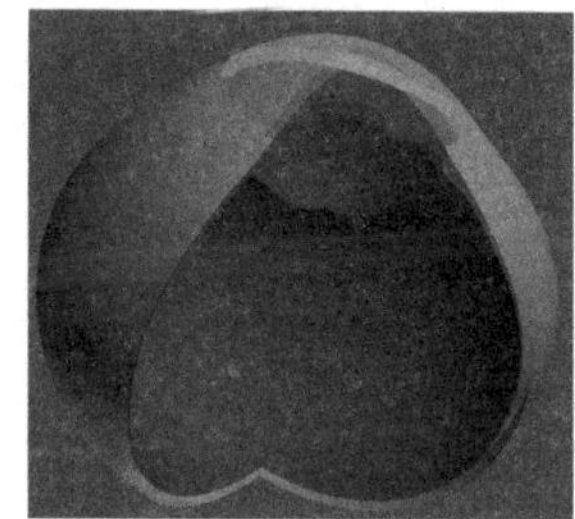

Figure 2. Eye model generated by a shape parameter network.

References

[1]　J Seevinck, M Scerbo, L Belfore, L Weireter, J Crouch, Y Shen, F McKenzie, H Garcia, S Girtelschmid, E Baydogan, E Schmidt. "A Simulation-Based Training System for Surgical Wound Debridement." Medicine Meets Virtual Reality 2005, IOS Press, pp. 491-496.

[2]　J Crouch, J Merriam, E Crouch. "Finite Element Model of Cornea Deformation." Medical Image Computing and Computer-Assisted Intervention (MICCAI '05), pp. 591–598.

Medicine Meets Virtual Reality 15
J.D. Westwood et al. (Eds.)
IOS Press, 2007

Real-Time Smoke and Bleeding Simulation in Virtual Surgery

Stefan Daenzer [a], Kevin Montgomery [b], Rüdiger Dillmann [c] and
Roland Unterhinninghofen [d]

[a] *National Biocomputation Center, Stanford University, stefan.daenzer@gmail.com*
[b] *National Biocomputation Center, Stanford University, kevin@biocomp.stanford.edu*
[c] *Institute of Computer Science and Engineering, Universität Karlsruhe (TH),*
dillmann@ira.uka.de
[d] *Institute of Computer Science and Engineering, Universität Karlsruhe (TH),*
uhhofen@ira.uka.de

Abstract. We present a particle-based smoke simulation and a particle-based fluid simulation in an interactive environment with rigid and deformable objects. Many smoke and fluid simulations offer high physical and visual accuracy, but the underlaying models are to complex to run in real-time while performing soft-tissue simulation, collision detection, and haptic device support at the same time. Our algorithms are based on simple models that allow the surgery simulation to run in real-time.

Keywords. Smoke Simulation, Fluid Simulation, Surgery Simulation, Particle System, Render-to-Texture

Introduction

In the surgical training field, surgery simulators play a great role, especially for minimally invasive surgery. The training effect of surgical simulators has been proofed by many studies [6][3][5]. Smoke and fluid simulations enhance the quality of the simulation and enable a surgical simulator to simulate a great variety of surgical tasks, such as cauterizing, cutting, rinsing, and suction-cleaning. However, the quality of the visual effects is limited by performance issues.

1. Related Work

There are many approaches to simulate the behavior of fluids and gases. Grid based techniques, such as surface and height field methods were used by Miller and Kass [8] to simulate the surface of waves in water of varying depth. Using a height field to represent the fluid surface. Later, Raghupathi [14] used a similar method to simulate the behavior of accumulated fluids in in real-time. Another grid based approach was done by Foster and Metaxas [4], including complex fluid behavior such as rotational eddies, splashing and vorticity as well as interaction with rigid obstacles. This method solves the full

Navier-Stokes equations in three dimensions on a grid with low resolution. Stam [16] introduced a new technique to solve the Navier-Stokes equations more efficiently on a grid. The method is extremely stable, regardless of the timestep between two iterations. Stam used his method to simulate smoke in real-time.

The big disadvantages of grid based techniques are the limitations in interaction with deformable and interactive models. If the environment changes, the grid has to be recomputed, which is very time consuming.

Particle systems are another approach of fluid simulation, introduced by Reeves [15]. Uncoupled particle systems, where no interactions between the particles are simulated, are used for smoke and blood-drop simulations by Andersson [1]. Coupled particle systems, where the particles interact with each other, are used by Miller and Murta [13] to simulate splashing and dripping behavior of fluids.

Smoothed Particle Hydrodynamics (SPH) is another particle based approach, where a continuous density field from a set of particles is computed and then visualized, rather than visualizing every particle on its own. SPH was used by Teschner et. al. [9] and Gross et. al. [10] to simulate the interaction of water with solid bodies almost in real-time.

2. Methods

We developed techniques to simulate and visualize smoke, blood, and water in our surgical simulation environment. Sections 2.1, 2.2, 2.3, 2.4, 2.5 and 2.6 will give an overview of the techniques we used, followed by a description of how we use these techniques in 2.7, 2.9 and 2.8.

2.1. Particle System

Our particle system consists of three components: particles, forces, and sources. Particles are described by coordinates in three dimensional space, a velocity vector, and a mass. Forces influence the velocity vector of the particles. Several types of forces can be added to the particle system. Constant Forces like gravity, position or time dependent forces like force fields and springs, as well as velocity dependent forces like drag. Sources handle the creation of particles. A source has a position in three dimensional space, a release velocity vector, and a release rate. Particles are generated by a source using stochastic methods. This adds a certain randomness to the particle's release velocity vector and the particle's release rate. The trajectory of each particle is governed by Newton's Second Law of Motion using a stepwise solver.

2.2. Spherical Billboarding

Spherical billboarding is a technique to adjust the orientation of an object, usually that the object faces the camera. Billboarding can be used to cut back the number of polygons of a model displayed on the screen by replacing the model with a two dimensional texture.

2.3. Collision Detection

A fast and interactive collision detection algorithm is a fundamental component of our particle system. We used a fast ray-triangle collision detection algorithm by Möller and

Trumbore [11] to detect intersections of particles with objects in the scene. This algorithm computes the barycentric coordinates of a ray-triangle intersection point. The algorithm also culls back facing triangles for efficiency.

We developed a subdivision algorithm to speed up the collision detection furthermore. Once a ray intersects a triangle that belongs to an object in the scene, a topological subdivision of the triangles belonging to the object is performed. Further collisions are only checked between the ray and the triangle that the ray intersected with and the triangles aligned with this triangle.

2.4. Collision Response

When particles collide with surrounding objects, a collision response algorithm is needed. If a particle's trajectory intersects a triangle of an object, the penetration depth d is given by equation 1, where $\vec{r}$ is the complete trajectory of the particle and $\vec{r_1}$ is the fraction of the trajectory that lies outside of the object.

$$d = |\vec{r}| - |\vec{r_1}| \tag{1}$$

The trajectory of a particle after a resolved collision $\vec{res}$ is given by equation 2,

$$\vec{res} = |(\vec{n} \times \vec{g}) \times \vec{n}| * d \tag{2}$$

where $\vec{n}$ is the normal vector of the triangle, and $\vec{g}$ is the gravity vector. If $\vec{res}$ intersects with another triangle, the collision response algorithm is repeated.

2.5. Texture Atlas Generation

We used the modeling tool Blender3D [2] to create models. Blender3D supports a texture atlas generation technique called Least Squares Conformal Maps (LSCM) published by B. Levy [7]. LSCM is a texture mapping method that keeps texture stretch and deformations minimal. The model to be textured is decomposed into charts, each chart is parameterized and packed into texture space. LSCM is a quasi-conformal parametrization method based on a least-squares approximation of the Cauchy-Riemann equations.

2.6. Render-to-Texture

We used the WGL_ARB_render_texture OpenGL extension for rendering to textures and the WGL_ARB_pbuffer OpenGL extension for off-screen rendering. We used these techniques to render to the texture of the models, created with Blender3D.

2.7. Smoke Simulation

For our smoke simulation, we use a specialized version of the particle system described in section 2.1. The time since creation of the particle is used to simulate the volatilization of smoke over time. This time is mapped to the opacity of each particle. The particles are visualized as textured quads using a texture mapping technique with spherical billboarding described in section 2.2.

2.8. Particle-Based Fluid Simulation

To be able to simulate more interactive and more realistic bleeding we developed a new particle-fluid simulation. This technique uses the particle system described in section 2.1 to simulate free moving blood and water drops in the scene. The blood and water drops are visualized as spheres. The ray-triangle collision detection in section 2.3 is used to detect collisions between the particles and the objects in the scene and we resolve the collisions with the algorithm stated in section 2.4. When a particle collides with an object, the render-to-texture technique described in section 2.6 is used to render blood trails on the surface of the model, or to erase the blood trails form the models surface. If a blood particle collides with a model, a red circle is drawn onto the texture of the model. If a water particle collides with a model, a transparent circle is drawn onto the texture of the model. This way we can achieve that blood particles leave blood trails behind, and that water particles erase those blood trails.

2.9. Pooling

We use a liquid surface model which represents a fluid pool at the bottom of the scene. The liquid surface model is visualized as an animated fluid surface using a Perlin Noise function. The height of the fluid pool is calculated as follows. If the y coordinate of a fluid particle (where y is the vertical) is lower than the y coordinate of the liquid surface model, the volume of the particle is added to the volume of the liquid surface model, and the surface level is raised accordingly.

3. Results

We have integrated our algorithms into the SPRING surgical simulation framework and we have set up scenarios to show the capabilities of our simulations. We set up a scenario with a soft-tissue simulated model of a gallbladder consisting of 500 vertices and 1000 triangles and a rigid, textured box with 16 vertices and 28 triangles. The texture rendered to had a size of 256×256 pixels. We ran the simulation on an Intel Xeon CPU with 3.06 GHz and 2 GB RAM. The graphics chip was NVIDIA Quadro FX 1000 with 128 MB video memory. The OS was Windows Server 2003. The simulation ran with about 35 fps.

Figure 1 shows the model of a bleeding gallbladder. Note how the blood drops leave a blood trail on the surface behind. In figure 2 the bleeding cuts are cauterized. Figure 3 shows the rinsing of the gallbladder. Note how the blood trails on the surface get washed away by the water drops. In figure 4 the pooled blood is cleaned up by a suction device.

4. Acknowledgements

We want to thank the guys from SUMMIT at Stanford University, Craig Cornelius Ph.D., Sean Kung, Robert Cheng, Leroy Heinrichs M.D., Ph.D., and Parvati Dev for their support throughout our research.

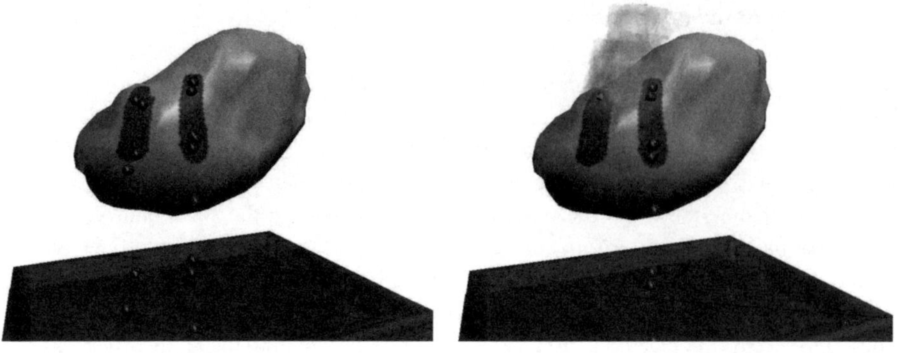

Figure 1. Bleeding gallbladder

Figure 2. Cauterizing of the wounds

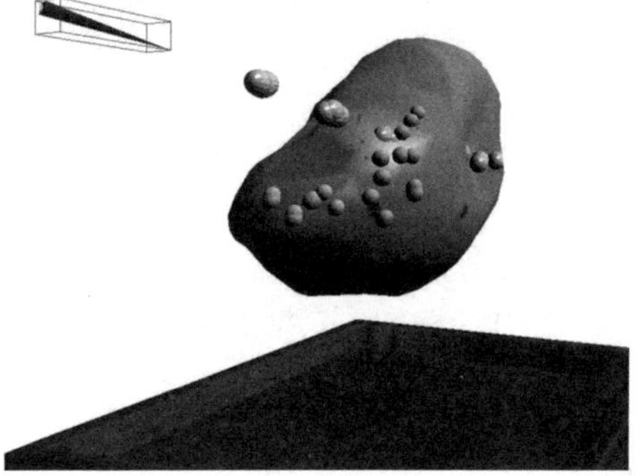

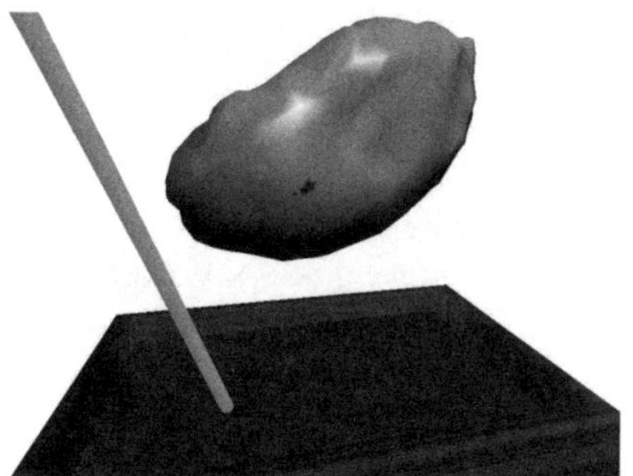

Figure 3. Rinsing of the gallbladder

Figure 4. Removing the pooled blood

References

[1]   Lars Andersson. Real-time fluid dynamics for virtual surgery. Master's thesis, Chalmers University of Technology, 2005.

[2]   Blender3D. http://www.blender.org, 2006.

[3]   M. Downes, M. Cavusoglu, W. Gantert, L. Way, and F. Tendick. Virtual environments for training critical skills in laparoscopic surgery. *In Medicine Meets Virtual Reality*, pages 316–322, 1998.

[4]   Nick Foster and Dimitri Metaxas. Realistic animation of liquids. *Graphical models and image processing: GMIP*, 58(5):471–483, 1996.

[5]   McClure N McGuigan J. Gallagher AG, Richie K. Objective psychomotor skills assessment of experienced, junior, and novice laparoscopists with virtual reality. *World Journal of Surgery*, 21(11):1478–1483, 2001.

[6]   Bendix J Bardram L Rosenberg J Funch-Jensen P. Grantcharov TP, Kristiansen VB. Randomized clinical trial of virtual reality simulation for laparoscopic skills training. *The British Journal of Surgery*, 91(2):146–150, 2004.

[7]   B. Levy, S. Petitjean, N. Ray, and J. Maillot. Least squares conformal maps for automatic texture atlas generation. 2002.

[8]   G. Miller M. Kass. Rapid, stable fluid dynamics for computer graphics. *SIGGRAPH Conference Precedings*, pages 49–57, 1990.

[9]   M. Gross M. Mueller, D. Charypar. Particle-based fluid simulation for interactive applications. *Proceeding of 2003 ACM SIGGRAPH Symposium on Computer Animation*, pages 194–201, 2003.

[10] M. Teschner M. Mueller, S. Schirm. Interactive blood simulation for virtual surgery based on smoothed particle hydrodynamics. *Journal of Technology and Health Care*, 12(1):25–32, 2004.

[11] Tomas Mller and Ben Trumbore. Fast, minimum storage ray-triangle intersection. *journal of graphics tools*, 2(1):21–28, 1997.

[12] K. Montgomery, C. Bruyns, J. Brown, S. Sorkin, F. Mazzela, G. Thonier, A. Tellier, B. Lerman, and A. Menon. Spring: A general framework for collaborative, realtime surgical simulation. 2002.

[13] Alan Murta and James Miller. Modelling and rendering liquids in motion. 1999.

[14] L. Raghupathi. Simulation of bleeding and other visual effects for virtual laparoscopic surgery. *Master thesis*, 2002.

[15] W. T. Reeves. Particle systems - a technique for modeling a class of fuzzy objects. *SIGGRAPH Computer Graphics*, 17:359–376, 1983.

[16] Jos Stam. Stable fluids. *SIGGRAPH Computer Graphics Proceedings*, pages 121–128, 1999.

Medicine Meets Virtual Reality 15
J.D. Westwood et al. (Eds.)
IOS Press, 2007

Modeling Isotropic Organs Using Beam Models for the Haptic Simulation of Blunt Dissections

Vishal DALMIYA[1], Guillermo RAMIREZ[2] and Venkat DEVARAJAN[1]
[1]*Department of Electrical Engineering, University of Texas at Arlington*
[2]*Department of Civil Engineering, University of Texas at Arlington*

Abstract. Haptic modeling of organs using existing approaches is still not realistic or real time. We propose and develop the mathematical foundation of a new approach to modeling organs using beams. Beams are well known entities in Civil and Structural engineering. We develop their mathematical properties in the context of organ simulation. The real time advantage arises from the fact that a single beam implementation eliminates hundreds, if not thousands of mass springs from the traditional mass spring models and, thousands of polygons from the finite element method. Even more importantly, our derivation is valid for large deformation. Most previous work has developed equations only for small deflections. Large deformation is important because we set out to simulate blunt cutting which requires models for large deflections. Our new model, when simulated and compared with an FEM model provides comparable accuracy.

Keywords. Beam, Large Deformation, Blunt Dissection

Introduction

Dissection is defined as the separation of tissues with haemostasis [6]. It consists of visual and tactile elements and, tissue manipulation and instrument maneuverability. These are combined to develop a suitable space for viewing and handling target structures.

A variety of mechanisms have been used to divide tissue and enable haemostasis. They all involve some form of physical energy being applied to the appropriate tissue. The amount of energy required for dissection depends on the type and constituency of the tissue. The properties of tissues may vary in different directions and for different disease states. This in totality influences the choice of the modality for dissection.

The ideal dissection technique requires a modality that can accomplish meticulous haemostasis and will be tissue-selective without causing inadvertent tissue damage. It must be safe for both the patient and the surgical team when in regular use and, when inactive in storage. In this respect, built-in safety measures are mandatory. An ideal dissecting modality should be efficient in both power delivery and in space requirement.

Endoscopic dissection and manipulation of tissue within a confined space requires a two handed approach: one assisting and one dissecting. A passive assisting instrument (usually a grasper) provides counter traction and exposure for the active dissecting instrument. The active instrument may be non-energized (e.g. scissors and scalpel) or energized with electricity (diathermy), ultrasound or light energy.

Our interest is in the simulation of blunt cutting in a trainer. Our work with the mass spring models gives us a good perspective on its use and its shortcomings. It is the shortcomings that led us to the viewing of a beam model as a completely novel approach to organ modeling. We believe the reason this has not been proposed before is because of the classic problem of the lack of sufficient interaction among scientific disciplines. Civil and Structural engineers have for decades studied beams, plates etc. The associated mathematical modeling, although complicated, do offer some very attractive properties which we believe will be useful for modeling organs.

Methods

In the following, we describe our work in beam modeling in relation to simulation of organs. We first derive an expression for the vertical deflection of a beam when a force is applied. In Figure 1, the term v_c denotes the vertical deflection of the beam at a particular position x of the beam. The beam is anchored at the left end. The deflection at the point A is taken to be zero as it is fixed. Also the slope at A is zero (always true for cantilever type beams). W_P is the work done by the external force P as revealed from equation (5). The *Rayleigh-Ritz* approximate energy method [1] states that the change in strain energy is equal to the change in external work done. Thus we equate the small change in energy due to the external work done to the small change in the strain energy due to bending. After some algebraic manipulation, we evaluate the v_c. The equations derived are valid for large deformation and no approximations have been made for small deformations.

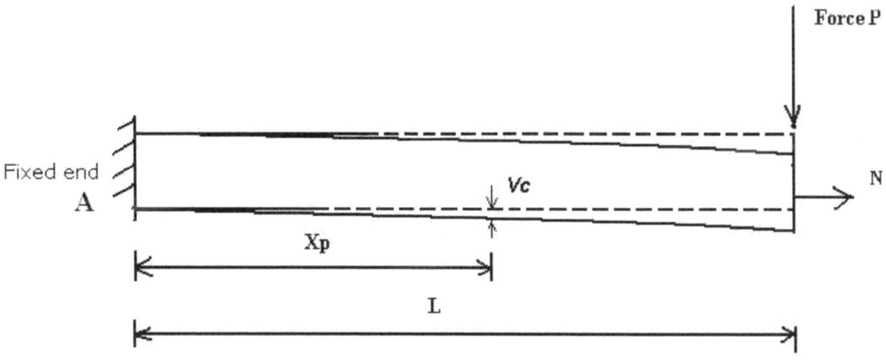

Figure 1. A simple bent beam

Some details of the derivation are presented here. At first we derive the total work done due to the external work done the force P at a distance $x_p = L$

The equation for the vertical deflection (v_c) of the beam is assumed to be parabolic (second order polynomial) in nature which could provide a good approximation to give accurate results in large deformation range. Thus,

$$v_c = a_0 + a_1 x + a_2 x^2 \quad\text{...(1)}$$

Where v_c is the vertical displacement at a distance x from the origin and a_0, a_1 and a_2 are the constants to be derived.

Since in this particular case, we have the vertical displacement and slope both equal to zero at x = 0, both a_0 and a_1 turn out to be zero. That is,

$$x = 0 \Rightarrow v_c = 0 \Rightarrow a_0 = 0 \quad\text{..........................(2)}$$

$$x = 0 \Rightarrow \frac{dv_c}{dx} = 0 \Rightarrow a_1 = 0 \quad\text{.............................(3)}$$

In general we have,

$$\frac{dv_c}{dx} = 2a_2 x \ \text{ and } \ \frac{d^2 v_c}{dx^2} = 2a_2 \quad\text{.....................(4)}$$

The small change in the work done W_P is therefore given by the following equation:

$$dW_p = 0.5d\left[-P\left(a_2 x_p^2\right)\right] = -0.5PL^2 d(a_2) \quad\text{.............(5)}$$

Now we calculate the work done by the normal force N (which we have assumed to be of the order of P so that x varies from 0 to L) acting on the cross-section of the beam at one end. The beam stretches along the longitudinal direction based mainly on this force. The total work done can be derived with approximate coupling (indicated by the integral term) as the following equation [1]:

$$W_N = W_A - 0.5N \int_0^L \left[\left\{1+\left(\frac{dv_c}{dx}\right)^2\right\}^{\frac{1}{2}} - 1\right] dx \quad\text{.....................(6)}$$

where A is the area of cross section, E is the Young's modulus and L is the length of the beam and W_A is the energy due to stretching. The integral can be derived as

$$\int_0^L \left[\left\{1+\left(\frac{dv_c}{dx}\right)^2\right\}^{\frac{1}{2}} - 1\right] dx = \left[\frac{L}{2}\sqrt{(2a_2 L)^2 + 1} + \frac{1}{4a_2}\log\left[2a_2 L + \sqrt{(2a_2 L)^2 + 1}\right]\right] - L \quad\text{.................(7)}$$

Finally, the small change in the work done by the normal force N acting on the cross-section of the beam is given by

$$dW_N = -0.5N \left[\frac{\frac{2L^3 a_2}{\sqrt{(2a_2L)^2+1}} - \frac{1}{4a_2^2}\log\left[2a_2L+\sqrt{(2a_2L)^2+1}\right]}{+\frac{1}{2a_2}\left[\frac{L}{2a_2L+\sqrt{(2a_2L)^2+1}}\right] + \frac{L^2}{\sqrt{(2a_2L)^2+1}\left[2a_2L+\sqrt{(2a_2L)^2+1}\right]}} \right] da_2 + dW_A \ldots\ldots(8)$$

Now we evaluate the strain energy stored in the beam due to bending. The energy stored due to bending denoted by U is approximately (as the component of P responsible for bending decreases with deformation) determined by the following [1]:

$$U = 0.5 \frac{1}{2EI_z} \int_0^L M_z^2 \, dx \ldots\ldots\ldots\ldots\ldots\ldots(9)$$

The term M_z, again can be evaluated for large deformation as

$$M_z^2 = (EI_z)^2 \frac{\left(\dfrac{d^2 v_c}{dx^2}\right)^2}{\left[1+\left(\dfrac{dv_c}{dx}\right)^2\right]^3} \ldots\ldots\ldots\ldots(10)$$

where M_z is the bending moment of the beam and I_z is the moment of inertia. Substituting M_z, we get the bending energy U as follows

$$U = 0.5 \frac{1}{2EI_z} \int_0^L (EI_z)^2 \frac{\left(\dfrac{d^2 v_c}{dx^2}\right)^2}{\left[1+\left(\dfrac{dv_c}{dx}\right)^2\right]^3} \, dx \ldots\ldots(11)$$

which after integration reduces to

$$U = 0.5 EI_z a_2 \left[\frac{3}{8}\tan^{-1}(2a_2L) + \frac{5}{4}\frac{a_2L}{(1+(2a_2L)^2)}\right]\ldots(12)$$

Now, a small change in strain energy after partial differentiation is given by (since the internal strain energy stored due to stretching is also W_A)

$$dU = dW_A + 0.5 EI_z \left[\frac{3}{8}\tan^{-1}(2a_2L) + \frac{a_2L}{4}\frac{(13+12L^2 a_2^2)}{(1+4a_2^2 L^2)^2}\right] da_2 \ldots(13)$$

Now we have the small change in energy due to the work done by the external force P and N given by Eq. (5) and Eq. (8) respectively and, the change in the strain energy U given by equation Eq. (13). By the Rayleigh–Ritz [1], we have:

$$dU = dW_P + dW_N ....(14)$$

This model for the large deformation can be extended for the simulation of blunt dissection (see Figure 2) where the beam like tissue, fixed at two ends is stretched (large deflection) to such an extent that it punctures. At any point of time we know the total amount of external force acting on the tissue at the point of application. We can pass the magnitude of force into Eq. (14) to find the appropriate deformation and then can set a threshold value of strain for the blunt dissection to take place.

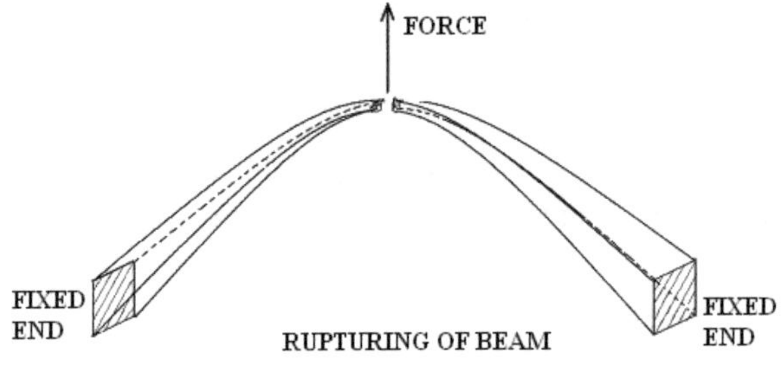

Figure 2. Blunt Dissection

Results

For the typical simulation results (see Figure 3 and Figure 4), the length of the beam is taken to be 1 inch, diameter 0.5 inch, Young's modulus as 1600 psi, shear modulus 650 psi (the stiffness of the tissue is compared with the properties of a soft rubber in the absence of real data), Poisson ratio 0.4 and for different values of P and N, the deformation at $x = 1$ inch is compared between our method (Beam Model) and FEA – the non real time gold standard for accuracy. The average error calculated was 8.29% (Figure 3). This is much more accurate than any mass spring model.

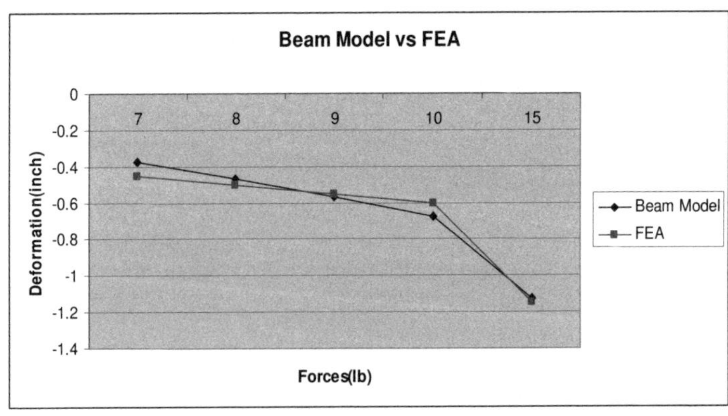

Figure 3. Comparison of accuracy of deformation between beam model and Finite Element Analysis

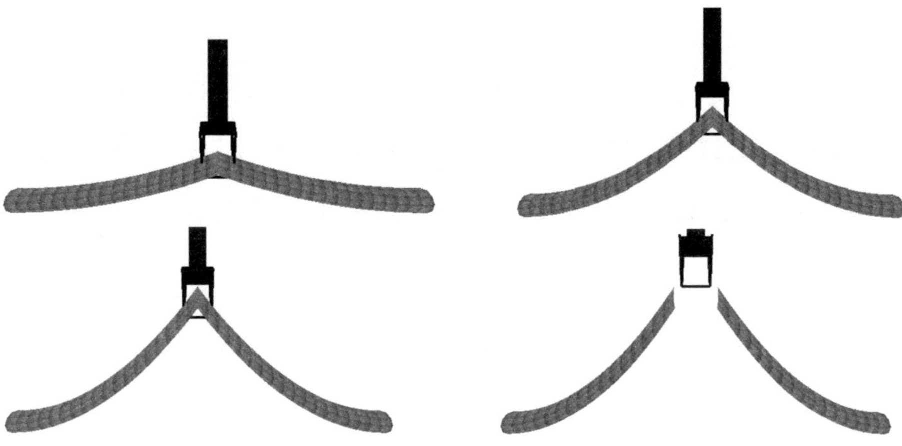

Figure 4. Simulation of Blunt Dissection

Discussion

With the use of our beam model, computation burden in simulating large deformation and blunt dissection will be much less than any other conventional method because once we calculate the deformation of the axis of symmetry all other points can be evaluated using a transformation matrix [See our companion paper in ref 5] instead of computing stiffness matrix [3] or per node analysis [4].

The numerical solution for the complex Eq. (14) works real time with less than 10 iterations to converge.

We believe that in our future work, we can improve the accuracy of our model using an additional constraint on the beam that is specific to its simulation of blunt dissection.

References

[1]   *Advanced Strength and Applied Stress Analysis*, Richard G. Budynas, 2nd Edition, Mc Graw Hill Book Co., 1999.

[2]   De S. and Bathe K. J., *The method of finite spheres*, Comp. Mechanics,Vol 25, Pg(s): 329-345, 2000.

[3]   Di Giacomo T. and Magnenat-Thalmann N., *Bi-layered mass-spring model for fast deformations of flexible linear bodies*, IEEE 16th International Conference on Computer Animation and Social Agents, Pg(s):48 – 53, 2003.

[4]   Berkley J., Turkiyyah G., Berg D., Ganter M. and Weghorst S., *Real-Time Finite Element Modeling for Surgery Simulation: An Application to Virtual Suturing*, IEEE transactions on Visualizations and Computer Graphics, Vol 10, Pg(s);314 – 325, 2004

[5]   Dalmiya Vishal, Tandon Sumit, Mohanraj Pradeep and Devarajan Venkat, *Determination of key and driving points a beam model for the simulation of tissues*, MMVR 15, 2007.

[6]   Dr.Tyrone Peter Sangster. M.D; C.P.H; D.G.S, *An overview of laparoscopic dissection modalitie*, http://www.laparoscopyhospital.com/dissection.htm.

Medicine Meets Virtual Reality 15
J.D. Westwood et al. (Eds.)
IOS Press, 2007

Determination of Key and Driving Points of a Beam Model for Tissue Simulation

Vishal DALMIYA, Sumit TANDON, Pradeep MOHANRAJ and Venkat DEVARAJAN

Department of Electrical Engineering, University of Texas at Arlington

Abstract. The simulation of catheter, guide wire, rigid tissues, muscles and blood vessels using conventional methods like mass spring model and FEM are computationally expensive. The former is comparatively faster than the latter but less accurate. Earlier, we proposed a new method of simulating of tubular organs using deformable beam models [3]. This method is not only accurate but also promises to be faster than mass-spring model for the simulation of tissues. This paper focuses on an important aspect of this approach - the determination of key and driving points of a beam model.

Keywords. Beam Model, Curve Fitting, Organ modeling, parametric modeling

Introduction

We have proposed a new method of object modeling based on representation of objects using sets of equations, deformation modeling based on concept of deformable beams based on the determination of key and driving points on the beam model [3]. This method is not only accurate but also promises to be faster than mass-spring model for the simulation of tissues. This paper focuses on the determination of key and driving points of the beam model.

Methods

The key points of a cross-section of an organ are defined as the important points on the edge of a cross-section while the driving point is the centroid of a cross-section of the beam.

We create a model of a tubular organ (Figures 1 and 2) using a 3D graphics modeler. We then take images of cross-sections at equal intervals and find their boundary points. These points lie on a closed loop. To avoid the computation requirement of spline-fitting, we divide the points into two halves to obtain two open curves. We fit two 6th order polynomials to the two sets of points. Thus the cross-section is represented as a pair of equations. We recalculate the location of the boundary points using these equations along with the centroid (driving point). If the RMS error between consecutive cross-sections is less than a threshold, one cross section can be discarded. If the cross-section of the organ does not change over a certain length, no information needs to be stored for that length of the organ.

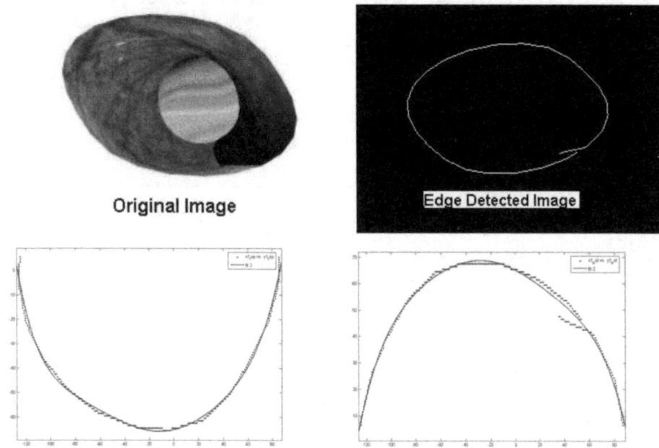

Figure 1. Processing of Image for fitting equations to cross section

Equations (1) and (2) used to curve fit the two parts of the cross section are:

$$y = 4.251e(-11)x^6 + 3.716e(-9)x^5 - 2.582x^4 - 5.553e(-6)x^3 + 0.005028x^2 + 0.1202x - 65.07$$

$$y = 4 - 3.043e(-11)x^6 - 3.841e(-9)x^5 + 7.16e(-8)x^4 + 2.792e(-5)x^3 - 0.003318x^2 - 0.2413x + 65.11$$

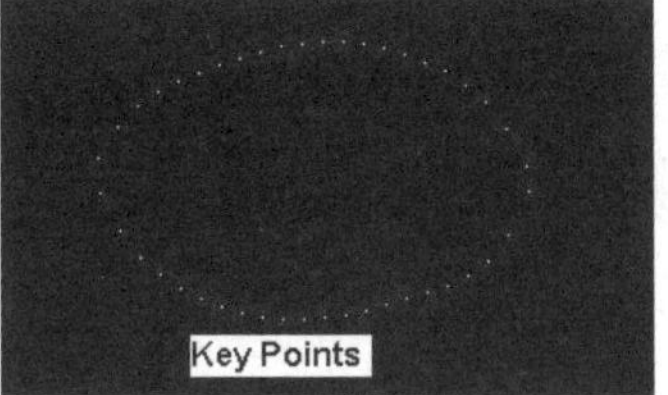

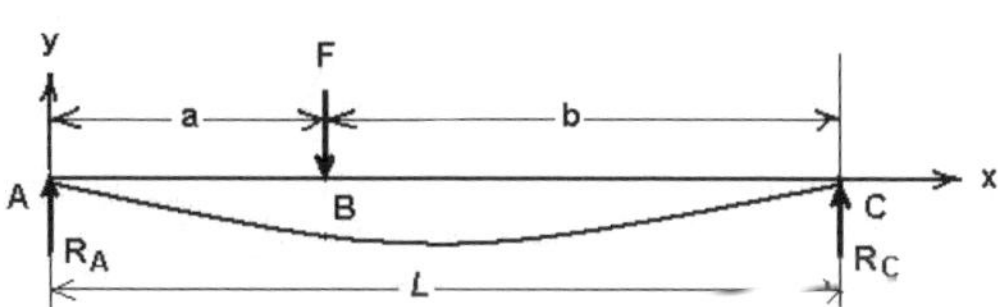

Figure 2. Key Points for the cross section　　　　　**Figure 3**. Beam undergoing deformation

We can use standard equations of a beam to calculate the deformation caused by interaction between a surgical tool and the soft tissue of the organ. [See Figure 3] [2]

$$(v_c)_{AB} = \frac{Fbx}{6EIL}\left(x^2 + b^2 - L^2\right)\cdots(3)$$

$$(v_c)_{BC} = \frac{Fa(L-x)}{6EIL}\left(x^2 + b^2 - 2Lx\right)\cdots(4)$$

Results

An irregularly shaped organ model was first created with 22 cross-sections. Curves were fitted to each cross-section. Depending on the RMS error between consecutive curves, 6 cross-sections were discarded as unnecessary [see Table I] and the organ model was reconstructed with the driving points (obtained from the equations fitted to the cross-section) of the remaining 16 slices. It was found that the reconstructed model was visually accurate and the change in volume was about 1.35%.

With a RMS error threshold of 10 units (Table1), slices 2, 3, 4, 5 can be approximated by slice 1. However, due to a large difference between the curves fitted to slices 1 and 6, slice 6 cannot be discarded. Again, slice 7 can approximate slice 6 but not 8. Also, only 511 vertices were used to recreate the entire object when all 22 cross-sections were used. The number of vertices required reduced to 336 when 6 cross-sections were discarded.

Slice A	Slice B	RMS Error between curves fitted to Slice A and Slice B
1	2	2.98
1	3	9.51
1	4	8.97
1	5	8.76
1	6	22.43
6	7	7.13
6	8	16.15

Table 1 RMS Errors between slices

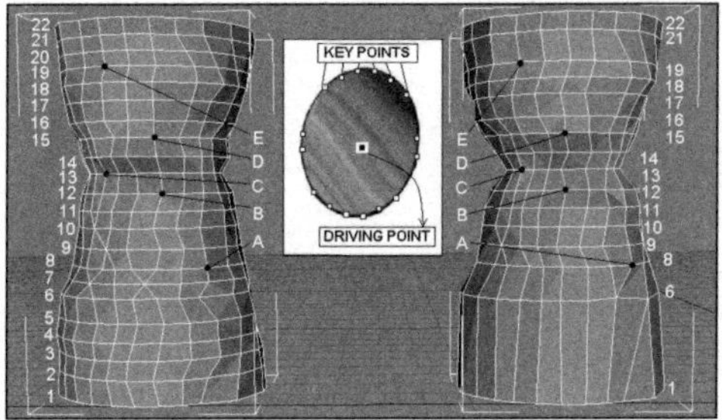

Figure 4 Models created using all the cross sections (left), a typical cross section (middle) and, the model after discarding some of the cross sections (right side)

Discussion

We have proposed and implemented a novel approach of organ modeling which requires keeping track of less number of points during virtual reality simulation. This may result in faster rendering and a better real-time experience. We have also shown that the idea of representing an organ model by a set of equations rather than a collection of points is quite accurate and the reconstructed object is visually accurate and has similar volume too.

References

[1]   Beylot, P., Gingins, P., Kalra, P., Magnenat Thalmann, N., Maurel, W., Thalmann, D. and Fassel, J., "3D Interactive Topological Modeling using Visible Human Dataset", in Eurographics '96, Blackwell Publishers, pp. C33-C44, 1996.
[2]   *Advanced Strength and Applied Stress Analysis*, Richard G. Budynas, Second ed. McGraw-Hill. 1999
[3]   Dalmiya V., Ramirez G., Devarajan V., "Modeling Isotropic Organs Using Beam Models for the Haptic Simulation of Blunt Dissections", Submitted to MMVR15, 2007.

Medicine Meets Virtual Reality 15
J.D. Westwood et al. (Eds.)
IOS Press, 2007

CIELab and sRGB color values of *in vivo* normal and grasped porcine liver

Smita DE[1], Aylon DAGAN[1], Phil ROAN[2], Jacob ROSEN[2], Mika SINANAN[2], Maya GUPTA[2], Blake HANNAFORD[2]

[1]*Dept. of Bioengineering,* [2]*Dept. of Electrical Eng., Univ. of Washington, Seattle, WA*

Abstract. Surgical simulators are excellent training tools for minimally invasive procedures but are currently lacking in realistic tissue rendering and tissue responses to manipulation. Accurate color representation of tissues may add realism to simulators and provide medically relevant information. The goal of this study was to determine feasible methods for measuring color of *in vivo* tissue, specifically liver, in a standardized color space. Several compressions were applied to *in vivo* porcine liver. Three methods were then used to determine the CIELab and/or sRGB colors of normal and damaged liver. Results suggest that there are significant differences between normal and damaged liver color.

1. Introduction

Minimally invasive surgical (MIS) techniques provide a number of patient benefits such as shorter hospital stays, decreased pain, and smaller scars. Surgical simulators have been developed to help surgeons train in MIS procedures and offer a number of advantages over traditional methods. Despite great potential, surgical simulators are still in a largely developmental stage [1]. Much effort is being devoted to improving the visual and haptic (force feedback) realism of simulators. Visual feedback is crucial as it provides 70% of our sensory input [2]. Therefore, it is important to accurately represent the effects of tissue manipulation in simulators such that trainees become accustomed to what occurs *in vivo*. Many current simulators tend to use approximate representations of organs and only illustrate consequences of gross errors (i.e. cutting a blood vessel) such that rough handling of tissues that may cause less severe injury may not be apparent to the trainee.

Color is a significant aspect of visual input and can provide medically relevant information. It has been used in other fields such as dermatology and dentistry to describe tissue pathology and aesthetics [3]. Monitors typically use device-dependent RGB, though many newer monitors utilize sRGB [4], a standardized color space. CIELab is also a standardized color space that is designed to be perceptually linear so that Euclidean distance in CIELab space is linearly related to human judgments of color differences. CIELab colors are described by 'L' for lightness, 'a' for the green to magenta spectrum, and 'b' for the blue to yellow spectrum.

Our goal was to develop a methodology that will allow for recording of accurate colors within an *in vivo* surgical field using a standard color space to allow for reproducibility. Such data could be used to improve the realism of tissue representation in simulators. We aimed to measure potential color differences between normal tissue and grasper-manipulated tissue, as basic manipulation with graspers can cause tissue damage [5]. Our methodology included three techniques that were tested on *in vivo* porcine liver: CIELab estimation based on digital image, direct measurement with a spectrophotometer, and subjective visual validation. Several pilot experiments were done to determine an appropriate methodology. The results of one animal experiment using the revised methodology are reported here.

2. Methods

Adult female pigs were placed under full anesthesia and a laparotomy was performed. A motorized endoscopic grasper was used to apply compression stresses within the previously determined range typical of MIS to the edge of the liver [6]. Three methods to assess the color changes were performed within five minutes of stress application.

Digital Image Estimation: Based on pilot studies, a printed color chart was created with 48 colors that encompassed the expected color range of unstressed (normal) and stressed liver. Endoscopic lighting was used to illuminate the tissues from five inches away to mimic a laparoscopic setting. The color chart was photographed next to the injured tissues using a Canon PowerShot A80. Images from the experiments can be found on brl.ee.washington.edu/~sde/. CIELab values of the color chart patches were measured using a Spectrolino spectrophotometer. Average RGB values of the color chart patches and grasped and normal liver were measured in the digital images. The device-dependent RGB color values were transformed to device-independent CIELab color values using a regularized local linear regression trained on the known (RGB, CIELab) color pairs for the color chart patches [7].

Direct Spectrophotometry: The spectrophotometer probe was wrapped in clear plastic wrap to protect it from surgical site fluids and directly placed on normal and damaged tissues to measure their CIELab values. This method was only used in pilot studies so no results are presented here.

Subjective Validation: CIELab values measured in the pilot studies were transformed to the sRGB color space. Colors within the range of the measured values were displayed on an sRGB monitor. Three experts chose the best match between colors displayed on the screen and colors of the tissues under endoscopic lighting.

3. Results

Preliminary results of the digital image estimated CIELab values are given in Table 1. Student t-tests for 'L,' 'a,' and 'b' showed significant differences between normal and grasped tissues ($p < 0.05$). The table also contains corresponding sRGB values to the estimated mean CIELab values.

Table 1: CIELab (mean ± standard deviation) and sRGB (mean) values from Digital Image Estimation

	L ± S.D.	a ± S.D.	b ± S.D.	R	G	B
Normal	35.6 ± 0.78	40.5 ± 1.89	13.9 ± 0.98	140	53	75
Stressed	15.1 ± 0.33	-2.52 ± 0.42	10.6 ± 0.37	36	39	29

Ranges of sRGB parameters of monitor colors identified by experts during the *in vivo* experiments are shown in Table 2.

Table 2: sRGB ranges from Subjective Validation.

	R	G	B
Normal	93-120	47-56	62-80
Stressed	96-120	44-56	55-70

4. Discussion

Three methods were tested for measurement of tissue colors *in vivo*. Pilot studies allowed for technique refinement and insight into which methods are most appropriate.

Digital image estimation was the most technical and user independent method, and similar estimation methods are standard in color management for printers. However, the estimations were only as accurate as the color chart allowed since the colors of interest should ideally be encompassed within the range of the color patches in the color chart. In addition, a continuing challenge is resolving differences in illuminants since the illumination of the spectrophotometer is not identical to the endoscopic light. Direct spectrophotometry was the simplest of the methods but had potential problems. Pressure from placing the probe on the tissue caused visible blanching of the tissue during measurement. Also, the *in vivo* setting may cause light from the probe to scatter rather than reflect back from the tissue leading to less saturated colors. This method will not be used further in this project. Subjective validation was the most relevant technique as the purpose of this study is for colors on simulator monitors to closely match what trainees will see in real surgeries. Other than subjectivity, a difficulty with this method was its dependence on what colors were shown on the monitor. Choices could be updated routinely based on subsequent experiments in order to obtain a narrower, more accurate range of sRGB values.

We have developed a methodology for accurate measurement of organ surface color with respect to the human observer. Preliminary results indicate that digital image estimation was sensitive enough to distinguish differences between normal tissue and damaged tissue, and subjective validation was appropriate based on our end goal. When transformed, the measured CIELab colors for normal tissue match closely with the sRGB range from the subjective validation. These two described approaches will be used to measure organ colors with statistically significant sample sizes.

5. References

[1] M. S. Richard, World Journal of Surgery V25, 1484 (2001).
[2] A. H. Meier, C. L. Rawn, T. M. Krummel, J. Am. Coll. Surg. 192, 372 (2001).
[3] C. Balas, IEEE Trans. Biomed. Eng 44, 468 (1997).
[4] M. Stokes, M. Anderson, S. Chandrasekar, R. Motta. A Standard Default Color Space for the Internet - sRGB. http://www.w3.org/Graphics/Color/sRGB . (1996).
[5] S. De et al., 2006 International Conf. on Biomedical Robotics and Biomechatronics. (IEEE/RAS-EMBS, Pisa, Italy, 2006), pp. 823-828.
[6] J. D. Brown, thesis, University of Washington (2003).
[7] M. R. Gupta, 2005 International Conf. on Image Processing. (IEEE, Genova, Italy, 2006), pp. 968-971.

Medicine Meets Virtual Reality 15
J.D. Westwood et al. (Eds.)
IOS Press, 2007

A Scalable Intermediate Representation for Remote Interaction with Soft Tissues

Dhanannjay Deo[1]*, Suvranu De[2], Shivkumar Kalyanaraman[3]
Rensselaer Polytechnic Institute, Troy, NY

Abstract. A scalable, internet aware "intermediate representation" has been developed for remote interactive simulation of large deformable models. Further a networked computational environment is presented in which commodity computers tele-connect to remote high end servers using real-time protocol to utilize their processing power to enable highly realistic and detailed simulation of surgical scenarios. This proposed intermediate representation ("hive" (set) of computational nodes associated with surgical tool tip) can be tuned to the computational capacity of the client computer and is also scalable to the quality of the available network resources (bandwidth, delay, delay jitter) for the connection between client and server.

1. Introduction

In physics-based surgery simulation the modeling of the interaction of surgical tools with soft biological tissues in *real time* is a formidable task since real time graphical rendering requires an update rate of 30Hz, whereas real time force update using a haptic interface device such as a Phantom requires a much higher rate of 1 kHz. For realistic organ geometries and tool-tissue interactions, solving coupled and possibly nonlinear sets of partial differential equations at this rate becomes infeasible on personal computers using even the fastest of algorithms that we have developed [1] that scale linearly with the number of degrees of freedom of the system. Hence, moving to massively parallel computation platforms is necessary.

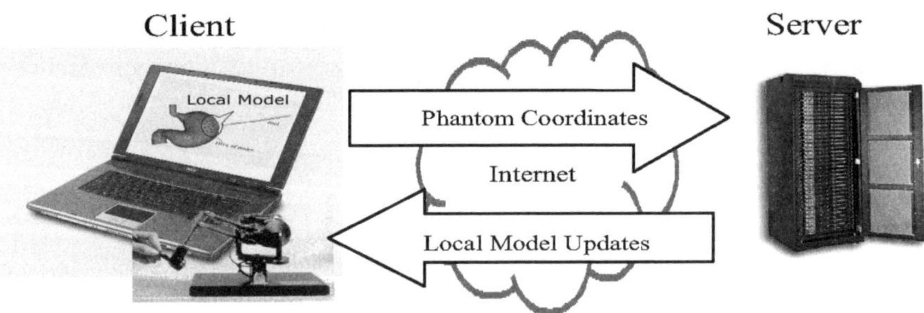

Figure 1 Remote interaction with soft tissues

Since the intended end users for the surgery simulators are surgeons and residents who have access to personal computers, it is important to develop a networked

---

[1] deod@rpi.edu* , [2] des@rpi.edu, [3] shivkuma@ ecse.rpi.edu

computational environment where these personal computers can connect seamlessly to remote high end servers and provide the smooth and rich end user experience which is easily manageable by currently available commodity hardware.

However, haptic interactions with slowly simulated deformable bodies (or remotely simulated in this case) are known to have stability issues due to delays [2]. In addition, it is necessary to overcome packet losses, variable bandwidths due to different capacities and varying during runtime due to TCP-friendly congestion control and variable delay and delay jitter while trying to achieve time critical communications with the server over the internet during runtime. Existing network middlewares for remote haptic interactions like [5] have not proposed any particular strategy to deal with this problem. We, in this paper are proposing a *local representation algorithm* to overcome these network issues for real time physics-based multimodal surgery simulation over the internet opening up exciting possibilities of highly realistic and detailed simulation of surgical scenarios.

<u>Client Side Processing</u>	<u>Server Side Processing</u>
• Continuously sends phantom™ motion (position and velocity) information to server, if the difference is two successive values exceeds *just noticeable difference.* • Computes and renders forces and deformation based on the local representation as described in [1] (a hive "set" of computational nodes associated with the underlying geometric mesh)	• Receives phantom motion information from client • Determines the optimum distribution of nodes (local representation) from the current & predicted motion of tool-tip and organ geometry database • Sends the updated representation if it differs from the current local representation already dispatched to client

2. Remote Surgery Scenario

In an earlier work, we have developed a novel mesh-free computational technique; the "Point-Associated Finite Field (PAFF)" approach [1] in which the organs are represented as collections of particles with overlapping finite influence zones which coordinate their motion during interaction and deformation. When the PAFF is to be used with massive human anatomy models obtained from the visible human project dataset [3] on massively parallel computers, the entire computational representation of the simulated scenario cannot be imported or processed on the client pc in real-time. Therefore A "hive" (set) of computational of nodes associated with the tool tip is maintained at the client for computation of the deformation and the reaction force. The server, which simulates the complete scene at high resolution receives all *noticeable* motion updates of the tool, and updates the local representation at client based on the underlying organ geometry in the current vicinity of the tool tip.

The local representation is also *scalable* to the class of the available internet connection, characterized by available bandwidth, round trip delay, delay jitter, packet loss rates, between client and server, size of local representation which depending on the number of nodes in local representation, the precise definition of node positions and the frequency of sending updates all of which are selected by the program runtime form the available class of connection. The maximum number of computational nodes the client pc can handle in real-time is also limited by the processor speed, given the maximum number of nodes that can be processed, the representation can also allow for differential accuracies of the surgical scene with desired local refinements by intelligent redistribution of nodes over the regions of "action".

3. Results and conclusion

The technique discussed is tested for simulation of scenarios involving multiple organ models obtained from the visible human project dataset [3].

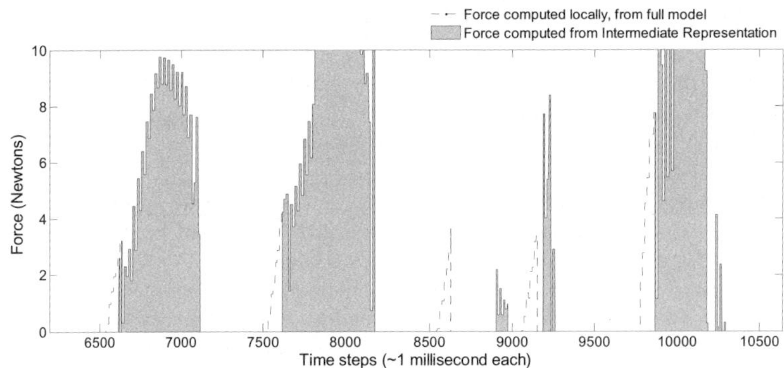

Figure 2 Plot of reaction force computed at the surgical tool tip.

The objective of the proposed local representation is to mask the delays and give a smooth interaction experience to the end-user to the extent possible. In figure 2, it can be seen (between time steps 6500 and 7000) that when the user interaction is consistent and focused around the same region, as is the case normally, the force computed from intermediate representation (dotted line) lags behind the one computed using the entire model on the client machine (solid line) but when the client receives the appropriate local model, the result closely matches the desired force curve. However, if the user interaction is in very short spurts of time (around time step 8500 in Figure 2), the interaction stops even before the correct local representation is obtained and the delay in the client-server communications cannot be masked.

A scalable, *internet aware* "intermediate representation" scheme has been developed for remote simulation of large scale virtual surgery. This will enable end users to utilize processing power from remotely located supercomputing hubs to run interactive surgery simulations.

4. References

[1] De, S.; Lim, Y.; Manivannan M.; Srinivasan M, Physically Realistic Virtual Surgery using the Point-Associated Finite Field (PAFF) Approach, , Presence: Teleoperators and Virtual Environments, Vol. 15, No. 3, pp 294-308, June 2006.
[2] Barbagli, F.; Salisbury, K.; Prattichizzo, D., Dynamic local models for stable multi-contact haptic interaction with deformable objects,; HAPTICS 2003. Proc. 11th Symposium on, pp.109–116
[3] M. J. Ackerman, The Visible Human project, Proceeding of MMVR Conference, pp.5-7, 1994.
[4] Q. Cai, V. Liberatore, and M. C. Cavusoglu, GiPSiNet: An Open Source/Open Architecture Network Middleware for Surgical Simulations.. In Proceedings of Medicine Meets Virtual Reality XIV (MMVR'06), pp. 316-371.

Medicine Meets Virtual Reality 15
J.D. Westwood et al. (Eds.)
IOS Press, 2007

Physics-based stereoscopic suturing simulation with force feedback and continuous multipoint interactions for training on the da Vinci ® surgical system

Dhanannjay Deo[1], Suvranu De[1], Tejinder P. Singh[2]

[1]*Advanced Computational Research Lab, Rensselaer Polytechnic Institute, Troy, NY*
[2]*Department of Surgery, Albany Medical College, Albany, NY*

Abstract. In this paper we present a 3d stereoscopic, bimanual surgical suturing system with a realistic thread model, and physics based force feedback training surgical residents at Albany medical college for the use da Vinci® surgical system. A novel algorithm is developed to calculate tissue deformations at multiple points due to both the frictional pull resulting from the passage of the thread through the tissue, and the additional forces applied by both hands of the user on the thread or tissues, enabling, for the first time, continuous sutures and knot tying with force feedback. Two Phantom Premium 1.0 (Sensable Technologies) are used for force feedback. Planar system's dual monitor based stereo vision system is used for simultaneous rendering of left and right eye views facilitating 3D rendering,

Keywords. Suturing simulator, physically based tissue interaction, realtime force feedback, bimanual, knot tying, multiple contact tissue interaction.

Introduction

Surgical suturing is an essential component of most surgical procedures ranging from laparoscopic microsurgeries to open wound stitching and is therefore an important feature of any part-task or full-scale surgical simulator. In this work we are interested in training of surgical residents at the Albany Medical College for operation on the da Vinci ® robotic surgical system [1]. This system employs a 3D vision system for enhanced depth perception and excellent hand-eye coordination.

The state of the art suturing simulators [2, 3] lack realistic algorithms for thread-tissue interaction and the resulting force feedback from both tissue elasticity and friction. In this paper, we develop a bimanual surgical suturing system with realistic thread model that overcomes these critical problems and can be used for both intermittent and continuous suturing. The simulations are displayed using a stereoscopic visio-haptic system to enable enhanced depth perception during knot tying.

Present algorithms only allow the needle or forceps to interact with the soft tissue. The suture then follows the needle and passes through the tissues passively without interaction. We have overcome this serious problem by developing a novel algorithm to calculate tissue deformations at multiple points due to both the frictional pull resulting from the passage of the thread through the tissue, and the additional forces applied by both hands of the user on the thread or tissues, enabling, for the first time, continuous suturing with force feedback.

1. Soft Tissue Modeling

In an earlier work, we have developed a novel meshfree computational technique; the point-associated finite field (PAFF) approach [4] for real time surgical simulation in which the organs are represented as collections of particles with overlapping finite influence zones which coordinate their motion during interaction and deformation. In this paper we present a surgical suturing algorithm that can be used with this model.

2. Thread Modeling

The suture is modeled as a series of rigid cylindrical links connected to each other at nodes by rotational degrees of freedom [2]. The thread motion was calculated using the *follow the leader* algorithm. which can update the positions of all links when the new positions of one or two leaders are specified. In the current context, the leading nodes are the ones which are controlled by the Phantom ™ cursor.

Collision detection and response schemes, extended from [2], are most vital from the point of view of knot tying stages of suturing simulator. A bounding sphere hierarchy is maintained for each suture, and is used for quick collision detection

---

```
For iteration from 1 to maximum iterations
    For each incremental displacement from 0 to follower displacement
            in current time step
        Update the thread according to follow the leader routine
            by displacing follower by one increment
    If self / mutual collision detected
        Return colliding pairs for response
    Else
        If the maximum displacement of any link is more than
                the link diameter
            Half the size of each increment
            Continue
        End
    End
Next iteration
```

Figure 1 Algorithm for iterative refinement in the follower displacement for stable collision detection

between sutures. Collision between individual links is determined by computing the closest distance between their axes and comparing them to the sum of their radii.

It is necessary for stable knot formation that the suture does not interpenetrate during knot tying. However, if large displacements (compared to the link diameter) are applied to the leader, the sutures may be collision free in the initial and final configurations, but they cross each other during the motion. This can lead to collapse of the knot. Hence it is required to apply displacements to the leaders in steps, iteratively reducing the step size if required until no link moves large enough to cross over in single motion step. The algorithm is presented in figure1.

The individual collisions between links were resolved in [2] by moving colliding links away from each other by a distance slightly greater than the link diameter. This slight gap created helps in motion of the suture thread in the next cycle of motion update.

3. Major Steps for the Suture-Tissue interaction

From the implementation standpoint the process of suturing can be conveniently separated into different steps which we discuss below.

1. **Position and orient** – A curved needle is attached to the leader. The suture thread follows the needle freely, neither thread nor the needle being in contact with the tissue. Surface models of needle and the tissue are continuously checked for overlap at every cycle of force update using the SWIFT++ package from Geometric Algorithms for Modeling, Motion, and Animation (GAMMA) group at UNC [6].

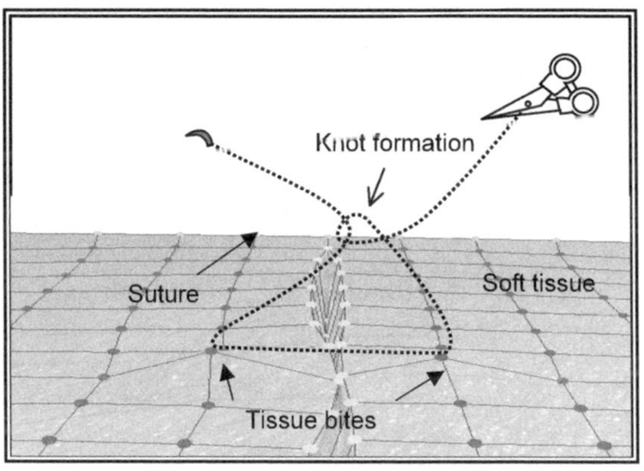

Figure 2 Schematic diagram for suturing procedure

2. **Bite the tissue-** In this step, the needle pierces the tissue and the suture passes through. The tissue is considered "bitten" (pierced) if the needle tip collides with the tissue model and the needle is at the correct angle i.e., making less than 30 degrees with the surface normal at the point of contact and exerts a contact force, computed using the physics-based PAFF model [4], greater than the *bite_threshold*. Only then will the suture enter the point of interaction following the needle. If the tissue is not bitten, the tissue deforms according to the displacement imposed by tool and corresponding reaction forces are rendered to the user. Though collision is detected for the solid curved needle, the tissue piercing is possible only through the tip in the current scenario.

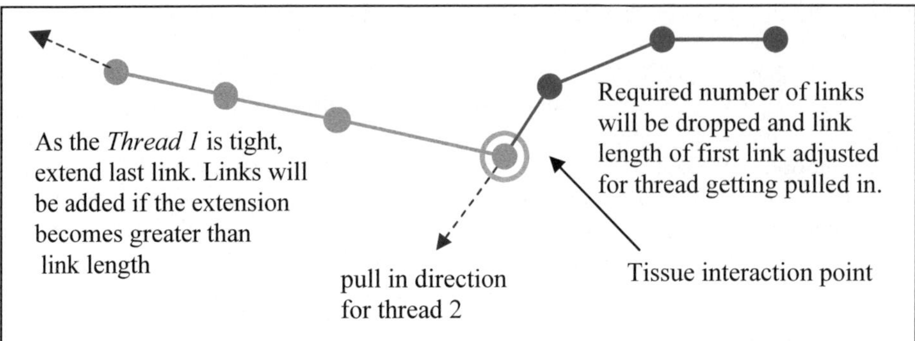

Figure 3 Threads at thread-tissue interaction

3. **Pull the suture** – At this stage, the suture is passing through at least one bite, as long as the thread pull exceeds a force greater than *friction threshold.* We have not performed studies on the friction properties of soft tissues. However, it is straightforward to incorporate such data into the model at this stage. The thread model used is capable of animating thread with only two leaders with arbitrarily specified new coordinates. In the beginning of the simulation, one end of the suture is associated with the needle, whereas the other end is held in a gripper. But as the suture starts passing through one or more thread-tissue interaction points, it becomes necessary to split the single suture into multiple thread identities at these points of interaction and update each suture segment by the position of its two end-nodes constrained. The mechanism by which the end conditions are handled at a tissue-interaction point are shown in figure 3. For calculation of final deformations for the tissue, the displacements calculated at each tissue-bite (grab point) are superimposed at the end.

4. **Re-Bite the tissue** – The same procedure of biting the tissue is repeated at the other side of the wound.

5. **Knot Positioning** - When the surgeon needs to tie a knot, the sutures have to be positions using two different Phantoms.

6. **Knot tightening** - When the suture is in position, and the two ends pulled apart, due to collision response, the knot gets tightened until a configuration in which the two ends of the sutures cannot be pulled further. Then the knot as defined by the colliding links in the knot configuration is treated as a single identity.

The algorithm for updating the thread configurations and calculation of reaction forces and tissue deformations during tissue-suture interaction is summarized in figure 4.

The maximum force rendering capacity of the Phantom is 8.5 N, so in the current simulation the tissue properties are adjusted so as to get reaction forces in the range of 0-6 N. This has the significant effect on the way forces are sensed while simulating multiple thread-tissue interactions. As described earlier, the friction resistance is exerted at every tissue bite, and if the maximum possible value of force is set too low in comparison with tissue stiffness, the corresponding deformations of tissues which are vital for closing the wound are not observed, and if the value of this frictional pull is set high, then some frictional resistance is exhibited at each tissue bite and hence the maximum force the device can render is limited. We have set the value of frictional resistance to 16% of the maximum allowable force which facilitates up to 6 tissue bites.

For each new tool tip position
    Update the position of the suture grabbed by the Phantom
    If maximum iterations of suture update over without success
        Knot is formed, update rest of the sutures.
    End
    For each thread starting with the one connected to needle
    If the thread is tight i.e. (thread length > the distance between the constraints)
        If the (force from tissue < force threshold)
            Deform the tissue render computed force
        Else (force = force threshold)
            Calculate Deformation = from force threshold
        Extend the thread length, add nodes if required
            Update the position of the connecting node from the next thread
    Else
        Allow free motion of the needle and thread
    Next thread
    If the thread is last

Figure 4 Algorithm for thread-tissue interaction

---

4. Stereo Rendering

Planar system's dual monitor based stereo vision system is used for simultaneous rendering of left and right eye views facilitating 3D rendering. Users have to wear polarized glasses so that only left eye view is visible to the left eye and right eye view is visible to right eye.

The result is a high quality 3d perception of the suturing scenario by the user, which represents the 3d vision system offered by the da Vinci surgical system. This type of 3d rendering is immensely helpful at the time of forming a knot where exact perception of depth is vital.

5. Results

In our implementation, a realistic wound model is texture mapped onto a physics-based PAFF tissue model. A bimanual suturing system is used with one hand manipulating the needle and the other either holding the forceps or the other end of the suture during knot tying. Some additional features of the simulator for improved realism include rupture of the suture if the applied force exceeds 6N and possible tearing of the tissue if the force exceeds critical values.

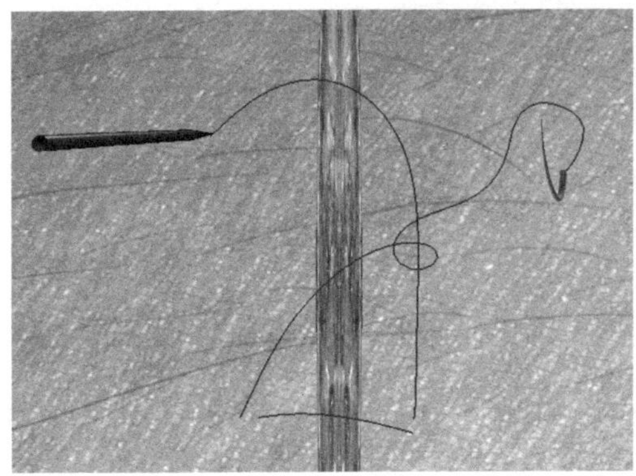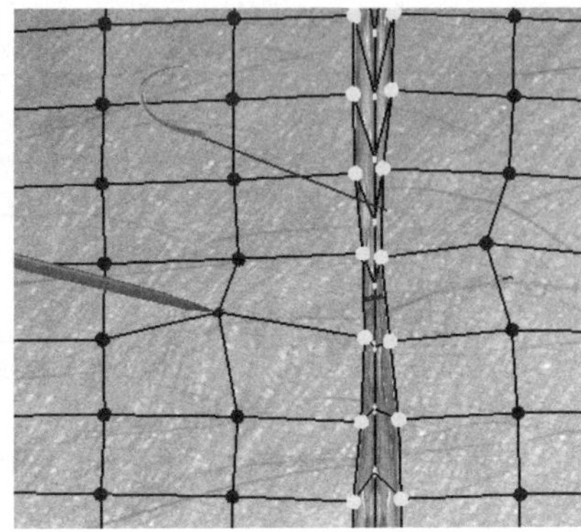

Figure 5 Screenshots from working simulator

6. Conclusion

A stereoscopic suturing simulator is presented for training surgical residents to use the da Vinci® surgical system. The novel contribution of this paper is the development of algorithms for interaction of the suture with physics-based tissue and the resultant force feedback. The algorithm also allows multiple point interaction and realistic knot tightening.

References

[1] The da Vinci telerobotic surgical system: the virtual operative field and telepresence surgery. Ballantyne GH, Moll F. Surg Clin North Am. 2003 Dec;83(6):1293-304

[2] Real-time Knot Tying Simulation Brown J., Latombe J-C, Montgomery K, The Visual Computer, vol. 20 (2-3), pages 165-179 May 2004.

[3] Two-Handed Next Generation Suturing Simulator, Lindblad AJ, Turkiyyah GM, Sankaranarayanan G, Weghorst SJ, Berg D., Proceedings of MMVR 12 conference

[4] Physically Realistic Virtual Surgery using the Point-Associated Finite Field (PAFF) Approach, De S, Lim Y, Manivannan M, Srinivasan MA, Presence: Teleoperators and Virtual Environments, June 2006, Vol. 15, No. 3, Pages 294-308,

[5] Lindblad, A.J., Turkiyyah, G.M., Sankanaranayanan, G., Weghorst, S.J. and Berg, D. (2004). Two-handed next generation suturing simulator. In J.D. Westwood et al. Proceedings of MMVR 2004.

[6] S. A. Ehmann and M. C. Lin. Accurate and fast proximity queries between polyhedra using convex surface decomposition. Tech. Report TR01-012, Department of Computer Science, Univ. of North Carolina, 2001.

Medicine Meets Virtual Reality 15
J.D. Westwood et al. (Eds.)
IOS Press, 2007

A Web-Based Teamwork Skills Training Program for Emergency Medical Teams

Eleen B. ENTIN, Jason SIDMAN, Gilbert MIZRAHI, Barry STEWART, Fuji LAI
Aptima, Inc, Woburn, MA
Lisa NEAL, *eLearn Magazine*
Colin MACKENZIE, Yan XIAO, *University of Maryland School of Medicine*

Abstract. T-TRANE is a scenario-based teamwork skills training program for emergency medical teams that uses web-enabled collaborative technologies. The program assumes students are skilled in clinical techniques but have minimal formal knowledge of teamwork. By providing training that focuses on teamwork skills in emergency medical settings, the program is designed to rapidly increase team proficiency. The program is comprised of information about and examples of teamwork skills, and scenario-based training exercises that provide practice in strategies to promote teamwork such as conducting pre-planning and debriefing sessions. T-TRANE is comprised of four modules, with both live (synchronous) interactive sessions and self-paced (asynchronous) sessions that students can complete at their convenience within scheduled intervals. The program includes an Instructor's Guide that provides the designated instructor the necessary support to conduct the training. The approach used in this program can be adapted to any domain in which distributed teams will benefit from pre-deployment training.

Keywords. Teamwork, distributed training, e-learning, emergency medicine, teamwork skills, debriefing

1. Background

Effective emergency medical treatment is comprised of both individual and team performance. While individual medical practitioners receive extensive training in clinical taskwork, they have had less experience learning about and applying teamwork skills in a collaborative environment in which there is a high degree of task interdependence and therefore a high need for team coordination. Furthermore, the high-pressure, time-constrained environment in which medical teams operate is replete with threats to teamwork such as equipment failure, limited resources, ad-hoc team formation, and so on, but in most cases the only existing training is on the job where newcomers are thrown together and expected to function as a team. Rapid deployment teams, such as crisis response teams and expeditionary medical support (EMEDS) teams, who may come from a variety of different organizations and locations, are deployed to a remote location where they must rapidly take effective action as a team under stressful conditions. A distributed training program conducted before teams are deployed could increment their effectiveness as a team.

To fill the need for training both co-located and distributed teams, we have developed Teamwork Training and Remote Assessment in a Networked Environment (T-TRANE), a web-based online course to teach teamwork skills to military and civilian emergency medical practitioners. The course assumes students are skilled in clinical techniques but have minimal formal knowledge of teamwork. Using networking technology, teams can be trained while they are in their home bases or even while they are en route to their deployed location. By providing training during either a distributed or co-located preparatory period, T-TRANE increases team proficiency and efficiency as quickly as possible.

In this paper we explain the pedagogical approach underlying the T-TRANE program, describe the components of the program, and discuss the results of an evaluation of the program.

2. Method

2.1 Pedagogical Approach Underlying T-TRANE

T-TRANE is grounded in the principles of scenario-based learning in which operationally realistic scenarios are used to engage the student in actively forming links between classroom and real-world applications of key concepts. Scenarios place students in a particular context, and encourage them to think about cause and effect [1]. To encourage active learning, T-TRANE uses two types of scenarios: videos from the Trauma Resuscitation Unit at the University of Maryland Medical School and textual scenarios developed with close guidance from Air Force personnel with extensive firsthand experience with trauma. The authenticity is crucial for the scenarios to resonate with students. The realism of the video clips reinforces the importance of the teamwork skills being studied more effectively than any other means since students can see the consequences of poor teamwork.   Using medical experts to provide commentary on aspects of teamwork captured in the videos can personalize the course by introducing a practicing clinician who has experienced real challenges to teamwork. It can also increase satisfaction and enjoyment, even in a "serious" application, through human narrative and storytelling [2].

T-TRANE is also grounded in principles of multimodal learning. An expansive set of literature emphasizes the importance of presenting information in a way that considers the structure of memory [3].   Multi-format presentations ensure accommodation of learning style differences by providing alternative information sources. Some of the multimedia features of the T-TRANE program are:

- textual definitions and scenarios
- video clips from a Trauma Resuscitation Unit that offer real-world examples of good and poor teamwork
- audio recordings of expert responses to question about teamwork in scenarios

T-TRANE is different from other teamwork skills training programs in that it does not require the presence of a trained instructor. Instead, the program includes an Instructor's Guide that provides the designated leader, who is assumed to be an experienced medical professional with the necessary support to conduct the training. Another innovative feature is the use of peer leaders, students in the class who assist the instructor by integrating and providing feedback on the other students' work for a given module. To support this responsibility each peer leader receives a Peer Leader's Guide focused on the module to which he or she is assigned.

2.2 Description of the Training Modules

To account for the busy schedules of medical personnel, T-TRANE is designed to be completed in approximately five to six hours, and incorporates both asynchronous and synchronous training sessions. Asynchronous sessions can be completed by the students at their convenience within a specified time period. Synchronous sessions are "live" sessions conducted over the web in which participants can interact via voice-over-IP as they progress through a module. Students are required to reserve the same block of time, but may participate from any location rather than having to travel to a co-located classroom.

Figure 1 shows the home page for the T-TRANE program with a notional training schedule. An **introductory session** is held to get the students set up and comfortable with the on-line technology. The students connect to a brief (half hour or less) session in which each student has a chance to speak and to make any necessary adjustments to his or her microphones and volume.

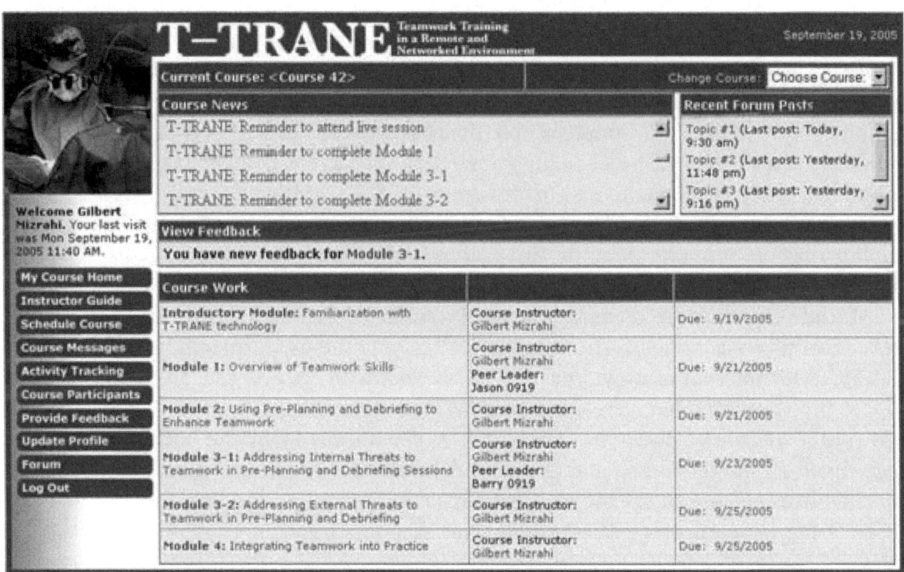

Figure 1. T-TRANE Course homepage, including module descriptions and schedule

Module 1, an asynchronous module, is an introduction to the course and is designed to promote formal learning on teamwork skills. Students are presented with an overview of the entire course and the motivation for the course. The module introduces students to five teamwork skills that support team effectiveness: leadership, communication, team orientation, back-up, and monitoring [4].   Good and poor examples of each skill are illustrated through videos of actual emergency room cases and through anecdotes both from the medical domain and from other teamwork-dependent domains such as flight navigation. Following the explanation and examples of the five teamwork skills, the students are asked to describe a situation they have experienced in which teamwork was lacking.

The section on teamwork skills is followed by an explanation of how internal threats (which arise from the interpersonal dynamics of the team) and external threats (which arise from factors outside the team itself) impact effective teamwork, and on the use of pre-planning and debriefing as strategies for improving teamwork. To apply this information, the students expand on the situation they previously shared by describing it in terms of internal or external threats and how it could have been addressed in a debriefing session. The students' responses are submitted to the peer leader for Module 1, who summarizes the class members' responses and comments upon them. Finally, the students are asked to post on the Discussion Form another situation in which teamwork failed and to read the responses that the other students submit to the forum. The Forum provides students with an opportunity to continue interesting discussions and share ideas even after the session has ended.

In **Module 2**, a synchronous module, students learn in more depth about two strategies for promoting teamwork: pre-planning sessions and debriefing sessions. The class views a videotaped scenario and responds to questions posed by the instructor about the teamwork skills displayed in the scenario. The students then participate in a simulated debriefing session based on the scenario. Debriefing sessions are crucial for providing an opportunity to learn from mistakes. Students are presented with strategies for dealing with teammates in a congenial and professional manner, while maintaining focus on using the material in the debriefing to aid future planning. In addition, the role play allows students to discuss their reactions to a stressful situation and the actions they would take to improve teamwork in the future. Students can be assigned a role other than their usual role (e.g., a nurse assigned to the role of surgeon) in order to promote a broader perspective of teamwork.

Figure 2 shows an example of a video-based scenario used in Module 2. The closed caption option provides text of the audio. As shown in Figure 2, the instructor interface includes notes for each slide displayed at the bottom.

Module 3, which is completed asynchronously, uses scenarios that illustrate and help students reflect on specific teamwork skills and the use of planning and debriefing to cope with internal and external threats to teamwork. Some scenarios are based on video clips, while others are generated as authentic stories in textual format. After answering questions about the teamwork skills displayed in the scenarios, students participate in simulated pre-planning and debriefing sessions based on these scenarios by submitting responses to the peer leader for the module. The peer leader's feedback helps them to learn more about their own responses and those of their classmates. Further, the peer leader, through reading and responding to classmates' responses, develops an even deeper understanding of the teamwork concepts under discussion.

Module 4, another synchronous module, is designed to reinforce what was learned in the course and discuss the experiences students have had implementing teamwork skills as part of their practice as well as students' observations of good and poor teamwork. It includes experts' examples of situations in which effective teamwork was instrumental. Students can discuss strategies they learned in the course that they plan to use in the future.

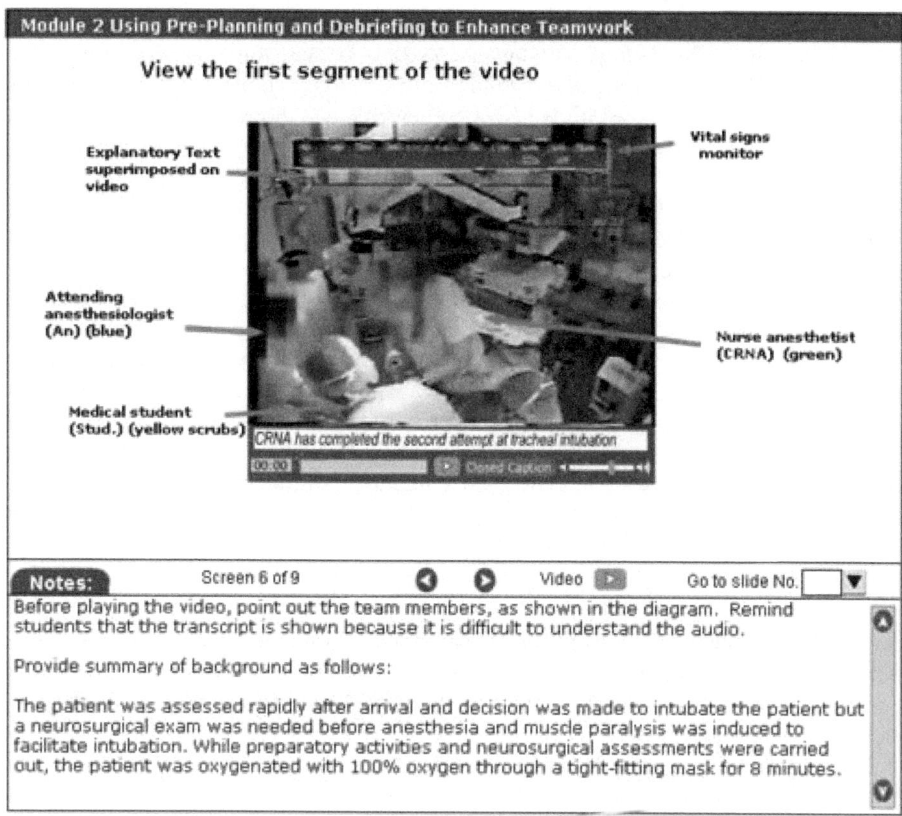

Figure 2. Example screen from T-TRANE Module 2, including labeling of key players in the scenario as well as notes available in the instructor's view

2.3 Evaluation Procedure

Three groups of medical professionals, including both civilian and military personnel, participated in the training program evaluation. Both student and instructor roles within the course were filled by participants. At the end of the course, participants completed a survey that probed their reactions to components of the training program and their assessment of the effectiveness and utility of the program as a whole. The survey included statements rated on a 7-point Likert scale and open-ended questions.

3. Results

Participants found the T-TRANE course to be engaging (M=5.4). They reported that T-TRANE provided them with an enhanced understanding of teamwork skills (M=5.3), and that they would be able to apply those skills in their future work (M=5.7). A majority (77%) of the participants said that they had a better understanding of how to conduct an effective debriefing. All participants agreed that T-TRANE would be valuable to others in their profession (M=5.9). Those who served as instructors reported that the Instructor's Guide provided sufficient guidance for serving in that role (M=6.3), confirming that the Guide is comprehensible and thorough.

When asked to list three things about T-TRANE they would not change, participants identified the interactive nature of T-TRANE, the use of real-life examples, and the self-paced nature of the asynchronous modules. This finding supports our pedagogical approach. The interactive nature of the course as well as the use of real-life examples were intended to make the course engaging, and they appear to have done so. While participants commented that they enjoyed the interactive sessions, in terms of scheduling they appreciated the self-paced nature of the asynchronous sessions. When asked what aspects of T-TRANE they would change, the primary factor participants recommended was improving the quality of the videos. In terms of when the training would be most useful, the military participants responded that the program would be most helpful before they came for on-site training and were thrust into intensive courses that consumed a great deal of time and mental energy.

4. Discussion and Conclusions

Overall, the participants' subjective assessments of the training were positive and attest to the value of the program. The extent to which this training will carry over into their teamwork in clinical settings requires a longer evaluation period, and must be addressed in subsequent work.

The pedagogical approach and technological components used in the T-TRANE program can readily be reused in different domains in which teams work together in intensive and stressful environments. Because it is delivered over the web, the program can be used for training both distributed and co-located teams.

Acknowledgements

This work was supported by a contract from the U.S. Air Force. The views, opinions and/or findings contained in this report are those of the authors and should not be construed as an official Department of the Air Force position.

References

[1] Neal, L., Miller, D., and Perez, R., 2004. Online Learning and Fun. *eLearn Magazine*. from www.elearnmag.org/subpage/sub_page.cfm?article_pk=12265&page_number_nb=1&title=FEATURE %20STORY.

[2] Braun, N. (2002). Storytelling & Conversation to Improve the Fun Factor in Software Applications. Workshop paper at CHI 2002 Conference on Human Factors in Computing Systems, http://www.zgdv.de/zgdv/departments/z5/Z5Publications/2002_04/index_html_en.

[3[Mayer, R.E. (1997). Multimedia Learning: Are We Asking the Right Questions? *Educational Psychologist, 32*, 1-19.

[4] Sims, D.E., Salas, E., & Burke, C.S. (2004). Is there a "Big Five" in teamwork? 19th Annual Conference of the Society for Industrial and Organizational Psychology, Chicago, IL.

Medicine Meets Virtual Reality 15
J.D. Westwood et al. (Eds.)
IOS Press, 2007

Virtual Reality for Robotic Laparoscopic Surgical Training

Matthew J. FIEDLER [a], *Shing-Jye CHEN [a], Timothy N. JUDKINS [a], Dmitry OLEYNIKOV [b], and Nick STERGIOU [a]

[a] *HPER Biomechanics Lab, University of Nebraska at Omaha, Omaha, NE*
[b] *Dept of Surgery, University of Nebraska Medical Center, Omaha, NE*
**shingjychen@mail.unomaha.edu*
http://www.unocoe.unomaha.edu/hper/bio/home.htm

Abstract: Virtual reality (VR) simulation has been used to improve training for manual laparoscopy and to give surgeons superior performance in the operating room. However, VR has not been used to train surgeons in robotic laparoscopy. *Subjects*: Five students of the University of Nebraska Medical Center (UNMC) and the University of Nebraska at Omaha gave consent according to UNMC ethical guidelines. *Experimental protocol*: Subjects performed with the Da Vinci robotic surgical system 5 trials for each of two tasks (Bimanual Carrying, BC; Needle Passing, NP). Each task was performed first in the actual robotic operating environment and then in VR. The data analysis included time to task completion, instrument tips distance traveled and the corresponding speed, and range of motion of the elbow flexion and extension of each subject. *Results*: The BC and NP tasks were not significantly different between the two environments with respect to robot tip speed and the elbow range of motion for both arms. Time to task completion and distance traveled were significantly different between the two environments for both tasks. Survey results showed that subjects partially agreed that it was easy to adapt to VR and felt comfortable manipulating the robot controls in VR. They also suggested that they would like to have VR as part of their regular training. Our preliminary efforts showed promise that our VR environment is valid and it can be used for training of robotic laparoscopy. However, the differences identified need to be further explored and point to the need to further improve our VR simulation.

Keywords. Virtual reality, laparoscopy, surgical robot, daVinci, surgical training

Background

Virtual reality (VR) simulation has been used to improve training for manual laparoscopy and to give surgeons superior performance in the operating room [1, 2]. However, to date there has never been a VR developed to train surgeons involving robotic laparoscopic surgery (Robotic daVinci Surgical System; dVSS; Intuitive Surgical Inc.). Our study presents preliminary efforts to develop a VR training environment for robotic laparoscopy. In addition, we compared our prototype VR environment to the actual environment, the dVSS, using simple tasks (needle passing and bimanual carrying) to determine the validity of the simulation.

Tools and Methods

Subjects: Five right hand dominant experienced daVinci users were recruited from the University of Nebraska Medical Center (UNMC) and the University of Nebraska at Omaha. Each subject signed a consent form according to UNMC ethical guidelines.

Tasks/Experimental protocol: Subjects performed two tasks: bimanual carrying (BC), and needle passing (NP). The tasks were performed in both the actual and the VR environments. The tasks were cyclical in nature and were designed to mimic actual laparoscopic tasks that require significant bimanual coordination. In the real environment BC task as in Figure 1a, the subject was first instructed to simultaneously pick up a 15 x 2 mm plastic piece (one each with left and right robotic graspers) from metal caps (30 mm in diameter) and then to place them in two other metal caps 60 mm away. The subjects reciprocated bimanual carrying movement five times in succession in one trial. A total of five trials were collected. After the real environment task was completed, a VR simulated BC task was performed as in Figure 1b. In the VR environment, the subject also performed five trials.

For the real environment NP task, the subjects were first instructed to use the right dominant arm to pick up a 26 mm surgical needle from a fixed location and then pass it through 6 consecutive 8mm in diameter holes of a latex tube for one trial. The tube was 14 cm in length. When passing through each hole, the left grasper picked up the passing needle. After the completion of five trials in the real environment, the VR simulated NP task was performed. In the VR environment, the subject also performed the same reciprocal passing movements between the two graspers.

Virtual Reality Construction: The VR environment for each task was developed using Webots 5.1.8 software (Cybertronics, Ltd, Switzerland). Each VR task was driven with kinematic data streamed in real-time from the daVinci robot's operating console through data acquisition software (LabVIEW 8.1, USA). The daVinci's instruments and each task's environment were modeled as 3D objects using SolidWorks (USA). In the BC VR simulation (see Figure 1b), virtual grasping and release of the target plastic pieces were based upon touch sensor information built-in between the instrument tip and the plastic target pieces. When both virtual instrument tips simultaneously touched the targets in each cup, the VR environment signified discrete events to relocate the targets to other cups. Reciprocal touching the target in the cups simulated the bimanual carrying movement in the actual robotic operation environment. In the NP VR simulation, a design of the built-in sensor touch between the instrument tip and virtual targeting hole on tube simulated the needle passing and retrieval. To view each VR task in the daVinci surgeon console, a virtual laparoscopic camera was built to project the virtual task to the viewing area of the console as a 3D stereoscopic image.

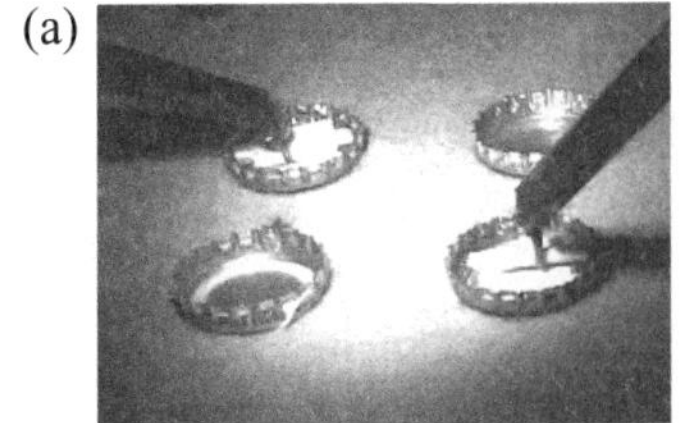
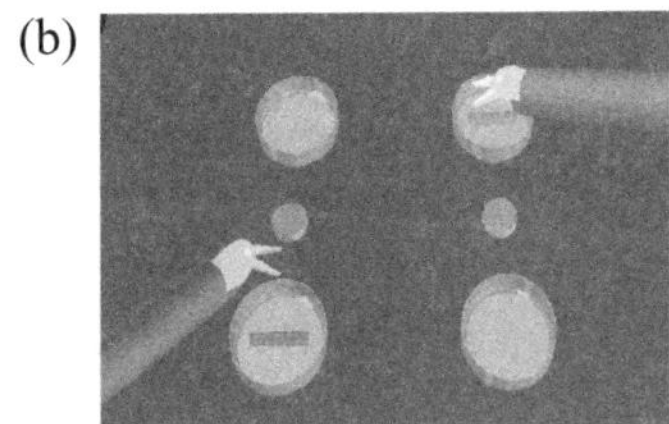

(a)   (b)

Figure 1. Robotic laparoscopic bimanual carrying task in a). Actual, b) VR environment

Data Collection and Analysis: Kinematics of the dVSS was collected at 100 Hz using the Application Programmer's Interface provided by the manufacturer. Elbow flexion and extension angles of each subject were also collected at 1000Hz using electrogoniometers (Biometrics, Ltd. USA). Analysis included time to task completion, instrument tip distance traveled and the corresponding speed, and range of motion of the elbow. Paired *t*-tests were used to compare the VR and the actual environment. Each subject was also asked to complete a written survey.

Results

The BC and NP tasks were not significantly different between the VR and actual environments with respect to the robot tip speed and the elbow range of motion for both arms (see Figure 2). However, time to task completion and distance traveled were significantly different between the VR and the actual environments for both tasks. Results of the written survey showed that subjects partially agreed that it was easy to adapt to VR and felt comfortable manipulating the robot controls in VR. They also suggested that they would like to have VR as part of their regular training.

Conclusion

Our preliminary findings showed that a promise of the developed VR environment can be potentially implemented for training of robotic laparoscopy. However, the differences in the time to task completion and the distance travel of the instrument tips suggest a need of improving the current VR environment. In future study, studies will be conducted to examine the effects of training between VR and actual environments in robotic laparoscopy[1].

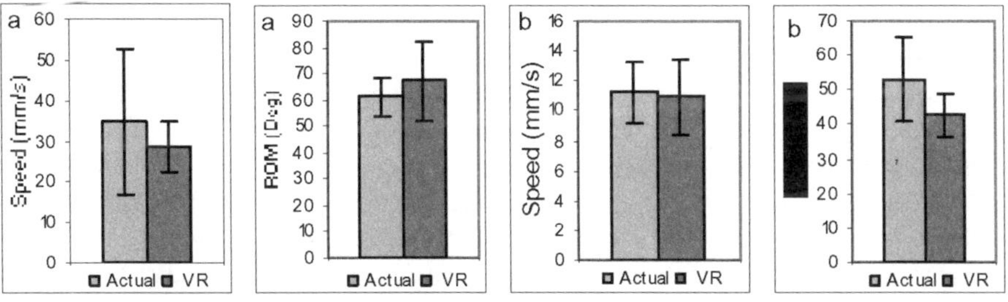

Figure 2. Tip speed and Range of Motion for a) BC and b) NP tasks, $p > .05$

REFERENCES
[1]   Aggarwal et al., Am J Surgery, 191:128-133, 2006.
[2]   Gallagher et al., Ann Surgery, 241:364-372, 2005.

---

[1] Supported by the Nebraska Research Initiative.

Medicine Meets Virtual Reality 15
J.D. Westwood et al. (Eds.)
IOS Press, 2007

Validation System of MR Image Overlay and Other Needle Insertion Techniques

Gregory S FISCHER [a], Eva DYER [a], Csaba CSOMA [a], Anton DEGUET [a], and Gabor FICHTINGER [a]

[a] *Engineering Research Center, Johns Hopkins University, Baltimore, MD*

Abstract.

In order to develop accurate and effective augmented reality (AR) systems used in MR and CT guided needle placement procedures, a comparative validation environment is necessary. Clinical equipment is prohibitively expensive and often inadequate for precise measurement. Therefore, we have developed a laboratory validation system for measuring operator performance using different assistance techniques. Electromagnetically tracked needles are registered with the preoperative plan to measure placement accuracy and the insertion path. The validation system provides an independent measure of accuracy that can be applied to varying methods of assistance ranging from augmented reality guidance methods to tracked navigation systems and autonomous robots. In preliminary studies, this validation system is used to evaluate the performance of the image overlay, bi-plane laser guide, and traditional freehand techniques.

Keywords. validation system, augmented reality, image overlay, mri, needle placement, percutaneous procedures, image guided surgery

Introduction

A comparative validation environment is necessary for an efficacious analysis of CT/MRI guided assistance techniques to be used in needle placement procedures. Clinical equipment is prohibitively expensive and often inadequate for precise validation. Precise measurement of placement accuracy by MRI is greatly limited by paramagnetic needle artifact and lack of distinct small targets. Scanner time cost can exceed $500/hour making statistically significant trials impractical. Therefore, we have developed a laboratory validation system for measuring operator performance of different assistance techniques. The validation system can be applied to varying methods of assistance ranging from augmented reality guidance methods to tracked navigation systems and autonomous robots.

Preliminary accuracy assessment of our MR image overlay system has been performed, but the excessive cost of scanner time has thwarted a large-scale study of the accuracy of this system. Therefore, an off-line validation system has been created in order to study needle placement accuracy; in particular we look at the accuracy of the image overlay and compare it to that of other insertion guidance methods. This system will also provide a means to study the trajectory and gestures throughout the insertion procedure in addition to the endpoint accuracy. The study of hand gestures for each of these methods will provide useful information that can be used to help minimize the number of re-insertion attempts needed, as each re-insertion causes significant discomfort to the patient. This system ensures a less resource exhaustive and more accurate means by which to validate needle insertion procedures.

In this paper, we describe the validation system shown in Fig. 2, and its use for comparative analysis of the virtual image overlay, the bi-plane laser guide and unassisted freehand techniques. The image overlay displays CT/MR images and a virtual needle guide over the patient [1] and is calibrated such that the overlay a MR or CT image and virtual needle guide appears to be floating inside the patient in the correct size and position as shown in Fig. 2(a,c). The bi-plane laser guide uses intersecting transverse and adjustable parasaggital laser planes to mark the trajectory of insertion [2], as shown in Fig. 2(b,d).

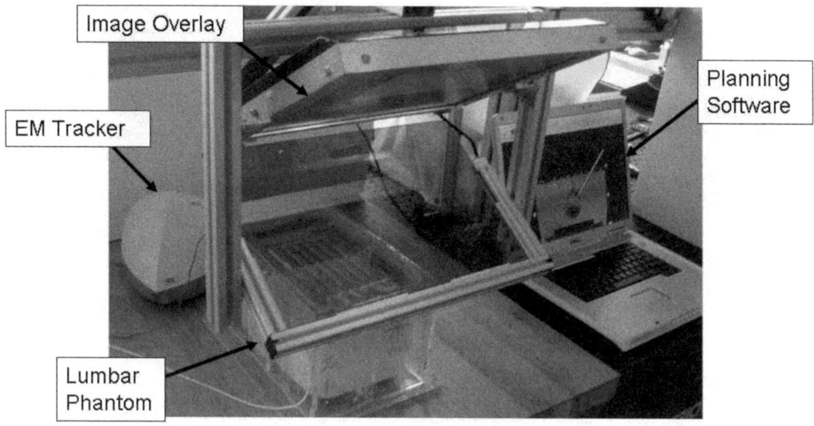

Figure 1. The validation environment shown with the image overlay system.

1. Validation System

Electromagnetic (EM) tracking (Aurora, Northern Digital, Waterloo, Ontario) is utilized to provide the position of the tip and orientation of the shaft of an instrumented needle as described in [3]. All necessary components must be registered with one another in order to track the needle with respect to the preoperative plan generated on the MR/CT images. The components of the system include: the Aurora EM Tracker, a tracked needle, the tracked phantom, the MR/CT images used for pre-operative planning and the AR guidance system. The system is shown in Fig. 1.

1.1. Phantom Design

A human cadaver lumbar spine phantom was designed to mimic the anatomy of a patient and aid in the process of registration. Lumbar vertebrae and simulated intravertebral discs are placed in proper alignment are embedded into a layered tissue mimicking gel (SimTest, Corbin, White City, OR) of two different densities emulating fat and muscle tissue. The gel phantom with lumbar spine is placed into an acrylic enclosure which was accurately laser-cut with 24 different pivot points spread over four sides for rigid-body registration. Stereotactic fiducial markers (MR-Spots, Beekley, Bristoll, CT) were placed on the phantom in precisely positioned laser-cut slots. The markers were placed in a 'Z' shape pattern on three sides allowing for automatic registration between anatomical images and the phantom. The acrylic enclosure was designed such that different phantoms can be placed inside it for studying other procedures.

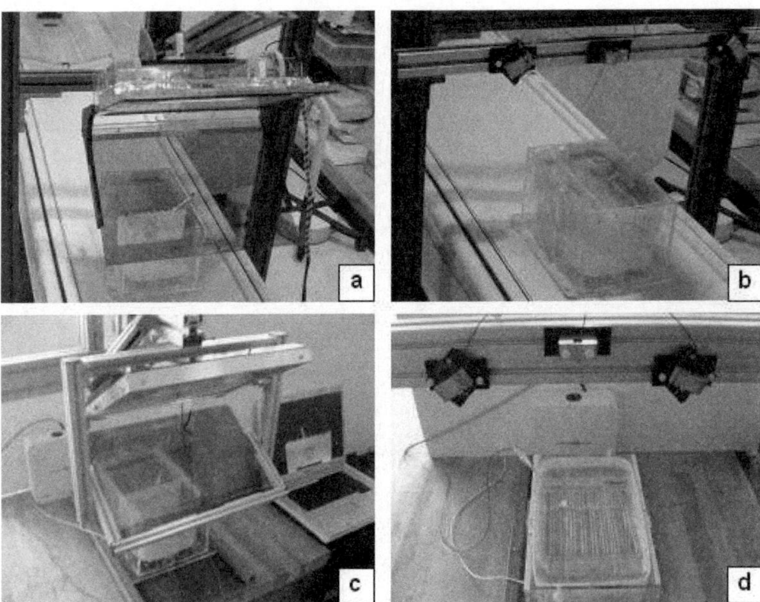

Figure 2. Image overlay (a,c) and bi-plane laser guide (b,d) AR needle placement systems with spine phantom. MR scanner feasibility trials (a,b) and laboratory validation system with tracked needle (c,d).

1.2. MR Image Registration

In order to register preoperatively obtained MR or CT images (and their respective pre-operative plans) to their corresponding physical space, techniques similar to those described in [4] are used. The Z-frame registration uses three stereotactic fiducial markers in the shape of a 'Z' on each of the left, right, and bottom faces of the phantom (Fig. 4). Axial images are taken near the center of the phantom; the locations of other images of the phantom are known with respect to this reference. The central image is used for registration, where the nine fiducial markers are segmented by applying an adaptive threshold and morphological operations to the image. The centroid of each marker was then found and the position of each marker with respect to the Dicom image was recorded into a set of nine points. After the nine distinct points were identified, the transformation from the scanner's image space to the phantom's coordinate system was computed. The RMS error incurred in the image to phantom space registration for a typical MR image was 1.26mm.

1.3. Electromagnetic Tracker Registration

The NDI Aurora EM tracking system is used to localize an instrumented needle with respect to the phantom. A 6 degree-of-freedom (DOF) reference tool is fixed to the phantom and a calibrated pointer tool is used for rigid-body registration of the phantom to the tracker. Data was obtained by pivoting about the 24 pre-defined divot points with the pointer. These points were used for registration between phantom coordinate system and that of the EM tracker by finding the transformation which aligns the known point locations obtained from the mechanical design specifications with the collected data points. The RMS error incurred in the rigid-body registration was 0.93mm. Fig. 3 illustrates the placement of the fiducial markers in the image and phantom space.

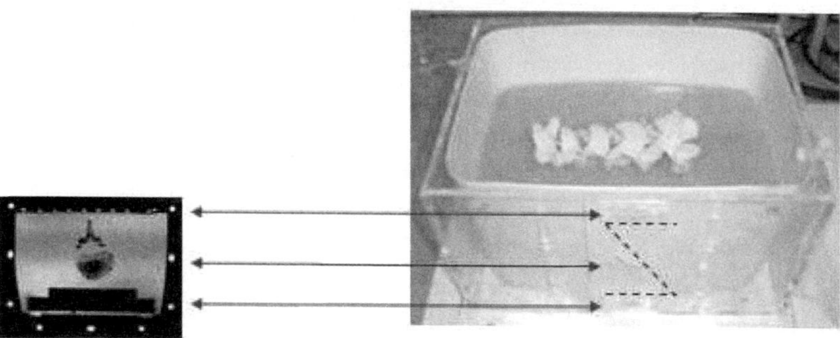

Figure 3. Phantom design showing spine partially embedded in gel and fiducial markers both on the phantom and their corresponding MR image.

This registration process requires only 5-10 minutes and is necessary only when the 6-DOF reference body tool is repositioned on the phantom. The rest of the registration process is automatic. Once both steps in registration are complete, an instrumented needle may be tracked as it maneuvers along a planned path within the phantom. To maximize the system's accuracy, future efforts will include distortion mapping and error compensation as described in [5].

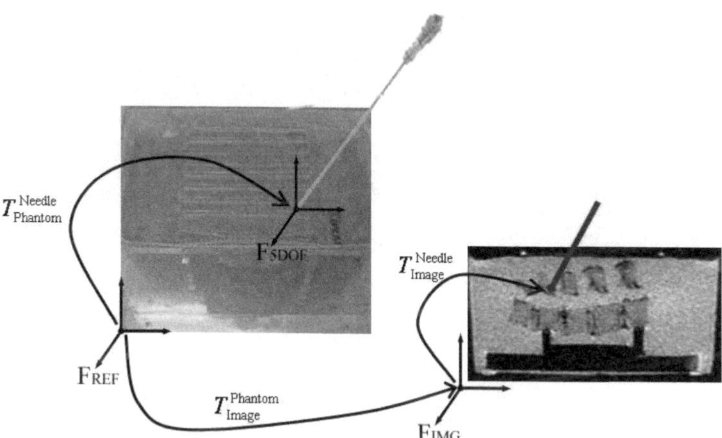

Figure 4. Frame transformations for the registration process shown on the spine phantom and its corresponding MR images. The tracked needle is represented in the original image space where the preoperative plan was made.

2. Experimental Methods

Prior to beginning trials, numerous needle paths were created in the EasySlice planning software that the author's have developed and is described in [1]. The software stores the insertion and target points for each planned path as well as the angle of insertion needed to accurately reach the desired target. For each of the three needle insertion methods (image overlay, bi-plane laser guide and freehand interventions) presented, subjects were randomly assigned three different paths in three different axial MR slices. The entire insertion attempt was recorded with the tracking software. The software then provides insertion and target point error, both in and out of the image plane. Needle axis orientation error is also computed. Simple forms of gesture tracking are now provided, including distances from the trajectory during insertion and the number of re-insertion attempts.

2.1. Results

To demonstrate workflow, four needle insertions were performed with each technique in a clinical MRI environment. As expected, accuracy could not be assessed due to large artifacts as shown in Fig. 5(a). In the validation testbed, the measured needle trajectories were graphically overlaid on the plan and targeting MR image as shown in Fig. 5(b). Twenty insertions were performed with each technique. Position and orientation errors were measured. Initial analysis showed that the results correlate with direct validation performed using fluoroscopy described in [2]. The image overlay's mean error in the image plane was 1.4mm and 2.5^o with standard deviations of 0.5mm and 1.9^o respectively. The laser guide's average error was 1.8mm and 2.0^o (1.2mm and 1.8^o standard deviation), and freehand produced average errors of 2.0mm and 5.2^o (1.4mm and 2.3^o standard deviation).

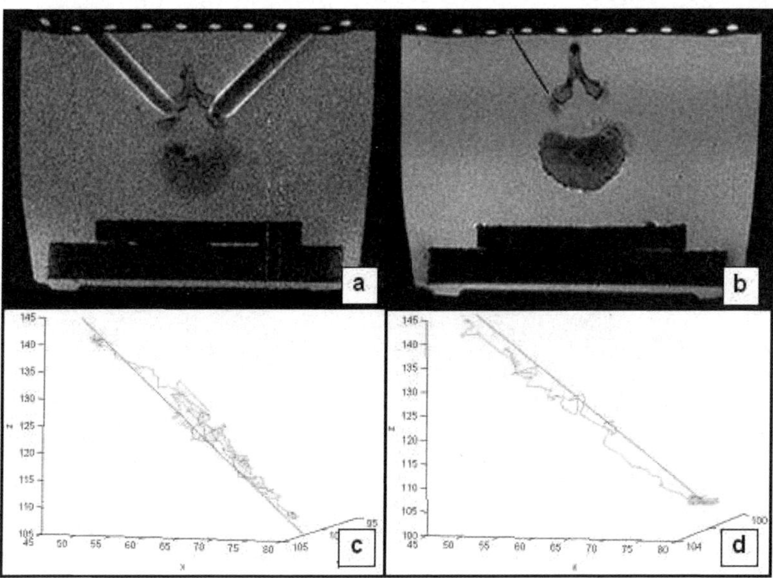

Figure 5. Typical results from an MR image (a) and a tracked path (b). Logged trajectory showing multiple corrections (c) and direct path (d).

3. Discussion

Initial assessments of the image overlay, laser guide, and freehand needle insertions were performed with the validation system. Experiments with experienced radiologists are currently underway. Future experiments will provide independent, large scale accuracy assessment of needle insertion procedures using commercial surgical navigation systems, image overlay, laser guidance, and traditional techniques. The goal is to quantitatively compare placement accuracy, consistency, and other important characteristics such as the needle trajectories throughout the entire placement procedure.

In typical needle placement procedures, the interventionalist will often probe the patient's anatomy until the desired target is reached. This probing action can result in a great deal of discomfort to the patient as well as significant bruising to the area. Analysis of the needle trajectory can provide information about the number of insertion and repositioning attempts that were made during an intervention. Fig. 5(c) illustrates a trajectory that resulted from repeated reinsertions and Fig. 5(d) shows an insertion with minimal repositioning attempts. This information enables researchers to study the systems' ability to minimize discomfort to the patient during the procedure. We intend to use gesture tracking techniques similar to those described in [6].

We also hope to implement the tracking system in clinical trials within a CT scanner, while utilizing the gesture tracking information given by the system for planning interventions. Future applications of this system may also include: providing realtime accuracy and position feedback to a user in vivo and evaluating the accuracy of needle placement procedures in clinical training settings. Applications of this system may also be extended further into autonomous robotic systems and many other augmented reality systems.

Acknowledgements

Partial funding for this project was provided by NSF Engineering Research Center Grant #EEC-97-31478, Siemens Corporate Research and William R. Kenan, Jr. Fund.

References

[1]   Fischer GS, Deguet A, Schlattman D, Taylor RH, Fayad L, Zinreich SJ, Fichtinger G. MRI image overlay: applications to arthrography needle insertion. Studies in health technology and informatics - Medicine Meets Virtual Reality 14, 2006; 119:150–155.

[2]   Fischer GS, Wamsley C, Zinreich SJ, Fichtinger G. Laser-Assisted MRI-Guided Needle Insertion and Comparison of Techniques. Int Soc for Comp Asst Orthopaedic Surg, Jun 2006.

[3]   Wood BJ, Zhang H, Durrani A, Glossop N, Ranjan S, Lindisch D, Levy E, Banovac F, Borgert J, Krueger S, Kruecker J, Viswanathan A, Cleary C. Navigation with Electromagnetic Tracking for Interventional Radiology Procedures: A Feasibility Study. J Vasc Interv Radiol. 2005; 16:493-505.

[4]   Lee S, Fichtinger G, Chirikjian GS. Novel algorithms for robust registration of fiducials in CT and MRI. J Med Phys 2002;29(8):1881Ű1891.

[5]   Fischer GS, Taylor RH. Electromagnetic Tracker Measurement Error Simulation and Tool Design, In Proceedings of Medical Image Computing and Computer Assisted Intervention. Med Img Comp & Comp Asst Int. 2005; LNCS 3750:73-80.

[6]   Lin HC, Shafran I, Murphy T, Okamura AM, Yuh DD, Hager GD. Automatic Detection and Segmentation of Robot-Assisted Surgical Motions. In Proceedings of Medical Image Computing and Computer Assisted Intervention. Med Img Comp & Comp Asst Int. 2005; LNCS 3749:802-810.

Medicine Meets Virtual Reality 15
J.D. Westwood et al. (Eds.)
IOS Press, 2007

Ultrasound and needle insertion simulators built on real patient-based data

Clément Forest[1], Olivier Comas[1], Christophe Vaysière[2], Luc Soler[1],
Jacques Marescaux[1]

(1)Ircad/EITS, Strasbourg, France (2)CMCO, Strasbourg, France

We present here the state of our work on medical simulators. We have developed several patient-based training simulators for ultrasound examination and ultrasound guided needle insertion. These simulators are built upon a method already described in MMVR in 2005 that allows to automatically create new cases from a 3D medical image (CT or MRI) They use indifferently one or two force feedback devices Omni from Sensable. Simulated procedures include hepatic biopsy, radiofrequency thermal ablation, prenatal examination and amniocentesis. An automatic evaluation informs users of the correctness of their gesture. First early validations with young residents have been started.

KEYWORDS: Ultrasound simulation, amniocentesis, radiofrequency, force feedback, …

Introduction

Ultrasonography is a non invasive technique that is widely used in a large range of procedures, for instance pre-natal diagnosis or tumor detection. Its use also becomes every day more essential for intra-operative needle insertion guiding. However, this technology, and especially its use for intra-operative guiding, is challenging to master for young residents. Main causes are the difficulty of interpretation of resulting images and the problem of coordinating hands according to those images. The aim of this research is to provide medical residents with realistic simulators for the training of ultrasound and ultrasound guided needle insertion procedures, in replacement of already existing mannequin-based ultrasound trainers.
This paper is the continuation of a previous work we presented at MMVR in 2005[1].

Ultrasound Simulation Technique

The technique for ultrasound simulation is based on the real time processing of a volumetric medical image, currently a CT-scan or a MRI. According to the position of a virtual transducer, that image is sliced and an automatic segmentation is performed to distinguish between air, bones and soft tissues. Using that segmentation, several images are computed to model noise, absorption and diffraction of the ultrasound wave. Those images are finally combined into the final simulated ultrasound image. For a more precise description of the method, interested persons can refer to [1]. It is to note that this process is fully automatic and no manual preprocessing of the medical image is necessary. The whole method has been recently patented.

One of the main interests of this method is its ability to use already existing medical images. Indeed, CT-scan Dicom images can be inserted as they are into the simulator and are directly usable. For MRI images, some precautions a have to be taken due to the high variability of that modality but the principle is similar. For that reason, new simulated cases corresponding to real anatomies can be obtained easily, facilitating for instance the pooling of pathological cases into a library for educational purposes. Furthermore, the introduction of new cases being done automatically, the method becomes also usable for pre-operative planning.

Existing prototypes

As planed in [1], we have integrated our method into a set of educational simulators, named HORUS (*Haptic Operative Realistic Ultrasound Simulator*). These simulators can use indifferently one or two force feedback devices (currently Omni from Sensable, see Figure 1). One is used to manipulate the ultrasound transducer and the other stands for the needle. For more realism, a dummy US- transducer handle can be plugged in place of the default Omni stylus.

These prototypes are all built upon a common framework we developed at IRCAD. This framework makes an intensive use of multithreading (GUI, haptics, physical simulation, US simulation, …). To improve future soft tissue deformation capabilities we planed to integrate the SOFA framework (http://www.sofa-framework.org/) during the next year. Prototypes run under Windows on almost any laptop or desktop computer with a modern graphic card.

All those prototypes have been developed in strong collaboration with US specialists, radiologists and obstetricians.

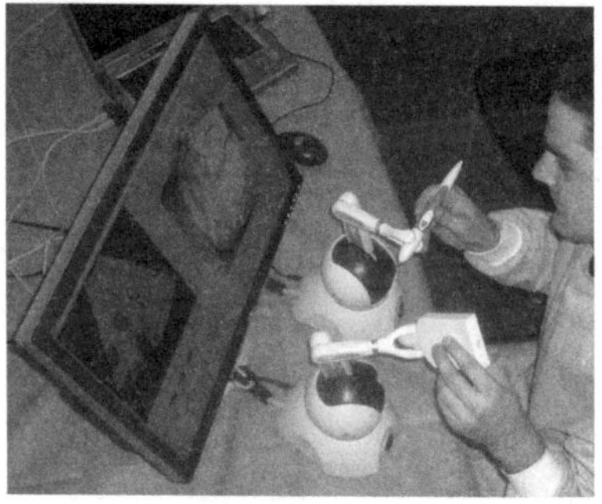

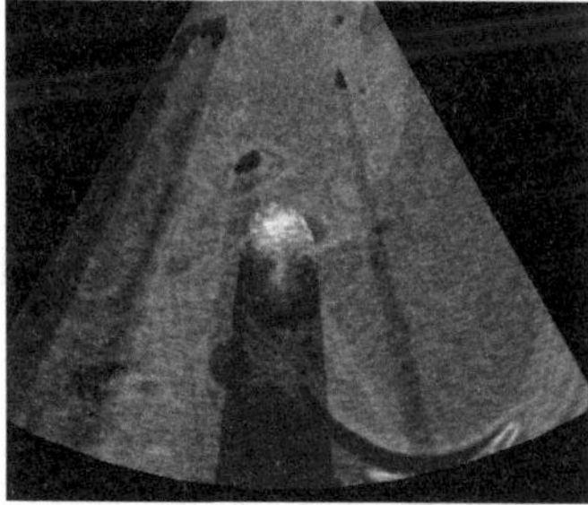

Figure2: Simulated thermal ablation

Figure1: External view of the simulator with the two force feedback devices.

Biopsy and radiofrequency simulator

This first prototype is dedicated to hepatic biopsy and radiofrequency thermal ablation. Five different cases are proposed: three biopsies and two radiofrequencies. All cases are built from real injected CT-scans. The purpose for the user is to proceed with the given operation correctly and without touching any vital organ with the needle. The needle and zone being burnt can be seen in the ultrasound view (see Figure 2).

Once completed, an automatic evaluation is done to estimate the correctness of the gesture (distance to the target, safety of the path, percentage of the tumor burnt, …). Several difficulty levels are proposed, one of them providing a transparency mode which appeared to be useful to improve beginners' understanding of the relation between transducer position and the corresponding ultrasound image (see Figure 3).

Obstetric Simulator

The simulation method has also been adapted to obstetrics. For this application we are using MRI images (T2) instead of CT-Scans[2]. We developed a prototype of the simulator that can be used for both prenatal examination training and amniocentesis simulation[3]. The fetus and placenta have been reconstructed manually and can be seen in a transparency mode (see Figure 4). For the prenatal examination, an automatic evaluation checks the precision of the transducer position for different classical measures (head, abdomen, …), the presence of several anatomical markers in the image and the correctness of the measured value. For the amniocentesis, the evaluation tool checks the success of the gesture.

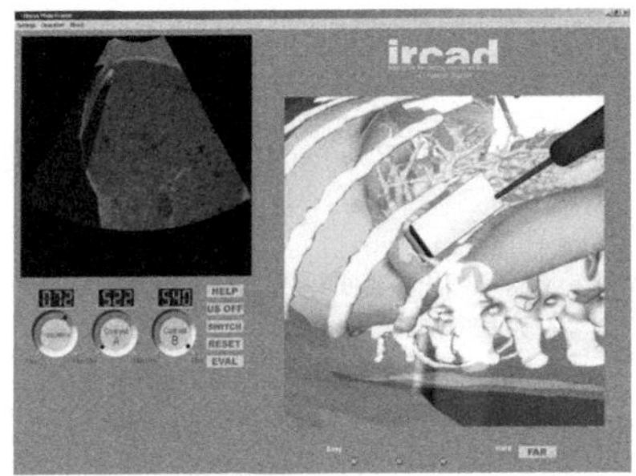

Figure3: Screenshot of the hepatic simulator showing the transparency mode.

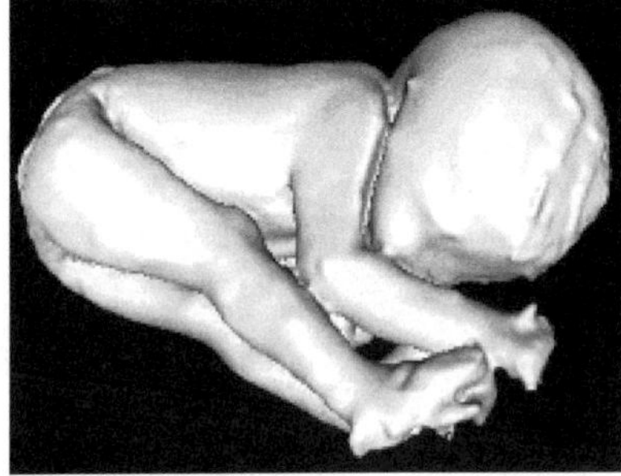

Figure 4: View of the reconstructed fetus. Validation

HORUS has been used during 2005-2006 at IRCAD by 8 medical students. After a month of a daily one hour training with the hepatic simulator, students were asked to manipulate the obstetric simulator they had never seen before, and to describe the fetus and draw its position. Then they had to localize several organs. All tests were successful. Feedback from the students was that they appreciated very much to use the simulator and they reported it helped them to understand better real US-images when encountered in medical services. The same experimentation will continue in 2007.

A more ambitious validation protocol is currently in advanced discussion for the obstetric/prenatal version of the simulator. The purpose will be to show that this simulator can be used to differentiate between amniocentesis experts and non experts.

Future work

An early prototype for a patient-based epidural simulator has been developed in collaborations with anesthetists. That prototype allows to use a modified epidural kit plugged on the force feedback Omni device in place of the default stylus.
An adaptation of the HORUS simulator including patient breathing simulation has also been developed. This prototype uses the technique presented in [4] in order to generate a deformation field that can be applied directly to the original medical image.
Finally, there are some projects to adapt the simulator to new medical fields (cardiology, emergency, …).

Prizes and distinctions

The hepatic version of HORUS has been awarded the second prize of the Sensable Developer Challenge in August 2005.
A start-up project based on this simulator has been awarded by the French Research Ministry and by the French Innovation Agency (ANVAR) at the 8th Competition for Start-up of Innovative Technologies. The creation is planed for early 2007.
That project also won the first prize of the European Young Entrepreneurs Award in October 2006.

Bibliography

[1] A. Hostettler et al. Real-time ultrasonography simulator based on 3d ct-scan images. MMVR 2005 191-193
[2] C. Vayssière et al. A virtual reality system based on patient imaging data for handson simulation of ultrasound examination. In International Fetal Medical Surgical Society, 2006.
[3] C.Vayssière et al. A virtual reality system based on patient imaging data for hands-on simulation and automatic evaluation of ultrasound examination and amniocentesis In Society for Maternal Fetal Medicine, 2007
[4] Real Time Simulation of Organ Motions Induced by Breathing:, A. Hostettler et al. ISBMS 2006 LNCS 4072 Springer pp9-18

Medicine Meets Virtual Reality 15
J.D. Westwood et al. (Eds.)
IOS Press, 2007

Use of a Virtual Human Performance Laboratory to Improve Integration of Mathematics and Biology in Sports Science Curricula in Sweden and the United States

GARZA D[a], BESIER T[a], JOHNSTON T[a], ROLSTON B[a], SCHORSCH A[a],
MATHESON G[a],
ANNERSTEDT C[b], LINDH J[b], RYDMARK M[b]
[a] Stanford University, United States
[b] Göteborg University, Sweden

Abstract. New fields such as bioengineering are exploring the role of the physical sciences in traditional biological approaches to problems, with exciting results in device innovation, medicine, and research biology. The integration of mathematics, biomechanics, and material sciences into the undergraduate biology curriculum will better prepare students for these opportunities and enhance cooperation among faculty and students at the university level. We propose the study of sports science as the basis for introduction of this interdisciplinary program. This novel integrated approach will require a virtual human performance laboratory dual-hosted in Sweden and the United States. We have designed a course model that involves cooperative learning between students at Göteborg University and Stanford University, utilizes new technologies, encourages development of original research and will rely on frequent self-assessment and reflective learning. We will compare outcomes between this course and a more traditional didactic format as well as assess the effectiveness of multiple web-hosted virtual environments. We anticipate the grant will result in a network of original faculty and student research in exercise science and pedagogy as well as provide the opportunity for implementation of the model in more advance training levels and K-12 programs.

Keywords. Biomechanics, human performance, sports science, virtual reality

Introduction

New technologies and advances in computational power have revolutionized biomedical research, bringing together such diverse fields as biology, math, physics, engineering, and computer science. However, the teaching of modern biological science has remained relatively unchanged. Frequently, undergraduates majoring in the biological sciences are required to take separate, basic courses in physical sciences

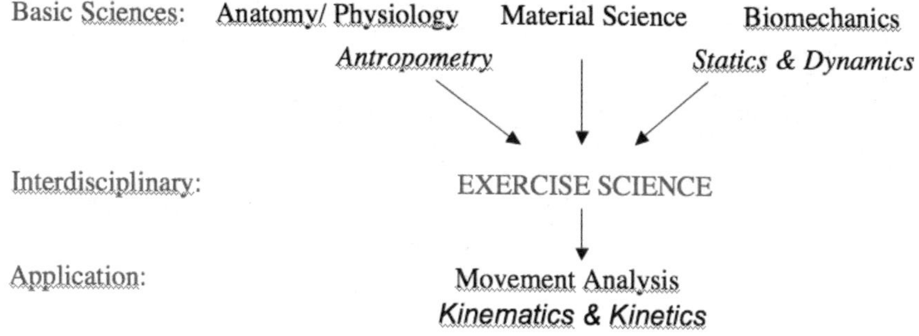

Figure 1. Multidisciplinary approach to sports science

and mathematics, but are never asked to use those principles in a meaningful study of biology.[1]　As a result, in the face of burgeoning graduate programs in interdisciplinary fields such as bioengineering [2], they enter as biologists with some math and mechanics background who must now rapidly synthesize these fields to advance to their degree. We believe it is both possible and advantageous for students majoring in the biological sciences to begin this synthesis at the undergraduate level. This will encourage increased collaboration among the different departments at the university level and prepare our students to excel in opportunities at the graduate level.

We propose that an ideal subject for this interdisciplinary approach is sports science. As shown in Figure 1, the various components of sports science (injury, rehabilitation, and performance) can be described in the context of biomechanics, anatomy, cellular physiology, and material science. Faculty involved in this project are working collaboratively to integrate each of these fields into a unified approach to sports science, with initial emphasis on the ability of students to analyze the dynamic movements involved in sport.

A prototype virtual laboratory (Figure 2) was held in April 2006 via web connection between students at Göteborg and Stanford and yielded important results; the diverse backgrounds of the participating students resulted in lively exchanges and original approaches to problem solving. However, the limitations of real-time live laboratory subjects were readily apparent. The use of virtual subjects would allow for students to exert immediate control over subjects in a variety of scenarios without the limitations of language or difficulty with speed of internet connection.

Two courses are being developed at Stanford and Göteborg respectively to implement this new pedagogical design. Commencing Spring 2007, the courses will follow identical curricula and will be taught simultaneously to allow for real-time interaction. Our goal is to avoid the secularization of faculty into their individual departmental approaches and develop a consistent multidisciplinary approach. Although it is frequently difficult to apply quantitative methods to living systems, exercise science, with its emphasis on motion and adaptation, is an ideal candidate for this application and is a field with which all faculty in this project have been involved. Cooperation among faculty members will serve as a model for undergraduate learning and give the students access to experts from a variety of fields.

Lundberg Labs (Göteborg)	Wallenberg Center (Stanford)

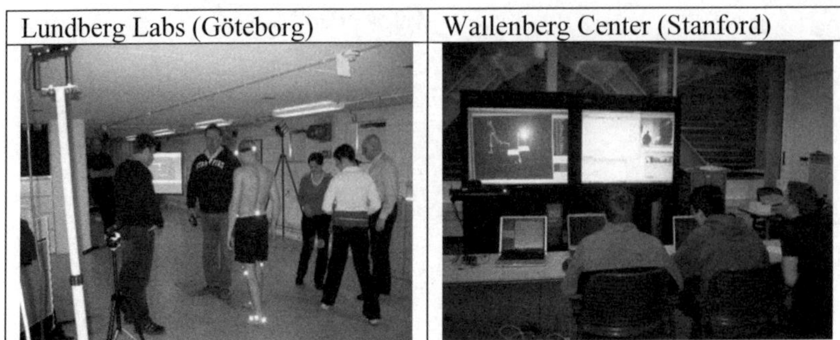

Figure 2. Prototype virtual laboratory at Göteborg (left) and Stanford (right)

Methods

Evaluation of whether the new pedagogical design improves learning outcomes and student satisfaction will be based on a control group of 40 students taking a traditional didactic course covering identical content at Stanford Spring 2006. Learning outcomes are assessed by objective examinations of student knowledge of the educational goals agreed upon by faculty. Student satisfaction and perception of learning are assessed by surveys that are distributed in paper form Spring 2006 and will be integrated into the interface for a reflective student blog in Spring 2007. Identical examination tools and surveys will be used for all courses and students. During Fall and Winter 2006, we will develop appropriate assessment tools to integrate into the course for crossover studies that will occur within the 5-week time period. These crossover studies will examine the effectiveness of web-based virtual experiments versus on-site lab experimentation and group work. Participating experts from the School of Pedagogy at Göteborg and Learning Design Technology at Stanford will work closely to ensure that course design meets the requirements for generating valid data in so short a time.

Finally, we are introducing a unique, year-long assessment of both faculty and student approach to our design to be conducted by graduate level students at Göteborg and at Stanford. Through an ethnographic research approach [3] with triangulation of data they will look upon the process, where student understanding is being challenged through different theories of learning and applied knowledge, and students are continuously active and problem-solving. Acting as an objective observer of the process through written and videotaped recordings, the graduate students will generate a record of the yearlong process that can be further analyzed for years to come. This process has previously been validated through work at the Göteborg School of Sport Science. [4]

References

1   Harris TR. Annual report on the VaNTH ERC, 2001.http://www.vanth.org/Annual_Report3.pdf
2   Harris TR, Bransford JD, Brophy SP. Roles for learning sciences and learning technologies in biomedical engineering education: A review of recent advances. Ann Review Biomedical Engineering 4:29-48, 2002.
3   Hammersley, Martyn & Atkinson, Paul. Ethnography: Principles in Practice. London: Routledge, 1995.
4   Kjerland, G. Teaching Education in Exercise Science as Learning and Social Practice. Göteborg University Dept of Education, 2005. (Submitted for Publication)

Medicine Meets Virtual Reality 15
J.D. Westwood et al. (Eds.)
IOS Press, 2007

In Vitro Skin-Tissue Experiment for Increased Realism in Open Surgery Simulations

Paul D GASSON and Rudy J LAPEER[1]

School of Computing Sciences, University of East Anglia, Norwich, NR4 7TJ, UK

Abstract. In-vitro uniaxial stress tests were conducted on samples of healthy human skin, obtained as a result of plastic surgical procedures. Pairs of test strips were cut from each sample to assess the effects of local orthotropy. Each strip was then subjected to constant strain-rate tensile testing, to observe its stress/strain behaviour. Typical maximal values for Young's modulus were found to be approximately 15.3MPa and 3.48Mpa for Langer-aligned and perpendicular test strips, respectively.

Keywords. In-vitro, Uniaxial, Stress, Skin, Orthotropy

Introduction

Our work attempts to accurately simulate the mechanical behaviour of human skin for open surgery procedures, such as skin flap-repair for facial reconstruction. Skin, and other biological soft tissue, exhibits complex material properties, making it a challenge to model accurately in interactive applications. There have been many attempts to simulate soft tissues with a range of methods, including various Mass-Spring-Damper models [1], Finite Elements [2,3] and others such as Tensor-Mass models [4,5]. We wish to compare various models from these categories, to determine an optimum solution for skin-tissue simulation. As part of this ongoing work, we have conducted stress tests on samples of human skin to assess its response to rapid stretching.

Although there is general acceptance of skin's mechanical behaviour (non-linear viscoelasticity and anisotropy), there is little consensus on its specific material properties. This is due to the variation of skin behaviour across the body and between different individuals. Additionally, the methods and types of experimental tests, used to observe these properties, has great influence on the results obtained. In-vivo testing [6,7] allows skin to be tested in its natural physiological state but introduces complex boundary conditions, which must be accounted for. In-vitro testing [8,9] is simpler to conduct but care must be taken to ensure that test samples are properly hydrated and maintained in a state close to in-situ conditions. We chose to conduct in-vitro experiments to avoid the aforementioned boundary condition problems.

---

[1]Corresponding author, email: rjal@cmp.uea.ac.uk

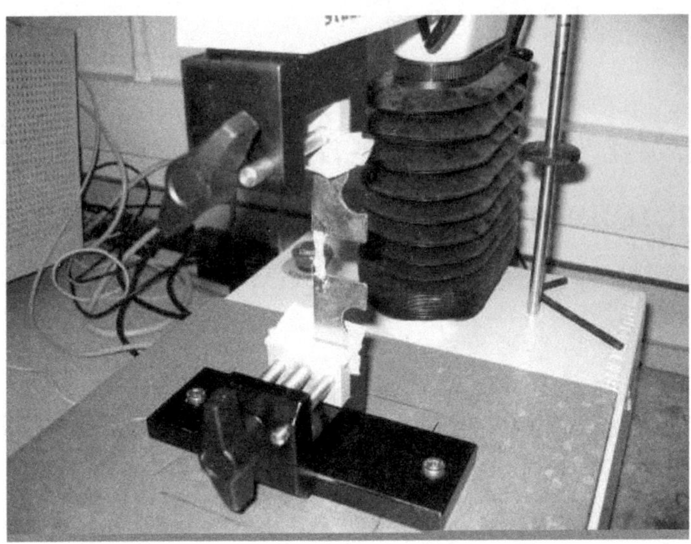

Figure 1. Test strip mounted in test machine.

1. Methodology

Skin samples were obtained from healthy patients undergoing plastic surgery. Each sample was cut to provide a pair of test strips, with one strip aligned coincident to local Langer line direction and the other oriented perpendicular to the first. This enabled the observation of local orthotropic behaviour. A twin-bladed scalpel was used to ensure that strips of consistent width were produced. Thickness measurements were made with a lightly sprung thickness gage, whilst unloaded length was determined using the stress testing machine's in-built length scale. Tests were conducted on a programmable uni-axial stress testing machine (Stable Micro Systems Texture Analyzer), as shown in Figure 1. This device allows for computer controlled application and measurement of strains and loads to a high accuracy. Each strip was held longitudinally between a pair of clamps and subjected to tensile stress testing using constant strain-rate cycles.

2. Results and Discussion

For these tests, extension rates of $2.0 \times 10^{-2} mms^{-1}$ were used. Test strips were extended from a resting strain of 0.0 to failure. Figure 2 shows an example stress-strain plot of a pair of test strips cut from the same sample. Maximal values of Young's modulus for the Langer-line aligned and perpendicular test strips were found to be approximately 15.3MPa and 3.48MPa respectively. The shape of the curves suggests that a hyperelastic model such as a Mooney-Rivlin or Ogden material is capable of modelling the material responses observed. Further tests will be conducted in the future that will include a range of strain-rates to mimic typical surgical gesture rates. Viscoelasticity and response to biaxial testing will also be explored.

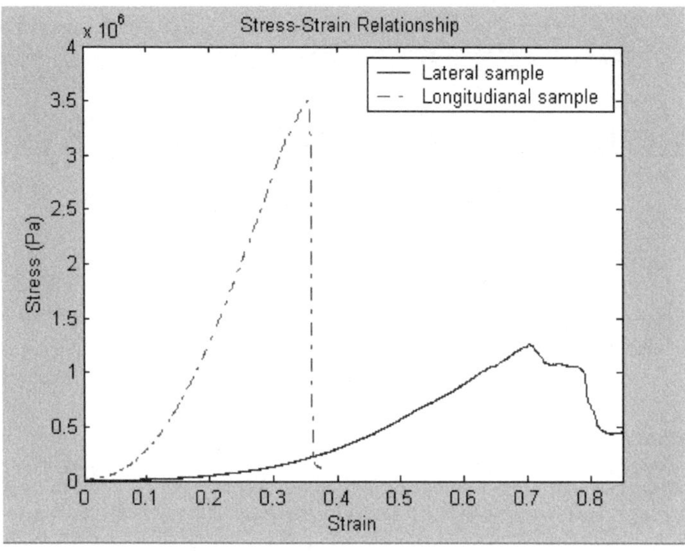

Figure 2. Stress-strain plot for orthogonal strips from one sample.

References

[1]   Gasson P., Lapeer R.J. and Linney A.D., "Modelling techniques for enhanced realism in an open surgery simulation"', MediViz/IV04 Conference Porceedings, IEEE Computer Society, 2004,pp. 73-78.

[2]   Wu X., Downes M., Goktekin T. and Tendick F., "Adaptive nonlinear finite elements for deformable body simulation using dynamic progressive meshes", Eurographics 2001, Vol.20, No. 3, pp. 349-358.

[3]   Szekely G., Brechbuhler Ch., Hutter R., Rhomberg A., Ironmonger N. and Schmid P., "'Modelling of soft tissue deformation for laparoscopic surgery simulation"', Medical Image Analysis 4, 2000, pp. 57-66.

[4]   Cotin S., Delingette H. and Ayache N., "A hybrid elastic model allowing real-time cutting, deformations and force-feedback for surgery training and simulation"', Visual Computer Journal, Vol 16, No. 8, 2000, pp. 437-452.

[5]   Picinbono G., Delingette H. and Ayache N., "Non-linear anisotropic elasticity for real-time surgery simulation", Graphical Models 65 2003, pp. 305-321.

[6]   Diridollou S., Patat F., Gens F., Vaillant L., Black D., Lagarde J.M., Gall Y. and Berson M., "In vivo model of the mechanical properties of the human skin under suction", Skin Research and Technology 2000, vol. 6, pp. 214-221.

[7]   Hendriks F.M., Brokken D., Oomens C. W. J. and Baaijens F. P. T. "Influence of hydration and experimental length scale on the mechanical response of human skin in vivo, using optical coherence tomography", Skin Research and Technology 2004, Vol 10, pp. 231-241.

[8]   Har-Shai Y., Bodner S.R., Egozy-Golan D., Lindenbaum E.S., Ben-Izhak O., Mitz V. and Hirshowitz B., "Mechanical properties and microstructure of the superficial musculoaponeurotic system. Plastic and Reconstructive Surgery 98, pp. 59-70.

[9]   Silver F.H., Freeman J.W. and DeVore D., "Viscoelastic properties of human skin and processed dermis", Skin Research and Technology 2001, Vol 7, pp. 18 - 23.

Medicine Meets Virtual Reality 15
J.D. Westwood et al. (Eds.)
IOS Press, 2007

Game Design in Virtual Reality Systems for Stroke Rehabilitation

Daniel GOUDE[1,2], Staffan BJÖRK[1], Martin RYDMARK[2]
[1] *Department of Computer Science, Chalmers & Göteborg University, Sweden*
[2] *Mednet, Institute of Biomedicine, Göteborg University, Sweden*

Abstract. We propose a model for the structured design of games for post-stroke rehabilitation. The model is based on experiences with game development for a haptic and stereo vision immersive workbench intended for daily use in stroke patients' homes. A central component of this rehabilitation system is a library of games that are simultaneously entertaining for the patient and beneficial for rehabilitation [1], and where each game is designed for specific training tasks through the use of the model. Contact: *daniel@goude.se*.

Keywords. Game design patterns, stroke rehabilitation, therapy, virtual reality.

1.   Introduction

Developing games for rehabilitation requires professional skills from both the medical and game design field. This is difficult since it entails communication between different professions within one design process, something that has been pointed out as one of the main challenges for modern design [2]. This is mainly due to the fact that more of designers' work has traditionally been done alone, but the increasing complexity of design today has made this impossible. The challenge is further made more difficult as the game industry, being a young industry, has yet to codify its design knowledge, and that most game designers are self-taught and therefore lack a common design language. To address this challenge, Game Design Patterns [3] has been developed as a design tool to facilitate communication regarding game design. As per the original design pattern concept by Alexander et al. [4] within architecture, each of these patterns provides a concise description of a potential design choice with possible consequences and variations. The patterns are connected to each other as the presence of one pattern may guarantee the presence of another (more general) pattern, or one pattern may describe a way to vary another pattern. Although each pattern includes an introductory description that can be comprehended without knowledge of any other pattern, this does not in itself support easy points of reference to other knowledge fields. To overcome this we have created a model which documents mappings between game design patterns and a taxonomy of rehabilitation tasks.

2.   Model for supporting rehabilitation training games

The taxonomy we chose to use focuses on neurological impairments, stroke rehabilitation exercises and rehabilitation goals and was created based on treatment recommendations and guidelines [5, 6]. On the basis of the individual entries in the taxonomy, related game design patterns were identified from an established collection [3]. By theoretically exploring gaps in this mapping, as well as analyzing games designed for specific entries, new patterns are discovered and documented. This leads to an iterative process where patterns suggest game designs and game designs suggest new patterns. The result is a conceptual model that supports game idea generation, task design and categorization of existing games in relation to stroke rehabilitation (Figure 1).

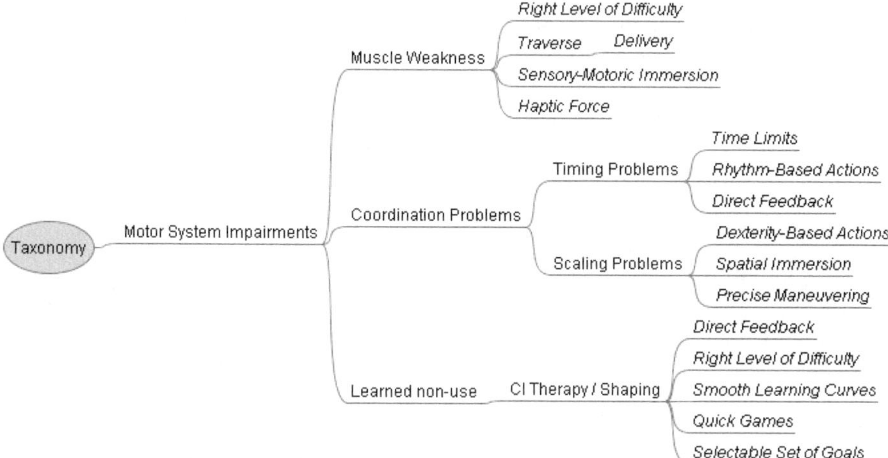

Figure 1. A subset of the taxonomy. Game Design Patterns italicized.

3. Example training games

A customized VR framework linked to a haptic workbench was used to prototype and implement training games based upon the patterns. A part of this collection of games is presented below (Figure 2), in which games are created by varying a core game through adding specific game design patterns (Table 1).

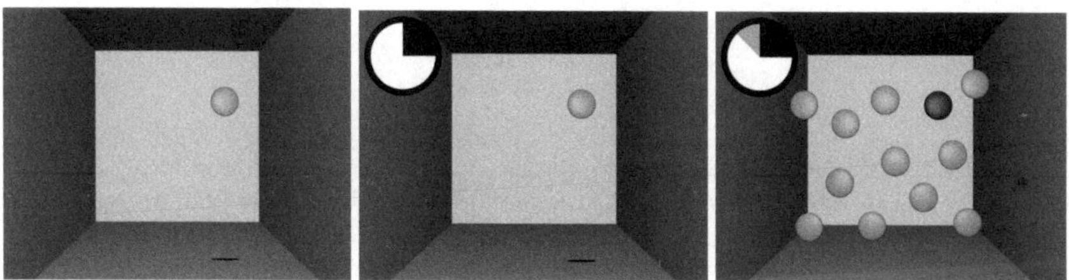

Figure 2. Upper extremity training game protoypes.

Table 1. Design stages of an upper extremity training game

Variation	Patterns (in additions to those of the previous variations)
1	*Haptic Targets, Traverse, Visibility Indication, Assessment Distribution*
2	*Time, Status Indicators*
3	*High Score List, Levels, Color Indication, Right Level of Difficulty*

Currently, about twenty games based on the taxonomy have been produced, including upper extremity reaching exercises, neglect assessment, and coordination-training activities. Since the games have a minimalist style (due to the ease of playing required by the target audience), the design choices included have become very visible. This has led to new patterns being added to the collection as well as allowing new games to easily be created as variations of other games. These variations provide a range of activities that can be used to personalize a rehabilitation session since the patterns in all variations have specific training tasks mapped to them.

4. Discussion & Conclusions

We believe that the ability to clearly communicate ideas between medical professionals and game designers is vital. Our initial experiences with applying Game Design Patterns to VR stroke rehabilitation warrant further investigation since they provide neutral definitions based on interaction in games – not on professional gaming industry jargon or one particular research field. Presently, we are focusing on refining the development model. More model-based games should be designed, with concurrent expansion of the pattern library. The associations between patterns and treatments need to be verified, and the taxonomy requires expansion; only a subset of stroke symptoms and treatments has yet been considered.

Creating applications for VR rehabilitation is associated with significant effort. This may be due to a lack of field-specific models, methodologies and tools [7]. We believe that in-house development of rehabilitation games is valuable when full control of the development process is needed. However, future research directions include investigating how the model can be used for analyzing and modifying existing commercial and Open Source games in the context of stroke rehabilitation.

This work is supported by VINNOVA (research grant 2004-02260).

References

[1] Broeren J, Dixon M, Stibrant Sunnerhagen K, Rydmark M. Rehabilitation after Stroke Using Virtual Reality, Haptics (Force Feedback) and Telemedicine. Proceedings of MIE2006.
[2] Jones CJ. Design Methods. John Wiley & Sons, Inc. 1982 (third edition).
[3] Björk S, Holopainen J. Patterns in Game Design. Charles River Media. 2004. ISBN 1-58450-354-8.
[4] Alexander C et al. A Pattern Language. Oxford University Press, New York. 1977.
[5] Shumway-Cook A, Woolacott MH. Motor Control: Theory and Practical Applications. Lippincott Williams & Wilkins. 2000 (second edition). ISBN 068330643X.
[6] Taub E et al. A Placebo-controlled Trial of Constraint-Induced Movement Therapy. Stroke. 2006;37(4):1045-9.
[7] Rizzo A., Kim GJ. A SWOT Analysis of the Field of Virtual Reality Rehabilitation and Therapy. Presence: Teleoperators & Virtual Environments. 2005;14(2):119-146.

Medicine Meets Virtual Reality 15
J.D. Westwood et al. (Eds.)
IOS Press, 2007

The Red DRAGON: A Multi-Modality System for Simulation and Training in Minimally Invasive Surgery

Scott GUNTHER MSME [a], Jacob ROSEN PhD [b,c]
Blake HANNAFORD PhD [b,c], Mika SINANAN MD PhD [c,b]
[a] *Department of Mechanical Engineering*
[b] *Department of Electrical Engineering*
[c] *Department of Surgery*
University of Washington, Seattle WA
URL: http://brl.ee.washington.edu
e-mail:<gunthers,rosen,blake,mssurg>@u.washington.edu

Abstract. With the development of new technologies in surgery, minimally invasive surgery (MIS) has drastically improved the way conventional medical procedures are performed. However, a new learning curve has resulted requiring an expertise in integrating visual information with the kinematics and dynamics of the surgical tools. The Red DRAGON is a multi-modal simulator for teaching and training MIS procedures allowing one to use it with several modalities including: simulator (physical objects and virtual objects) and an animal model. The Red DRAGON system is based on a serial spherical mechanism in which all the rotation axes intersect at a single point (remote center) allowing the endoscopic tools to pivot around the MIS port. The system includes two mechanisms that incorporate two interchangeable MIS tools. Sensors are incorporated into the mechanism and the tools measure the positions and orientations of the surgical tools as well as forces and torques applied on the tools by the surgeon. The design is based on a mechanism optimization to maximize the manipulability of the mechanism in the MIS workspace. As part of a preliminary experimental protocol, five expert level surgeons performed three laparoscopic tasks – a subset of the Fundamental Laparoscopic Skill (FLS) set as a baseline for skill assessment protocols. The results provide an insight into the kinematics and dynamics of the endoscopic tools, as the underlying measures for objectively assessing MIS skills.

Keywords. Minimally Invasive Surgery, Laparoscopy, Spherical Mechanism, Markov Models, Fundamental Laparoscopic Skills, Objective Skill Assessment

1. Introduction

Within the last two decades, minimally invasive surgery (MIS) has revolutionized the surgical field. Traditional surgical procedures utilize incisions designed to allow the maximum exposure of the operation location. In contrast, MIS procedures make use of small incisions, one centimeter or less, to allow cameras and surgical instruments to be inserted into the body cavity through air-tight ports. This significantly decreases the amount of tissue trauma for the patient as well as limiting the amount of pain, drastically improving the cosmetic effects of surgery, and allowing much shorter hospital stays.

Unlike traditional surgeries, MIS does not allow the surgeons to directly see the operation; cameras inserted through the body cavity display the procedure on video monitors instead. Also, a new set of surgical tools are used that requires specific skills. As a result, a new set of skills are required to be known for an optimal usage of this technique.

The Blue DRAGON, which is based on a four bar mechanism, was the first generation of the system that was previously utilized to record the kinematics and the dynamics of MIS using an animal model [1]. Data acquired by the Blue DRAGON was used to develop and objectively assess surgeons' methodology for MIS using Markov models [2]. The data collected by the Blue DRAGON system also defined the workspace of the two endoscopic tools. Given a clear definition of the MIS tools' workspace, a new generation of the system known as the Red DRAGON was developed based on a spherical mechanism which was design and optimized in order to minimize the footprint of the system in the surgical site [3]. Both the four bar mechanism of the Blue DRAGON and the spherical mechanism of the Red DRAGON have a remote centers which are located at the intersection of the mechanisms' rotation axes. This characteristic allowed the incorporation of position sensors into the mechanism to track the rotation and the translation of the MIS tools with respect to their ports without creating interferences at the tool/port interface. The main objective of this paper is to describe the development of the Red DRAGON utilizing a spherical mechanism for tracking two tools in a MIS setup.

2. Method

2.1. Design

The port in MIS limits the six Degrees of Freedom (DOF) of any surgical tool to only five DOF including tool tip manipulation. The design of the Red DRAGON is based on a spherical mechanism with a remote center of rotation that is located at the midpoint of the abdominal wall cross-section or any other layer simulating it. The two DOF spherical linkage allows the attached tool to move its tip along a two-dimensional sphere with a center located at the port. Three more DOF were added to the system to allow linear translation along the tool's long shaft, rotational motion along the same axis, and opening and closing of the tool's handle.

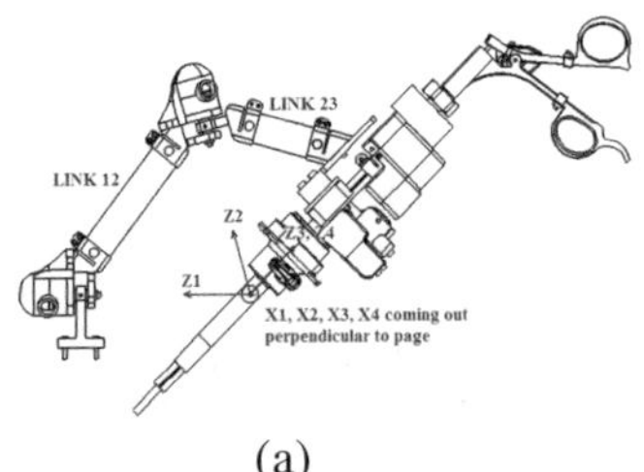

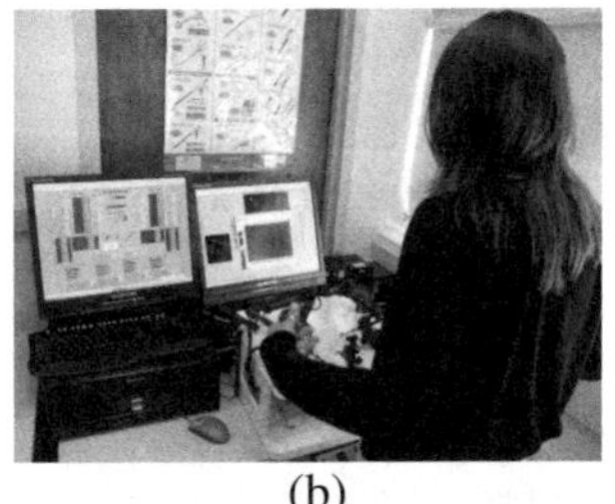

(a)   (b)

Figure 1. The Red DRAGON (a) the Left side mechanism and the associated coordinate system (b) A full assembly of the system with the endoscopic tools

Position sensors were incorporated into the links of the mechanism along with a multi-axis force sensor located in the proximal end of the tool and a force sensor located at the handles of the MIS instruments. The sensors were connected to a PC utilizing USB-based data acquisition cards for acquiring the data. A graphical user interface (GUI) developed in Labview incorporated a graphical display of the data as well as a video stream of the endoscopic camera. The data along with the video screen were recorded for offline analysis. The software converts the signals received from the data acquisition cards back into either the tool's angular or linear displacement calculated from conversion factors found by testing performed on each of the sensors. The GUI also includes a virtual representation of the tools with an overlay of the velocity vectors as well as a three-dimensional representation of the force and the torque vectors.

2.2. Manipulator Kinematics

The Red DRAGON is a serial spherical mechanism comprised of five DOF defined by two joint rotations, the surgical tool translation and rotation, and the tool handle's opening/closing. The system geometry was defined as three joints and two links (Figure 1a). To specify the position and orientation of the tool, Denavit-Hartenberg (D-H) parameters [4] were assigned to the mechanism joints. The z-axis of each frame was aligned with the axis of rotation or the direction of linear translation, pointing out from the sphere, and positioned at the center of the mechanism. From this parameter setup, Eq. (1) was used to calculate the transformation matrices between each of the frames where the angular motions of the joints were denoted as θ_i, the relative position as p_x, p_y, and p_z, the link angles as α_{i-1}, and the sine and cosine functions as 'S' and 'C', respectively.

$$
{}^{i-1}_{i}T = \begin{bmatrix}
C\theta_i & -S\theta_i & 0 & p_x \\
S\theta_i C\alpha_{i-1} & C\theta_i C\alpha_{i-1} & -S\alpha_{i-1} & p_y \\
S\theta_i S\alpha_{i-1} & C\theta_i S\alpha_{i-1} & C\alpha_{i-1} & p_z \\
0 & 0 & 0 & 1
\end{bmatrix}
\tag{1}
$$

The forward kinematics maps the mechanism joint configuration defined by its DOF (θ_1, θ_2, θ_3, d_4), to the position of the tool tip and the orientation of the tool. The forward kinematics enables the surgical tool tip tracking that is the key to the data acquisition and later on to the objective skill assessment algorithms. Using the joint parameters and transformation matrices, the coordinate transformations from the base of the tool to each joint and tool tip were calculated. The transformation from the base frame to the tool tip frame was calculated using Eq. (2).

$$
{}^{0}_{4}T = {}^{0}_{1}T\, {}^{1}_{2}T\, {}^{2}_{3}T\, {}^{0}_{4}T
\tag{2}
$$

This matrix can be dissembled into a rotation and position denoted in Eqs. (3) and (4), respectively.

$$\,^{0}_{4}R = \begin{bmatrix} r_{11} & r_{12} & r_{13} \\ r_{21} & r_{22} & r_{23} \\ r_{31} & r_{32} & r_{33} \end{bmatrix} \tag{3}$$

where

$$
\begin{aligned}
r_{11} &= -C\alpha_{12}S\theta_1(C\theta_3S\theta_2 + C\theta_2C\alpha_{23}S\theta_3) + C\theta_1(C\theta_2C\theta_3 - C\alpha_{23}S\theta_2S\theta_3) \\
&\quad + S\theta_1S\theta_3S\alpha_{12}S\alpha_{23} \\
r_{12} &= -C\theta_1C\theta_3C\alpha_{23}S\theta_2 + C\alpha_{12}S\theta_1S\theta_2S\theta_3 - C\theta_2(C\theta_3C\alpha_{12}C\alpha_{23}S\theta_1 + C\theta_1S\theta_3) \\
&\quad + C\theta_3S\theta_1S\alpha_{12}S\alpha_{23} \\
r_{13} &= -C\alpha_{23}S\theta_1S\alpha_{12} - C\theta_2C\alpha_{12}S\theta_1S\alpha_{23} - C\theta_1S\theta_2S\alpha_{23} \\
r_{21} &= C\theta_2C\theta_3S\theta_1 + C\theta_1C\theta_3C\alpha_{12}S\theta_2 + C\theta_1C\theta_2C\alpha_{12}C\alpha_{23}S\theta_3 - C\alpha_{23}S\theta_1S\theta_2S\theta_3 \\
&\quad - C\theta_1S\theta_3S\alpha_{12}S\alpha_{23} \\
r_{22} &= C\theta_1C\theta_2C\theta_3C\alpha_{12}C\alpha_{23} - C\theta_3C\alpha_{23}S\theta_1S\theta_2 - C\theta_2S\theta_1S\theta_3 - C\theta_1C\theta_3S\alpha_{12}S\alpha_{23} \\
r_{23} &= C\theta_1C\alpha_{23}S\alpha_{12} + C\theta_1C\theta_2C\alpha_{12}S\alpha_{23} - S\theta_1S\theta_2S\alpha_{23} \\
r_{31} &= C\theta_3S\theta_2S\alpha_{12} - C\theta_2C\alpha_{23}S\theta_3S\alpha_{12} - C\alpha_{12}S\theta_3S\alpha_{23} \\
r_{32} &= -C\theta_2C\theta_3C\alpha_{23}S\alpha_{12} + S\theta_2S\theta_3S\alpha_{12} - C\theta_3C\alpha_{12}S\alpha_{23} \\
r_{33} &= C\alpha_{12}C\alpha_{23} - C\theta_2S\alpha_{12}S\alpha_{23}
\end{aligned}
$$

and

$$
P = \begin{bmatrix} P_x \\ P_y \\ P_z \end{bmatrix} = \begin{bmatrix} d_4(C\alpha_{23}S\theta_1S\alpha_{12} + C\theta_2C\alpha_{12}S\theta_1S\alpha_{23} + C\theta_1S\theta_2S\alpha_{23}) \\ -d_4(-S\theta_1S\theta_2S\alpha_{23} + C\theta_1C\alpha_{23}S\alpha_{12} + C\theta_1C\theta_2C\alpha_{12}S\alpha_{23}) \\ d_4(C\theta_2S\alpha_{12}S\alpha_{23} - C\alpha_{12}C\alpha_{23}) \end{bmatrix} \tag{4}
$$

The Jacobian Matrix was determined for the Red DRAGON mechanism as a way to map the angular and linear velocities measured by the sensors incorporated into the Red DRAGON mechanism to the angular and linear velocities of the surgical tool, most notably the tool tip. By expressing the end-effector angular and linear velocities with respect to the tool frame ($\,^{4}\omega_4$ and $\,^{4}v_4$) in terms of the system's Jacobian matrix, a closed form solution, Eq. (5), was found in terms of the input joint velocities ($\dot{\theta}_1, \dot{\theta}_2, \dot{d}_4$).

$$
\begin{bmatrix} \,^{4}\omega_{4x} \\ \,^{4}\omega_{4y} \\ \,^{4}v_{4z} \end{bmatrix} = \begin{bmatrix} -S\alpha_{12}S\theta_3 & 0 & 0 \\ S\alpha_{12}C\alpha_{23}C\theta_3 + C\alpha_{12}S\alpha_{23} & S\alpha_{23} & 0 \\ 0 & 0 & 1 \end{bmatrix} * \begin{bmatrix} \dot{\theta}_1 \\ \dot{\theta}_2 \\ \dot{d}_4 \end{bmatrix} \tag{5}
$$

2.3. Testing Protocol

The Fundamentals of Laparoscopic Surgery (FLS) education module created by the Society of American Gastrointestinal and Endoscopic Surgeons (SAGES) is used for testing the Red Dragon. Three tasks are currently being studied including object manipulation, suturing, and dissecting. Out of a thirty subject protocol including surgical residents at different levels of their five training stages (R1-R5), data was collected from five expert level surgeons from the University of Washington Medical

Center.　Markov Modeling analysis will be further applied to objectively assess surgical skills [5].

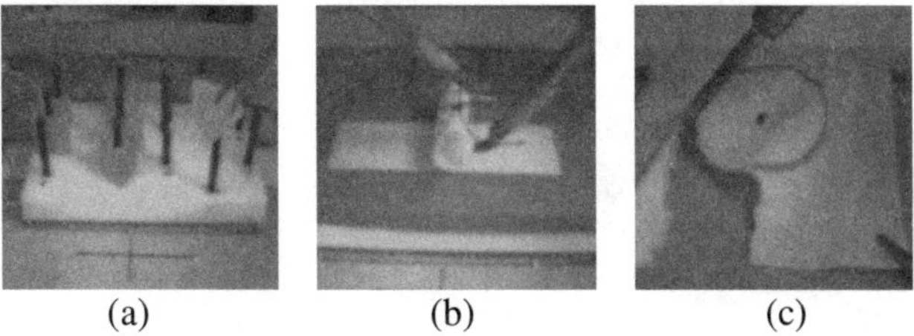

(a)　　　　　　　　(b)　　　　　　　　(c)

Figure 2. Subtasks of the FLS system used skill testing with the Red DRAGON: (a) object manipulation, (b) suturing, and (c) dissecting

3. Results

Typical raw data of forces torques and tool tip position was plotted in 3D graphs showing the kinematics and the dynamics of the left and the right endoscopic tools measured by the Red DRAGON while performing the FLS tasks (Figure 3). The forces and torques (F/T) can be described as vectors with an origin at the center of the sensor and a coordinate system aligned with the tool coordinate system. These vectors are constantly changing both their magnitudes and orientations as a result of the F/T applied by the surgeon's hand on the tool while interacting with the models. The F/T displayed as vectors can be depicted as arrows attached to the origin that are changing their lengths and orientations as a function of time. Figures 3a and 3b describe the traces of the tips of these vectors as they were changing during the surgical procedure. In a similar fashion the traces of the tool tips positions were plotted in Figure 3c.

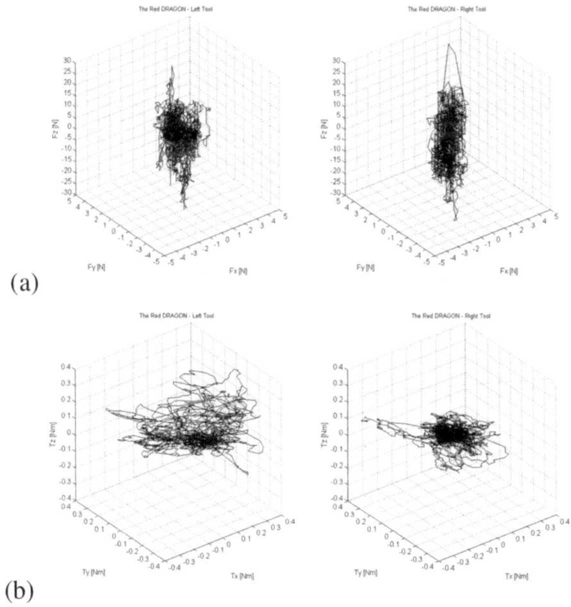

(a)

(b)

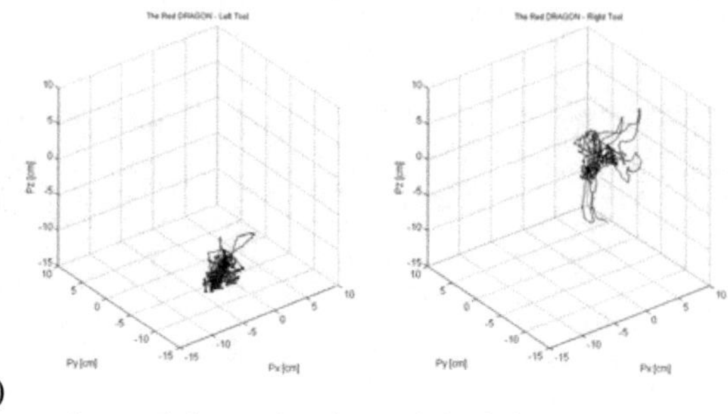

(c)

Figure 3. The kinematics and dynamics data of the left and the right endoscopic tools measured by the Red DRAGON during a suturing procedure (For coordinate system definition see Fig. 1) - (a) forces; (b) torques (c), and tool tip position.

4. Discussion

The Red Dragon provides a multi-modal training system for MIS. Physical models, virtual models, and real animal models, can all be used with the same system. Using the system with these various modalities provides a means to study translation of skill from a simulation environment to a real animal model. Further analysis using Markov Models will allow objective assessment of MIS skills [2] and the ability to use the system for credentialing and continuing education programs in MIS.

References

[1]   Rosen, J.; Brown, J.; Chang, L.; Barreca, M.; Sinanan, M.; Hannaford, B., "The Blue DRAGON – A System for Measuring the Kinematics and Dynamics of Minimally Invasive Surgical Tools In Vivo," *Proceedings of the 2002 IEEE International Conference on Robotics & Automation*, pp. 1876-1881, 2002.

[2]   Rosen J., J. D. Brown, L. Chang, M. Sinanan B. Hannaford, Generalized Approach for Modeling Minimally Invasive Surgery as a Stochastic Process Using a Discrete Markov Model, IEEE Transactions on Biomedical Engineering Vol. 53, No. 3, March 2006, pp. 399 - 413

[3]   Lum, M.; Rosen, J.; Sinanan, M.; Hannaford, B., "Kinematic Optimization of a Spherical Mechanism for a Minimally Invasive Surgical Robot," *Proceedings of the 2004 IEEE International Conference on Robotics & Automation*, pp. 829-834, 2004.

[4]   Craig, J., *Introduction to Robotics*, Reading, MA: Addison-Wesley, 1986.

[5]   Rosen, J.; Hannaford, B.; Richards, C.; Sinanan, M., "Markov Modeling of Minimally Invasive Surgery Based on Tool/Tissue Interaction and Force/Torque Signatures for Evaluating Surgical Skills," *IEEE Transactions on Biomedical Engineering*, vol. 48, pp. 579-591, 2001.

Medicine Meets Virtual Reality 15
J.D. Westwood et al. (Eds.)
IOS Press, 2007

155

The Effect of Degree of Immersion upon Learning Performance in Virtual Reality Simulations for Medical Education

Fátima GUTIÉRREZ MS III[1], Jennifer PIERCE MS III[1], Víctor M. VERGARA, Ph.D[2]
Robert COULTER, M.A.[1], Linda SALAND, Ph.D.[1], Thomas P. CAUDELL, Ph.D.[2],
Timothy E. GOLDSMITH, Ph.D.[3], Dale C. ALVERSON, M.D.[1]
*[1]School of Medicine, [2]School of Engineering, [3]Department of Psychology,
University of New Mexico, Albuquerque, New Mexico 87131 U.S.A.*

Abstract. Simulations are being used in education and training to enhance understanding, improve performance, and assess competence. However, it is important to measure the performance of these simulations as learning and training tools. This study examined and compared knowledge acquisition using a knowledge structure design. The subjects were first-year medical students at The University of New Mexico School of Medicine. One group used a fully immersed virtual reality (VR) environment using a head mounted display (HMD) and another group used a partially immersed (computer screen) VR environment. The study aims were to determine whether there were significant differences between the two groups as measured by changes in knowledge structure before and after the VR simulation experience. The results showed that both groups benefited from the VR simulation training as measured by the significant increased similarity to the expert knowledge network after the training experience. However, the immersed group showed a significantly higher gain than the partially immersed group. This study demonstrated a positive effect of VR simulation on learning as reflected by improvements in knowledge structure but an enhanced effect of full-immersion using a HMD vs. a screen-based VR system.

Keywords. Virtual Reality, Medical Simulation, Education, User Interface, Knowledge Structure.

Introduction

Virtual reality (VR) allows medical students to be immersed in lifelike situations where they can learn without suffering the consequences that may occur due to lack of experience. With VR, students are offered a type of training that would otherwise be impossible to achieve. VR training is especially important in medical education where students are expected to learn how to react in high-risk situations where human lives are potentially at stake. Developing ways to increase student competence and understanding of these issues is an ongoing pursuit in medical education as attempts to decrease medical errors and improve quality of care have been brought to the forefront of curricula in medical schools across the country [1], [2]. Simulations have been used as a method to enhance learning, training, and assessment of competence [3]-[5]. Several studies have been carried out under the auspices of Project TOUCH (Telehealth Outreach for Unified Community Health), a multi-year collaboration between The University of Hawaii and The University of New Mexico. Previous TOUCH investigations determined whether medical students could work as a team within a virtual problem-based learning environment. The study concluded that team performance within the VR environment was as good as in real life team sessions [6]. Another study investigated whether medical student learning could be objectively demonstrated within VR training. The study found evidence of significant learning as a function of a single VR training experience [7]. Despite a long-standing interest in VR training, few studies have measured learning effects in different VR environments. Using first-year medical students as the study subjects at the University of New Mexico School of Medicine the students were randomly divided into two groups; one group used a fully immersed VR environment using a head mounted display (HMD) and another group used a partially immersed (computer screen) VR environment. The study aims were to determine whether there were significant differences within and between the two groups as measured by changes in knowledge structure before and after the VR simulation experience.

1. Materials and Tools

1.1. The Study Population

Twenty five volunteers were obtained from the first year medical school class at the University of New Mexico during their neuroscience block and randomly divided into two groups: Fully-immersed, where participants wore a stereoscopic head-mounted display, or partially-immersed, where participants interacted with the VR simulation via a computer monitor. Both groups used a joystick for navigation, locomotion and manipulation of objects within the VR simulation. Each group used the same problem-based case. Informed consent was obtained from each participating student.

1.2. The Flatland Platform

Flatland served as the software infrastructure [8]. It is an open source visualization/VR application development environment, created at The University of New Mexico. Flatland allows software authors to construct, and users to interact with, arbitrarily complex graphical and aural representations of data and systems. It is written in C/C++ and uses the standard OpenGL graphics language to produce all graphics. Flatland is designed to integrate any position-tracking technology. A tracker is a multiple degree of freedom measurement device that can, in real time, monitor the position and orientation of multiple receiver devices in space, relative to a transmitter device. In the standard immersive Flatland configuration, trackers are used to locate hand held wands and to track the position of the user's head. Head position and orientation are needed in cases that involve the use of head mounted displays or stereo shutter glasses. The events within the virtual environment are controlled by an Artificial Intelligence (AI) engine. This AI engine was a forward chaining IF-THEN rule based system that specifies the behavior of objects in the VR world. The rules governing the physiology of the avatar were obtained from subject matter experts. The rules were coded in a C computer language format as logical antecedents and consequences. The AI loops over the rule base, applying each rule's antecedents to the current state of the system, including time, and testing for logical matches. Matching rules are "fired," modifying the next state of the system. Time is a special state of the system that is not directly modified by the AI, but whose rate is controlled by an adjustable clock. Since the rate of inference within the AI is controlled by this clock, the user (or student) is able to speed up, slow down, or stop the action controlled by the AI. This feature allows a user to learn from his/her mistakes by repeating a scenario.

1.3. The Virtual Environments

In the fully immersed virtual reality environment, students wore a head-mounted display with trackers and used a joystick for hand movement, which allowed the students a sense of presence within the virtual environment. The interactions between user and virtual environment were controlled by a joystick equipped with a six degree of freedom tracking system, buttons, and a trigger. The user could pick up and place objects by moving the virtual hand and pulling the wand's trigger. Participants were able to examine the virtual patient by independently controlling their viewpoints and motion within the virtual world. In this fully-immersed environment, the student could see only the virtual world.

In the partially immersed VR environment, a student did not wear a head-mounted display, but saw the patient on a computer screen and used a mouse to rotate the viewpoint. The navigation and manipulation of objects within the virtual environment occurred by using a joystick, similar to the fully-immersed environment. Students were still able to examine and interact with the virtual patient, although, they were also aware of the outside environment (see Figure 1).

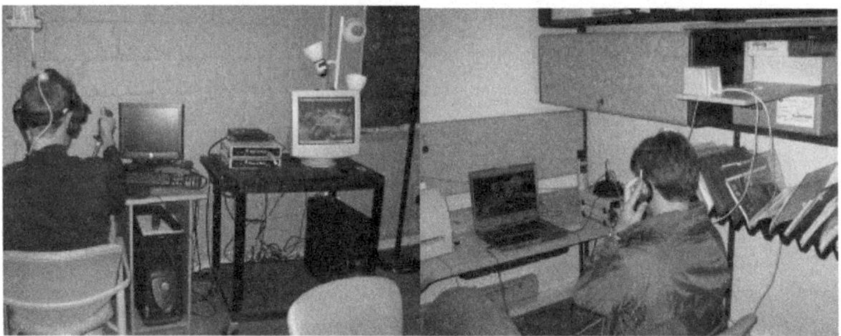

Figure 1. Student using Full Immersion vs. Partial Immersion

2. Procedures and Methods

2.1. Experimental Procedures

Participants were tested individually After reading and signing a statement of informed consent, students were oriented to the VR equipment. After the orientation, the students were directed to a web site where they filled out a demographic questionnaire and then watched an instructional video on the use of the VR equipment. The web site also contained links to interactive, labeled diagrams of the VR equipment and links to head-injury reference materials such as brain section diagrams, schematics, short video animations and textual information. When the students were finished watching the video, they were allowed to view additional reference materials and to practice using the VR equipment until they felt comfortable in locomotion, navigation and manipulation objects. The students were then directed back to the web site for step-by-step instructions for the experiment. Before starting the experiment, students were given a knowledge assessment test that consisted of rating the relatedness of 72 pairs of concepts critical to the case, 36 of which were previously defined to be related by a experts and 36 unrelated. The terms were selected by having subject matter experts identify the most important concepts related to a traumatic head injury involving an epidural hematoma. The students participating in the VR were immersed in a scenario where they were the first responders in an automobile accident that involved head trauma. Next, they read a web-based, textual orientation to the clinical scenario and, based on this, they were asked to complete a list of known and anticipated problems. Then they were given 30 minutes to enter the virtual environment (see Figure 2) and to perform a physical exam on the virtual patient.

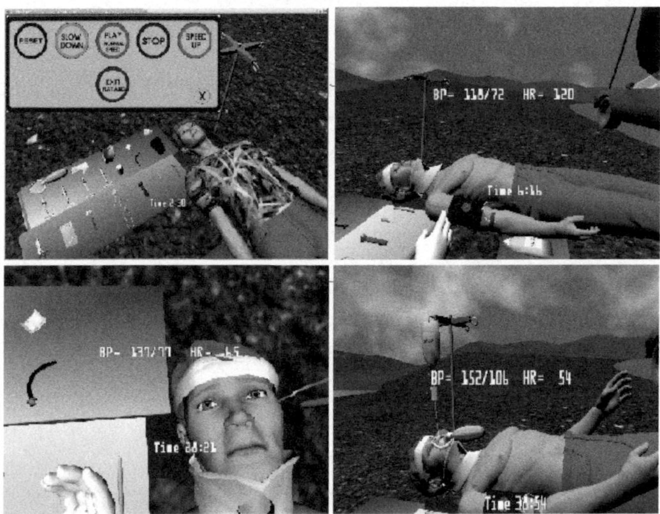

Figure 2. A depiction of what the students saw in the virtual environment

After performing the physical exam, participants read a summary of the expected physical exam findings and were then able to treat the patient as they chose. Next, they read a case conclusion, explaining the virtual patient's injuries, follow-up or confirmatory studies, and the expected actions to be taken once the patient arrived at an ER. Finally, the participants completed the knowledge assessment exercise a second time.

2.2. Learning Evaluation Method

VR learning was evaluated by having the students perform the relatedness ratings task both before and immediately following VR training [9], [10]. The Pathfinder scaling algorithm was then applied to each student's pre and post-learning ratings to derive two knowledge structures. Previously, a group of subject matter experts had rated the relatedness of the hematoma concepts, and Pathfinder was used to derive a single expert knowledge structure.   This expert knowledge structure was then used as a gold standard against which to compare the students' knowledge structures. A similarity score, ranging from 0 to 1, was used to compare how close the student's knowledge structures were to the expert's. VR learning would be reflected by higher similarity scores after the VR experience than before. In addition, the difference between VR learning of the fully-immersed and partially-immersed groups was evaluated by examining changes in students' knowledge structures.

2.3. Statistical Analysis

Knowledge acquisition and impact on learning of the VR simulation was examined by measuring changes in knowledge structure. Knowledge structures of the students were compared to the expert knowledge structure-using Pathfinder to determine similarity coefficients before and after VR experience and then between the two training groups. If learning is occurring, the student's knowledge structure should correlate more strongly with the expert's knowledge structure after the experience. Power analysis determined that sample size of 20 (10 in each group) will achieve 80% power to detect a difference of 0.08 between pre-test and post-test scores with an estimated SD of 0.12 and a significance level of 0.05 using a paired t-test. The similarity scores of the two student cohorts, fully-immersed and partially immersed, before and after the VR experiments were compared using analysis of variance where full-immersion vs. partial immersion was the independent variable.

3. Results

There were a total of 25 students who completed training, 13 students who were fully immersed and 12 students who were partially immersed. Pathfinder was computed on each student's raw ratings to derive a knowledge network. These networks were then compared to the expert knowledge network using a method that produces a similarity index (s) that varies from 0 to 1. The mean similarity scores are shown in Table 1.

Table 1. Mean similarity scores (and standard deviations)

	Pre	Post
Fully Immersed	.49 (.08)	.69 (.13)
Partially Immersed	.56 (.11)	.64 (.12)
Means	.52 (.10)	.67 (.13)

A 2x2 repeated measures analysis of variance was performed with pre vs. post simulation experience as a within-subjects variable and fully vs. partially immersed as a between-subjects variable.   There was a significant interaction between groups and time, $F(1,23)=4.548$, $p=0.044$, indicating that the difference between pre and post similarity scores for the fully immersed group was different from the pre/post difference for the partially immersed group. The overall pre/post difference was also significant, $F(1,23)=30.734$, $p<0.001$, but the overall group difference (fully vs. partially immersed) was not significant $F(1,23)=0.05$. Matched pairs t-tests were then performed comparing pre and post simulation scores for the two groups separately. The difference for the fully immersed group was highly significant t(12)=5.115, p<0.001 and the difference for the partially immersed group was also significant t(11)=2.625, p=0.024.

4. Conclusion

The results showed that both groups benefited from the VR simulation training as measured by the significant increased similarity to the expert knowledge network after the training experience. However, the immersed group showed a significantly higher gain than the partially immersed group. This study demonstrated a positive effect of VR simulation on learning as reflected by improvements in knowledge structure but an enhanced effect of full-immersion using a HMD vs. a screen-based VR system. Future studies should be developed to understand better the reasons for those differences.

References

[1]   Windish, D.M., Paulman, P.M., et.al. Do clerkship directors think medical students are prepared for the clerkship years? *Academic Medicine*; 79: 56-61, 2004

[2]   Committee on Quality of Health care in America. Crossing the quality chasm: A new health system for the 21st century. *Institute of Medicine*, Washington, D.C, National Academy Press, 2001

[3]   Winn, WD. A conceptual basis for educational applications of virtual reality. *Human Interface Technology Laboratory Technical Report TR-93-9*. Seattle, WA: Human Interface Technology Laboratory, University of Washington; August 1993

[4]   Champion, H.R. and Higgins, G.A.Meta-Analysis and Planning of SIMTRAUMA:Medical Simulation for Combat Trauma Training. *USAMRMC TATRC Report*; No.00-03, 2000

[5]   Satava, R.M. and Jones, S.B. The Future is Now: Virtual Reality Technologies. In: *Innovative Simulations for Assessing Professional Competence: from Paper-and-Pencil to Virtual Reality*. Tekian A, McGuire CH, McGaghie WC and Associates (eds) University of Illinois at Chicago, Department of Medical Education; (12): 179-193, 1999

[6]   Alverson DC, Saiki SM Jr, et al.. Distributed immersive virtual reality simulation development for medical education. Journal of International Association of Medical Science Educators; 15:19-30, 2005

[7]   Stevens SM, Goldsmith TE, et.al.. Virtual Reality Training Improves Students' Knowledge Structures of Medical Concepts. in Medicine Meets Virtual Reality 13; The Magic Next Becomes the Medical Now, Volume 111 Studies in Health Technology and Informatics Edited by: James D. Westwood, Randy S. Haluck, Helene M. Hoffman, Greg T. Mogel, Roger Phillips, and Richard A. Rob. IOS Press, Amsterdam, The Netherlands; 519-525, 2005

[8]   Caudell TP, Summers KL, et. al. A Virtual Patient Simulator for Distributed Collaborative Medical Education. Anat Rec (Part B:New Anat) 270B:16-22, 2003

[9]   Johnson PJ, Goldsmith TE et al.. Structural knowledge assessment: Locus of the predictive advantage Pathfinder-based structures. *Journal of Educational Psychology*; 86:617-626, 1994

[10] Schvaneveldt RW (Ed.). Pathfinder Associative Networks: Studies in Knowledge Organization. Norwood, NJ. Ablex; 1990

Medicine Meets Virtual Reality 15
J.D. Westwood et al. (Eds.)
IOS Press, 2007

Experiences of Using the EndoAssist–Robot in Surgery

Nina HALÍN, M.Sc. *, Pekka LOULA, PhD, Prof. *, Pertti AARNIO, MD, PhD, Prof. **
* Tampere University of Technology, Pori, Finland ** Satakunta Central Hospital

Abstract. EndoAssist is a robotic camera-holding device controlled by the operator's head movements. Operations on forty-nine patients undergoing laparoscopic surgery were made using the robotic assistant. The aim of our project was to find out how using an EndoAssist-robot influences the operating times in contrast to using human assistant. A further aim was to collect the surgeons' experiences of using the robot. In this paper we describe the results of our project.

Keywords. EndoAssist, robot, surgery

Introduction

The role of the human camera holder during laparoscopic surgery can be quite boring and even tedious. It also keeps indispensable personnel from other duties. [1] Robotic camera holders provide steady camera movement and view during laparoscopic surgery. The EndoAssist (Armstrong Healthcare, United Kingdom) was developed to allow the surgeon complete autonomy over the laparoscopic surgical view without the need for manipulation by an assistant. EndoAssist is a robotic camera-holding device controlled by the operator's head movements. This study assesses its introduction into clinical practice. Operations on forty-nine patients undergoing laparoscopic surgery were made using the robotic assistant. The aim of our project was to find out how using an EndoAssist-robot influences the operating times in contrast to using human assistant. A further aim was to collect the surgeons' experiences of using the robot. In this paper we describe the results of our project.

1. Tools and methods

Minimally invasive surgery has been shown to offer many advantages to general surgical patients.[2] General benefits to patients include decreased post-operative pain, shorter hospital stays and earlier resumption of normal activities.

Normally, the operating team consists of one or two surgeons and one surgical nurse. As the surgeon generally needs to use instruments with both hands during the operation, the endoscope shaft must be held in place and oriented by an assistant to follow the work of the surgeon. Increasing cost pressure within the health care system has promoted the development of robotic systems able to replace personnel. Robotic technology offers devices to perform the role of the person holding the camera. The human hand becomes tired after a few hours, but a robotic hand will always be steady.

EndoAssist is a freestanding laparoscopic camera manipulator controlled by infrared signals from a headset worn by the operating surgeon. A sensor is placed on the laparoscopic video monitor, which tracks and indicates the direction of head movement. The surgeon wears a head-mounted optical transmitter and as the surgeon moves his head, a receiver box detects the direction. The movement in the indicated direction can then be initiated and terminated with a foot control.[3] A light-emitting diode arrow on the sensor confirms the intended direction of camera movement. The robotic arm can be moved in the left, right, up and down directions. For in and out zoom, surgeon depresses the foot pedal a second time to change the settings and then looks down to zoom in and up to zoom out. The EndoAssist robot is shown in figure 1.

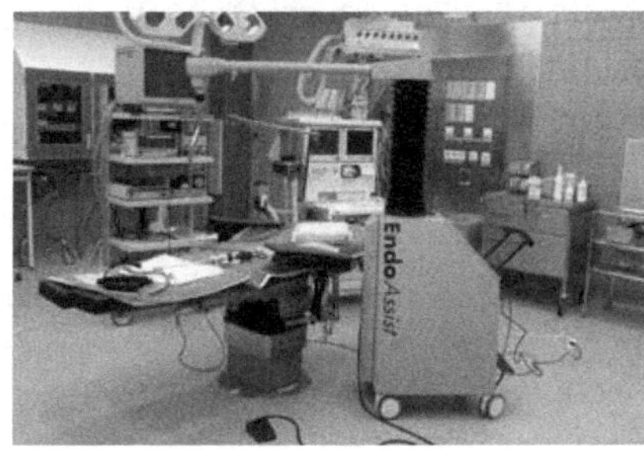

Figure 1. The EndoAssist robot.

2. Results

During our study two surgeons practised using EndoAssist. After three months we started to collect test data. We collected the operation times from forty-nine laparoscopic operations and the surgeon filled in a questionnaire after the operation. Twenty-seven of the operations were laparoscopy cholecystectomies, sixteen were fundoplications, one hernia repair and three other operations. The aim of this study was to compare operating times between human assisted and robotic-assisted surgical operations. For times with human assisted operations, we took the comparative data of similar operations from an electronic operation record system.

Considering operation times at cholecystectomies, they were nearly the same +/-10minutes in both human assisted and robotic-assisted operations. With robot the mean operation time was 1 hour twenty-six minutes and with human assistance it was 1 hour seventeen minutes. However, in fundoplications, the mean operation time (~2h 3min) using a robot was noticeably shorter than with human assistant (~3h 49min). These results showed that most tasks were completed more quickly with the EndoAssist than with human assistance. The mean operation time was nearly one hour shorter using the robot assistant than human assistant. Further, camera positioning was significantly steadier with robot assistance. The Theatre teams also learnt how to set up the robot without difficulty. The assistant nurse was able to concentrate on her/his work without having to hold the camera. We found the design to be very practical, confirming previous clinical studies.[1] The Surgeons' opinions were quite positive and they were very satisfied with EndoAssist. They said for example, that the robot is easy to use, it works technically very well and that the robot improves working ergonomics.

3. Conclusion

This study compared robot assistant with human assistant. The results of our study support the feasibility of using the robotic system in routine and advance endoscopic operations. EndoAssist proved to be a practical and stable substitute for a human camera holder, which has the potential to improve the efficient use of theatre time and free the camera assistant for more productive work. The advantages of the EndoAssist include its accurate response and ability to provide the surgeon with complete control of the desired operative view without replying on an assistant. Its disadvantages include its quite large profile, lack of a table-mounted design and the need for pedal activation. The EndoAssist has been used in Satakunta hospital for endoscopy operations. Our research is still going on and we will get more experiences and results.

References

[1]   Aiono S, Gilbert JM, Soin B, Finlay PA, Gordan A: Controlled trial of the introduction of a robotic camera assistant (EndoAssist) for laparoscopic cholecystectomy. Surg Endosc 2002; 16:1267-1270

[2]   Hance I, Rockall T, Darzl A: Robotics in Colorectal Surgery. Dig Surg 2004; 21:339-343

[3]   Ballester P, Jain Y, Haylett KR, Stone R, McCloy RF: Comparison of task performance of the camera-holder robots EndoAssist amd Aesop. SUrg Laparosc Endosc Percutan Tech 2003;13;5;334-338

Medicine Meets Virtual Reality 15
J.D. Westwood et al. (Eds.)
IOS Press, 2007

Comprehensive 3D Visual Simulation for Radiation Therapy Planning

Felix G. HAMZA-LUP[a,1], Ivan SOPIN[a] and Omar ZEIDAN[b]
[a]Computer Science, Armstrong Atlantic State University, Savannah, GA 31419
[b]M. D. Anderson Cancer Center Orlando, FL 32806

Abstract. External beam radiation therapy is concerned with the precise and accurate delivery of radiation for cancer treatment. Highly-collimated beams are generated in a linear accelerator, consisting of several hardware components that move around the patient in a complex geometry to allow radiation target the tumor from every possible angle. The complex arrangements of the hardware components may give rise to collisions among the components or between the components and the patient. We present a premiere Web-based 3D visual simulator that enables early detection of collision scenarios based on the accurate 3D representation of a specific linear accelerator model and volumetric patient-specific CAT scan data.

Keywords. Radiation Therapy, 3D Simulation, Web 3D.

Introduction

External beam radiation therapy is the precise use of high-energy radiation to treat cancer. About 50-60% of cancer patients are treated with radiation at some time during their disease [1]. A radiation oncologist may use the radiation generated by a machine for non-invasive treatment procedures. Radiation is generated by a linear accelerator (LINAC), consisting of three components: the gantry (rotates around the horizontal axis), the table (translates on the axes and rotates in the horizontal plane) and the collimator (rotates and shapes the radiation beam) as illustrated in Figure1.

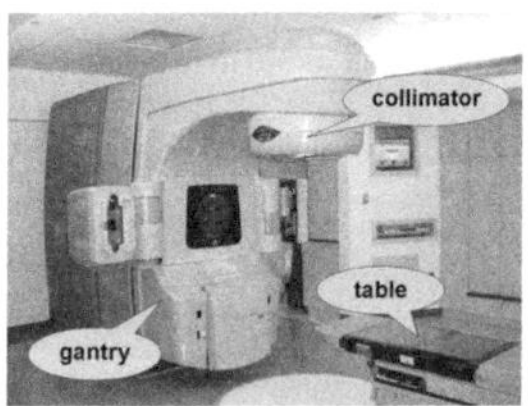

Figure 1. Varian 23iX Trilogy™ Linear Accelerator

1. Problem and Related Work

The complex relative orientations of the LINAC components may cause collisions with the components themselves or between the components and the patient. In addition,

---

[1] Felix G. Hamza-Lup, Ph.D.: Computer Science Department, School of Computing, Armstrong Atlantic Sate University, Savannah, GA 31419; E-mail: felix@cs.armstrong.edu.

LINAC head attachments and various patient immobilization devices may contribute as additional sources of collisions. Therefore, a radiation treatment planner may generate a seemingly optimal plan, only to result in a collision when a "dry run" (i.e. an execution of the plan without radiation for collision checking) is executed. This is a serious problem as it may cause significant delays to the patient treatment since the plan has to be revised and re-approved to account for these unforeseen collisions. Additional time and resources must be invested to adjust or to create an alternative treatment plan.

Analytical methods for collision detection have been proposed in the past as a means to improve the planning process [2, 3]. Even though mathematically accurate, these methods are based on the hardware rotational and translational numerical values disregarding LINAC and patient-specific geometry. The existing 3D simulations of the LINAC system have major limitations; they involve only generic patient body representations [4, 5] and do not use accurate three-dimensional graphical models of the LINAC components [4].

Our contribution combines the integration of a highly accurate representation of a specific LINAC model (i.e. Varian 23iX Trilogy™) and the integration of patient-specific CAT (Computed Axial Tomography) scan data in a Web-based simulation system that enables collaboration with remote experts during treatment planning or teaching sessions. A brief description of the system follows.

2. Web-based 3D Radiation Therapy Simulator

Employing the X3D standard [6] and considering the lessons learned from a previous implementation of the simulator [7], we have developed a Web-based 3D simulator, employing the laser scan model of a Varian 23iX Trilogy™ and a 3D surface reconstruction from patient-specific CAT scans as illustrated in Figure 2.

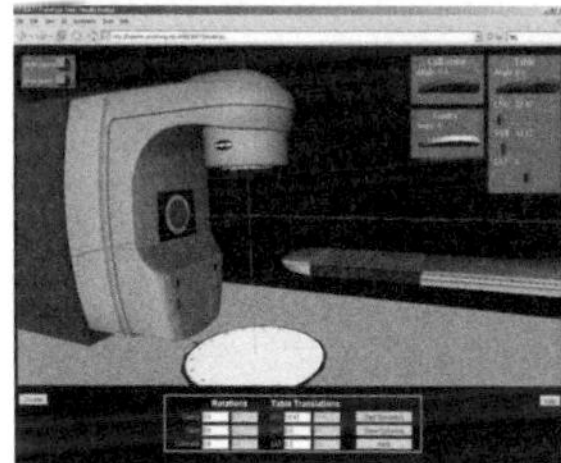
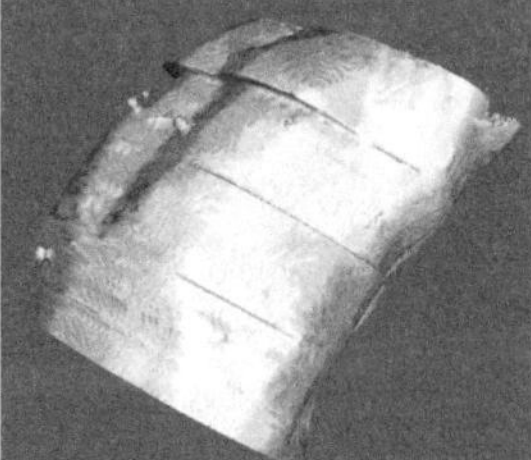
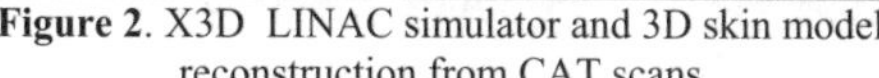
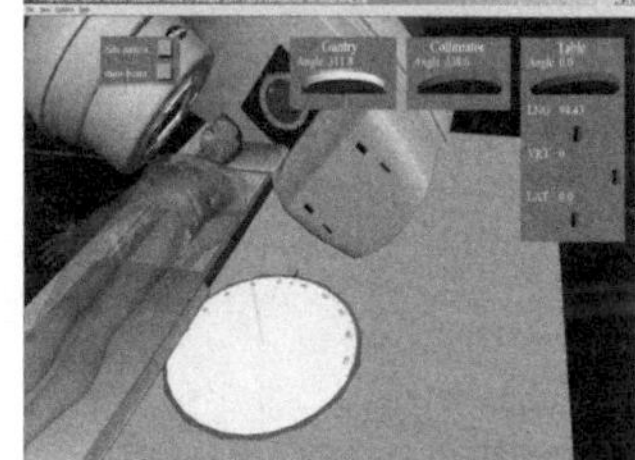

Figure 2. X3D LINAC simulator and 3D skin model reconstruction from CAT scans

Figure 3. Simulator with patient specific data

We optimized the marching cubes algorithm [8] to obtain a patient-specific 3D skin surface model. Several steps were necessary to process the laser scans of the LINAC into an optimized polygonal model. The decimation algorithm of the polygonal model was particularly important as it improved the rendering speed of the Web-based application.

The simulator (Figure 3) provides an intuitive floating graphical user interface (GUI) to control the angles and locations of the LINAC's parts. The user may rearrange the GUI components to avoid occlusion of important objects. Volumetric slides and scrolls keep operations simple and naturally fit in the 3D scene. The user can also show/hide the patient and the radiation beam by turning designated switches on/off. The system has a distributed functionality and can easily be shared among researchers and medical personnel at remote locations.

3. Assessment

We have deployed the system on a secure web site and allowed the medical personnel from M. D. Anderson Cancer Center, Orlando, to remotely access the simulation. As an objective test of collision scenarios, we asked radiation therapy technicians to simulate a plan that contains collisions among the system components. The preliminary assessment using visual inspection from different angles (illustrated in Figure 4) provides an early validation for the accuracy of the simulator (i.e. centimeter accuracy).

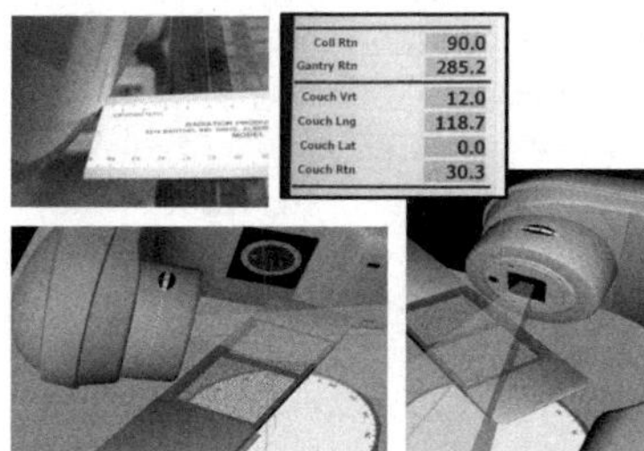

Figure.4 Visual Collision Validation

4. Conclusion and Future Work

We have presented a 3D simulation system that improves the planning process for radiation therapy. The system can be used to detect/predict possible collisions between LINAC components for a given patient and eliminate the need for backup plans, saving planning time. It also enables planners to explore variant and unconventional gantry-couch-collimator combinations of for treatment that may give rise to better quality plans.

We are exploring other methods to generate high-resolution 3D data to add various components to the existing LINAC model. We are also exploring new automatic collision detection algorithms based on polygon intersections. The collision criteria will be pre-determined by the planner as a single parameter such as the closest distance allowed between any two surfaces.

References

[1]   Radiological Society of North America [www.radiologyinfo.org], "Radiation Therapy", 2006.
[2]   I. Beange and A. Nisbet, "A collision prevention software tool for complex three-dimensional isocentric set-ups", British Journal of Radiology, vol.73, pp.537-541, 2000.
[3]   C. Hua, J.Chang, and K.Yenice, "A practical approach to prevent gantry-couch collision for linac-based radiosurgery", Medical Physics, vol.31, pp. 2128-2134, 2004.
[4]   M. F. Tsiakalos, E. Scherebmann, and K. Theodorou, "Graphical treatment simulation and automated collision detection for conformal and stereotactic radiotherapy treatment planning", Medical Physics, vol.28, pp.1359-1363, 2001.
[5]   A. Beavis, J. Ward, P. Bridge, R. Appleyard, and R. Phillips, "An Immersive Virtual Environment for Training of Radiotherapy Students and Developing Clinical Experience", American Association of Physicists in Medicine, vol. 33, pp. 2164-2165, 2006.
[6]   Web3D Consortium (online: http://www.web3d.org/), "What is X3D?", 2006.
[7]   F. Hamza-Lup, L. Davis, and O. Zeidan, "Web-based 3D Planning Tool for Radiation-Therapy Treatment", 11th Intl. Symposium on 3D Web Technology, pp.159-162, April 18-21, Columbia, Maryland, 2006.
[8]   W. E. Lorensen and H. E. Cline, "Marching cubes: A high resolution 3D surface construction algorithm", 14th Annual Conference on Computer Graphics and Interactive Techniques, 1987.

Medicine Meets Virtual Reality 15
J.D. Westwood et al. (Eds.)
IOS Press, 2007

Haptic Interface Module for Hysteroscopy Simulator System

Matthias HARDERS [a,1], Ulrich SPAELTER [b], Peter LESKOVSKY [a],
Gabor SZEKELY [a] and Hannes BLEULER [b]

[a] *Virtual Reality in Medicine Group, Computer Vision Lab, ETH Zurich, Switzerland*
[b] *Laboratoire de Systemes Robotiques, Institut de Production et Robotique, EPF Lausanne, Switzerland*

Abstract. A fundamental element of a surgical simulator system aiming at high fidelity is the surgical instrument to be used by the simulation. The input device, as well as haptic feedback from the system should resemble the real environment. In this paper we describe all elements of the haptic interface module developed for a hysteroscopy simulator.

Keywords. haptic interface, surgical simulation, hysteroscopy

Introduction

The focus of our current endeavors is the development of a highly realistic simulator for training of hysteroscopic interventions. In this respect, the sense of presence plays an important role in the training effect, which can be achieved. To enable user immersion into the training environment, the interaction metaphors should be the same as during real surgery. Therefore, an actual surgical instrument has been modified in order to allow natural control of the intervention. Moreover, a haptic mechanism providing force-feedback and allowing complete removal of the instrument has been integrated.

In previous work, a number of specialized interfaces have been built within the context of surgical simulation. Proprietary input devices, e.g. [2], as well as setups connecting endoscopic instruments to commercial haptic devices, e.g. [5], have been developed. Apart from this, specialized hardware for endoscopic procedures is also commercially available [1,4]. The focus of the majority of these devices is laparoscopic intervention. Nevertheless, some projects aiming at hysteroscopy have also been carried out [3]. This work has later on been continued by Immersion, resulting in the Hysteroscopy AccuTouch simulator system.

While workspace and surgical gestures performed in laparoscopy are similar to those in hysteroscopy, most of the developed rather generic devices are not appropriate for our purpose. The necessary angular workspace for a typical hysteroscopy (pitch, yaw $< 55^O$, roll $\approx \pm720^O$) is in general larger than for laparoscopy (pitch, yaw $< 45^O$, roll $< \pm 360^O$). In addition in hysteroscopy the relevant anatomy is very close to the surgery tool insertion point. Therefore, hysteroscopy simulation has to start right after instrument insertion. In generic haptic interfaces the surgical tool is either fixed to the device and is

---

[1] Correspondence to: mharders@vision.ee.ethz.ch

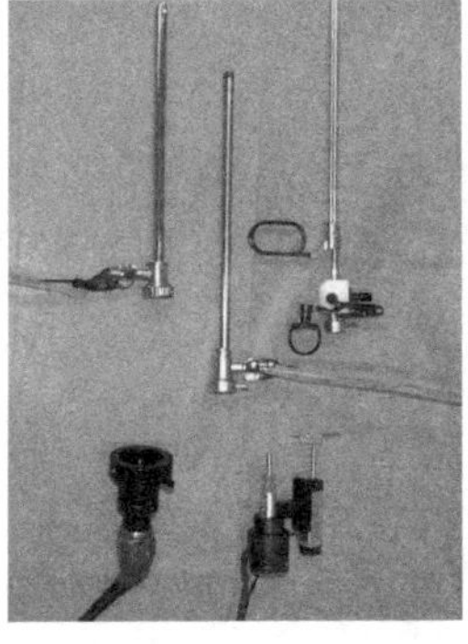
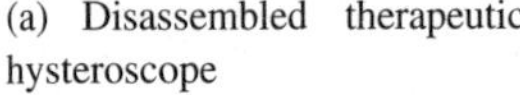
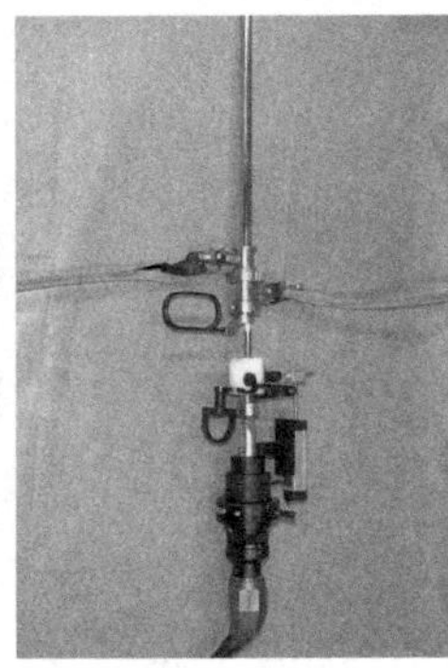
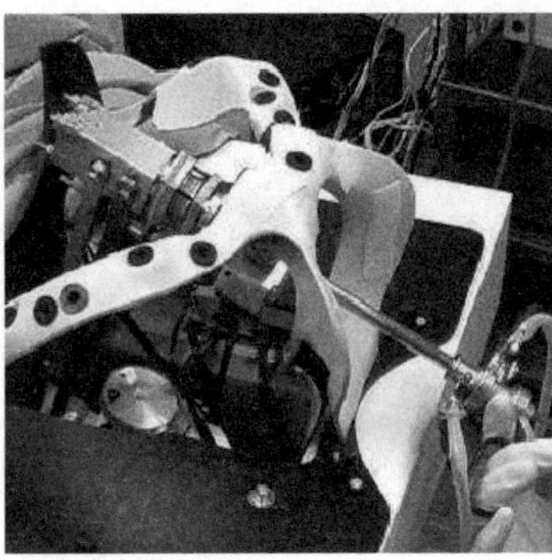

(a) Disassembled therapeutic hysteroscope

(b) Assembled tool

(c) Hysteroscope inserted into haptic mechanism

Figure 1. Therapeutic hysteroscope equipped with sensors

not removeable or a minimum insertion length is necessary (> 50mm), which is too long to simulate anatomies located close to the insertion point (> 25mm). This motivates our development of a dedicated device for hysteroscopy simulation, which also allows for easy integration into the confined space of the patient mannequin.

Haptic interface module

The first element of the device is the adapted original therapeutic resectoscope. Sensors have been integrated to provide tracking of the linear displacement of the loop electrode handle as well as the positions of the fluid in- and outflow valves. Camera focus and rotation are tracked as well. Signal and power cables of the sensors are hidden in the unused fluid tubes or standard instrument cables. Furthermore, the surgical instrument can be completely assembled and disassembled into its usual components. Force-feedback is generated by a haptic mechanism, into which the tool can be seamlessly inserted. The system has a parallel 2-DOF structure providing a remote center of motion architecture for rotations around a pivoting point, and a serially attached 2-DOF manipulator for linear and rotational tool actuation. Inertia is reduced by fixing the actuators of the parallel structure to the base. The mechanism has no singularities within the half-spherical workspace. The manipulator can transmit pitch and yaw torques up to 0.5Nm, roll torques of 0.02Nm and linear forces of 2N. The hardware is shown in Figure 1.

To generate force-feedback we follow a point-based haptic proxy paradigm [6]. This technique is applied to single, as well as multiple interaction points. Collisions are detected based on a spatial hashing approach [7]. The objects in the simulation have a dual representation. Tetrahedral meshes are used for collision detection and deformation calculation, while surface meshes are employed for visualization and local proxy update. The connection of the external device to the simulation is controlled by a device manager module in the system framework. The haptic device is run on a separate machine, which is linked to the simulation machine via a 100 MBit Ethernet UDP socket connection. The simulation runs on our current hardware at about 250Hz. To avoid any instability, a local model is used on the haptic client side. The update rates of the haptics loop are generally >1kHz.

Specialized control schemes minimize parasitic effects and thus increase haptic rendering realism. The static continuous model proposed in [8] allows for easy parameter

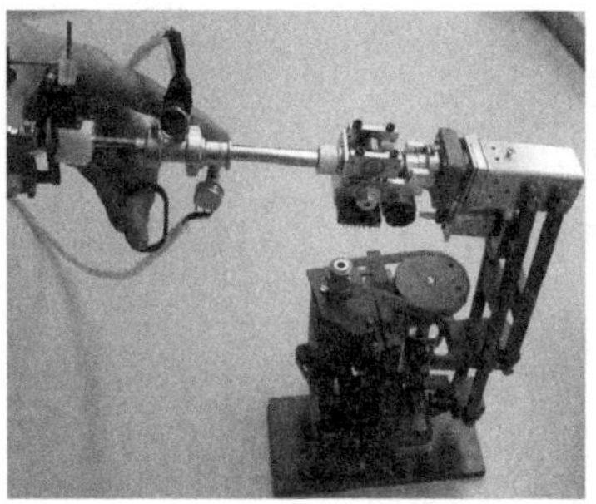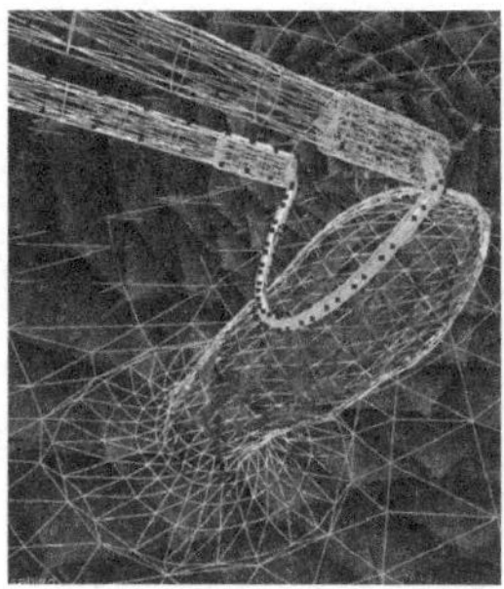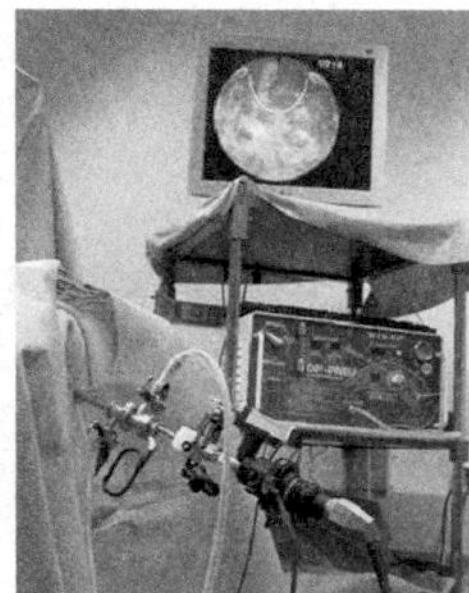

(a) Completely assembled haptic interface　(b) Example scene with meshes　(c) View of complete setup

Figure 2. Elements of haptic interface module.

identification and performs well in the low velocity range. In order to take dynamic friction effects into account, we extend the proposed continuous model by a switching strategy. According to the velocity and the sign of the acceleration, different parameter sets are applied in the friction model equation. Furthermore, device weight is compensated by a model-based approach.

Conclusion

In order to provide an immersive training setup, several elements have been developed for the haptic interface module of our simulator system. To enable user immersion into the training environment, the interaction metaphors are the same as during the real intervention. The final elements of the haptics module are depicted in Figure 2.

Acknowledgements

This research has been supported by the NCCR Co-Me of the Swiss National Science Foundation. The authors would like to thank all developers of the hysteroscopy simulator project.

References

[1]　Immersion Inc. *http://www.immersion.com* , 2006.

[2]　U. Kuehnapfel, H. Krumm, C. Kuhn, M. Huebner, and B. Neisius. Endosurgery simulations with KISMET: A flexible tool for surgical instrument design, operation room planning and vr technology based abdominal surgery training,. In *Proc. Virtual reality World'95*, pages 165–171, 1995.

[3]　K. Montgomery et al. Surgical simulator for hysteroscopy: a case study of visualization in surgical training. *VIS '01: Proceedings of the conference on Visualization '01*, pages 449–452, 2001.

[4]　Xitact SA. *http://www.xitact.com.* , 2006.

[5]　G. Szekely et al. Virtual reality-based simulation of endoscopic surgery. In *Presence*, volume 9, pages 310–333, 2000.

[6]　Diego C. Ruspini, Krasimir Kolarov, and Oussama Khatib. The haptic display of complex graphical environments. In *Computer Graphics (SIGGRAPH 97 Conference Proceedings)*, pages 345–352. ACM SIGGRAPH, 1997.

[7]　M. Teschner, B. Heidelberger, M. Mueller, D. Pomeranets, and M. Gross. Optimized spatial hashing for collision detection of deformable objects. In *Proceedings of Vision, Modeling, Visualization VMV03*, pages 47–54, November 2003.

[8]　C. Makkar, W.E. Dixon, W.G. Sawyer, and G.Hu. A new continously differentiable friction model for control system design. *International Conference on Advanced Intelligent Mechatronics*, pages 600–605, July 2005.

Medicine Meets Virtual Reality 15
J.D. Westwood et al. (Eds.)
IOS Press, 2007

Comparative Visualization of Human Nasal Airflows

Bernd HENTSCHEL [a,1], Christian BISCHOF [b] and Torsten KUHLEN [a]

[a] *Virtual Reality Group, RWTH Aachen University, Germany*
[b] *Institute for Scientific Computing, RWTH Aachen University, Germany*

Abstract. The use of computational fluid dynamics allows to simulate a large number of different variations of a general flow phenomenon in a reasonable amount of time. This lays the foundation for large scale comparative studies. However, in order to be able to compare the simulation results effectively, advanced comparison methods are needed. In this paper we describe a set of techniques for the comparison of flow simulation results. All methods are integrated in a virtual reality based prototype and facilitate the interactive exploration of the data domain. As a specific application example the described techniques are used to compare different human nasal cavity flows to each other.

Keywords. Comparative visualization, virtual reality, nasal airflow

1. Introduction

The human nose consists of a system of various cavities in the frontal part of the skull. It has to satisfy a variety of different functions, among others moistening, tempering and cleaning the inhaled air. The fulfillment of these functions mainly depends on the flow field inside the main nasal cavity, which in turn is shaped by the cavity's complex internal geometry. If this geometry is malformed, e.g., by hereditary deformity or serious injury, nasal respiration can be impaired. This may result in a serious loss of life quality and can therefore require surgical intervention. Unfortunately, long term success rates of such surgeries are by no means satisfactory. The main goal of the interdisciplinary project underlying this work is to establish a fundamental understanding of the complex process of nasal respiration. In order to achieve this, we want to numerically predict the flow field inside the nose, and its relation to geometric changes. Ultimately, we strive to integrate this knowledge into a computer assisted surgery system, which should lead to minimally invasive treatment and increased overall success rates.

In order to reach this goal, a detailed, model-based analysis of the nasal flow has been carried out. In this study general, objective criteria should be derived, which on the one hand quantify the quality of a given nasal cavity's flow field, and on the other hand help to predict the outcome of a surgical intervention. The fundamental results gained

---

[1]Corresponding Author: Bernd Hentschel; Virtual Reality Group, Center for Computing and Communication, RWTH Aachen University, Seffenter Weg 23, 52074 Aachen, Germany; E-mail: hentschel@rz.rwth-aachen.de.

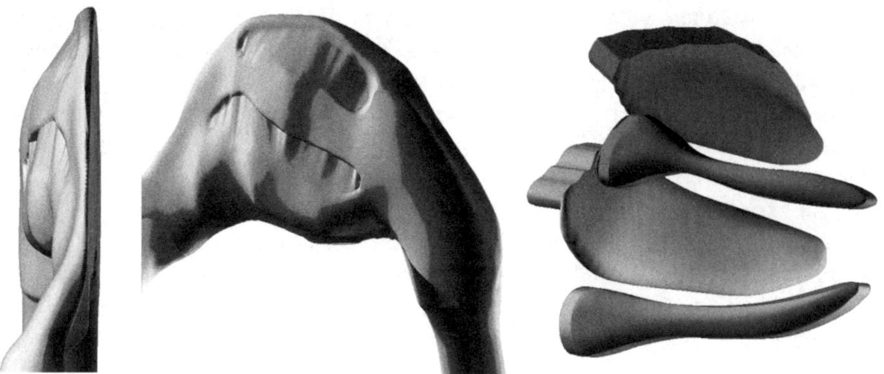

Figure 1. The computational model of the nasal cavity with its components. Left and center: The outer hull of the main nasal cavity. Right: The models for lower and middle turbinate and the cartilage spurs.

from the model-based study will be transferred to patient-specific data sets in a second project phase.

The nose model consists of several modules matching the nose's main anatomical components. These modules can be assembled in different combinations in order to simulate the airflow for a variety of different geometrical configurations. The main parts of the model, shown in Figure 1, are the nasal cavity's outer hull, the middle and the lower turbinate, and two cartilage spurs, which adhere to the side of the septum. In order to assess the effect of each of these components on the nasal airflow, several simulations have been performed with varying model configurations and input parameters. The resulting data sets have to be compared to each other, in order to assess how the different nasal cavity geometries affect the flow field. A manual, purely image-based comparison of all the results is very tedious and time consuming. Therefore, we devised a set of visualization techniques, which are used to assess the differences of the various data sets more efficiently. In order to overcome problems of occlusion and information overload, which arise, amongst others, from the complex three-dimensional shape of the nasal cavity, these methods rely on virtual reality techniques. Stereoscopic projection and direct interaction allow us to quickly convey meaningful results and to provide an intuitive interface for data exploration. All methods described in this paper are part of the VRhino software framework described in [1]. For the illustration of the techniques described in this paper, we will use only two example configurations of the nasal cavity: the empty configuration, designated NC_{000}, which is made up of only the outer hull, and the full configuration NC_{111}, which includes the entire set of modules.

The rest of this paper is structured as follows: First we briefly review related work in the field of comparative flow visualization. Section 3 then describes our own comparison methods and the way in which we embed them into a virtual reality based analysis tool. Finally, we conclude our paper with a brief summary and remarks on future work.

2. Related Work

Comparison methods are generally categorized into three main groups. The simplest form is image-based comparison, where only the final 2D renderings of two or more data sets are compared to each other. This can be done manually or by using automated algorithms, which quickly point out key differences. However, this approach is not applicable in virtual environments, since the user's view onto two different data sets would have to be locked in order to create comparable imagery. We found this to be too much of a limitation. In contrast, data based comparison techniques, which make up the second category, directly compare the underlying data sets using some kind of similarity measure. The results can be processed by follow up visualization algorithms. Examples can be found in [2]. Finally, feature-based comparisons use flow features computed from the original raw data, e.g., streamlines [3] or critical points [4,5], and compare these primitives to each other. This can be done using either a side-by-side view or by overlaying the features in a single view [6]. Approaches from the two latter categories allow for an interactive inspection of the comparison results from different points of view and are therefore suited for a virtual reality based comparison.

Nasal airflow has been the subject of other studies before [7,8]. In contrast to these, our analysis is not directly based on real patient data, but rather uses a generalized, anatomically correct model of the nasal cavity. Although the use of real-world patient data seems to be beneficial at first sight, the results gained by this approach are prone to patient-specific anatomic deformities. For a detailed description of the fluid mechanical results gained from our model-based study, we refer to [9,10].

3. Comparison Methods

Before we describe the comparison algorithms themselves, we will briefly introduce two additional categories into which we group comparison techniques. This additional separation has proven to be useful, when desinging the methods, as well as specific interaction techniques for them.

The first of these dimensions is the scale at which a given technique compares the input data. Here we distinguish between global and local scale. A global technique conveys a general understanding of similarities and differences throughout the entire data domain, whereas a local technique allows to selectivly compare data in a small subset thereof. The second dimension considers the degree of necessary user interaction. Automatic techniques require minimal user input and can therefore often be used to precompute comparison data. In contrast, interactive techniques depend on highly variable user inputs during the visualization process itself. Thus, results cannot be precomputed.

When comparison data is separately derived from each of the input data sets, this results in one or more visualization primitives for each data set. There are two possibilities to handle this problem. On the one hand, the derived data can be shown side by side using two different views. On the other hand one can use a single integrated view. This concept of data overlaying is adopted for the rest of this paper. If a comparison technique results in one or more visualizaion primitives, e.g., arrow glyphs, for each of the two data sets, we use color coding to distinguish between the two.

3.1. Data Based Comparison

The first two comparison techniques introduced here directly take the raw data as input. In order to gain a global understanding of the differences between two data fields, we

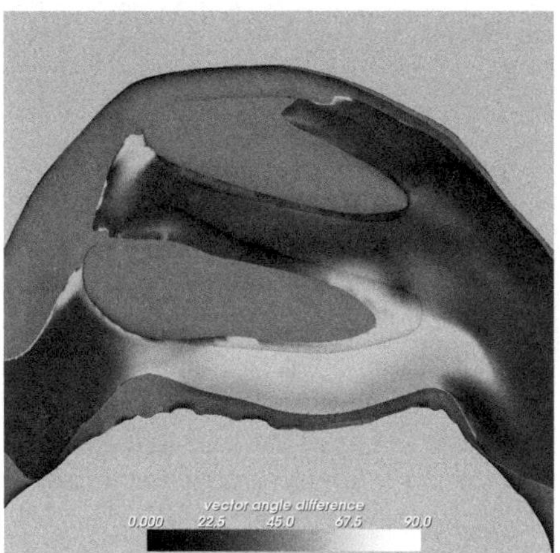
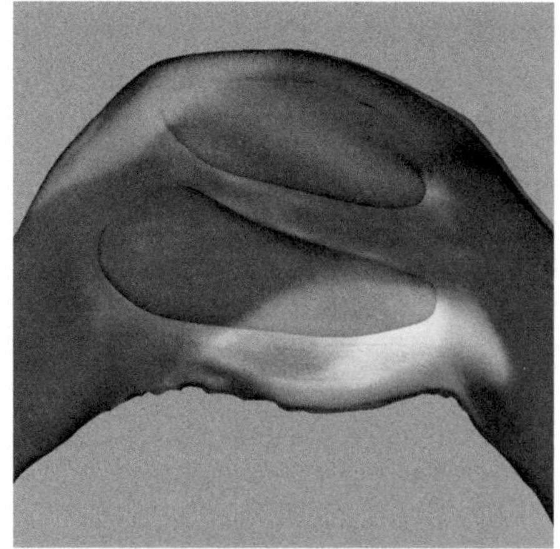

Figure 2. Two different visualizations of the angle difference metric for the NC_{000} and the NC_{111} configurations. Left: Analyzing the metric scalar field using a semi-transparent cut plane parallel to the septum. Right: Direct volume rendering highlighting regions with an angle derivation greater than 45 degrees. In both cases the NC_{111} geometry is shown as context.

implemented a set of difference metrics. Such a metric is a mapping $\sigma : \mathbb{R}^n \times \mathbb{R}^n \mapsto \mathbb{R}$. It takes as input one n-dimensional data tuple for each input data set and yields a scalar quantifying the degree of similarity between the two attribute sets. On the one hand this technique can be used in a straightforward fashion to compare single attributes, e.g., the pressure values, to each other. On the other hand it can be used to formulate more complex similarity measures incorporating more than one data field at a time. Technically, the data tuple for the first input point is taken directly from a grid point of the first input data set while the second tuple is obtained by interpolation in the second data set. Points at which the comparison is impossible, e.g., because the position lies within a turbinate which is only included in one of the two data sets, are marked as invalid and are extracted before later visualization. In order to allow for a meaningful interpretation of the results, the data range of the valid points is saved along with the comparison data. The results for various metrics are precomputed prior to interactive exploration. Analysis is done using standard scalar field visualization methods, e.g., using cut planes or direct volume rendering, as shown in Figure 2. Both images clearly show the region of major flow differences below the lower turbinate. Moreover, the volume rendering image shows another region of difference in the frontal part of the nasal cavity, while the flow between the turbinates is quite similar.

The second data based comparison method complements the first one in that it is used to interactively inspect local differences in the underlying vector fields. This is done by providing an interface for direct probing, which can be done very intuitively in virtual environments using a six-degrees-of-freedom input device. Different types of probing icons are available, as shown on the left hand side of Figure 3. Each icon contains two kinds of special nodes. First, there is a set of probing positions, i.e., positions at which the vector fields are interpolated. Second, each icon has several interaction handles, which are used to move around or scale the icon, respectively. Handles typically coincide with probing points. The probed velocity vectors are displayed using color coded arrow glyphs, where the color indicates from which data set the respective glyphs have

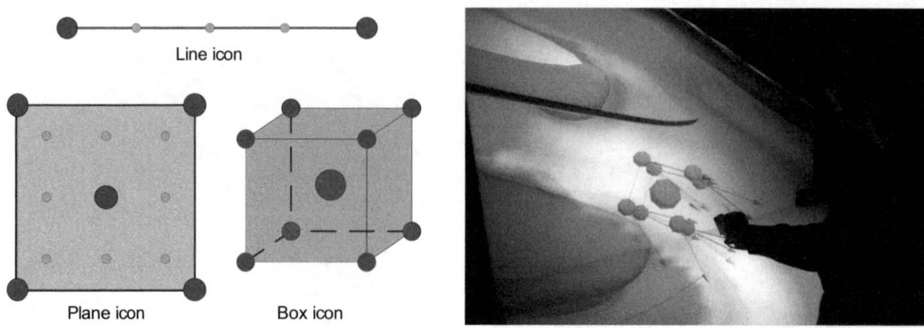

Figure 3. Left: Illustration of the different icons available for direct probing of the vector fields. Dark grey spheres indicate interaction handles for moving and scaling the icon, while light grey spheres indicate probing positions. Right: A user interactively compares two data sets using a box style probe icon.

been obtained. The right hand side of Figure 3 shows a user, who probes a vector field interactivley using a box probe icon.

3.2. Feature Based Comparison

One problem with data-based comparison is, that the complexity of analyzing the comparison data always scales directly with the size of the raw input data. Therefore, it can become tedious in itself. Feature extraction in general provides a more abstract, condensed visualization, leading to a significant reduction of data size. Consequently, it is beneficial to compare features to each other in contrast to comparing the raw data itself. A particularly interesting technique is the visualization of vector field topologies as introduced in [11,12].

From the location of critical points, i.e., the points at which the velocity magnitude equals zero, insights about a flow field's general structure can be gained. Comparing two distributions of critical points for two different data sets consequently points out main regions of difference. Although the two critical point sets under comparison may look completely different, this technique is useful, since the regions around a critical point in either data set can be analyzed in more detail, e.g., by using the data based probing approach described in the previous section.

4. Conclusion and Future Work

In this paper we have presented a set of virtual reality based techniques for an interactive comparison of flow fields. The methods have been developed with a specific use case in mind, namely the analysis of the human nasal cavity. While the current prototypical implementation, as discussed in this paper, already helped during the analysis, there are still some issues that need to be addressed.

As stated in Section 2, there are more sophisticated topology-based comparison methods, which try to quantify the similarity between two vector fields directly. This has been shown for two dimensional data sets in [4] and extended to three dimensions in [5]. We plan to incorporate such advanced techniques, because they do not only give a qualitative impression of similarity but rather provide quantitative information. Another venue for this research would be the use of techniques from information visualization, e.g., histograms and scatterplots, which enable the user to efficiently identify differences in data space. Finally, we would like to design and perform formal user studies in order to actually quantify the effectiveness of the given comparison methods themselves as well as the integration into an immersive environment.

Acknowledgements

This work has kindly been funded by the German Research Foundation (DFG) under grant WE 2186/5. The authors would like to thank their cooperation partners from the Institute of Aerodynamics, RWTH Aachen University, and the university hospitals of Aachen and Cologne for their valuable input during the design and implementation of the described techniques.

References

[1] Bernd Hentschel, Torsten Kuhlen, and Christian Bischof. VRhino II: Flow Field Visualization inside the Human Nasal Cavity. In *Proceedings of IEEE VR 2005*, pages 233–236, 2005.

[2] K. Kim and A. Pang. A Methodology for Comparing Direct Volume Rendering Algorithms Using a Projection-Based Data Level Approach. In *Proceedings of the Joint Eurographics/IEEE TVCG Symposium on Visualization '99*, pages 87–98, 1999.

[3] Vivek Verma and Alex Pang. Comparative Flow Visualization. *IEEE Transactions on Visualization and Computer Graphics*, 10(6):609–624, November/December 2004.

[4] Yingmei Lavin, Rajesh Batra, and Lambertus Hesselink. Feature Comparisons of Vector Fields Using Earth Mover's Distance. In *Proceedings of IEEE Visualization '98*, pages 103–109, 1998.

[5] Rajesh K Batra and Lambertus Hesselink. Feature Comparisons of 3-D Vector Fields Using Earth Movers Distance. In *Proceedings of IEEE Visualization '99*, pages 105–114, 1999.

[6] Hans-Georg Pagendarm and Frits H. Post. Studies in Comparative Visualization of Flow Features. In Gregory M. Nielson, Hans Hagen, and Heinrich Müller, editors, *Scientific Visualization, Overviews, Methodologies, Techniques*, chapter 9, pages 211–227. IEEE Computer Society, 1997.

[7] Wolfgang Müller-Wittig, Gunter Mlynski, Ivo Weinhold, Uli Bockholt, and Gerrit Voss. Nasal Airflow Diagnosis - Comparison of Experimental Studies and Computer Simulations. In *Proceedings of Medicine Meets Virtual Reality 2002*, pages 311–317. IOS Press, 2002.

[8] Brendan C. Hanna, John K. Watterson, Neil Bailie, and Jonathan Cole. Virtual Nasal Surgery - A New Dimension in Rhinological Surgery Planning. In *Proceedings of the 35th AIAA Fluid Dynamics Conference and Exhibit*, Toronto, Ontario Canada, June 6-9 2005.

[9] Ingolf Hörschler, Matthias Meinke, and Wolfgang Schröder. Numerical simulation of the flow field in a model of the nasal cavity. *Computers & Fluids*, 32:39–45, 2003.

[10] Ingolf Hörschler, Christoph Brücker, Wolfgang Schröder, and Matthias Meinke. Investigation of the Impact of the Geometry on the Nose Flow. *European Journal of Mechanics-B/Fluids*, 25(4):471–490, 2006.

[11] James L. Helman and Lambertus Hesselink. Visualizing Vector Field Topology in Fluid Flows. *IEEE Computer Graphics and Applications*, 11(3):36–46, 1991.

[12] Al Globus, Creon Levit, and Thomas Lasinki. A Tool for Visualising the Topology of Three-Dimensional Vector Fields. In Gregory M. Nielson and Larry Rosenblum, editors, *Proceedings of IEEE Visualization '91*, pages 33–40, 1991.

Medicine Meets Virtual Reality 15
J.D. Westwood et al. (Eds.)
IOS Press, 2007

A Blending Technique for Enhanced Depth Perception in Medical X-Ray Vision Applications

Frida Hernell[a,b,c,1], Anders Ynnerman[a,b] and Örjan Smedby[a,b,c]
[a] Center for Medical Image Science and Visualization, Linköpings universitet
[b] ITN/VITA, Linköpings universitet, [c] IMV/Radiology, Linköpings universitet

Abstract. Depth perception is a common problem for x-ray vision in augmented reality applications since the goal is to visualize occluded and embedded objects. In this paper we present an x-ray vision blending method for neurosurgical applications that intensifies the interposition depth cue in order to achieve enhanced depth perception. The proposed technique emphasizes important structures, which provides the user with an improved depth context.

Keywords. X-ray vision, depth perception, MRI, neurosurgical planning

1. Introduction

Visualizing occluded objects with augmented reality can be of great navigational aid during neurosurgical interventions, for instance, to localize a tumor in preoperative Magnetic Resonance (MR) images. The two most common methods for this "x-ray vision" are to create a "virtual hole" in the real occluding object or to give an illusion that the real object is semi-transparent [1-3]. A common problem in x-ray vision systems is the lack of clear depth perception when hidden objects become visible [1-2, 4-5]. One of the reasons for this is that the most important human depth cue, interposition, becomes contradictory since we know that near objects cannot be occluded by far objects. In this paper we present a novel x-ray vision blending technique for MRI data that strengthens the interposition depth cue in order to enhance the depth perception. The proposed technique emphasizes structures close to the observer while homogenous surfaces become transparent.

2. Methods

Inner structures of a CT volume can be visualised with preserved context using a technique described by Bruckner et al. [6]. We have modified this algorithm to enable its deployment in augmented reality. We make use of real parameters, captured with a camera and our blending algorithm is performed in a single pass ray casting scheme on the GPU, Eqs. 1 and 2.

---

[1] Corresponding Author: Frida Hernell, Center for Medical Image Science and Visualization, Linköpings universitet/US, SE-581 85 Linköping, Sweden. E-mail: frida.hernell@cmiv.liu.se

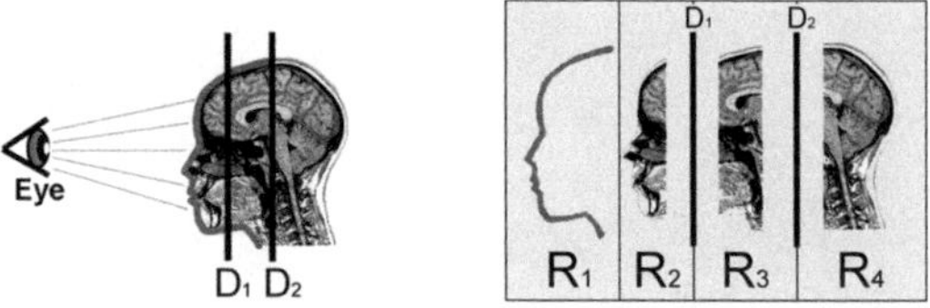

Figure 1. Illustration of the regions with different opacity properties.

To create an illusion that parts of the head are translucent, Eq. (3) is used to determine the opacity of each pixel in the video-captured image. Eq. (3) is based on properties of the point where the ray intersects with the skin surface, P_0, (Figure 1, R_1). These properties include the 2D gradient magnitude, $\|g_{Pxy}\|$, of the captured image, the distance between P_0 and the eye point, E, normalized to the range [0..1], and a measure ρ_{xy} of how centered the sample point is in a 2D projection of the head. K_t and k_s are constants (comparable to the description in [6]) and R is a function that clamps the values to the range [0..1].

$$\alpha_i = \alpha_{i-1} + \alpha(P_i) \cdot (1 - \alpha_{i-1}) \tag{1}$$

$$c_i = c_{i-1} + c(P_i) \cdot \alpha(P_i) \cdot (1 - \alpha_{i-1}) \tag{2}$$

$$\alpha(P_0) = R\left(\left\|g_{P_{xy}}\right\| + \rho_{xy} \cdot k_b\right)^{\left(k_t \cdot (1 - \|P_0 - E\|)\right)^{k_s}} \tag{3}$$

$$\alpha(P_i) = R\left(\left\|g_{P_i}\right\| \cdot \varphi \cdot k_a + \rho_{xy}^{\ k_t}\right)^{\left(k_t \cdot (1 - \|P_i - E\|) \cdot (1 - \alpha_{i-1})\right)^{k_s}} \tag{4}$$

$$\alpha(P_i) = \alpha_{tf}(P_i) \tag{5}$$

The user defines two depths in the volume (Figure 1, D_1 and D_2). The segment located between the skin surface and D_1 is transparent, region R_2 in Figure 1. Sample points between the two user-specified depths (Figure 1, R_3) are processed with an opacity function that intensifies important structures in order to enhance the depth perception further, Eq. 4. Homogenous areas in this region become transparent. The terms introduced in Eq. 4 are the 3D gradient in the MR volume, g_{Pi}, the angle, φ, between the gradient, g_{Pi}, and the viewing direction, the opacity of the previous sample point, α_{i-1}, and a constant, k_a, that amplifies inner structures. Beyond the furthest user defined depth, region R_4 in figure 1, the opacity rapidly increases to 1.0, as in Eq. 5.

3. Results

To evaluate the blending method basic registration and tracking methods were used. The initial registration was adjusted manually and the tracking was performed using the ARToolkit [7] and optical markers. For a surgical environment testing high-end registration and tracking methods may prove more suitable. The data used in this evaluation was a T1-weighted 3D MRI volume of 256×256×176 voxels and a video stream captured using a simple web camera with a resolution of 800×600 pixels. Figure 2 shows an example of the presented blending technique. A soft transition between the photo and the MRI volume is created while structures are accentuated to emphasize the interposition depth cue.

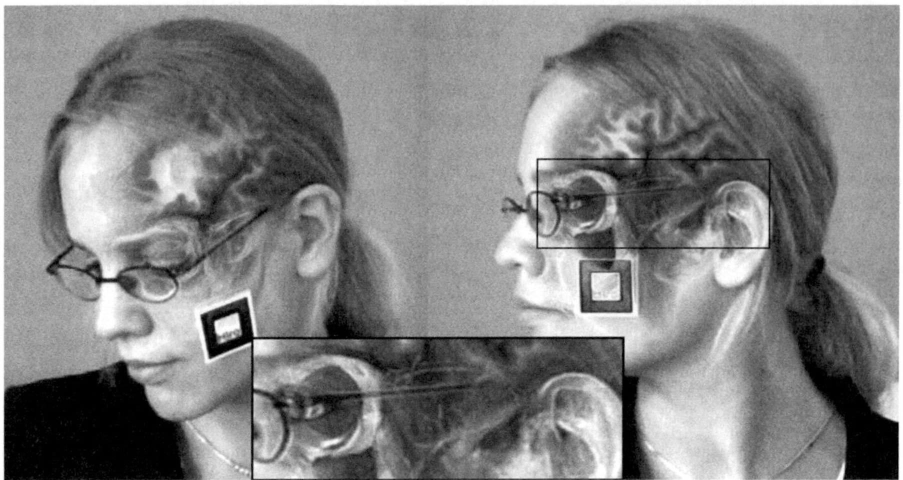

Figure 2. Results of the blending algorithm. Note the transition from opaqueness to transparency, of the ear and the spectacle frame, in the enlargement square.

4. Conclusions

The blending technique described in this paper gives the user visual information about the object hierarchy and therefore the interposition depth cue becomes less contradictory. Understanding of the spatial relations increases even more when the user interacts with the depth parameters and the level of visible structures. Interactions also introduce other depth cues, such as motion parallax. It should be noted that adding other depth cues into the method, e.g. realistic lighting and shadowing, might enhance the depth perception even further.

The preliminary visual results appear promising and in future work, we will evaluate the clinical impact of the presented method. Since the method is quite general, it can also be applied in other augmented reality applications where information about hidden objects is available.

References

[1]   Furmanski, C., R. Azuma, and M. Daily. Augmented-reality visualizations guided by cognition: Perceptual heuristics for combining visible and obscured information. in Mixed and Augmented Reality, ISMAR. 2002. Darmstadt, Germany.

[2]   Livingston, M.A., et al. Resolving Multiple Occluded Layers in Augmented Reality. in Mixed and Augmented Reality, ISMAR. 2003. Tokyo, Japan.

[3]   Bane, R. and T. Höllerer. Interactive Tools for Virtual X-Ray Vision in Mobile Augmented Reality. in Mixed and Augmented Reality, ISMAR. 2004. Arlington, VA.

[4]   Bulthoff, I., H. Bulthoff, and P. Sinha, Top-down influences on stereoscopic depth-perception. Nat Neurosci, 1998. 1(3): p. 254-7.

[5]   Ellis, S.R. and B.M. Menges, Localization of virtual objects in the near visual field. Hum Factors, 1998. 40(3): p. 415-31.

[6]   Bruckner, S., et al. Illustrative Context-Preserving Volume Rendering. in Proceedings of EuroVis 2005. 2005.

[7]   Billinghurst, M., "ARToolKit", Human Interface Technology Laboratory and Center for Environmental Visualization, University of Washington.

Medicine Meets Virtual Reality 15
J.D. Westwood et al. (Eds.)
IOS Press, 2007

Surgery on the Lateral Skull Base with the Navigated Controlled Drill Employed for a Mastoidectomy (Pre Clinical Evaluation)

M. Hofer [a,d,1], R. Grunert [d], E. Dittrich [d], E. Müller [a,d], M. Möckel [d], K. Koulechov [b], M. Strauss [b], W. Korb [d], T. Schulz [c], A. Dietz [a,d], T. Lüth [b], G. Strauss [a,d]

[a] *BMBF-Innovation Center Computer Assisted Surgery ICCAS, University of Leipzig*
[b] *Institute for Micromedicine-MiMed, Technical University of Munich*
[c] *University Hospital, Neurosurgery Department, University of Leipzig*
[d] *University Hospital, ENT Department / Plastic Surgery, University of Leipzig*

Abstract. Patients who are treated with a mastoidectomy usually suffer from an inflammation of the petrosal bone. The intervention is a time consuming landmark based surgery and usually performed with a powered drill. Delicate risk structures must be respected. Navigated Control (NC) describes the control for a power driven instrument which is controlled by a surgeon and additionally controlled according to the position of the instrument relatively to a deliberated position known from a preoperatively segmented work space which excludes risk structures. The force of a drill can be regulated by the principle of NC. Following results were received: 1. Risk structure segmentation is feasible 2. The drill and a phantom can be registered. 3. With NC the resection is faster, more accurate and with no risk structures damage. 4. The phantom is suitable.

Keywords. Navigation, Navigated Control, Petrosal Bone, Mastoidectomy

1. Background

Patients who are treated with a mastoidectomy usually suffer from an inflammation of the petrosal bone. The intervention is a time consuming landmark based surgery and usually performed with a powered drill (figure 1). The difficulty in this type of surgery is the identification and, therefore, the protection of risk structures such as the facial

---

[1] Mathias Hofer
Innovation Center Computer Assisted Surgery (ICCAS)
University of Leipzig
Philipp-Rosenthal-Strasse 55
04103 Leipzig, Germany
Tel: +49-341-9712005   Fax: +49-341-9712009
Mathias.Hofer@medizin.uni-leipzig.de

nerve, the sigmoid sinus, the inner ear, the organ of equilibrium and the lateral skull base with an immense time effort in order the trace them [1].

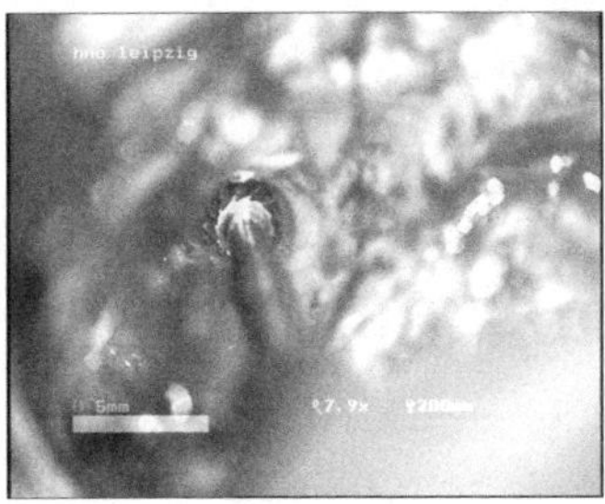

Figure 1. Microscopic view of the intervention site

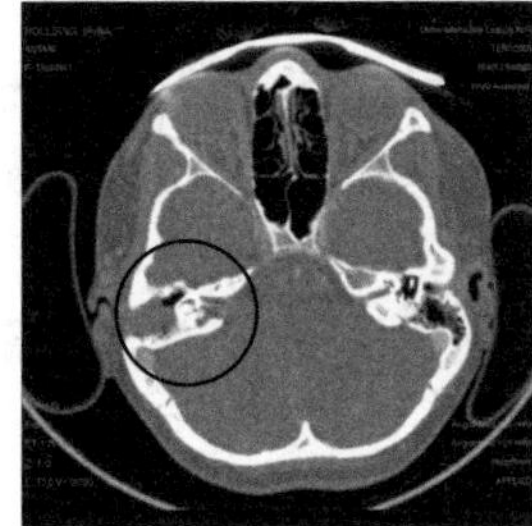

Figure 2. CT scan of the intervention site

A co-morbidity of 2-6% is described for the operation. Surgeons use high resolution CTs to study patient anatomy for procedure planning (figure 2). However, navigation on the lateral skull base has not yet been established. Navigated Control (NC) describes the control for a power driven instrument which is controlled by a surgeon and additionally controlled according to the position of the instrument relatively to a deliberated position known from a preoperatively segmented work space which excludes risk structure [2]. The force of a drill can be regulated by the principle of NC [3].

1.1. Technical Problems

For applying the principle of navigated control for surgery on the lateral skull base, it becomes necessary to overcome the following problems:
- A sure risk structure detection or segmentation within the imaging is mandatory for segmentation of the workspace in demarcation to the risk structures.
- A robust drill and patient/phantom registration is mandatory in order to achieve reproducible accuracy. However, the registration process must be practicable.
- A suitable phantom must be found, which allows measurement under reproducibility conditions [4].

1.2. Hypothesis

The resection with NC is faster, more accurate and with no risk structures damage.

2. Tools and Method

The ICCAS Electronic Head-Phantom (ElePhant) was used for evaluation. This phantom is generated with a rapid prototyping method (3D print) based on original patient data. Different petrosal bone models can be reproducibly connected to a receptacle. They contain the following important risk structures: Facial nerve, horizontal semicircular canal and sigmoid sinus.

Their damage through the instrument can be opto-electronically quali- and quantified. Two principles are employed: 1. Risk structures are represented by an electric conducting alloy (molting temperature 96°C). 2. Risk structures are represented by fiber optics. The risk structures are connected to a data acquisition card (National Instruments, Austin, Texas, USA). A with LabView 7.1 (National Instruments, Austin, Texas, USA) programmed Program controls the process and analyses it. There are objective evaluation criteria like number of damages, type of damaged risk structure, grade of damage and time course which can be used for statistical analyses. Throughout the simulation process, the damage of risk structures are represented graphically and acoustically (figure4).

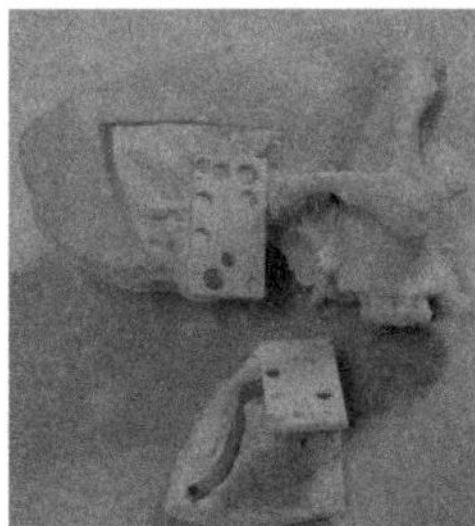

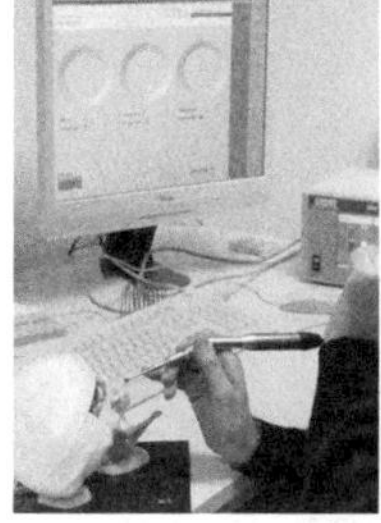

Figure 3. Phantom with exchangeable petrosal bone models (risk structures inherent)

Figure 4. Control monitor

The phantom bears a dental splint for registration. CT scans of the phantom after routine clinical protocol are performed. Workspace segmentation is done in the navigation data corresponding to a mastoidectomy. The segmentation was performed by an experienced ear surgeon: All risk structures laid outside the allowed workspace (figure 5).

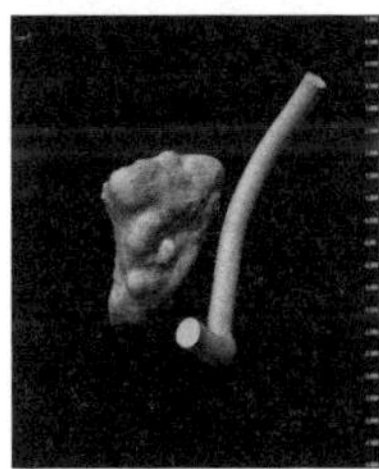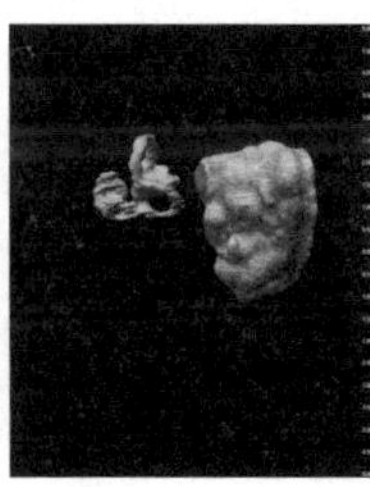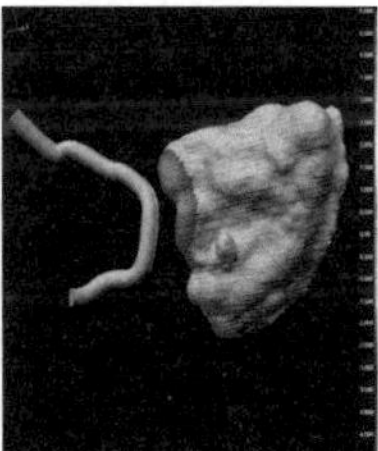

Figure 5. Distance mastoidectomy to risk structure

An optical navigation system (MiMed, TU Munich, Germany) is connected to a control unit (MiMed, TU Munich, Germany) which controls the drive of a 3.8mm diameter drill (Karl Storz GmbH, Tuttlingen, Germany). The drilling was performed on 15 different petrosal bone models executed by 5 inexperienced test persons and 5 experienced ear surgeons. The test persons were asked to perform a mastoidectomy according to the planned workspace.

The resections were divided into three different groups:

Group 1: **Inexperienced** test persons 5 mastoidectomies **with NC** (they were ask to drill until the system´s shut off)

Group 2: **Experienced** Ear-Surgeons 5 mastoidectomies **without NC**. (Navigation data was represented; the workspace volume could be seen, but free hand resection)

Group 3: **Experienced** Ear-Surgeons 5 mastoidectomies **with NC**. (They were ask to drill until the system's shut off)

Through the whole process the drill was controlled by a foot pedal in a conventional way. There was no automatic resection, however when NC was in use there is an automatic shut off when reaching the work space boarders. The phantom position during the investigation was equivalent to a surgical intervention (figure 6).

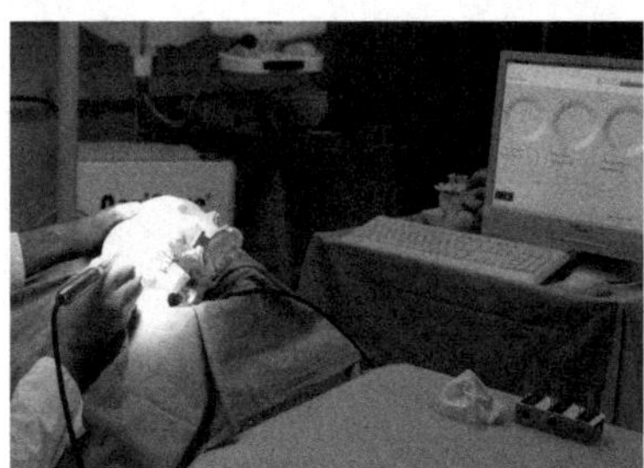

Figure 6. Investigation setup

Investigated were the following parameters: Resected volume, time and number and grade of damage. After the procedure the petrosal bone models were CT scanned and subsequently analyzed with measuring software (Polyworks®, Mimics®).

3. Results

In the CT scan of the petrosal bone models the sigmoid sinus, horizontal semicircular canal and facial nerve could be detected as risk structures. A workspace respecting the structures and corresponding to a mastoidectomy could be segmented. This process required 17minutes. The drill and phantom could be registered and tracked. Resection times were:

Group 1: Ø 2009.8 s
Group 2: Ø 715.0 s
Group 3: Ø 817.6 s

The resected volume was correlated to the required time:

Group 1: Ø 6.61mm^3/s
Group 2: Ø 9.6mm^3/s
Group 3: Ø 10.1mm^3/s

Comparing the planned workspace to the implemented resection led to the following results:

Group 1: resected +7.4% more than planned
Group 2: resected -39.9% less than planned
Group 3: resected -34.0% less than planned

There was no risk structure damage with NC. Without NC one mechanical damage of 20% of the facial nerve was registered.

4. Conclusion

The segmentation of a mastoidectomy within the petrosal bone models is possible. Registration of the drill and the phantom was technically solveable. A planned cavity can be realized corresponding to a planned mastoidectomy (figure 5). With NC the drilling speed increases. With NC inexperienced test persons drilled with an elevated accuracy in accordance to the planned volume for lack of alternative information on how a mastoidectomy has to be performed. It seemed the experienced test persons tended to make their own decision about the extension of the resection due to their clinical expertise. Although they were asked to follow the segmented volume presented on the navigation system, they resected with and without NC noticeably less than planned. However, employing NC led to fewer complications and to a more extensive resection (group 1 and 3). The phantom is very close to clinical practice (in anatomy and haptics, not in texture). Possibly, the damage of the facial nerve in group 2 might not have occurred on cadaver specimen or patients still due to a certain lack of realism. The investigation was performed with a modified system initially designed for a NC-shaver in para nasal sinus surgery, for example the drill tip was registered, but the actual drill sphere should be registered. In an ongoing second technical trial a NC-mastoid specific hardware is used for evaluation. With this specified setup, clinically satisfactory results are expected. From a clinical perspective the <u>maximum</u> deviation for the resection must be below 2mm. If this is feasible, the authors will propose an ethics committee approval for clinical testing.

The authors believe that lateral skull base surgery with NC has a great potential for safe risk structure protection, a morbidity reduction, a reduction in intervention time and also in a relief of strain for the surgeon. That is for an intervention (mastoidectomy) which is conducted about 50 times per year in the ENT department of the university hospital of leipzig. As mentioned in literature regarding Navigated Control: The change in the technical setup for NC in the operating room is minimal, since the fundamental systems are already integrated. The actual surgery remains nearly unchanged in its procedure [5].

Promotion and Sponsors

This treatise is supported by means from the European Fund for Regional Evolution (EFFRE), the German Ministry of Education and Research (BMBF), the Saxon Ministry of Science and the Fine Arts (SMWK), the Alfried Krupp zu Bohlen und Halbach-Stiftung und the Deutsche Forschungsgemeinschaft (DFG). The Karl Storz GmbH & Co. KG, Tuttlingen, Germany kindly provided the surgical systems and technical support.

References

[1]   T. Van Havenbergh, E. Koekelkoren, D. De Ridder, P. Van De Heyning, J. Verlooy,Image guided surgery for petrous apex lesions,Acta Neurochir (Wien),145(2003),737-42; discussion 742.

[2]   J. Glagau, O. Schermeier, A. Hein, T. Lüth, R. Kah, D. Hildebrandt, J. Bier 2002. Navigated Control in der Dentalen Implantologie. Leipzig.

[3]   K. Koulechov, T. Lueth 2004. A new metric for drill location for Navigated Control in navigated dental implantology. Elsevier,.

[4]   G. Strauss, M. Hofer, W. Korb, C. Trantakis, D. Winkler, O. Burgert, T. Schulz, A. Dietz, J. Meixensberger, K. Koulechov,Genauigkeit und Prazision in der Bewertung von chirurgischen Navigations- und Assistenzsystemen. Eine Begriffsbestimmung,HNO,54(2006),78-84.

[5]   M. Hofer, G. Strauss, K. Koulechov, M. Strauss, S. Stopp, A. Pankau, W. Korb, C. Trantakis, J. Meixensberger, A. Dietz, T. Luth,Establishing navigated control in head surgery,Stud Health Technol Inform,119(2006),201-6.

Medicine Meets Virtual Reality 15
J.D. Westwood et al. (Eds.)
IOS Press, 2007

185

Localized Virtual Patient Model for Regional Anesthesia Simulation Training System

John HU[a,1], Yi-Je LIM[a], Neil TARDELLA[a], Chuyin CHANG[a], Lisa WARREN[b]
[a] *Energid Technologies Corporation*
[b] *Massachusetts General Hospital*

Abstract. This paper presents the progress made in the development of a localized virtual patient model for regional anesthesia simulation training system by Energid Technologies. In our on-going project, a feasible engineering virtual patient model has been designed to capture the reflexive responses during nerve block stimulation. Our model combines advanced technologies in tissue deformation, motor nerve stimulation model, and haptic feedback rendering.

Keywords. Regional anesthesia, virtual patient model, tissue deformation, haptic feedback, nerve block, reflexive response

1. Introduction

Over the past decade, the use of peripheral nerve blocks for intraoperative and postoperative analgesia, or pain control, has become increasingly popular [1]. Though nerve block procedures present fairly low risk in a hospital setting, the same may not be true on the battlefield—where severe trauma cases are prevalent and properly trained pain management specialists in high demand. There is a need for all military anesthesiologists to undergo training for the administration of peripheral nerve blocks, yet currently no suitable curriculum or training system exists. Energid Technologies is developing a natural, immersive virtual environment, incorporating haptic, visual, and auditory feedback [2]. Anesthesiologists will use an untethered needle and syringe in simulated procedures. This will be achieved through a novel vision-based tracking system and innovative device for generating haptic feedback during needle insertion, needle injection, and palpation.

Regional anesthesia simulation has the same challenge in virtual patient modeling as surgical simulation does [3]. To have a realistic simulation for nerve stimulation in regional anesthesia simulation, it is important to have a good localized virtual patient model to capture the reflexive behaviors and perception. Under contract with the Telemedicine & Advanced Technology Research Center (TATRC), Energid Technologies is developing a novel localized virtual patient model for regional anesthesia simulation that includes anesthesia phenomena, tissue deformation, and muscular-skeletal motion induced by nerve stimulation.

Our localized virtual patient model uses a 3D virtual patient model (from Zygote) with accurate anatomic structures including accurate nerves, vessels, muscular-skeleton,

---

[1] Corresponding Author: John Hu, Ph.D., Energid Technologies Corporation, 124 Mount Auburn Street, Suite 200 North, Cambridge, MA 02138; E-mail: jju@energid.com.

and tissue. We visualize the complications of nerve blocks using a scene graph, a special high-speed data structure for graphical representation. By means of a neuro-muscular-skeletal model, we simulate muscle contraction, tweaking, and limb motion under nerve stimulation. Our model also covers neural sensory functions that link with auditory feedback. A meshless based tissue deformation modeling technique supports realistic force response as well as visual deformations in real time during needle insertion [4].

In this paper, we present our design and implementation of a localized virtual patient model for regional anesthesia simulator. We show the simulation results of needle insertion for femoral nerve block procedure, the novel design of a neuro-muscular-skeletal model for local patient modeling, muscle contraction and tweaking phenomena, and the sensory functions in a femoral block procedure. The haptic, visual, and auditory perceptions are simulated through the localized patient model we developed in regional anesthesia simulation.

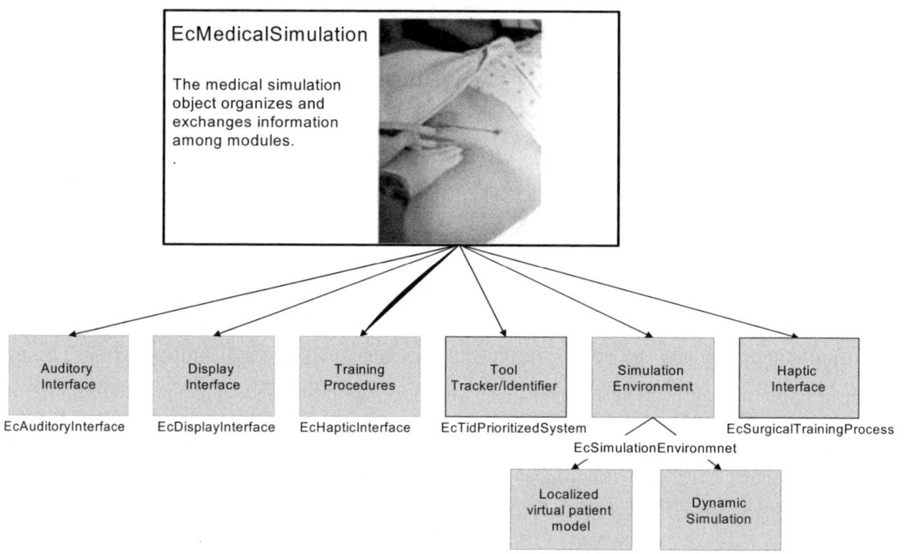

Figure 1: The relationship among the simulation and the top-level modules. The system is described with XML, allowing modules to be exchanged for different surgical procedures.

2. Development of Regional Anesthesia Simulator

We have been developing a realistic regional anesthesia training simulator. We use 3D machine vision algorithms to track hand and anesthesia instrument movements using video cameras. This is coupled with an innovative untethered haptic feedback device that imposes simulated force on free-moving needles for the regional anesthesia simulator. Our design, illustrated in Figure 1, allows any module to be easily exchanged. This design is configured using the Extensible Markup Language (XML), a method for creating text-based languages for computer understanding. Each of the modules shown in Figure 1 can be exchanged through XML. The design is well suited to interface with SCORM compliant contents [5].

Our software architecture is organized into six modules with the simulation environment further decomposed into two additional modules. Each module shown in Figure 1 can connect to any implementation that meets its interface. This organization allows the easy exchange of functionality using XML.

3. Development of Localized Virtual Patient Model

In this research, we have investigated and defined a localized patient model for the regional anesthesia simulator. Complete live human patient models are not available for research and simulator development today. Building a complex whole body virtual patient model is an extraordinary development effort. In order to have a complete regional anesthesia simulator, we focused on developing an efficient method to model the virtual patient reactions. This is especially important in the case of stimulator based nerve block procedures where a stimulator is used to identify needle proximity to the nerve.

We have defined the following functions for the regional anesthesia simulator: 1) high-fidelity anatomical structures required to develop the proposed nerve block procedures (i.e., Brachial Plexus block and Femoral nerve block), 2) vascular information, 3) complications of nerve blocks (possible hematoma, nerve injuries, systemic toxicity or intravascular injections), 4) neural-sensory information [6], 5) neural-muscular-skeletal movement [7], 6) visualization of the above behaviors, and 7) simulation of the voice / speech feedback. We have focused mainly on the trainee-stimulator interaction at the beginning. For the femoral nerve block case, for instance, we primarily consider the needle proximity to key landmarks throughout its insertion path. The simulation will take local nerve stimulation signals and generates an appropriate muscle contraction. The muscle stimulation force may be considered as a pure disturbance force source in the model. The sensory nerve reacts to the stimulation accordingly, and it influences the adjacent muscle/motor nerve directly.

3.1 Anatomic Structure

Figure 2 shows a partial anatomic structure of our 3D virtual patient model from Zygote (www.zygote.com). It has accurate nerves, vessels, muscular-skeletal structure information for our regional anesthesia procedure. The quality of visualization was achieved using Energid viewer.

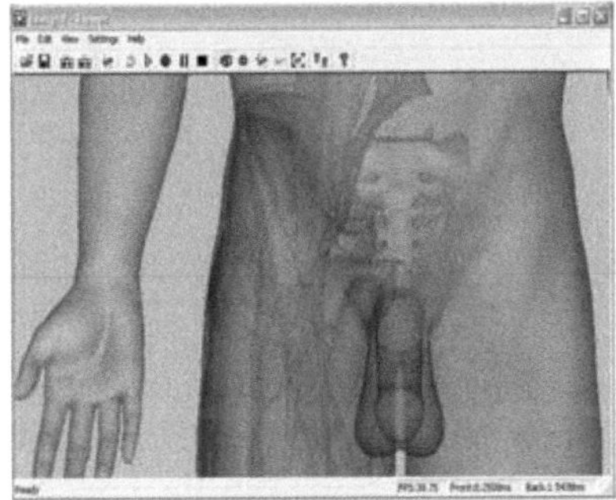

Figure 2: A partial anatomic structure of virtual patient model in Energid's viewer display.

3.2 Nerve Block Complications

The anesthesiologist's familiarity with anatomy, block technique, and potential complications are the most important determinants of the procedure's success. We have defined the immediate complications and the appropriate response for the success nerve block and used to assess the performance of participants. With our advanced rendering methods based on Open Scene Graph, we visualize the complications of nerve blocks, such as bleeding, tissue irregularities, swelling, shock, and so on, in our simulator.

3.3 Neuro-Muscular-Skeletal Movement

Effective muscle modeling requires taking into account the muscles specific contractile properties. The forces induced in the muscle (depending on its length and shortening velocity) must be modeled by considering their actual fiber-oriented distribution through the volume as well as for their resulting force at the tendon extremity.

We have designed a muscular skeletal model for motor reflexive responses during a nerve block procedure. Figure 3 shows the muscular-skeletal leg model (left). A mechanical lumped-parameter model of the human muscle representing the mechanical phenomena involved in a real muscle contraction has been constructed according to the Hill muscle model [8] for our motor-muscle-skeletal movement simulation (Figure 3, right). Though the proposed approach may be convenient in practice for simulating muscle contraction, its appropriateness for effectively representing the mechanical behaviors should be verified. Given the complexity of the muscle, the determination of the individual muscle forces from the joint efforts is an indeterminate problem. Therefore, we will perform an optimization analysis and force prediction for parameter estimation of the mechanical model with experimental investigations.

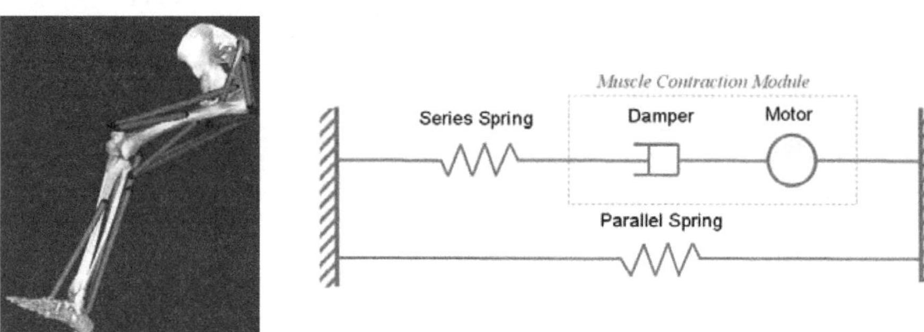

Figure 3: Muscular-skeletal model. On the left is a muscular-skeletal model for a lower extremity and on the right shows muscle modeling. Using Hill's three-element muscle model [8], a mechanical lumped parameter model of muscle is shown in the right side.

3.4 Neural Sensory Functions

Use of a nerve stimulator has the advantages of continuous feedback and a definite endpoint for locating the nerve. When the motor nerve is not responding well, the nerve sensory feedback becomes most important in the regional anesthesia simulation. We are in the process to define the boundary of reaction region for a critical sensory nerve (see Figure 4). When a needle is inserted in a patient body, a redefined region of nerve sensing is used to generate sensory responses and reflexive body responses under the needle stimulation.

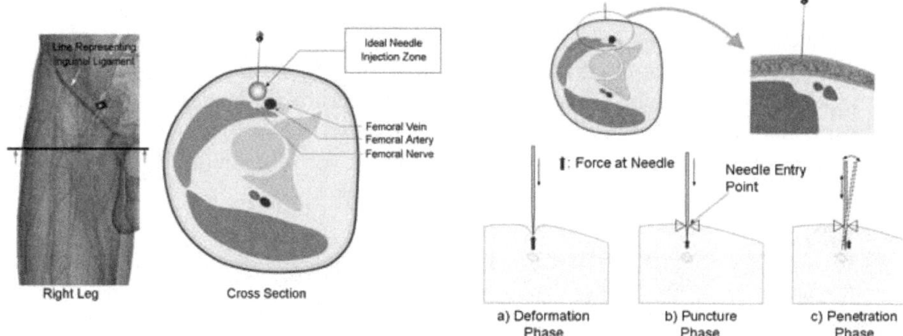

Figure 4: Boundary of reaction region for a critical sensory nerve, i.e., 'ideal needle injection zone'.

Figure 5: Distinct phases of needle insertion procedure

3.5 Real-time Tissue Deformation Modeling

With the goal of developing realistic simulation of the nerve block scenarios, we use a mesh-free physics-based computational technique for simulating the realistic force response as well as visual deformations in real time [4]. Unlike traditional mesh-based finite element methods (FEMs), large tissue deformations are particularly easy to handle since interpolation functions are compactly supported on spherical subdomains which may intersect and overlap and are not constrained to abut each other as they are in FEM. The insertion of the block needle is extremely complex and requires precision on the part of the anesthesiologist.

We compute the reaction force at the tip of needle and deformation profile before the primary puncture of tissue occurs using our mesh-free based computational scheme. The sudden drop in tip force will be observed after the maximum force. Upon puncture, the friction force will be dominant along the needle inside the tissue, and is due to friction, tissue adhesion, and damping. We characterize the following three distinct interactions between block needle and tissue and illustrate these three phases in Figure 5: a) deformation phase, b) puncture phase, and c) penetration Phase. During the penetration of block needle into tissue, the trainee may correct the insertion angle and path to find the proper drug injection site. We leave the measurement and quantification of the axial and bending forces acting on needle for our future study.

We have shown in Figure 6 a virtual needle insertion for the femoral nerve block. To illustrate the versatility of our rendering capability, the skin has been made transparent so the student can view exactly where the needle tip is located.

4. Conclusion and Future Work

In this research, we have established the software architecture of simulation and functional modules of localized virtual patient model. We have been successful in a simulation of real-time tissue deformation using a promising mesh-free algorithm. Our virtual patient model covers visualization of dynamic simulation in patient reflexive responses and the needle insertion process, and it also provides haptic rendering for force feedback. By measuring the needle proximity to various nerves, we accurately model the patient's expected physiological response. We store the database to simulate an accurate muscle contract and reaction, such as leg-kicking, caused by the corresponding nerves.

In this project, we are in the process of incorporating the articulated components in the virtual patient models. This will allow us to accurately model muscle twitching (such as the "dancing patella" seen during a femoral nerve block) as a function of needle tip to nerve proximity and stimulator current. We are continuing to implement our design in localized virtual patient model for the nerve stimulation and reflexive responses in the femoral nerve block procedure.

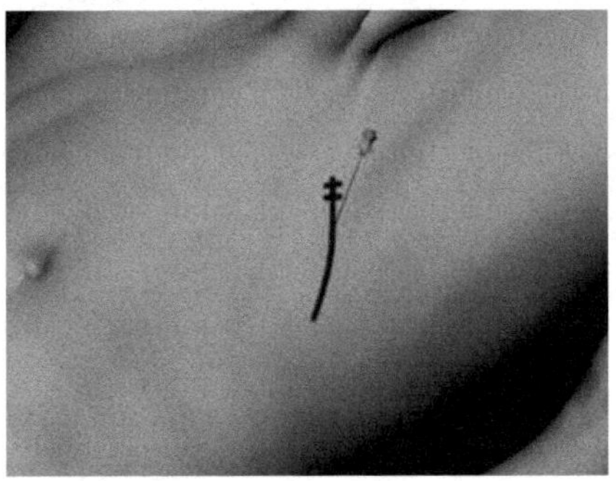 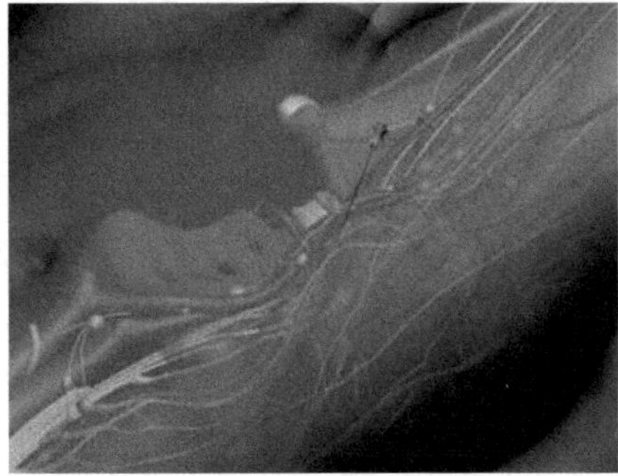

Figure 6: Needle insertion for the femoral nerve block. The right hand side shows where the needle is in proximity to femoral nerve and other structures.

Acknowledgements

The authors gratefully acknowledge the important support and guidance of Dr. Kenneth Curley. The work described above has been partially supported by the U.S. Army's Telemedicine and Advanced Technology Research Center through the direction of Dr. Kenneth Curley. The advice from Dr. Chester Buckenmaier and Dr. Scott Croll at Walter Reed Army Medical Center was also highly appreciated.

References

[1]   New York School of Regional Anesthesia: www.nysona.com.
[2]   Hu, J. SBIR Phase I Final Report of Regional Anesthesia Simulation for Training of Resident and Staff Pain Management Specialists, Contract W81XWH-06-C-0052, August 16, 2006.
[3]   A. Liu, F. Tendick, K. Cleary, and C. Kaufmann, A Survey of Surgical Simulation: Applications, Technology, and Education, *Presence: Teleoperators and Virtual Environments,* vol. 12, issue 6, Dec. 2003.
[4]   S. De, Y.-J. Lim, and M.A. Srinivasan, Point-Associated Finite Field (PAFF) Approach for Physically-based Digital Surgery, *Presence: Teleoperators and Virtual Environments,* 15 (3), pp 294-308, 2006.
[5]   P. Dodds and S. Thropp, SCORM 2004 2nd Edition Overview, *Advanced Distributed Learning,* July 22, 2004.
[6]   T. A. McMahon, Muscles, Reflexes, and Locomotion, *Princeton University Press,* Princeton, New Jersey, 1984.
[7]   G. Taga, A Model of the Neuro-musculo-skeletal System for Human Locomotion: I. Emergence of Basic Gait, *Biological Cybernetics,* 73:97-111.
[8]   A.V. Hill, The heat of shortening and the dynamic constants of muscle, *Proceedings of the Royal Society of London, Series B, Biological Sciences,* Volume 126, Issue 843, pp. 136-195, 24, 1938.

Medicine Meets Virtual Reality 15
J.D. Westwood et al. (Eds.)
IOS Press, 2007

Surface Exploration Using Instruments: The Perception of Friction

Cindy HUNG[a], Adam DUBROWSKI[b], David GONZALEZ[a], and Heather CARNAHAN[b,c,1]
aDepartment of Kinesiology, University of Waterloo
bDepartment of Surgery, University of Toronto
cDepartment of Occupational Science and Occupational Therapy & Toronto Rehabilitation Institute, University of Toronto

Abstract. The purpose of this study was to investigate the ability to discriminate friction during surface exploration using a finger and surgical instrument under normal vision and when vision was absent. Participants explored surfaces with either with the finger or with an instrument and rated the slipperiness. Results showed that the explorations with the instrument were estimated to be more slippery and less sensitive than those for the finger. There were no effects for visual condition. This study showed that novices who use instruments to make estimations of tissue slipperiness require practice and training in order to adequately perceive friction. Novices' reduced ability to perceive friction with instruments should be integrated into simulator design.

Keywords. touch, haptics, learning, slipperiness, motor control

1. Introduction

Understanding how instrument use can aid in discriminating surface friction has implications for the development of high fidelity simulation. Friction is defined as the minimal force used to initiate and maintain sliding of a given weight on a particular surface. Using the ratio of the tangential force to the normal force, and is perceived as slipperiness [1]. It is not clear how friction is perceived when using an instrument. Brydges et al. found that using tools can decrease tactile sensitivity during texture discriminations [2]. This deficit to the haptic system is compensated through monitoring the vibrations of the tools across a surface. However, this strategy cannot be used as an efficient source of information to construct perceptual estimations of slipperiness since texture and friction have different physical properties, triggering different haptic perceptions.

The focus on these haptic perceptions regarding instrument use can be useful in applied settings when indirect touch is relied upon. During laparoscopic surgery, blood or other tissues, may obstruct the surgeon's visual field requiring the

---

[1] Corresponding Author. Heather Carnahan, Department of Surgery, The Wilson Center, 200 Elizabeth St., 1 ES 559, Toronto, ON, Canada, M5G 2C4
Email: heather.carnahan@gmail.com

surgeon to rely solely on his or her tactile sensation through the instrument. While visual information has been shown to play an important role in texture discrimination, it is not clear what role vision plays in friction discrimination. This is important because many simulators use vision only to simulate haptic experiences.

1.1 Purpose & Hypotheses

The purpose of the present study is to investigate the ability to discriminate friction during object exploration using a finger and surgical instrument under normal vision and when vision is absent. It is hypothesized that friction will not be perceived well when a surgical instrument is used because there is an indirect contact between the explored surface and the receptors in the finger and that vision will not augment friction discrimination when exploring with a instrument.

2. Method

2.1 Apparatus & Procedure

Twelve right-handed undergraduates participated (7 females, 5 males, mean age = 22 years old). Glass microscope slides were explored either with no coating, or with spray glue (3M spray adhesive), liquid honey or personal lubricant (K-Y liquid). To measure exploration velocity, an Optotrak system was used to track a 2mm marker that was attached to either the nail bed of the index finger, or to the tip of the instrument. They were presented with the range of potential substances by exploring the two extreme surfaces (glue being the least slippery and lubricant being the most slippery), prior to the experiment. The explorations were made with both the right index finger and the tip of an instrument, using an 8 cm left to right sweeping motion (paced at 1 Hz with a metronome). The instrument used was surgical snaps, which is a metal, scissor-like instrument with a blunt end, designed for tissue exploration during surgical procedures. Participants were instructed to hold the surgical snaps at the base of their palm, with their index finger placed along the shaft of the instrument. Following each exploration, participants were instructed to rate the slipperiness of the surfaces on an 18 point visual analog scale [2,3]. There were two visual conditions in this experiment: vision and no vision. All trials of one visual condition were completed within a block and the order of visual conditions was counterbalanced across participants. Each of the four surfaces was explored randomly six times in each visual condition, with both the finger and the instrument. Thus, each participant completed a total of ninety-six trials.

2.2 Statistical Analysis

Data were analyzed in separate 2 probe (index finger, instrument) x 2 visual condition (vision, no vision) x 4 surface (glue, control, honey, lubricant), repeated measures analyses of variance (ANOVAs). Effects significant at $p < 0.05$ were further analyzed using Tukey HSD post hoc method for comparison of means.

3. Results

3.1 Perceptual Estimates

The coefficient of friction was highest for the glue (.24), intermediate for the plain glass (.10) and honey (.065) and lowest for the lubricant (.05). The explorations made by the participants with the instrument were estimated to be more slippery and less sensitive than those for the finger. When using the finger, participants judged the higher friction surfaces as least slippery, and the low friction surfaces were estimated to be more slippery (F (3, 33) = 50.69, p <.01). There were no statistically significant effects for visual condition.

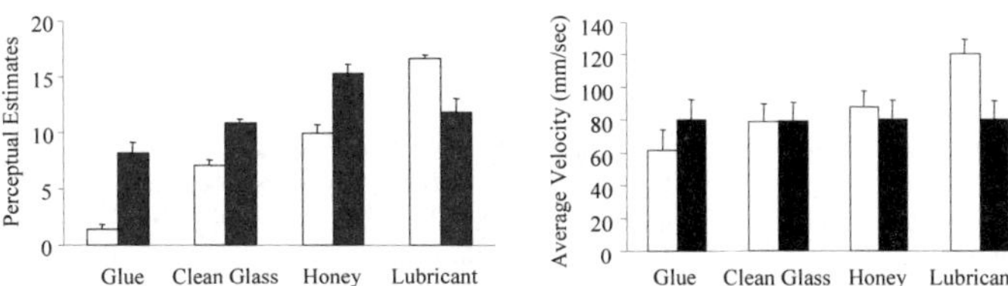

Figure 1. Perceptual estimates and average velocity of exploration for the finger (white bars) and the instrument (black bars), for each of the surfaces.

3.2 Average Velocity

The average velocities of the surface explorations were faster for the finger than the instrument. For the finger, the most slippery substance had the fastest average velocity; whereas the least slippery substance had the slowest average velocity. For the instrument, the average velocity during exploration was not statistically different F (3, 33) = 25.56, p <.01.

4. Discussion

The present study showed that the participants were able to accurately perceive surface friction using the finger and when using the surgical snaps, surface friction was not perceived as well. The removal of vision had no impact on the perception of slipperiness in either exploratory condition. Velocity was not used to make inferences about surface friction when exploring with the instrument, probably leading to the less accurate perception of slipperiness in comparison to exploring with the finger (where velocity cues were used). This study has shown that novices who use instruments to make estimations of tissue slipperiness require practice and training in order to adequately perceive friction. The ability of novices to perceive friction with instruments should be integrated into simulator design.

5. References

[1] G. Cadoret, G., A.M. Smith, Friction, not texture dictates grip forces during object manipulation, *Journal of Neurophysiology* **75** (1996), 1863-1869.
[2] R. Brydges, et al. Surface exploration using laparoscopic surgical instruments: The perception of surface roughness, *Ergonomics* **48** (2005), 874-94.
[3] A.M. Smith, et al. Role of friction and tangential force variation in the subjective scaling of tactile roughness, *Experimental Brain Research* **144** (2002), 211- 223.

Medicine Meets Virtual Reality 15
J.D. Westwood et al. (Eds.)
IOS Press, 2007

An Interactive, Cognitive Simulation of Gastroesophageal Reflux Disease

Bruce JARRELL[a], MD, Sergei NIRENBURG[b], PhD, Marjorie MCSHANE[b], PhD,
George FANTRY[a], MD, Stephen BEALE[b], PhD, David MALLOTT[a], MD,
John RACZEK[a]
[a] *University of Maryland School of Medicine*
[b] *University of Maryland Baltimore County*

Abstract. The Maryland Virtual Patient (MVP) Project seeks to create realistically functioning virtual humans endowed with automatic physiological and cognitive function that can be used in the training of medical personnel. Physiologically, the state of an MVP changes in response to internal pathophysiological stimuli and external stimuli, the latter initiated by either by the patient or the trainee. Cognitively, the MVP can communicate with trainees about current symptoms, lifestyle, history, adherence to prescribed treatments, etc. We will demonstrate simulation in the MVP environment using the example of patients suffering from gastroesophageal reflux disease (GERD).

Keywords. cognitive simulation, virtual patient, medical education

Introduction

Clinical decision making skills are developed through practice on live patients. We train our physicians using the mix of live patients available at the time of training and trust that the knowledge acquired by managing this cohort of patients will be sufficient to generalize to all patients. Even though this is a tried and true method, it has many drawbacks related to patient safety, lack of objective measures for competence, and the inconsistency of the learning experience with respect to types of diseases, variations in the presentation or course of the disease, and individual patient differences. We need more opportunities to expose our trainees to sufficient patient scenarios in order to foster mastery of the complex knowledge needed daily by practicing physicians.

Computer-based simulation is one way to address the shortcomings of current clinical training practices. For simulation to be effective, it must expose the student to virtual patients that demonstrate sophisticated, realistic behaviors; it must allow open-ended patient investigation by the student (learning through self-discovery); and it must provide each student with a population of patients suffering from a given disease, with each patient displaying clinically relevant variations on the disease theme. Such variations might involve the path or speed of disease progression, the profile and severity of symptoms, responses to treatments, and secondary diseases or disorders that affect treatment choices. If each student could independently manage the care of many such patients – especially in a context in which trial and error learning carried no risk – we hypothesize that the decision making skills of each student would develop faster than with traditional training methods alone. In the Maryland Virtual Patient (MVP)[1,2] project we are developing a simulation and tutoring environment to test this hypothesis.

Before launching full-scale work on this project, exploratory observational exercises were conducted with medical students at the University of Maryland School of Medicine to understand the specifications for effective interaction with a simulated patient [1].[3] In the exercises, the students managed several structured patients in electronic and manual simulations. All the exercises employed patient management problems used routinely in teaching and focused on high-level decision-making, such as the proposal and proof of an inference or the substantiation of an intervention. The most notable observations from this and a follow-up study of simulation for medical training were [1]:

- The simulation must accommodate trial and error patient management with multiple clinically plausible pathways to a solution.

- Changes in patient anatomy and physiology resulting from user action or disease processes over time must result in a consistent appropriate alteration of the state of the patient.

- The representation of time-related patient activities is critical for successful simulation, including allowing the user to "advance the clock" to the next phase of patient management.

In addition to these capabilities, the following are being incorporated into the MVP environment: chronic and acute disorders; simple and complex diseases; knowledge about well-understood and poorly-understood disease processes; knowledge spanning all levels, from gene to organism to population; complications of diseases and treatment modalities; and automatic tutoring. Among the most important conceptual aspects of MVP simulation is automaticity, which refers to the fact that the state of an MVP changes in a realistic way over time and in response to internal (physiological and pathological) and external (clinical and behavioral) stimuli.

Elicitation and Encoding of Knowledge

The MVP project centers on an ontology-based model of the physiological and cognitive processes affecting the virtual patient. We encode knowledge about biophysical functions that have clinical relevance in the maintenance of health, the production of disease, and the bidirectional transitions between these two states. When biomechanisms are known, they are modeled using causal chains. Where gaps exist in our knowledge of explicit biomechanisms, they are bridged in various ways – with non-biomechanistic knowledge from the literature, practical clinical knowledge, situational knowledge, observations, probabilistic methods, etc. This integration of implicit and explicit knowledge reflects precisely what a clinician employs when working with a patient. Further, the depth and granularity of this knowledge are determined by the demands of automatic function and realism. Thus, MVPs need not include every mechanism known to biology and clinical medicine.

---

[1] Patent pending.
[2] This research was supported by Department of Defense grant #17-03-2-001.
[3] The exercises were conducted under IRB Exemption No. BJ-090103 for the project entitled "Computer Simulation as an Aid to Enhancing Medical Education."

Diseases are modeled as changes in key property values over time. For each disease, a set number of conceptual stages is established, and typical values (or ranges of values) for each property are associated with each stage. Values at the start or end of each stage are recorded explicitly, with values between stages being interpolated. The disease model includes a combination of fixed and variable features. For example, although the number of stages for a given disease is fixed, the duration of each stage is variable; similarly, although the values for *some* physiological properties undergo fixed changes across patients, the values for other physiological properties are variable within a specified range. Therefore, on the one hand, each disease model is sufficiently constrained so that MVPs suffering from the disease must show appropriate physiological manifestations of it, while on the other hand, each disease model is sufficiently flexible to permit instances of MVPs to differ in clinically relevant ways, as selected by the author of each MVP instance.

Once an approach to modeling a given disease has been devised and all requisite details have been elicited, the disease-related events and their participants are encoded in ontologically-grounded scripts written in the metalanguage employed in the OntoSem environment.[4] Scripts represent typical sequences of events and their causal and temporal relationships. In other words, they encode how individual events hold well-defined places in routine, typical sequences of events that happen in the world, with a well-specified set of objects filling different roles throughout that sequence. For example, if the event is swallowing, there is only one animate participant (the swallower), but many other objects play necessary roles: various nerves and muscles act as instruments of peristalsis; the swallowed bolus is the theme of peristalsis-driven motion events; the stomach is the final destination of the bolus, and so on. Scripts normally contain subscripts and can be more or less fine-grained depending on the goals of the given simulation. Within the MVP project we have developed both domain scripts and workflow scripts. Domain scripts describe basic physiology, disease progression and responses to treatments, whereas workflow scripts model the way an expert physician would handle a case, thus forming the knowledge substrate for automatic tutoring.

The OntoSem ontology differs from others not only in its inclusion of scripts, but also in its rich inventory of properties, both attributes and relations (most other ontologies, e.g., UMLS [3], are actually hierarchical word nets rather than knowledge-rich ontologies). As we expand the OntoSem general-purpose ontology into the medical domain, we are incorporating, where possible, the terminology used by the Foundational Model of Anatomy [4].

Reasoning with Knowledge

MVPs are modeled as "double agents" with both physiological and cognitive functions. Physiologically, the state of an MVP changes in response to internal pathophysiological stimuli and external stimuli, the latter initiated either by the patient or the trainee. Cognitively, the MVP can communicate with trainees about current symptoms, lifestyle, history, adherence to prescribed treatments, etc. Structured knowledge in the disease model acts as input to the simulation engine. The simulation

---

[4] OntoSem is the implementation of the theory of Ontological Semantics, a theory originally developed for knowledge-rich text processing (Nirenburg and Rakin 2004).

can run in clinical mode, where patient symptoms and physiology are known only through questions and diagnostic tests, or in omniscient mode, in which all patient properties can be monitored throughout the simulation. As an example of automaticity in response to external interventions, students are permitted to prescribe any treatment available in the system at any time, with the MVP responding accordingly. If, for example, the student launches an inappropriate treatment, the MVP's state may or may not change, but certainly will not produce the intended result. Upon recognizing this undesirable result, the student can attempt to recover from the mistake, for example by withdrawing the treatment or introducing a different one. The effect of recovery attempts are interpreted relative to encoded knowledge and the current state of the MVP. The system does not exhaustively list all permutations of paths a trainee could take and all consequential responses of the MVP; instead, it relies on ontologically-grounded descriptions of basic physiology, disease processes, effects of treatments, and so on, so that the state of a given MVP at a given time will, quite literally, fall out of the underlying model.

Authoring Instances of MVPs

A cornerstone in creating a realistic MVP environment is providing for wide variation among instances of MVPs with a given disease. That is, the basic model of a disease includes all relevant tracks (i.e., paths of progression), and each track provides many choice points that differentiate cases. Among the many tasks carried out by the author of a disease model is the selection of properties to be tracked, their ranges of values, and the defaults for those values. Such a disease model is then concretized into a given patient instance by an instance author, who is typically a physician-teacher or disease specialist. The instance author determines the MVP's basic physiological properties, relevant lifestyle factors, the rate of progression of the disease, which path the disease takes at all possible furcations, the specific symptom profile at given times, and so on. This process has been reduced to an electronic multiple-choice questionnaire that takes little time to complete. The simplicity of authoring patient instances derives from the care taken to create the basic model of the disease, including delineating exactly which property values are available for individual parameterization and which ones are fixed for all patients experiencing the given stage of a disease. As soon as the values (or defaults) for all relevant properties are chosen, the patient instance is available for use.

Results

Knowledge Elicitation. The MVP project places significant demands on authors of disease models to render complex, multi-scale functions in a form that can be implemented computationally. The knowledge elicitation process is a collaboration between the model author and a knowledge engineer, who mediates between the physician and the programmer. Physicians must distill their extensive and tightly coupled physiological and clinical knowledge into the most relevant subset, and express it in the most concrete of terms. Not infrequently, they are also called upon to hypothesize about the unknowable, like the state of a patient experiencing a pre-clinical stage of disease, or the state of a patient after an effective treatment that is never, in real life, followed up by objective tests. Such hypotheses reflect the mental models of given experts, which might differ in subtle ways from those of other experts. However, such differences, we would suggest, have little bearing on the ultimate goal of this enterprise: to create MVPs whose behavior is sufficiently life-like to further specific teaching goals.

Disease Simulation. We chose to initially model esophageal disease because the esophagus is a relatively uncomplicated organ and because one of the symptoms of esophageal disease, chest pain, can cause significant diagnostic dilemmas with cardiac disease. Knowledge about the normal and abnormal anatomy and physiology of the esophagus was elicited from model authors and recorded. The two common mechanisms for gastroesophageal reflux disease (GERD) – a decreased Lower Esophageal Sphincter Pressure (LESP) and Transient LES Relaxation (TLESR) – and all relevant clinical forms of GERD were modeled. The latter included: non-erosive GERD; GERD with erosive esophagitis, stricture, Barrett's metaplasia and adenocarcinoma; and proximal GERD. In addition, diseases potentially associated with GERD, including scleroderma, Zenker's Diverticulum and achalasia, were modeled. For achalasia and scleroderma, which are diseases with a poorly understood esophageal pathophysiology, property values of the MVP change as a function of passing time, since the disease natural history can only be clinically observed rather than explained using causal chains. By contrast, for GERD, which has a well understood pathophysiology, the disease model is driven by causal chains that reflect current biomedical thinking.

Causal chain modeling is a particularly potent strategy that allows expanded opportunities for automatic function in virtual patients:

- A new disease can be generated as a side-effect of another disease: for example GERD is automatically initiated in any patient whose LESP drops below 10, which can occur due to scleroderma or after a successful surgical intervention for achalasia.

- The rate of progression of a disease can be automatically determined: for example, a patient with an LESP of 0 (after a successful Heller myotomy) will have a faster progression of GERD than a patient with an LESP of 9 (after a successful pneumatic dilation).

- The effects of interventions can be automatically determined: for example, whether GERD is progressing or healing is determined by the daily total time in acid reflux (TTAR). TTAR is determined by total time in reflux – which can be altered in some patients by changes in lifestyle, and by the acidity of the refluxed substance – which can be affected medication.

Upon testing, the MVP has functioned accurately, including reasoning effectively when responding to both expected and unexpected user actions.

Discussion

We have designed a simulation system that has demonstrated complex, automatic behavior. Thus far, it has a limited repertoire of esophageal physiology, pathophysiology, and clinical management for common esophageal diseases. In spite of the limited repertoire, we believe that MVPs represent a conceptual leap in the computer modeling of humans in the continuum of health and disease. MVPs display realistic function in simulations where they can be observed, interacted with, and treated by students. Variability of selected parameters permits a wide variety of instances of virtual patients to be created from the same ontologically-grounded disease model. We have honed our approaches to knowledge elicitation, script writing and incorporating scripts into the simulation engine. We are now positioned to test our hypothesis that trial and error management of MVPs can teach students the basics of clinical medicine as well as, or better than, bedside teaching or small group teaching. In fact, there is evidence that learning by working through computer-based scenarios can be very effective: for example, in the evaluation of the SHERLOCK II system, which teaches electronics troubleshooting, it was reported that technicians learned more from using this system for 24 hours than from 4 years of work in the field [5].

Two components are necessary for a trainee to learn clinical medicine: an inventory of patients showing clinically relevant variations of disease, and a tutor to guide the student (as necessary) and to validate that his or her success derives from accurate and sufficient knowledge. We have recently implemented the first version of the tutor for esophageal diseases.

Our work on tutoring has been informed by results from the CIRCSIM group, which has been pursuing automatic tutoring strategies for the diagnostics and treatment of the baroreceptor reflex. The current CIRCSIM-Tutor evolved from a system that offered students a dynamic mathematical model with no tutoring support into a system that offers tutoring without the dynamic mathematical model (results of certain scenarios were stored and are deemed sufficient for the given educational goals). The contrast with MVP is clear: for us, the autonomous functioning of MVPs is, and will remain, central, with tutoring being interpreted as a useful option alongside trial-and-error learning.

We are also currently working on incorporating natural language interaction into the system, with the current mode of interaction being menu-driven (that is, the trainee is presented with inventories of questions, diagnostic tests, treatments, hypotheses and diagnoses to choose from). The desire to incorporate natural language interaction into tutoring systems has been expressed by developers of many tutoring systems. Unlike others, however, our group has been working on knowledge-based natural language processing (NLP) for some twenty years. In fact, the OntoSem ontology, knowledge representation language, and many of the processors that are serving as a substrate for the MVP system were all originally developed for NLP applications. Therefore, we have confidence in our ability to incorporate natural language support into the MVP environment in the near term.

References

[1] D. Mallott, J. Raczek, C. Skinner, K. Jarrell, M. Shimko and B. Jarrell. 2005. A basis for electronic cognitive simulation: the heuristic patient. *Surgical Innovations* March, 12(1):43-9.
[2] S. Nirenburg and V. Raskin. 2004. *Ontological Semantics.* The MIT Press.
[3] O. Bodenreider. 2004. The Unified Medical Language System (UMLS): Integrating biomedical terminology. *Nucleic Acids Research* 32: 267-270.
[4] C. Rosse and J.L.V. Mejino. 2004. A reference ontology for bioinformatics: The Foundational Model of Anatomy. *Journal of Biomedical Informatics.*
[5] M. Evens and J. Michael. 2006. *One-on-One Tutoring by Humans and Computers.* New Jersey and London: Lawrence Erlbaum and Associates, Publishers.

Medicine Meets Virtual Reality 15
J.D. Westwood et al. (Eds.)
IOS Press, 2007

A Stable Cutting Method for Finite Elements based Virtual Surgery Simulation

Lenka JEŘÁBKOVÁ [a,1], Jakub JEŘÁBEK [b], Rostislav CHUDOBA [b] and
Torsten KUHLEN [a]

[a] *Virtual Reality Group, RWTH Aachen University, Germany*
[b] *Chair of Structural Statics and Dynamics, RWTH Aachen University, Germany*

Abstract. In this paper we present a novel approach for stable interactive cutting of deformable objects in virtual environments. Our method is based on the extended finite elements method, allowing for a modeling of discontinuities without remeshing. As no new elements are created, the impact on simulation performance is minimized. We also propose an appropriate mass lumping technique to guarantee for the stability of the simulation regardless of the position of the cut.

Keywords. Surgical simulation, finite elemets method, cutting, virtual reality

Introduction

Surgical simulation is an important field of application in virtual reality (VR). A virtual surgery trainer can not only help to improve the surgeons' skills, it also solves ethical issues related to training on animals or humans. Numerous surgical training systems have been developed in the last decade. The main requirement for a surgery simulator is the plausible deformation of the soft tissue in realtime and its interactive manipulation using various surgical instruments. The majority of current surgical simulators use the finite elements method (FEM) for tissue deformation. Simulation objects are represented using a volumetric mesh of tetrahedral elements. An interactive cutting simulation is an essential feature of a surgery trainer. However, the interactive progressive cutting of a deformable FEM mesh is a challenging problem. The number and quality of the FEM elements have a direct impact on the simulation performance and stability. Although a number of different approaches have been presented recently, the problems have not been solved satisfyingly.

1. Related Work

The methods for surgical cutting published so far require the FEM elements to be aligned with the cut. This is achieved either by constraining the cut to the borders of existing

---

[1]Corresponding Author: Lenka Jeřábková, Virtual Reality Group, RWTH Aachen University, Seffenter Weg 23, 52062 Aachen, Germany; E-mail: jerabkova@rz.rwth-aachen.de.

elements [1] at the cost of creating unpleasing visual artifacts, or by splitting the elements along the cut [2,3,4]. [5] generate a minimal set of new elements to replace the cut tetrahedron. The main drawback of this group of methods is the creation of small ill-shaped elements (slivers) leading to numerical instability of the simulation. To avoid the drawback of the previous methods, [6] snaps the nodes of the existing elements to the trajectory of the cut. Although no new elements are created, this method can still lead to degenerated elements, which are then detected and removed. Moreover, if the snapping distance is large, the parameters of the mesh have to be updated. [7] use a combination of snapping and subdivision. However, they only support nonprogressive cutting.

2. Contributions

Our approach is based on the extended finite elements method (XFEM) as proposed in [8]. The XFEM can effectively model discontinuity regions, e.g., cracks or cuts, within an FEM mesh. We prove the suitability of the XFEM method for interactive cutting of deformable objects as used in a surgery simulator. Instead of actually remeshing the FEM mesh during the cuttin process, discontinuous nodal enrichment functions are added together with new nodal degrees of freedom. As no new elements are created, the impact on simulation performance is minimized. We show, that for the linear tetrahedron, which is the most commonly used element in interactive FEM simulations, the enrichment operation does not require any other computations than determining the size of the dissected volumes. The remeshing based methods suffer from stability problems when small parts of the tissue are separated. The reasons for the instability are twofold. First, ill-shaped elements are created, and second, the masses of the new elements are very low. As in the XFEM method no new elements are created, no ill-shaped elements are added. The choice of an appropriate mass lumping technique is the key to a stable dynamic simulation using XFEM. We propose a mass lumping approach that guarantees the stability of the dynamic simulation regardless of the location of the cut.

3. Modeling Discontinuities using XFEM

In simple terms, the FEM approximates the displacement field using a mesh of elements connected at nodes. The deformation of the object is given by the displacement of the nodes according to the acting external and internal forces. In a VR simulation the applied forces change in time and the virtual objects have to react to them in real time. Therefore, the FEM has to be simulated dynamically. Mass and damping factors are added to the static deformation forces $\mathbb{K}\mathbf{u}$, in order to account for inertia and energy dissipation. The dynamic deformation is described by the following formula.

$$\mathbb{M}\ddot{\mathbf{u}} + \mathbb{D}\dot{\mathbf{u}} + \mathbb{K}\mathbf{u} = \mathbf{f}, \tag{1}$$

where $\mathbb{M}$ is the mass matrix, $\mathbb{D}$ is the damping matrix, $\mathbb{K}$ is the global stiffness matrix, $\mathbf{u}$ is the vector of nodal displacements and $\mathbf{f}$ is the external load. The left hand side of Equation 1 corresponds to the object's internal forces, whereas the right hand side corresponds to the external load.

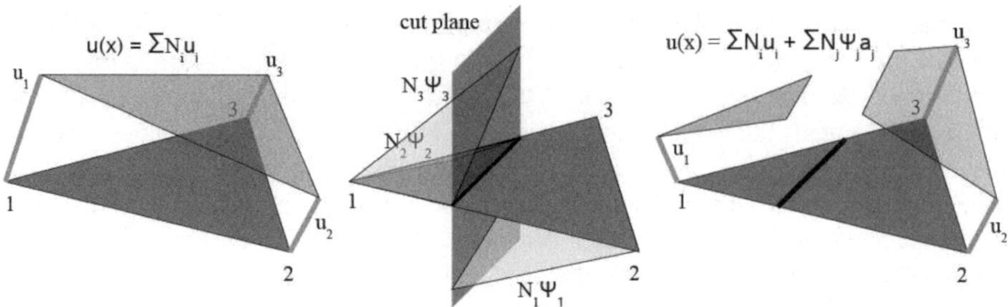

Figure 1. The effect of a discontinuous enrichment of a triangle element. In FEM, the nodal displacements are interpolated in order to get a continuous displacement within an element (left). The discontinuous enrichment functions (middle) lead to a discontinuous displacement field (right).

Element shape functions are used to interpolate the displacement within an element from the nodal displacements. The displacement of an arbitrary point x can be computed as

$$\mathbf{u}(x) = \sum_{i=1}^{n} N_i(x)\mathbf{u}_i \tag{2}$$

where n is the number of element nodes, N_i are the element shape functions and $\mathbf{u}_i$ are the displacements of the element nodes. For a linear tetrahedron, the shape functions are identical to the barycentric coordinates and the resulting displacement is a linear interpolation of the nodal displacements (Fig. 1 left).

When a discontinuity has to be added, the surrounding mesh nodes are enriched by an additional discontinuous function and the corresponding number of nodal degrees of freedom is added.

$$\mathbf{u}(x) = \sum_{i=1}^{n} N_i(x)\mathbf{u}_i + \sum_{j=1}^{m} N_j(x)\psi_j(x)\mathbf{a}_j \tag{3}$$

where m is the number of enriched nodes, N_j are the nodal shape functions of the added nodal degrees of freedom $\mathbf{a}_j$, $\psi(x)$ is the discontinuous enrichment function. The enrichment function can be any arbitrary discontinuous function provided that it is discontinuous over the crack or cut domain. Figure 1 shows the effect of a discontinuous enrichment of a triangle element in a three dimensional space.

The new nodal degrees of freedom $\mathbf{a}$ are added to the vector of displacements $\mathbf{u}$. The vector of forces has to be extended as well, in order to match the dimensions of the system, although the external load corresponding to the enriched degrees of freedom is zero. In the following sections, we will explain how the enriched stiffness and mass matrices are computed. The damping matrix is typically a linear combination of the stiffness and mass matrices.

3.1. The Enriched Stiffness Matrix

The stiffness matrix of the enriched element has the form

$$\tilde{\mathbb{K}}_e = \begin{bmatrix} \mathbb{K}^{uu} & \mathbb{K}^{ua} \\ \mathbb{K}^{au} & \mathbb{K}^{aa} \end{bmatrix} \tag{4}$$

where $\mathbb{K}^{uu}$ is the original element stiffness matrix, whereas $\mathbb{K}^{ua}$, $\mathbb{K}^{au}$ and $\mathbb{K}^{aa}$ correspond to the added degrees of freedom.

In oder to compute the enriched stiffness matrix for a general element, the products of partial derivatives of the shape functions have to be integrated over the subvolumes created by the cut. However, for the special case of a linear tetrahedral element, the formulas for the enriched stiffness submatrices turn out to be very simple. The only remaining unknowns, that have to be computed after the cut, are the volumes of the dissected parts V_1 and V_2. Depending on possible combinations of ψ_i and ψ_j, the matrices $\mathbb{K}^{ua}_{ij}$, $\mathbb{K}^{au}_{ij}$ and $\mathbb{K}^{aa}_{ij}$ take on the following values

	$\psi_i = -1$	$\psi_i = 1$	$\psi_j = -1$	$\psi_j = 1$
$\mathbb{K}^{ua}_{ij}$	-	-	$2\mathbb{K}^{uu}_{ij}\frac{V_1}{V}$	$-2\mathbb{K}^{uu}_{ij}\frac{V_2}{V}$
$\mathbb{K}^{au}_{ij}$	$2\mathbb{K}^{uu}_{ij}\frac{V_1}{V}$	$-2\mathbb{K}^{uu}_{ij}\frac{V_2}{V}$	-	-

	$\psi_i = \psi_j = -1$	$\psi_i = \psi_j = 1$	$\psi_i \neq \psi_j$
$\mathbb{K}^{aa}_{ij}$	$4\mathbb{K}^{uu}_{ij}\frac{V_1}{V}$	$4\mathbb{K}^{uu}_{ij}\frac{V_2}{V}$	0

3.2. Stable Mass Lumping

Similarly to the enriched stiffness matrix, the enriched mass matrix has the form

$$\tilde{\mathbb{M}}_e = \begin{bmatrix} \mathbb{M}^{uu} & \mathbb{M}^{ua} \\ \mathbb{M}^{au} & \mathbb{M}^{aa} \end{bmatrix} \tag{5}$$

where $\mathbb{M}^{uu}$ is the original element mass matrix, whereas $\mathbb{M}^{ua}$, $\mathbb{M}^{au}$ and $\mathbb{M}^{aa}$ correspond to the added degrees of freedom. We refer to [9] for the formulas of the consistent (non-lumped) mass matrices. Most numerical algorithms used to solve Equation 1 require the inversion of the mass matrix to compute the nodal accelerations. Therefore, the mass matrices are diagonalized using a technique called mass lumping. The main requirement for the lumped mass matrix is to conserve the kinetic energy of the element. The most widely used lumping technique for the non enriched part is the row summation. However, if this technique is applied to the enriched mass matrix, it can lead to instability of the simulation. If one of the subvolumes created by the cut is small, the situation is equivalent to creating sliver tetrahedra element using one of the methods referenced in section 1. An alternative lumping for the enriched part solves the problem. The submatrices $\mathbb{M}^{ua}_{ij}$ and $\mathbb{M}^{au}_{ij}$ are zero and $\mathbb{M}^{aa}_{ij}$ is defined as

$$\bar{\mathbb{M}}^{aa}_{ii} = \frac{m}{n}\frac{1}{V^e}\int_{V^e} (\psi_i(x))^2\, dV \tag{6}$$

where $\bar{\mathbb{M}}^{uu}_{ii}$ is the lumped mass matrix, m is the total mass of the element, n is the number of the element nodes and V^e is the volume of the element. ψ_i only takes on the value of 1 or -1, and thus

	$\psi_i = -1$	$\psi_i = 1$
$\bar{\mathbb{M}}^{aa}_{ii}$	$4\,\bar{\mathbb{M}}^{uu}_{ii}\frac{V_1}{V}$	$4\,\bar{\mathbb{M}}^{uu}_{ii}\frac{V_2}{V}$

Depending on the position of the cut, the enriched part of the mass matrix may contain zero elements, e.g., if V_1 or V_2 is zero, which seems to imply an infinite eigenfrequency of the system and thus leading to an instability. However, this is not the case, as at the same time, there will be corresponding changes to the stiffness matrix, pushing the eigenfrequency of the system towards zero. If the enriched stiffness and mass matrices had been implemented as described above, it would lead to a division of zero by zero during the simulation if one of the subvolumes V_1 or V_2 were zero. This problem occurs independently of the chosen implicit or explicit integration scheme. Therefore, we propose premultiplying of Equation 1 by the diagonal matrix $\mathbb{W}$, defined as

$$\mathbb{W}_e = \begin{bmatrix} \mathbb{I}^{uu} & \mathbb{O}^{ua} \\ \mathbb{O}^{au} & \mathbb{W}^{aa} \end{bmatrix} \tag{7}$$

where $\mathbb{I}^{uu}$ is an identity matrix covering the non enriched part of the system, $\mathbb{O}^{ua}$ and $\mathbb{O}^{au}$ are zero matrices and the elements of W^{aa} are

	$\psi_i = -1$	$\psi_i = 1$
$\bar{\mathbb{W}}^{aa}_{ii}$	$\frac{1}{4}\frac{V}{V_1}$	$\frac{1}{4}\frac{V}{V_2}$

The enriched rows of the stiffness and mass matrices are modified as follows

$$\bar{\mathbb{M}}^{aa}_{ii} = \bar{\mathbb{M}}^{uu}_{ii} \tag{8}$$

	$\psi_i = -1$	$\psi_i = 1$
$\mathbb{K}^{au}_{ij}$	$\frac{1}{2}\mathbb{K}^{uu}_{ij}$	$-\frac{1}{2}\mathbb{K}^{uu}_{ij}$

	$\psi_i = \psi_j$	$\psi_i \neq \psi_j$
$\mathbb{K}^{aa}_{ij}$	$\mathbb{K}^{uu}_{ij}$	0

These are the final forms we use to build the enriched mass and stiffness matrices. The resulting matrices are positive definite, and the mass matrix does not contain any zero elements. The eigenfrequency of the cut element not only never becomes infinite, but it is of the same order of magnitude as the eigenfrequency of the original non-enriched element regardless of the location of the cut.

4. Results

The XFEM-based approach is suitable for both, the partial incision and the total dissection of soft tissue without significant impact on the performance or stability of the simulation. The dimension of the stiffness matrix of an enriched element is twice the dimension of a standard element. Therefore, the time spent on evaluating the forces at an enriched element can theoretically be expected to be four times the time spent on a standard element. However, the real value is lower, depending on the deformation approach used, as the $\mathbf{f} = \mathbb{K}\mathbf{u}$ multiplication does not have to be the only computation involved. For example, if the corotational FEM method is used, a considerable amount of time is spent on computing the rigid rotation of each element. The total time spent on an enriched element is then only about 1.5-times the time spent on a standard element. This

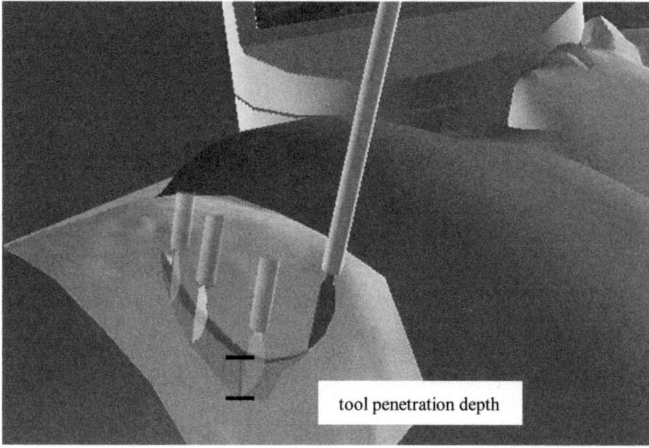

Figure 2. An interactively created surgical incision. The incision depth corresponds to the penetration depth of the cutting tool.

is a significant advantage of our method in comparison to methods based on remeshing that replace a cut element by 5-6, potentially bad shaped, new elements in average. An appropriate mass lumping technique is a key to the stability of the simulation.

The proposed technique has been integrated into a virtual surgery training framework, where it is used for interactive progressive cutting with force feedback. During an interactive surgical cut, a wound is modeled according to the position and penetration depth of the scalpel (Fig. 2). The opening of the wound is controlled by the FEM simulation.

References

[1] Stéphane Cotin, Hervé Delingette, and Nicholas Ayache. A hybrid elastic model for real-time cutting, deformations and force feedback for surgery training and simulation. *The Visual Computer*, 16(7):437–452, 2000.

[2] Daniel Bielser, Volker A. Maiwald, and Markus H. Gross. Interactive Cuts through 3-Dimensional Soft Tissue. In *Proceedings of the European Association for Computer Graphics 20th Annual Conference. Eurographics'99.*, volume 18/3, pages 31–38, September 1999.

[3] Gerrit Voss, James K. Hahn, Wolfgang Müller, and Rob Lindemann. Virtual Cutting of Anatomical Structures. In *Proceedings of Medicine Meets Virtual Reality*, pages 381–383, January 1999.

[4] Fabio Ganovelli, Paolo Cignoni, Claudio Montani, and Roberto Scopigno. Enabling Cuts on Multiresolution Representation. In *CGI '00: Proceedings of the International Conference on Computer Graphics*, page 183, Washington, DC, USA, 2000. IEEE Computer Society.

[5] Andrew B. Mor and Takeo Kanade. Modifying Soft Tissue Models: Progressive Cutting with Minimal New Element Creation. In *Proceedings of Medical Image Computing & Computer Assisted Intervention*, pages 598–607, 2000.

[6] Han-Wen Nienhuys and A. Frank van der Stappen. Supporting cuts and finite element deformation in interactive surgery simulation. Technical report, University of Utrecht, 2001.

[7] Denis Steinemann, Matthias Harders, Markus Gross, and Gabor Szekely. Hybrid Cutting of Deformable Solids. In *Proceedings of IEEE VR 2006*, pages 35–42, Los Alamitos, CA, USA, March 2006. IEEE Computer Society.

[8] Ted Belytschko and T. Black. Elastic crack growth in finite elements with minimal remeshing. *International Journal for Numerical Methods in Engineering*, 45(5):601–620, 1999.

[9] Goangseup Zi, Hao Chen, Jingxiao Xu, and Ted Belytschko. The extended finite element method for dynamic fractures. *Shock and Vibration*, 12(1):9–23, 2005.

Medicine Meets Virtual Reality 15
J.D. Westwood et al. (Eds.)
IOS Press, 2007

Visualization of Large-Scale Confocal Data Using Computer Cluster

Bei JIN,   Zhuming AI, Mary RASMUSSEN
bjin1@uic.edu   *zai@uic.edu*   *mary@uic.edu*
Virtual Reality in Medicine Lab   *University of Illinois at Chicago*

Abstract: A virtual reality system with remote computer cluster for interactive three-dimensional reconstruction and alignment of large confocal microscopy data is presented. It provides the flexibility and the accumulated power of computer cluster for this specific application.

1. Introduction

Laser scanning confocal microscopy (LSCM) is a tool for obtaining high-resolution images of specimens at various depths. Volume rendering technique has been used to interactively generate 3D reconstructions of the tumor microcirculation from multiple confocal sections [1], and it has been applied to the problem of comparing the vasculogenic mimicry (VM) and the microvascular density (MVD) in melanoma. [2] Because of the distortion between sections caused by cutting process, the manual alignment system in the virtual environment has been developed to correct the volumetric data [1]. However it can only handle small volumes because of the restriction of the graphic card texture memory. Meanwhile, an automated registration technique [3] has been developed, which can tile confocal slides together, thus the whole volume can be extent to 2000x2800x208 voxels. In the existing system, the original data is either down sampled to lower resolution, or only part of the volume is selected for 3D display. Investigators have to trade off between the covered area and the details of the structure. In this study, a volume rendering approach on a computer cluster is developed to break the limitation on the input volume size, thus provides significant improvement in accuracy and consistency of rendering acquired from serial paraffin sections.

2. Methods

Because of the rapid growing of both the speed and memory size of high-end PC graphics cards, large-scale volume rendering is increasingly being performed on low-cost PC clusters instead of expensive supercomputers. The goal of this study is to develop and implement a volume rendering system using a high-performance PC cluster server for high-resolution medical volumetric data visualization.

The user interface of the system is a client program of a client/server architect resides on a personal computer. It is meant to facilitate the local usage on the user's desktop without requiring specialized facility far away. Its low cost makes it easy to be widely deployed. It supports frame sequential stereo on a conventional CRT PC display, and utilizes gain controller for the 3D interface. A lower resolution version of the volume is rendered on the client desktop to provide an interface to control the volume's position and orientation. With the mouse button down, this rough volume will move according to the mouse's movement. Once the button is released, the current transformation matrix is sent to the remote PC cluster for high resolution rendering. The high resolution PC cluster rendering image will be streamed back to the desktop to replace the rough image until the button is pressed again.

The 20-node PC cluster is the main renderer for the distributed volume rendering system. The cluster includes one master node, one blending node, and multiple slave rendering nodes, each with the Nvidia Quadro FX 3000 graphics card. (Figure 1) The master node is the bridge between the remote client and the cluster. It can broadcast the transformation matrix to the slave rendering nodes, and send the final image from blending node back to the client PC over a gigabit network. The blending node's task is to collect the sub-images from the slave nodes, compositing them into the final full image. The slave rendering nodes mainly perform stereoscopic volume rendering simultaneously on the static sub-volumes they keep locally, and will update the rendering result whenever the transportation matrix is changed.

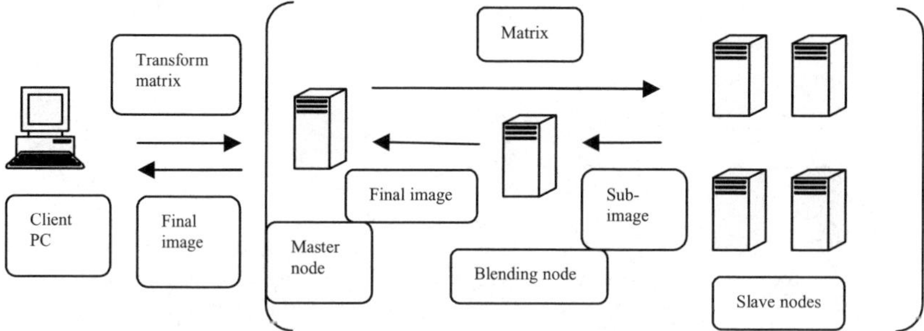

Figure1. the rendering system structure

The available 16 sections of volume data in size of 2000x2800x13 voxels each are distributed to 16 slave rendering nodes. Sort-last parallel 3D texture volume rendering is the basic algorithm used here to share the workload among the cluster nodes. And the rendering algorithm has been modified in color and alpha blending function according to the Porter Duff over operator [4], which can fit the associativity requirement of the cluster usage. This is critical in both volume rendering and image compositing steps to make sure that the blended image from sub-volume rendering are the same as the whole volume's rendering. The Porter Duff equation is as below [4]:

$$Aout = Afgd + (1 - Afgd) * Abkg$$
$$Cout' = Cfgd' + (1 - Afgd) * Cbkg' \qquad where\ C' = C * A$$

With the usage of cluster and the modification of blending function, the restriction on rendering volume size is eliminated. However the limitation on the number of pixel in each dimension still exists in the old method [1]. Although the size of 2000x2800x13 volume section is within the limit of the graphic card's memory, it can't be loaded into the graphics texture memory directly as a whole because the graphics card only accept 512 pixels in each dimension for one single texture. The rendering algorithm has been modified to have the ability to automatically create multiple smaller texture blocks that can be loaded into the memory. In this way, first the user can fully enjoy the flexibility on the volume shape. Secondly, for some special applications such as this confocal section alignment, each section is the best processing unit for individual cluster node. Time waste and complexity can be avoided in the matrix and image delivery and image compositing. Thirdly, the resource can be used more efficiently; only 16 nodes are needed if a 2000x2800x13 volume can be rendered. Otherwise, with dimensional limitation, at least 24 nodes have to be used.

The final image compositing has become the bottleneck of the parallel volume rendering method. The traditional CPU software approach is too slow even if it is parallelized by complicated algorithms. Special compositing hardware development is not applicable in every case. Here an OpenGL function is used in image compositing to take advantage of graphics card's speed, and also avoid special hardware requirement. The function glDrawPixel is used to add images into the frame buffer layer by layer sequentially after the rendering images from slave nodes are put in order back to front according to the sub-volume's position.

3. Result

The user need not compensate between the resolution and the data size with this system. The application can either display the large-scale data in full (figure 2), or interactively zoom in to a smaller area to view the detailed structure (figure 3). The red part in the image in the figures is MVD, and the green part is the VM pattern. (Fullcolor images is at http://plum.bhis.uic.edu:8080/zai)

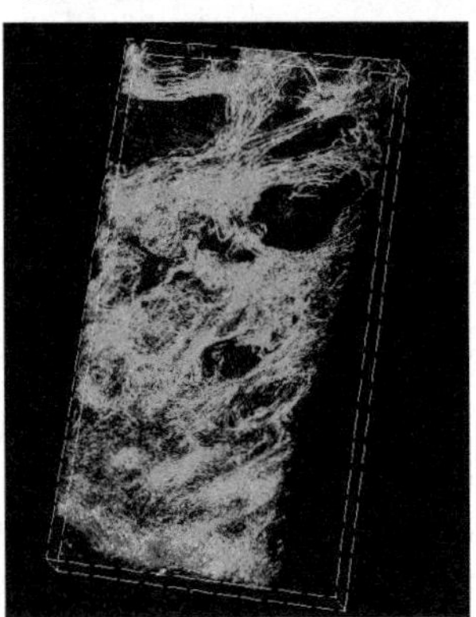

Figure 2. confocal full display

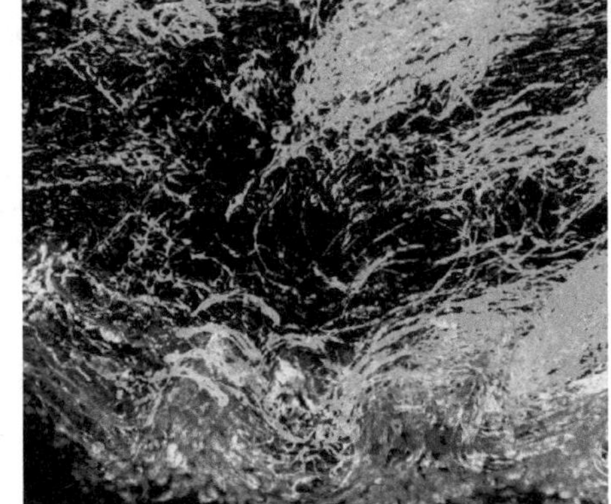

Figure 3. confocal detailed structure

4. Conclusion and Discussion

The cluster's volume rendering can clarify the full spatial configuration of the large scale pathological tissue data. And this system can also be extended to the visualization of other large-scale biological and medical volumetric data.

Reference
[1]	Ai ZM, Chen X, Rasmussen M, et al.: Reconstruction and exploration of three-dimensional confocal microscopy data in an immersive virtual environment, *Comput Med Imaging Graph* 2005;29:313-318
[2]	Chen X, Ai Z, Rasmussen M, et al.: Three-dimensional reconstruction of extravascular matrix patterns and blood vessels in human uveal melanoma tissue: preliminary findings. Invest Ophthalmol Vis Sci 2003;44(7):2834-40
[3]	Peter Bajcsy, Sang-Chul Lee, Amy Lin, et al: 3D Volume Reconstruction of Extracellular Matrix Proteins in Uveal Melanoma from Fluorescent Confocal Laser Scanning Microscope Images, *in Journal of Microscopy*, Blackwell Synergy, vol. 221(1), pp. 30-45, 2006.
[4]	PORTER T., DUFF T.: *Compositing digital images.* In Computer Graphics (Proceedings of SIGGRAPH84) (July 1984), vol. 18, pp. 253-- 259. 5

Medicine Meets Virtual Reality 15
J.D. Westwood et al. (Eds.)
IOS Press, 2007

209

A Haptic-enabled Toolkit for Illustration of Procedures in Surgery (TIPS)

Minho KIM [a,1], Tianyun NI [a], Juan CENDAN [b], Sergei KURENOV [b], and Jörg PETERS [a]

[a] *Dept. CISE, University of Florida*
[b] *Dept. Surgery, University of Florida*

Abstract. Good surgical training depends greatly on case experiences that have been difficult to model in software since current training technology does not provide the flexibility to teach and practice uncommon procedures, or to adjust a training scenario on the fly. The TIPS kit aims to overcome these limitations. To the expert, it presents visual and haptic tools that make illustrating procedures easy and can model unusual anatomic variations. For a non-specialist, it provides a locally customized learning environment and repeated practice in a safe environment. We used the toolkit to illustrate removal of the adrenal gland.

Keywords. medical illustration, haptic rendering, haptic authoring, teaching, virtual surgery training,

1. Introduction

Medical illustrations are the standard for publishing and documenting medical procedures in biological textbooks, teaching illustrations, instructional films, and legal proceedings involving medical documentation. Presently, the hurdles for taking descriptive text to illustration involve long hours between a trained medical illustrator and the documenting physician to illustrate even the simplest procedure. Subsequent "views" are generated by the illustrator with many attempts needing to be reworked before the results are satisfactory.

2. Tools and Methods

The toolkits' goal is to remove the intermediary and empower the *specialist surgeon as author* by placing advanced media conveniently at the surgeon's disposition. Like word processing software, but including haptic forces and 3D models, this allows the specialist to create customized instructional illustrations. The learner, typically a resident or non-specialist surgeon, can follow the instructions 'hands-on' by having the haptic stylus guide the hand (Figure 1, *left*) as key moments of a procedure are replayed in

---

[1]Correspondence to: SurfLab, Dept. CISE, CSE Bldg E325, University of Florida, Gainesville, FL 32611. Tel.: +1 352 392 1255; Fax: +1 352 392 1220; E-mail: {mhkim,jorg}@cise.ufl.edu.

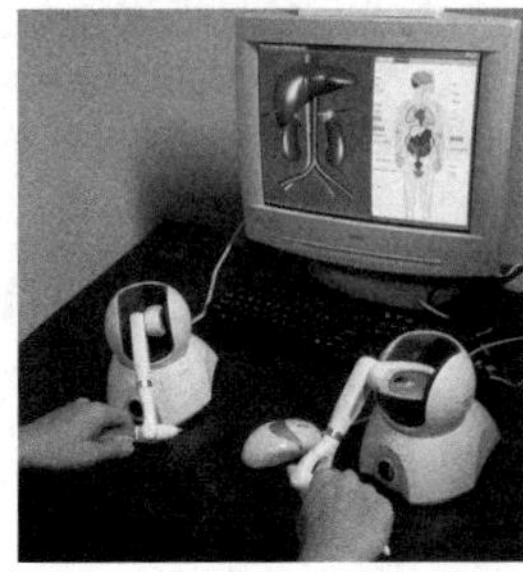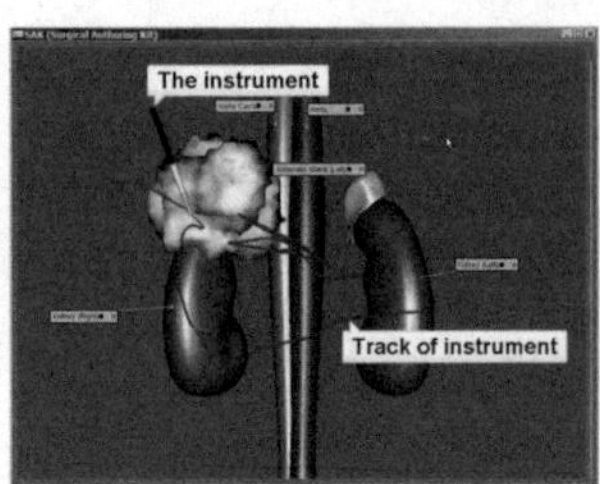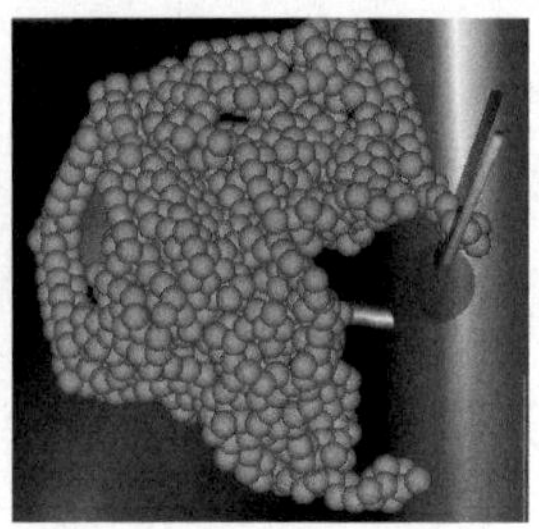

Figure 1. (*left*)Replay of (*middle*) 3D motion (red) to remove fatty tissue (*right*).

the virtual environment. At any point in the procedure, the illustration can be paused to explore the environment, and then continue or repeat the process until the skills are understood. Conversely, the learner's skills can be compared to the metrics laid down by the specialist.

Currently, TIPS modules are being validated by specialist surgeons at the Department of Surgery University of Florida. Modules and their associated metrics undergo peer review and are validated by a metric-driven validation of residents.

3. Results

3.1. The Authoring Kit

We created two types of the toolkit: an authoring toolkit and a learning toolkit. The authoring toolkit is an environment for a specialist surgeon to create a multimedia experience, and authoring consists of four stages.

The *Conceptual* stage consists of storyboarding and mapping steps to media. That is, the surgeon breaks the procedure into steps and decides on the simplest means of conveying the idea. In increasing order of complexity the available media are: (i) scanned sketch (Figure 2, lower left), (ii) photographic or textbook image (Figure 2, upper right), (iii) video of life procedure, (iv) animation, (v) haptic simulation.

In the *Anatomic Layout* stage the author populates the virtual 3D scene with objects from an extendable database of predefined 3D models (organs, vessels, surgical tools) and interactively generated fatty tissue (Figure 1, *middle*). When instantiating the objects, a simple interface allows adjusting their parameters: position (scaling, orientation), visual properties (base color, color when touched, transparency, etc.) and haptic properties (elasticity, extent of deformation). The properties are adjusted by touching the object with the haptic device and adjusting the value by mouse motion. Since typically, layouts will be downloaded from a database or shared from colleagues and then loaded, both conceptual and layout stages are not expected to be revisited frequently. Rather, a particular surgical scenario is established so that the main work reduces to creating variants by adjusting properties.

During the *Anatomy Exploration* stage, the author traverses the 3D anatomy, and modifies it - for example, by removing fatty tissue, or displacing organs and vessels in preparation for ligation, etc. The system records the 3D motion of the surgical procedure via a feedback stylus (see Figure 1, *left*).

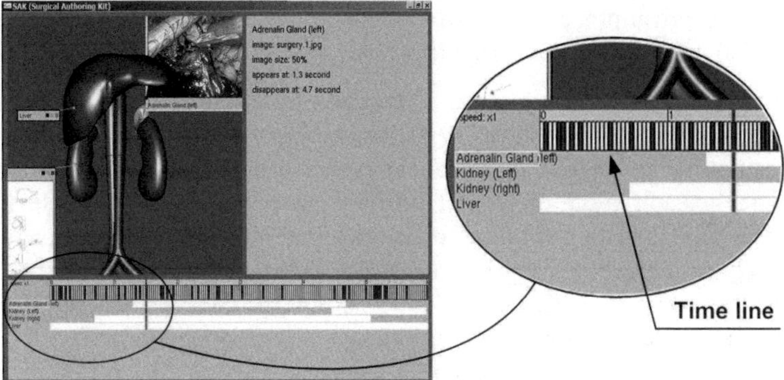

Figure 2. Editing the 'pop-up' time rail to add additional illustrations (e.g. recorded video, *top right*))

In the *Annotation* stage, the surgeon-author adds or deletes recorded motion sequences and adds other media using the timeline of the recorded motion (see Figure 2). This is similar to deleting or editing text on a page in a word processing or video-editing environment. Annotation is an important alternative to full simulation. The tags are non-occluding and attached to objects in the 3D scene. Each functions as a (computer) window and allows display of video clips, hand-drawn or book-scanned images and plain text.

3.2. The Learning Kit

The learning kit allows a non-specialist surgeon to retrace the recorded, annotated motion. In the *passive mode*, the haptic feedback interface guides the learner's hands along a specific path while the computer screen shows the authored 3D scenario. Tissue or material resistance is experienced from acceleration or deceleration of the author's hand motions and from the model settings. The replay can be adjusted to slow motion. An alternative view than the original can be selected.

While the author fixes the path, the forces that guide along this master path can be relaxed. In this *active mode*, the non-specialist can move more freely and make mistakes. The non-specialist's motion in the active mode is recorded for comparison.

3.3. Case Study: Removal of the Adrenal Gland

As a test, we illustrated *laparoscopic adrenalectomy*. Here, safe dissection of the fatty tissue to expose the adrenal vein requires (i) correct 3D motion, adapted to the highly variable layout of organs, vessels and fatty tissue; and (ii) application of appropriate force conveyed by the haptic device, to lift the vein free of the surrounding tissue in preparation for ligation (Figure 1, *left*). Rupturing the adrenal vein or neighboring vena cava could result in catastrophic hemorrhage.

The specific anatomic relationships between the adrenal gland and the surrounding structures deserve special attention. There is an adrenal gland on each patient's side; however, the relationship between the gland and the nearby organs differ significantly from cases to case. In particular, the vascular relationships are completely different between the right and the left gland. Each poses its unique challenges to the surgeon during surgery. At present there is no method for preparing for these anomalies and variations a priori. There is no road map for the surgeon, other than experience.

In the 3D surgical procedure illustration environment, we could emphasize and illustrate the following aspects in particular:

1. The right gland is attached via a short and frail vein to the largest vein in the body, the inferior vena cava (IVC). The adrenal vain is generally in a standard location but its wide to short caliber is particularly challenging for dissection. Undue tension in the process of surrounding the vein, prior to its ligation, can create brisk bleeding from the inferior-medial junction of the vein to the IVC. This type of bleeding can be catastrophic in the laparoscopic setting.
2. The procedure is applied behind the right lobe of the liver, and deserves a controlled environment for practicing.
3. The left gland also has its unique challenges. Although the vein on this side is longer and easier to manipulate, its location is more variable. The ability to construct multiple anatomic relationships, cover them with fatty tissues and impose dissection on the learner allows exploration of these relationships in a safe environment. The tail of the pancreas and the spleen must also be exposed to see the adrenal gland.

The Authoring kit allows representation of these relationships in a three-dimensional and tactile environment. These modalities are missing from videos and books. In particular, the authoring kit allows the author surgeon to, on the spot, create a number of variations. For example, there are a number of vascular relationships that are modeled simply by adjusting the gland (size, position, haptic feedback), relative position of the vessels and the distribution and character of the fatty tissue and covering peretoneum. The learning kit then allows a competent, but not expert, surgeon to review the procedure to prepare for surgery. The review reiterates the key anatomic relations and forces as defined by the expert.

4. Discussion and Future Work

A key point of our approach is that the specialist surgeon rather than a computer programmer will author the material. This makes the approach flexible and removes a level of indirection that easily leads to incorrect emphasis. This toolkit is not in competition but rather complements the rapidly advancing academic or commercial surgery training tools [1,2,3,4,5,6,7].

By placing the specialist surgeon at the center of the content generation, we follow a different paradigm. The toolkit brings together a number of state-of-the-art technologies: advanced graphics, both hardware (GPU acceleration of subdivision surfaces [8]) and software (novel surface representations, realtime shadows as depth cues, etc.) and makes judicious use of haptic measurement and feedback at key points of the illustration. Opensource development of the toolkit is expected to trigger further collaboration of computer and surgical specialists to develop libraries and shared repositories for continued education.

Acknowledgements

This research was made possible in part by NSF Grants DMI-0400214 and CCF-0430891.

References

[1] J. Berkley and G. Turkiyyah and D. Berg and M. Ganter and S. Weghorst.   Real-time finit element modeling for surgery simulation: An application to virtual suturin. *IEEE Transactions on visualization and computer graphics*, 10(3):314–325, May/June 2004.

[2] S. Cotin and H. Delingette and M. Bro-Nielsen and N. Ayache and J.M. Clement and V. Tasseti and J. Marescaux. *Geometric and physical Representations for a Simulator of Hapatic Surgery.* 1996.

[3] S.L. Dawson. A critical approach to medical simulation. *Bull Am Coll Surg*, 87(11):12–18, 2002.

[4] H. Delingette. Toward realistic soft-tissue modeling in medical simulation. In *in Proccedings of the IEEE*, volume 86, pages 512–523, March 1998.

[5] R.S. Haluck and T.M. Krummel. Computers and virtual reality for surgical education in the 21st century. *Arh Surg*, 135:12–18, 2000.

[6] J. Lenoir and P. Meseure and L. Grisoni and C. Chaillou. *A Suture Model for Surgical Simulation.* 2004.

[7] A. Liu and F. Tendick and K. Cleary. A survey of surgical simulation: applications, technology, and education. *Virtual Environ*, 12:599–614, December 2003.

[8] M. Kim and S. Punak and J. Cendan and S. Kurenov and J. Peters. Exploiting graphics hardware for haptic authoring. In *Proceedings of Medicine Meets Virtual Reality, Long Beach,CA*, volume 14, pages 255–260. Studies in Health Technology and Informatics (SHTI), IOS Press, Amsterdam, Jan. 2006.

Medicine Meets Virtual Reality 15
J.D. Westwood et al. (Eds.)
IOS Press, 2007

Non-Clinical Evaluation of the KAIST-Ewha Colonoscopy Simulator II

Woo Seok Kim[a], Hyun Soo Woo[a], Woojin Ahn[a], Kyungno Lee[a], Jang Ho Cho[a],
Doo Yong Lee[a], and Sun Young Yi[b]
[a]*School of Mechanical, Aerospace and Systems Engineering, KAIST
Daejeon, Republic of Korea*
[b]*Department of Internal Medicine, Ewha Womans University, Seoul, Republic of Korea*

Abstract. This paper presents non-clinical evaluation of the KAIST-Ewha Colonoscopy Simulator II. Thirty one engineering-major students with no medical background were divided into two groups after they had been given instruction on colonoscopy and its operation. The baseline evaluation showed that both groups were equivalent in the level of the colonoscopy skills. The simulation-trained group underwent training until they passed all the performance criteria established by colonoscopy experts. Results of final evaluation showed that the simulation-trained group noticeably improved their skills.

Keywords. Colonoscopy Simulator, Validation

Introduction

Colonoscopy has a relatively slow learning curve. Over 100 procedures are minimally required for competency [1]. Computer-based colonoscopy simulators have been developed to accelerate the learning curve, and reduce risk to patients [2-4]. As new training simulators are developed and introduced to the market, it is essential to asses the training efficacy of the developed simulators [5,6].

The KAIST-Ewha Colonoscopy Simulator II is extended from the previous version, jointly developed by KAIST and Ewha Womans University [4], to provide better realism, haptic feel, and various training scenarios. This paper reports that the developed simulator actually improves the targeted colonoscopy skills.

1. Method

For this study, three colon models, easy, intermediate, and difficult, are developed. The difficult model is constructed from CT data of an actual patient, and it contains loops and flexures. Easy and intermediate models are relaxed versions of the difficult model with less loops and flexures. These three colon models are evaluated by colonoscopy experts with experience of at least over 1000 procedures each. Performance during simulation by the experienced experts is used to establish criteria for training. The criteria includes dwelling time, air insufflation time, air suction time, red-out time, number of red-outs, the length of folded colon, and polyp-detection rate.

Figure 1 shows the design of this study. A total of thirty one engineering-major students participated in the study. They did not have any medical background, and were given instruction by a colonoscopy expert, on the operation of colonoscope and basic colonoscopy skills. The participants were, then, divided into two groups, simulation-trained (n=16) and control (n=15).

The both groups underwent a baseline evaluation using the easy colon model to make sure the uniformity of the two groups. Subjects in the simulation-trained group underwent training using the intermediate colon model. The simulation-trained group was required to practice repeatedly until they passed all the required criteria established by the colonoscopy experts. The both groups were evaluated using the difficult colon model after completion of the simulation-based training.

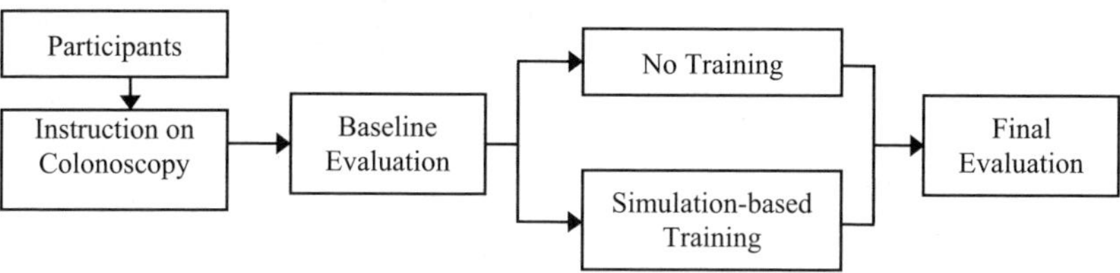

Figure 1. Design of the study

2. Results and Discussion

The two groups did not show any significant differences in all the performance criteria (p>0.05) during the baseline evaluation. Result of the final evaluation is shown in Table 1. Figure 2 shows the relative magnitude of the trained group as we set the magnitude of the control group at one for each performance criterion. The simulation-trained group shows better colonoscopy skills in terms of dwelling time, air insufflation time, air suction time, and the length of folded colon, compared to the control group. But both groups show high polyp-detection rate of over 85%. Time and number of red-outs do not show any meaningful difference, either. Although the subjects did not have any prior medical background, the developed simulator was generally effective in improving the targeted colonoscopy skills. Clinical evaluation is also being carried out to determine whether this acquired level of the skills can be transferred to colonoscopy to actual patients.

Table 1. Result of the final evaluation

Performance criteria	Simulation-trained group	Control group	p-value
Intubation time (sec)	136.50 (28.72)	264.44 (77.29)	0.000
Air insufflation time (sec)	0.00 (0.00)	2.39 (4.39)	0.037
Air suction time (sec)	21.24 (20.36)	7.16 (12.64)	0.029
Red-out time (sec)	3.30 (1.74)	4.09 (2.92)	0.364
Number of red-outs	5.75 (2.65)	7.20 (4.66)	0.292
Length of folded colon (mm)	1001.66 (21.31)	1030.19 (16.78)	0.000
Polyp-detection rate (%)	90.63 (16.11)	84.56 (15.85)	0.228

Note: Values in parentheses are standard deviations.

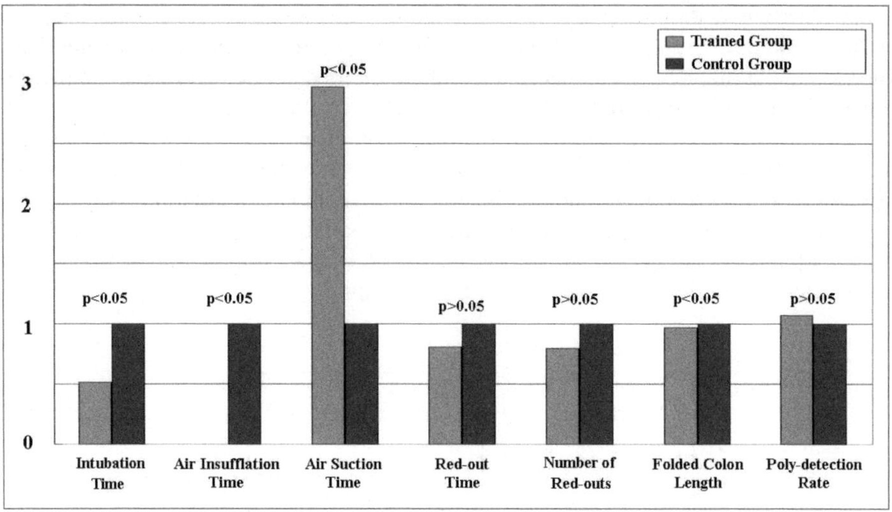

Figure 2. Comparison between the simulation-trained and the control groups

References

[1] P.S. Tassio, S.D. Ladas, I. Grammenos et al., "Acquisition of competency in colonoscopy: the learning curve of trainees," Endoscopy, vol. 9, pp. 702-706, 1999.

[2] K. Ikuta, K. Iritani, and J. Fukuyama, "Mobile virtual endoscope system with haptic and visual information for non-invasive inspection training," Proc. of the 2001 IEEE International Conf. on Robotics and Automation, Seoul, Korea, pp 2037-2044, 2001.

[3] O. Körner and R. Manner, "Implementation of a haptic interface for a virtual reality simulation for flexible endoscopy," Proc. 11th IEEE Symp. on Haptic Interfaces for Virtual Environment and Teleoperator Systems, Los Angeles, CA, pp 208-212, 2003.

[4] S.Y. Yi, H.S. Woo, W.J. Ahn, J.Y. Kwon, and D.Y. Lee, "New colonoscopy simulator with improved haptic fidelity, "Advanced Robotics, vol 20, no 3, pp. 349-365, 2006.

[5] A. Ferlitsch, P. Glauninger, A. Gupper et al., "Evaluation of a virtual endoscopy simulator for training in gastrointestinal endoscopy," Endoscopy, vol.34, pp. 698–702, 2002.

[6] R.E. Sedlack, J.C. Kolars, and J.A. Alexander, "Computer simulation training enhances patient comfort during endoscopy," Clinical Gastroenterology and Hepatology, vol. 2, pp. 348–352, 2004.

Medicine Meets Virtual Reality 15
J.D. Westwood et al. (Eds.)
IOS Press, 2007

217

A Pneumatic Haptic Feedback Actuator Array for Robotic Surgery or Simulation

Chih-Hung KING [a,b], Adrienne T. HIGA [a,b], Martin O. CULJAT [a,c],
Soo Hwa HAN [a,c], James W. BISLEY [d], Gregory P. CARMAN [a,b],
Erik DUTSON [a,c], and Warren S. GRUNDFEST [a,b,c,1]
[a]*Center for Advanced Surgical and Interventional Technology (CASIT)*
[b]*UCLA Henry Samueli School of Engineering and Applied Science*
[c]*UCLA Department of Surgery*
[d]*UCLA Department of Neurobiology*

Abstract. Robot-assisted minimally invasive surgery (MIS) offers improved range of motion over standard laparoscopic techniques, but is characterized by a total loss of haptic feedback, requiring surgeons to rely solely on visual cues. Pneumatic tactile displays have many advantages, including low mass, low cost, compact size, and adaptability. A pneumatic haptic feedback actuator array has been developed that is suitable for mounting unto surgical robotic tools. The balloon actuators consist of spin-coated thin-film silicone membranes and molded substrates with cylindrical channels. Human perceptual tests were conducted on balloon diameters ranging from 0.75 to 2.0 mm to determine the optimal size that can be effectively detected. The control system was programmed to sequentially inflate a single balloon to one of the three levels, 100% (full hemispherical deformation), zero, 50% (half deformation), and 0% (no inflation). Blinded subjects (n=5) were asked to determine which of the two inflation levels was higher. Test results suggest that balloon diameters greater than 1.0 mm can deliver high detection accuracy. This indicates that pneumatic balloon-based actuation is a viable solution for generating haptic feedback. In addition to surgical applications, many other fields such as virtual reality-based simulators and neuroprosthetics can benefit from this technology.

Keywords. Tactile display, haptic feedback, robotic surgery, pneumatic actuator

1. Introduction

Minimally invasive surgery (MIS) has revolutionized surgical care by decreasing the need for medication and shortening recovery times through the reduction of trauma to patients during operations [1,2]. Current surgical robots for MIS enable surgeons to operate remotely with improved range of motion, bringing their expertise in-theater to address critical needs such as those encountered in battlefield surgery. While surgical robots offer many benefits, they suffer from a total loss of haptic feedback, requiring surgeons to rely solely on visual cues during operations. This drawback has led to longer learning curves for surgeons, and has increased the chances of inadvertent surgical errors [3,4]. The addition of tactile information will enable surgeons to "feel"

---

[1] Correspondence to: Warren S. Grundfest, MD, warrenbe@seas.ucla.edu

tissue characteristics, appropriately tension sutures, identify pathologic conditions, and will enable expansion of MIS to other surgical procedures and simulations. It is proposed that the haptic feedback actuator, when integrated with a tactile sensor array mounted onto the tips of robotic graspers, can effectively translate tactile information to the surgeon's fingertips. The actuator can also provide virtual tactile information when implemented with surgical simulators.

Various haptic feedback actuator and system technologies have previously been explored, including piezoelectric, shape memory alloys, electromagnetic, and servo motors [5-9]. Pneumatically actuated tactile displays have also previously been described [10,11], but have not been implemented on surgical robotic systems. Pneumatic balloon actuation has various advantages, including surface conformation, compact size, and large deflection. In this paper, we present a modular and scalable pneumatically driven balloon-based actuator array suitable for mounting onto surgical robotic tools. This system uses the human sensory apparatus in the skin as a pathway for providing information to the brain. Human perceptual studies, which provide preliminary guidelines for determining the optimal balloon diameter, are also discussed.

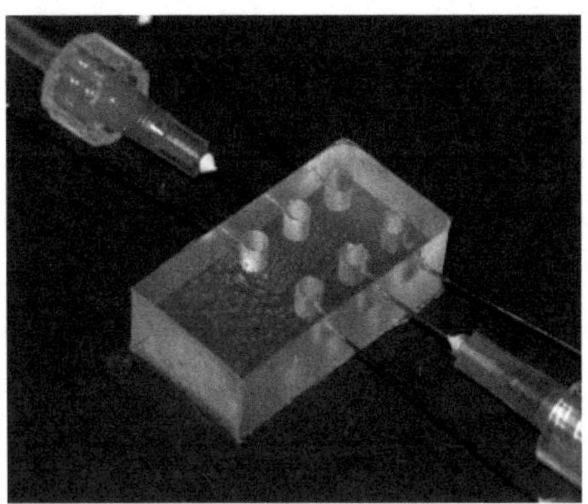

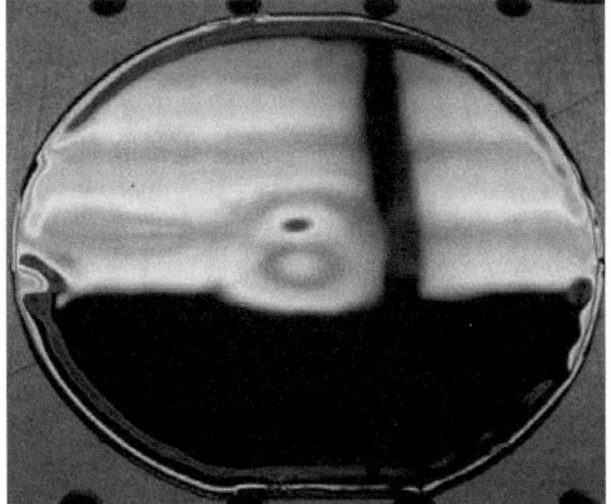

Figure 1. 3 x 2 pneumatic balloon actuator array   **Figure 2.** Thin-film silicone membrane on a wafer

2. Design and Methods

The pneumatic balloon actuators are constructed from thin-film silicone membranes and molded polydimethylsiloxane (PDMS) substrates (32 mm x 17 mm x 10 mm) with cylindrical channels (Figure 1). The flexible PDMS material has the advantage that it can conform to the shape of the fingers, and the highly elastic silicone membrane can be bonded to the PDMS substrate while expanding into balloons above each of the channels. The membrane was fabricated by spin coating silicone in liquid form on a silicon wafer. The spin coater (Headway EC101D) was used to control the thickness and uniformity of the membrane. A cured thin-film silicone membrane (~300 μm) is shown attached to a silicon wafer in Figure 2. Using this process, balloon actuators with diameters of 0.75, 1.0, 1.5, and 2.0 mm were fabricated with array sizes up to 3 x 2 elements.

The schematic of the control system to the balloon actuators is illustrated in Figure 3, consisting of a microcontroller and associated electronics, pressure regulators, an air source, and pneumatic tubing and fittings. The microcontroller (PIC16F877A, Microchip, Chandler, AZ) was programmed and controlled by a computer via the serial interface (RS-232) to: (1) receive control instructions from the operator, (2) determine the required inflation level of the balloon actuator, and (3) generate the corresponding analog control signals to the pressure regulators (Marsh Bellofram T3210), which in turn inflated the balloon actuators with proportional pressures.

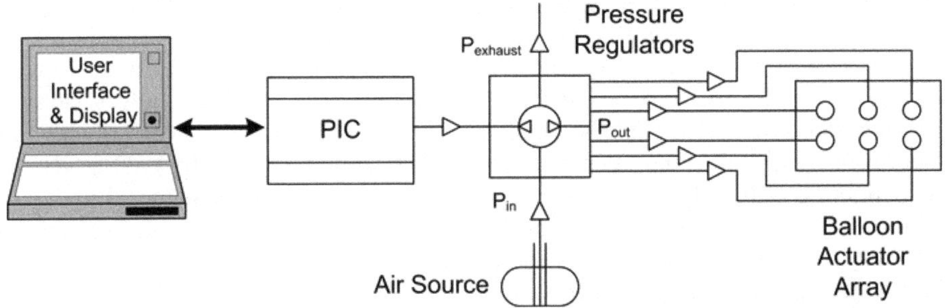

Figure 3. Schematic of the control system

Human perceptual tests were conducted for each of the existing balloon diameters to determine the optimal size that can be effectively detected. The control system was programmed to sequentially actuate a single balloon to one of three actuation levels based on the instruction of the operator. The three inflation levels used in this study were 100% (full hemispherical deformation), 50% (half deformation), and 0% (no inflation). There were six possible combinations of sequential actuation among the three inflation levels: 0-50, 0-100, 50-100, 100-50, 100-0, and 50-0. For instance, 0-50 represents the actuation sequence from 0% inflation to 50% inflation.

Five subjects (three men, two women, age range 23-40 years) participated in the study, and were trained to ensure that they were familiar with the haptic feedback system. Each subject was asked to perform one session for each of the four balloon diameters; for each session, the subject asked to perform 15 two-alternative forced choice trials, comparing two sequentially presented stimuli. The stimuli were presented over a 4 s period, were separated by a 100 ms delay, and had a < 100 ms inflation time. After each trial, the subjects had to inform the operator whether the first or second stimulus had more pressure. The 15 sequential actuation trials were selected pseudo-randomly from all of the possible combinations, with each combination repeated at least once. Subjects placed their index fingers in contact with the balloon actuators, and the same finger was used for the duration of testing. Accuracy was calculated based on the percentage of total correct responses divided by the total number of trials.

3. Results

Table 1 provides the results of the human perceptual tests. The total numbers of trials are different for each combination due to the pseudo-random selection of each trial sequence. Figure 4 shows the detection accuracy for each balloon diameter and each actuation combination. Combination 0-100 achieves the highest average accuracy (100%) of all six combinations. Responses for the 0.75 mm balloon diameters under combination 50-0 were the least accurate (50%) and were significantly worse than any other combination ($p<0.05$, χ^2 test). Combinations 0-50 and 50-0 accounted for 72% of total inaccurate responses. 92.3% of the inaccurate responses from combinations 0-50 and 50-0 were experienced with 0.75 and 1.0 mm diameter balloons. Overall, combination 50-0 had the lowest average accuracy (83%).

Average accuracy as a function of balloon diameter is shown in Figure 5. Average accuracy was directly proportional to balloon diameter, with the lowest average accuracy (86.4%) for the smallest balloon diameter (0.75 mm). This performance was significantly worse than that seen with the 1.5 and 2.0 mm balloons ($p<0.03$, χ^2 test). In the debriefing, subjects indicated that 0.75 and 1.0 mm balloon diameter tests required greater concentration than the 1.5 and 2.0 mm balloons. For balloons with 0.75 mm and 1.0 mm diameters, the average accuracy under combination 0-100 and 100-0 was 96.7%, whereas that of combination 0-50 and 50-0 was only 76.9%. These results indicate that it was significantly more difficult to determine more than two pressure levels in the 0.75 and 1.0 mm balloons ($p=0.001$, χ^2 test).

Table 1. Human Perceptual Test Results

Balloon Diameter	0.75 mm		1.0 mm	
Combination	**Number of Trials**	**Accuracy (%)**	**Number of Trials**	**Accuracy (%)**
0-50	12	83.3	13	84.6
50-0	14	50	13	92.3
0-100	12	100	11	100
100-0	15	93.3	15	100
50-100	12	91.7	13	100
100-50	10	100	10	90
Balloon Diameter	**1.5 mm**		**2.0 mm**	
Combination	**Number of Trials**	**Accuracy (%)**	**Number of Trials**	**Accuracy (%)**
0-50	13	100	12	100
50-0	14	92.9	14	100
0-100	11	100	11	100
100-0	14	100	16	93.8
50-100	13	92.3	12	100
100-50	10	100	10	100

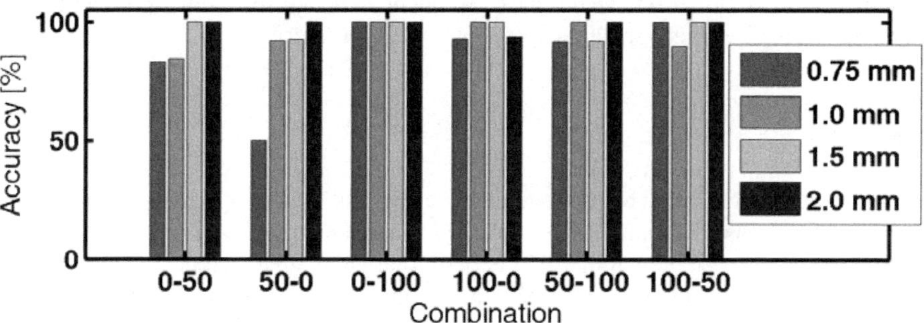

Figure 4. Detection accuracy of each balloon diameter and each combination of the sequential actuation.

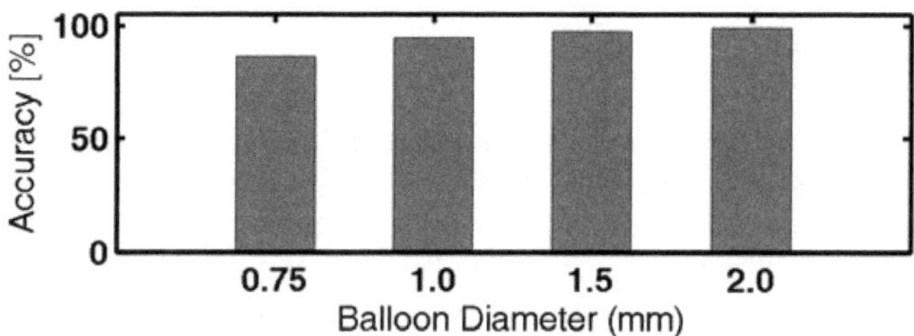

Figure 5. Average detection accuracy of each balloon diameter

4. Discussion

Balloons with diameters larger than 1.0 mm deliver high accuracy (>90%) in all sequential actuation combinations and no significant differences were seen in performance among any of the combinations. This result suggests that balloons with diameters larger than 1.0 mm can effectively deliver three or more levels of reliable tactile sensation, and that the number of detectable inflation levels increases with diameter. This observation is consistent with previous studies, which have demonstrated that a range of forces between 10 and 70 g wt can be estimated in solid spheres with radii as small 1.4 mm [12].

In addition to reduced accuracy of the 0.75 and 1.0 mm balloons, the requirement of increased concentration for sensing multiple inflation levels of these balloons might adversely affect task performance; by dedicating more effort to interpreting the feedback information, a user's concentration on the task may be interrupted.

The relationship between balloon diameters and the number of detectable inflation levels is an important factor in determining the optimal balloon diameter for a haptic feedback actuator. Ideally, an actuator that can generate a higher number of discreet levels will deliver more dynamic haptic feedback, allowing the tactile information to more closely resemble the actual sense of touch. However, larger balloon diameters limit the number of actuator array elements that can be organized in a fixed space, therefore decreasing spatial resolution. Future studies will focus on actuator miniaturization, fabrication techniques, frequency response, and optimization of balloon diameters, element spacing, array sizes, and geometries.

5. Summary

The presented pneumatic balloon actuator array has many advantages, including flexibility, low mass, compact size, scalability, and adaptability. Preliminary human perceptual tests have demonstrated that balloon diameters greater than 1.0 mm provide effective haptic feedback to the human index finger. When combined with a micro-sensor array and closed-loop pneumatic system and integrated onto robotic surgical instrumentation, surgical performance and training can be improved and enhanced. In addition to surgical applications, many other fields such as virtual reality-based simulators and neuroprosthetics may benefit from this technology.

6. Acknowledgements

The authors would like to thank Dr. E. Carmack Holmes for his support of this project, and Mr. Sam Y. Bae and Mr. Victor White of the Jet Propulsion Laboratory for their creativity and their contributions to this work. The authors most gratefully appreciate funding provided for this work by the Telemedicine and Advanced Technology Research Center (TATRC) / Department of Defense under award number W81XWH-05-2-0024.

References

[1]   Feussner H, Siewert JR, "Reduction of surgical access trauma: reliable advantages", *Chirug* 2001 Mar 72(3):236-44.

[2]   Jacobs JK, Goldstein RE, "Laparoscopic adrenalectomy: a new standard of care" *Ann of Surg,* 225(5): 495-501, 1997.

[3]   Sung GT, Gill IS, "Robotic Laparoscopic Surgery: A Comparison of the *da Vinci* and Zeus Systems," *Urology,* 58: 893-898, 2001.

[4]   Chapman WHH, Albrecht RJ, Kim VB, Young JA, "Computer-Assisted Laparoscopic Splenectomy with the da Vinci™ Surgical Robot." *J. Laparoendosc. Adv. Surg. Tech.,* 12(3): 155-159, 2002.

[5]   Hayward, V., Cruz-Hernandez, M, "Tactile Display Device Using Distributed Lateral Skin Stretch," in *Proc. of 8th Symp. On Haptic Interfaces for Virtual Environment and Teleoperator Systems, ASME IMECE2000,* 2000, pp. 1309–1314.

[6]   Kontarinis DA, Son JS, Peine W, Howe RD, "A tactile shape sensing and display system for teleoperated manipulation," in *Proc. IEEE Int. Conf. Rob. Autom.,* 1995, pp. 641–646.

[7]   Hannaford B, Trujillo J, Sinanan M, Moreyra M, Rosen J, Brown J, Lueschke R, MacFarlane M, "Computerized endoscopic surgical grasper," in *MMVR-98,* Jan. 1998, pp. 111-117.

[8]   Okamura AM, Webster RJ, Nolin JT, Johnson KW, and Jafry H, "The Haptic Scissors: Cutting in Virtual Environments," in *Proc. IEEE Int. Conf. Rob. Autom.,* 2003, pp. 828-833.

[9]   Taylor R, Jensen P, Whitcomb L et al, "A steadyhand robotic system for microsurgical augmentation," *Int. J. Robotic. Res.,* 1999;18:12.

[10] Moy G, Wagner C, Fearing RS. "A compliant tactile display for teletaction," in *ICRA 2000 IEEE Int. Conf. Rob. Automat.,* 2000, pp. 3409 - 3415.

[11] Caldwell,DG Tsagarakis N, Giesler, C, "An Integrated Tactile/Shear Feedback Array for Stimulation of Finger Mechanoreceptor", in *Proc. IEEE Int. Conf. Rob. Autom.,* 1999, pp. 287-292.

[12] Goodwin AW, Wheat WE, "Magnitude estimation of contact force when objects with different shapes are applied passively to the fingerpad," *Somatosens. Mot. Res.* 9:339-344, 1992.

Medicine Meets Virtual Reality 15
J.D. Westwood et al. (Eds.)
IOS Press, 2007

Virtual Simulation-Enhanced Triage Training for Iraqi Medical Personnel

Paul N. KIZAKEVICH[a], Andrew CULWELL[a], Robert FURBERG[a],
Don GEMEINHARDT[a], Susan GRANTLIN[a], Robert HUBAL[a],
Allison STAFFORD[a], COL R. Todd DOMBROSKI[b]
[a]*RTI International, Research Triangle Park, NC*
[b]*U.S. Army Medical Corps*

Abstract. Triage, establishing the priority of care among casualties in disaster management, is generally practiced using constructive tabletop or live exercises. Actual disasters involving multiple casualties occur rarely, offering little opportunity for gaining experience and competency assessment. When they do occur, response needs to be rapid and well-learned. In the Iraqi medical education environment where the need for triage is immediate, but the ability to stage practice is nearly impossible, blending didactic learning with simulation-based triage offers an alternative training methodology.

Keywords: Triage, patient simulation, virtual patients, disaster medicine

1. Introduction

As part of a U.S. Agency for International Development (USAID) project to enhance medical training in Iraq, we were asked to design and deliver a "Train-the-Trainer" curriculum in trauma triage. Mass casualty triage is the process of establishing the priority of care among multiple casualties to rationally allocate the use of limited resources. Like most time-sensitive, high-stakes cognitive skills that are rarely used, triage requires regular practice to maintain proficiency and confidence in decision-making. Actual disasters, such as explosions, hurricanes, or toxic exposures, occur so rarely that there is little opportunity for gaining experience. Constructive tabletop simulations are abstract mental exercises without direct patient interaction. The expense of obtaining, training, and moulaging multiple actors for live training exercises usually forces triage training to be incorporated into collective training exercises designed for the entire disaster response infrastructure. To provide an alternative methodology, including individual self-paced learning, we developed a blended didactic and simulation-based curriculum in multiple-casualty triage.

2. Methods

2.1. Virtual Patient Simulation

The triage simulation was developed by leveraging several virtual reality systems developed for medical care training, including trauma, bioterrorism, and chemical agent casualties, called Sim-Patient™.   The patient is an animated 3D character situated in a 3D scene (Figure 1).   The simulation includes 3D visual models of the full range of medical devices available to the student, including bandages, drugs, and monitoring devices.   The student can navigate and survey the scene, as well as interact (e.g., take a pulse) and converse with the virtual patient.

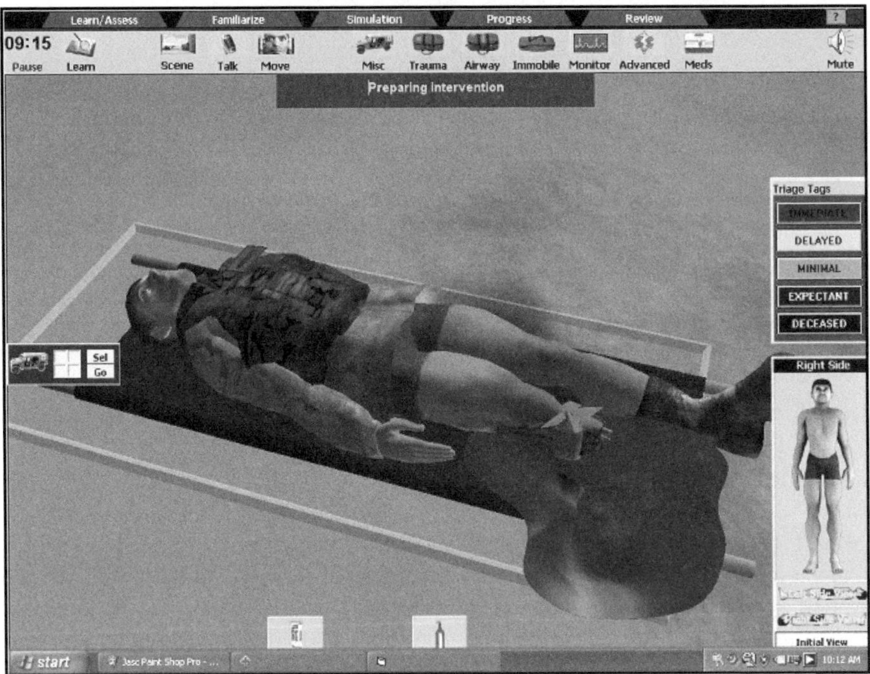

Figure 1. Single casualty in Sim-Patient trauma patient simulator.

Simulated patients have been developed for trauma, bioterrorism, and chemical casualties [1, 2] as well as mentally disturbed individuals and pediatric patients [3, 4]. The simulated patient can be configured for a practice session with a variety of injuries and will exhibit appropriate signs and symptoms that change with the evolving condition of the patient over time. Animations such as vomiting, tearing, coughing, seizure, and convulsions relate to physiological status and interventions. The patients have dynamic facial expression, gestures, body movement, and can portray anger, fright, confusion, or other emotions or behaviors based on cognitive, emotional, physiological, and pathological models.

The effects of various treatments are simulated by a physiological model. The physiological simulation integrates real-time cardiovascular, respiratory, and pharmacokinetic models.   A supervisory layer provides overall control of the simulation, controls the BODY™ physiology model (Advanced Simulation Corporation, Point Roberts, WA).

All of these add to the realism of the training by requiring that the student integrate knowledge of diagnostic processes with the search for and recognition of visual and audible symptoms, visual reinforcement of monitoring and treatment devices, and awareness of the changes in patient conditions over time. The dynamic visuals and audio increase the emotional involvement of the student.

2.2. Multiple-Casualty Triage Simulation

Sim-Patient was enhanced to support multiple-casualty scenarios. Each casualty has its own injury models, physiological simulation, and signs and symptoms that reflect changing physiological conditions. Figure 2 shows a multiple-casualty scenario in an urban environment, showing what might result from the explosion of an improvised explosive device (IED). Color-coded tags are used to triage each casualty, thereby designating the victim's priority of care. The triage tags are used within a four-level classification system (Immediate, Delayed, Minor, and Expectant) consistent with the Simple Triage and Rapid Treatment (START) triage method. Developed in the 1980's by the Newport Beach (CA) Fire Department and Hoag Memorial Hospital for use by civilian responders in the aftermath of earthquakes [5], the START method is universally recognized as a highly accessible and easy to use algorithmic approach to performing primary disaster triage [6]. Though START triage has come under attack in recent years, a retrospective review of over 1100 trauma patients triaged by different algorithms suggests that START triage is still a sensitive tool for predicting critical injuries [7].

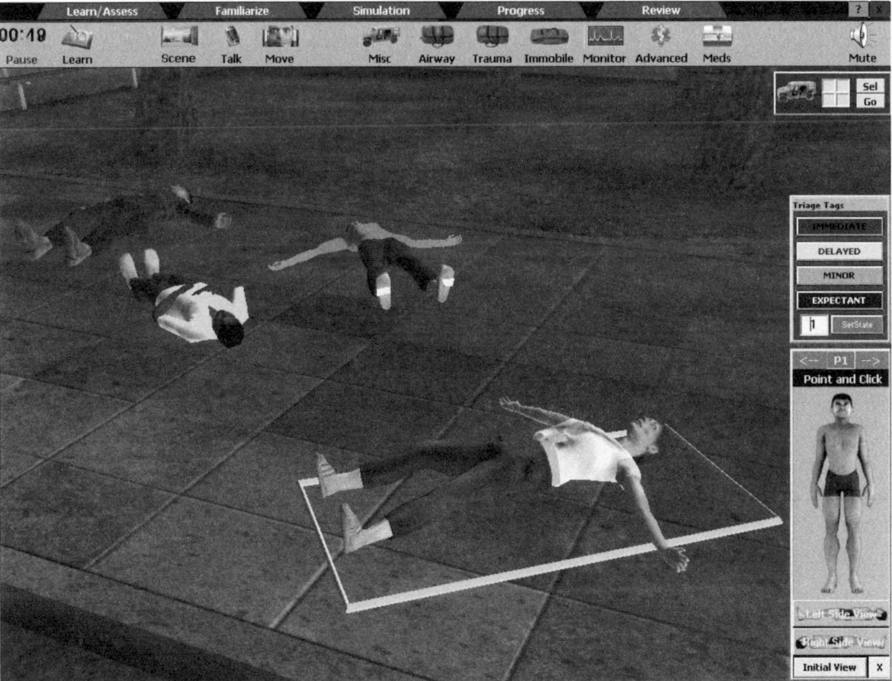

Figure 2. Sim-Patient Triage Simulation Trainer, showing multiple trauma casualties. Note the learning management tabs (top), toolbar resources (top), START triage tags (right), and transport management buttons (upper right).

2.3. Scenario Definition for Triage Training

Scenarios were initially developed for training U.S. military physicians in triage and initial care consistent with IED-related injuries. These scenarios provide an evolving medical situation with graphically intense casualties including amputations, penetrations, massive burns, chest wounds, blunt trauma. Since the medical conditions were dynamic, conducting triage for these patients was not a deterministic process. How the caregiver moves about and selects individual casualties would affect the 'correct' triage assessment. For example, while evaluating casualty "A", casualty "B" might deteriorate, evolving from an "Immediate" to an "Expectant" state. While this represents a realistic, evolving casualty situation, training scenarios with unstable patients may detract from effective learning and make it difficult to assess student performance.

To address this issue, we modified the simulator to provide casualties with stable physiological conditions according to defined triage learning objectives. Based on an analysis of the START algorithm, we identified seven assessment paths that might be followed before arriving at a triage determination (Figure 3). The Minor, Expectant, and Delayed categories each have a single path to triage classification. The Immediate triage tag category has four assessment paths, depending upon different critical conditions (i.e., airway, breathing, circulatory, and mental impairment).

To support triage training, 32 casualties were created with a spectrum of injuries and physiological conditions covering all of the 7 pathways. Eight scenarios were developed, with different mechanisms of injury, and 4 casualties were assigned to each scenario. One scenario was reserved for learning how to use the simulator, and the remaining seven configured for learning and practicing the START triage algorithm. These cases were designed to ensure that each path through the START triage algorithm is practiced at least 3 times by each trainee.

2.4. Student Feedback and After-Action Review

The simulation tracks the student's actions and compares them against the correct protocol path (Figure 3). At the end of each scenario, a chart presented the expected START-path (left pane) and the actions taken by the student (right pane) for each casualty in the scenario. For example, one of the first actions a first responder should take is to ask out loud for all 'ambulatory' casualties to walk to a separate area. These are the "walking well" and according to START can be tagged as Minor. Farther down the flowchart, the first responder should assess mental status, normally by asking the casualty to respond to simple commands. If the casualty is able to respond then the casualty is tagged as Delayed, otherwise the injured should be tagged as Immediate. A summary of the relevant physiological parameters are displayed for further guidance and review (bottom).

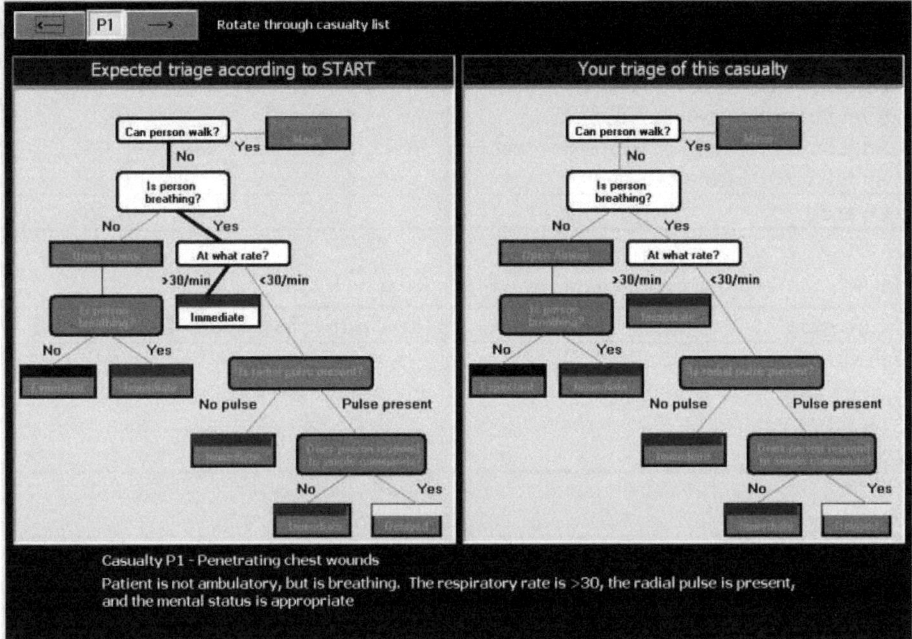

Figure 3. START algorithm used as an after action review (AAR). For stable casualties, the expected triage assessment (left) and the student's ongoing assessment (right) are presented and compared.

2.5. *Triage Course Curriculum and Delivery*

A comprehensive set of learning modules was developed comprising prehospital trauma care, the START triage methodology, how to use the Sim-Patient simulator, and how to employ Sim-Patient for training others. The latter module supported the Train-the-Trainer objective of the parent USAID program for Training Model Primary Providers The learning modules were developed in Microsoft PowerPoint format, and with annotated learning objectives and teaching points.

Twenty-two graphics-intensive laptop computers were configured with the Sim-Patient software and delivered to the Iraqi Ministry of Health (MOH) for use in the triage course, and subsequent turn-over to the planned Centers of Excellence for training of other medical personnel. In cooperation with the MOH, select physicians were recruited to attend one of two 2-day short courses on triage and using the Sim-Patient triage simulator. The two courses were conducted in July of 2006.

3. Results

Thirty-one physicians, identified by the MOH, participated in the blended didactic and simulation-based triage curriculum. Participants evaluated the curriculum using a questionnaire comprising qualitative measures (Likert-scale: strongly disagree=1 to strongly agree=5), and requests for comments according to several categories. The physicians were not followed after their participation, so assessment of transfer of learning was not possible. Summary statistics were developed for the qualitative measures and comments as follows:

Table 1. Qualitative measures of didactic presentation and simulation.

Category	Mean	Std. Dev.
Didactic Course & Presenter	4.36	0.43
Simulation Realism & Navigation	4.40	0.20
Simulation Content & Responsiveness	4.42	0.04
Simulation Learning Content	4.41	0.20
Overall	**4.38**	**0.36**

Table 2. Distribution of participant comments across all course elements.

Category	Count (%)	Pos/Neg (%)
Positive	56 (52%)	56 (93%)
Negative	5 (4%)	5 (7%)
Descriptive	4 (5%)	
Suggestive	43 (40%)	

4. Conclusions

A curriculum has been developed blending didactic training and case-based simulation for START triage training. The course has been given to a group of physicians with the goal of improving prehospital and emergency trauma care throughout Iraq. The participants' evaluations have been overwhelmingly favorable, with expressions of appreciation for the course and for being introduced to the START triage methodology. Several mentioned that they had been unaware of any formal trauma triage methodology. It has been suggested that this training, if made readily available to the first responders in Iraq, would make an immediate and measurable impact on the survivability of casualties in the field.

References

[1]   Kizakevich, P.N., M. L. McCartney, D. B. Nissman, K. Starko, and N. Ty Smith. "Virtual Medical Trainer: Patient Assessment and Trauma Care Simulator." Stud Health Technol Inform. 1998;50:309-15.

[2]   Weaver, A.L., P.N. Kizakevich, W. Stoy, J.H. Magee, W. Ott, and K. Wilson. Usability Analysis of VR Simulation Software. Stud Health Technol Inform. 2002;85:567-9.

[3]   Frank, G., Guinn, C., Hubal, R., Pope, P., Stanford, M., & Lamm-Weisel, D. JUST-TALK: An Application of Responsive Virtual Human Technology. Proceedings of the Interservice/Industry Training, Simulation and Education Conference, December 2-5, 2002, Orlando, FL.

[4]   Hubal, R.C., Deterding, R.R., Frank, G.A., Schwetzke, H.F., & Kizakevich, P.N. Lessons Learned in Modeling Pediatric Patients. Stud Health Technol Inform. 2003;94:127-30.

[5]   Super, G. START: a Triage Training Module. Newport Beach, CA; Hoag Memorial Hospital Presbyterian; 1984.

[6]   Benson, D.O., Keonig, K.L., Schultz, C.H. Disaster triage: START then SAVE—a new method of dynamic triage for victims of catastrophic earthquake. Prehosp Disaster Med. 1996; 11: 117-124.

[7]   Garner, A., Lee, A. Harrison, K. Schultz, C.H., Comparative Analysis of Multiple-Casualty Incident Triage Algorithms. Ann Emerg Med. 2001; 38(5): 541-548.

Medicine Meets Virtual Reality 15
J.D. Westwood et al. (Eds.)
IOS Press, 2007

Training and Assessment of Procedural Skills in Context using an Integrated Procedural Performance Instrument (IPPI)

R KNEEBONE, F BELLO[1], D NESTEL, F YADOLLAHI and A DARZI
Department of Biosurgery and Surgical Technology, Imperial College London

Abstract. The use of simulation in the training and assessment of procedural skills is widely acknowledged as a powerful and necessary alternative to the traditional apprenticeship model. However advanced, simulation on its own cannot provide the necessary conditions for holistic practice. The Integrated Procedural Performance Instrument presented in this paper combines simulated patients (SPs) with inanimate models, items of medical equipment or computer generated virtual models to recreate a panel of realistic scenarios, each addressing a combination of technical and non-technical clinical challenges. The result is a safe yet authentic clinical context which can be used for training and assessment. This novel use of simulation provides a patient-centred, learner-focused approach that builds up a composite picture of technical skills, communication skills and professional behaviours across a range of challenging clinical situations.

Keywords. Procedural skills, context-aware simulation, training and assessment

1. Background

Clinical procedures are a core component of healthcare practice. Current assessment focuses on technical skill, often using simulation ranging from inanimate models (e.g. venepuncture, intravenous infusion, urinary catheterisation) to advanced VR simulators (e.g. MIST, VIST [1], AccuTouch [2]). Likewise, training based on the traditional apprenticeship model and, more recently, utilising simulation, tends to disregard non-technical skills such as communication and other professional skills. In this paper we describe an Integrated Procedural Performance Instrument (IPPI) which combines physical or high level computer generated virtual models with simulated patients (SPs) to create a closer approximation to actual clinical situations. This innovative approach uses a panel of realistic scenarios, each addressing a combination of clinical challenges (technical and non-technical) relating to core procedures, together with a powerful computer-based remote assessment methodology that makes possible the provision of timely, personalised and focused feedback.

---

[1] Corresponding Author: F Bello, Dept. of Biosurgery and Surgical Technology, 10th Floor QEQM Building, St Mary's Hospital, Praed St, London W2 1NY, UK; E-mail: dorothy.F.Bello@imperial.ac.uk

2. Methods

Performing a clinical procedure requires a complex mixture of technical skill and professionalism. Effective communication is essential, both with the patient and with other members of the clinical team. Even a 'simple' task such as taking blood or giving an injection can pose considerable challenges if a patient is anxious, aggressive, confused or unable to speak the clinician's language. Appropriately empathic behaviour is essential [3] but may be overlooked during technical procedures. We have developed a scenario-based innovative approach to the teaching and assessment of clinical procedures, where technical skill and professional behaviour are given equal value. Scenarios combine simulated patients (SPs) with inanimate models (Fig. 1(a)), items of medical equipment (Fig. 1(b)) or computer generated virtual models (Fig. 1(c)) to create a safe yet authentic clinical context which can be used for formative and summative assessment [4]. In each case, the clinician performs the procedure on a model (thereby ensuring patient safety) while interacting with the 'patient' in an authentic way. A computer-based assessment methodology using commercially available surveillance cameras and networked videomonitoring technology allows assessors to observe and rate scenarios remotely, using desktop computers with on-screen buttons to control camera position and zoom. Candidates and SPs use handheld computers to input performance data. Data streams are integrated automatically, using on-screen rating software (the Imperial College Feedback and Assessment System, ICFAS) that generates a secure, web-based feedback site where each participant can access summary information about their performance and review videorecorded scenarios. The IPPI concept and remote rating system draw on literature relating to expertise, tutor support, workplace based learning and educational climate [5-7]. Learners are able to practise repeatedly within a safe environment that parallels the workplace, but where their needs are given priority.

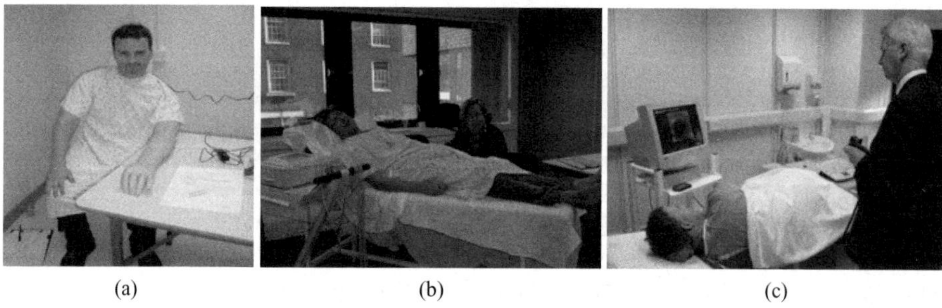

(a)   (b)   (c)

Figure 1. Sample patient-practitioner scenarios combining simulated patients with inanimate models (a), medical equipment (b) and endoscopy simulator (c).

3. Results

We have conducted a number of IPPI sessions with 12 and 8 scenarios, resulting in an excess of two thousand scenario episodes where over two hundred doctors in training have participated. Evaluation has included scenario realism scales, group interviews, SP role play questionnaires and direct observation. Interview and questionnaire data showed that the majority of candidates found IPPI to be a powerful and valuable learning experience. Many identified areas where they needed to refresh existing skills, develop new ones or better integrate their technical, communication and other professional skills.

4. Discussion and Conclusion

Our results demonstrate that IPPI is feasible for assessing clinical procedures, providing an overall picture of a clinician's procedural competence at a given level of challenge. ICFAS provides a high level of performance detail and supportive feedback, placing the patient's perspective at centre stage. Sampling data from a series of procedures offers a picture of a participant's performance across a range of domains. Equally, IPPI is a valuable training tool providing the necessary conditions for holistic practice, especially with challenging situations where patients may be disabled, angry, distressed or have other special needs.

The innovation of IPPI lies in its recreation of authentic context by combining models and simulation with SPs, presenting a range of challenges that can be useful for training and assessment. Our intention was to create an instrument which combines key elements of clinical practice and constructs a picture of competence across a range of important and commonly encountered clinical settings.

References

[1] http://www.mentice.com/
[2] http://www.immersion.com/medical/products/endoscopy/
[3] Larson EB, Yao X. Clinical empathy as emotional labour in the patient-physician relationship. JAMA 2005; 293(9):1100-1106.
[4] Kneebone R, Kidd J, Nestel D, Barnet A, Lo B, King R et al. Blurring the boundaries: scenario-based simulation in a clinical setting. Med Educ 2005; 39:580-587.
[5] Kneebone RL. Clinical simulation for learning procedural skills: a theory-based approach. Acad Med 2005; 80(6):549-553.
[6] Ericsson KA. Deliberate practice and the acquisition and maintenance of expert performance in medicine and related domains. Acad Med 2004; 79(10):S70-S81.
[7] Lave J, Wenger E. Situated learning. Legitimate peripheral participation. Cambridge: Cambridge University Press; 1991.

Medicine Meets Virtual Reality 15
J.D. Westwood et al. (Eds.)
IOS Press, 2007

Real-time Marker-based Tracking of a Non-rigid Object

Andreas KÖPFLE [a,b], Florian BEIER [a], Clemens WAGNER [b], Reinhard MÄNNER [a,c]

[a] *Institute for Computational Medicine, University of Mannheim*
[b] *VRmagic GmbH, Mannheim*
[c] *Department of Computer Science V, University of Mannheim*

Abstract. Real-time tracking of non-rigid objects for use in interfaces of VR-simulators is presented. Markers are attached to the objects and observed by several cameras with integrated image-processing hardware which extracts relevant marker data (centroid, area & color) in real-time. Data from the different cameras is then matched in the host PC to reconstruct the 3D positions. We present two approaches to this special matching problem because standard image feature based algorithms are not feasible for marker-based tracking. A model of the deformation is extracted from the reconstructed 3D point cloud and the simulation model is updated accordingly. Experiments with a prototype of a deformable eye interface for the ophthalmosurgical simulator EYESI show that latency, robustness and accuracy of the deformation tracking are adequate for application in VR simulators. The approach is extensible to other types of simulators where deformable tissue has to be tracked.

Keywords. optical tracking, real-time deformation tracking, non-rigid object, VR interface

Problem

Optical tracking systems are a key technology in human-computer interfaces of medical VR-simulators. They allow easy acquisition of the interaction with the simulated environment. To achieve the required low latency and real-time capability mainly marker-based approaches are used where well-detectable markers are attached to the objects. Current systems focus on the tracking of rigid bodies (e.g. surgical instruments) with a fixed setup of the attached markers [1]. However situations exist where interaction with deformable tissue is necessary. Approaches for tracking of non-rigid objects have been presented [2], but they are not applicable under the tight real-time and low latency conditions of an interactive simulator. For example, during a simulated ophthalmosurgical intervention it may be necessary to deform the eye interactively in order to get a better view on the retina through the lense. In this paper we present a deformable eye interface for the ophthalmosurgical simulator EYESI [3], which is needed to track deformation with sufficiently low latency to enable a realistic interaction with the simulated VR eye.

Methods

In our setup small CMOS cameras are mounted under the hemispherical artificial eye to observe the simulated operation area. Originally three cameras were used to increase precision and robustness of the reconstruction. The inner side of the eye is tagged by colored markers that get identified in the camera images. To fullfill the low-latency demands of real-time interaction and to reduce load on the simulator's main CPU, an FPGA-based coprocessor preprocesses the images. We implemented a new single-pass blob-segmentation algorithm that detects the markers in the image data on the fly and extracts relevant information like position, color, area and centre of gravity with a latency of well below 1ms. Extracted information of the distinct markers is then transmitted to the main CPU, where the data from different cameras has to be matched in order to reconstruct the markers' 3D positions and therefrom the objects.

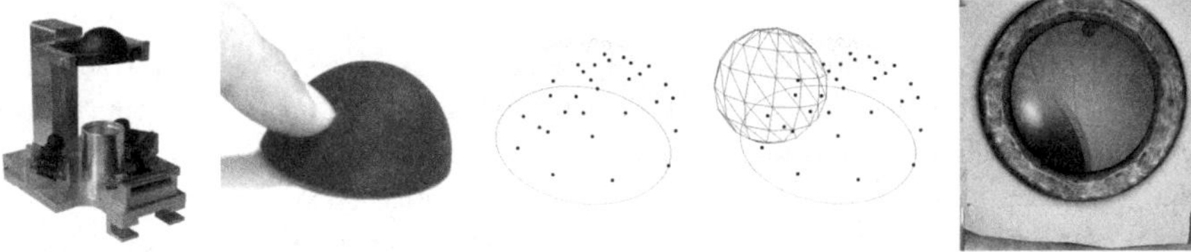

Figure 1. The eye interface setup, deformation of the artificial eye, point-cloud of reconstructed 3D markers with fitted deformation sphere and simulator view through the lense with the deformed retina in the lower left

The fundamental step for reconstruction is to identify matching images of each marker in the different camera views. To reduce the number of possible candidates the camera images are rectified pair-wise. Candidates for corresponding marker images have to fulfill the epipolar constraint, i.e. they need to be on or near corresponding epipolar lines. This standard technique in stereo reconstruction tremendously reduces the number of possible matches [4].

Further standard solutions to the remainig stereo matching problem are based on image features. As all markers have identical shape, these approaches are not suitable for marker-based reconstruction. Likewise due to the deformability of the object, resolving correlation ambiguities by fitting a known rigid 3D configuration is not feasible. An additional problem in our setup is that instruments or the deformed eye itself may occlude markers in one or more cameras. We present two different approaches for the basic marker matching and further methods for optimization of the reconstructed deformation model:

The first approach exploits the redundant information of the three camera setup by means of trifocal geometry [4]. In the process each stereo-reconstructed 3D marker candidate is validated by the third camera image. In some special cases though (where the marker arrangement is point-symmetric to the camera arrangement), false points may be reconstructed due to geometric ambiguities. These "phantom" markers are identified and removed in further processing steps described below.

Our second method uses a relational matching approach based on the PMF algorithm [5]. This uses the fundamental idea that matching points have a similar neighborhood of markers. A strength of match for each candidate pair is calculated by weighting these similarities in distance and angle with respect to a surrounding neighborhood in each camera image. This strength of match is optimized for the best fit between markers.

Once the matches are known the 3D marker positions are reconstructed via triangulation. Some falsely detected markers are filtered out by tracing the detected 3D points and setting an upper threshold to the allowed position delta. Other outliers may occur as the instruments or the deformed eye itself occlude some of the markers. To further detect and eliminate false markers a robust model of the deformation is needed. Using a-priori knowledge about the setup we model the scene as a halfsphere (the mechanical eye). All points deviating from the main halfsphere are considered for the deformation, which is modelled as a virtual second sphere intersecting the main halfsphere. Points deviating from these two spheres more than a certain threshold are marked as outliers and the deformation fit is repeated without them. The simulation is then updated with the coordinates of the deepest deformation point and the deformation depth.

Results

Experiments with a first prototype using approx. 40 markers on the eye interface showed a robust real-time detection of the deformation at an image acquisition rate of 30Hz. Latencies after camera read-out were measured as 2ms for the trifocal and approx. 9ms for the PMF approach. Both methods reconstructed more than 90% of markers correctly, which is sufficient for our application as falsely reconstructed 3D points can be detected and eliminated by the deformation model fit. We measured the accuracy by determining the depth and position of the deepest point of the deformation. Error of reconstructed position in angular coordinates was approx. 4-5% and the impression depth error < 1mm.

Conclusion and Discussion

We presented a first implementation for an optical tracking of deformable objects for surgical VR-simulators. The results concerning robustness, accuracy and latency are adequate for integration in the ophthalmosurgical simulator EYESI. The tracking setup yields fast, robust results while not imposing heavy processing demands on the main simulators CPU, leaving the majority of resources to simulation and graphics. Our first approach uses even less CPU resources, but demands at least a 3 camera setup. The second method is more resource intense, however it already works in a stereo camera setup. Both approaches can be extended to several other types of simulators where deformable tissue has to be tracked, e.g. the abdominal wall in a laparoscopy simulator.

References

[1]　R.J. Lapeer, M.S. Chen, J.G. Villagrana. *Simulating Obstetric Forceps Delivery in an Augmented Environment*. Proceedings of AMI/ARCS sattelite workshop of MICCAI 2004, pp. 1-10

[2]　N.A. Ramey, J.J. Corso, W.W. Lau, D. Burschka, G.D. Hager. *Real-time 3D Surface Tracking and Its Applications*. Proceedings of Computer Vision and Pattern Recognition Workshop 2004 (CVPRW'04) Volume 3 pp. 34

[3]　C. Wagner, M. A. Schill, R. Maenner. *Intraocular Surgery on a Virtual Eye*. Communications of the ACM. Vol. 45, No. 7 (2002), pp 45-49

[4]　R. Hartley, A. Zisserman. *Multiple View Geometry in Computer Vision*. Cambridge University Press, 2004

[5]　S.B. Pollard, J.E.W. Mayhew, J.P. Frisby. *PMF: A stereo correspondence algorithm using a disparity gradient limit*. Perception, 14:449-470, 1985

Medicine Meets Virtual Reality 15
J.D. Westwood et al. (Eds.)
IOS Press, 2007

A New Force-Based Objective Assessment of Technical Skills in Endoscopic Sinus Surgery

Toru Kumagai [a,1], Juli Yamashita [a], Osamu Morikawa [a] and Kazunori Yokoyama [b]

[a] *National Institute of Advanced Industrial Science and Technology, Japan*
[b] *Hana Clinic @ South Avenue, Japan*

Abstract. We propose objectively assessing endoscopic sinus surgery (ESS) skills by measuring the force applied to a patient model. We collected data on 16 subjects performing gauze packing task using a precise human nasal model with a six-degree-of-freedom force/torque sensor. Mann-Whitney's U test was used to analyze their performance. Intermediates (ESS: 10-50 cases) used significantly greater force than students or experts (ESS: over 150 cases) at the 5 % level. Maximum force improved only among experts. These results imply that young surgeons pay too little attention to force applied to patients or tissues.

Keywords. Objective assessment, technical skill, endoscopic sinus sugery

Introduction

Objective assessment is one key to effective surgical technical skills training. Recent attempts to assess surgical skills have involved measuring the forces exerted during procedures using virtual reality [1] or by employing instrument-installed force sensors [2]. We are developing a training system for endoscopic sinus surgery (ESS).

In this study we selected, as objective measures, maximum force (Fm) and average force (Fa) generated during instrument-to-patient contact, which we measured and evaluated during gauze packing (GP) into the ethmoidal sinus using a nasal model equipped with a force sensor (Figures 1 and 2). GP is the packing of gauze via the nasal cavity to ensure hemostasis or surface anesthesia, using forceps under endoscopic guidance. Appropriate packing pressure (PP) between the packed gauze and the lesion is necessary. The nasal mucosa

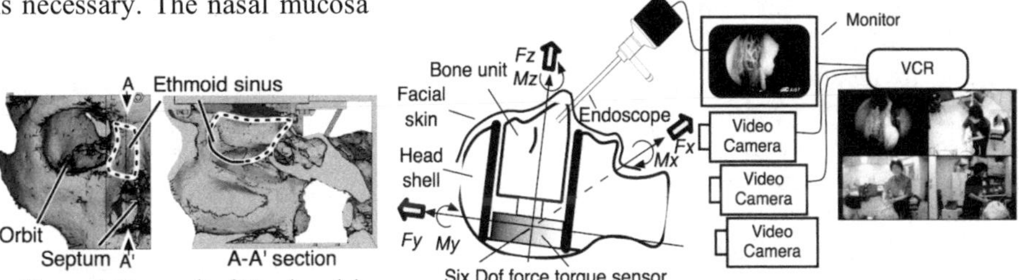

Figure 1. Bone unit of Nasal model.

Figure 2. Experiment system.

---

[1] Corresponding Author: Senior Research Scientist, Institute of Advanced Industrial Science and Technology (AIST), 1-1-1 Higashi, Tsukuba, Ibaraki 305-8566, Japan; E-mail: kumagai.toru@aist.go.jp.

en route to the lesion must be protected from abrasion by the instrument.

1. Tools and Methods

Fm and *Fa* applied during GP to the ethmoidal sinus were experimentally measured and compared among four groups of subjects.

The subjects were 16 volunteers (13 otolaryngologists and 3 medical students), classified according to experience: 3 Experts (Group E: ESS experience > 100 cases; PGY > 9 years), 6 Intermediates (Group I: ESS experience 10–50 cases; PGY, 3–10 years), 4 Beginners (Group B: ESS experience 0–2 cases; PGY, 0–10 years), and 3 students (Group S).

A nasal model with an open ethmoidal sinus (Figures 1 and 2), precisely reconstructed from CT images, was employed. A questionnaire survey had confirmed this model to be as useful as a cadaver for intranasal observation training [3]. The bone unit was separate from the head shell and supported by only a six-degree-of-freedom force sensor (Model IFS-67M25A 25-140, Nitta Corp., Japan). The force sensor detected the force and torque on the bone unit. Forces $(Fx^2 + Fy^2 + Fz^2)^{1/2}$ were recorded at 10Hz on a PC. The surgical instruments were a ø 4mm 0° rigid nasal endoscope (Shinko Optical Co., Ltd., Japan), a monitor (14 inch color CRT, Sony, Japan), forceps (Lucae, 17cm), and gauze (3cm x 40cm) moistened with 2ml water.

The subjects watched an instruction video on ethmoidal sinus anatomy, use of the instruments, and GP, and then performed GP on the right ethmoidal sinus of the nasal model. The force applied, completion time (*T*), endoscopic images, and images of the subjects were recorded.

2. Results

Mann-Whitney's U test was performed between Group E and the other groups for *T*, *Fm*, and *Fa* (Figure 3). The results of GP were evaluated by video observation. Good results (good) were obtained by Groups B, I, and E. In Group S, gauze projected from the ethmoidal sinus (poor).

3. Discussion

Origin of *Fm* was evaluated by video observation. In Group E, *Fm* of ~1.5–3N developed while confirming appropriate packing by pushing the packed gauze in the ethmoidal sinus. In Groups S, I and B (excluding two subjects with *Fm* of ~1.5–3N), the subjects frequently generated *Fm* of ~3–8N by instrument-to-model contact: a) Hitting due to interference between instruments or lack of tactical feedback for depth, b) Unnecessary pressure against the intra-

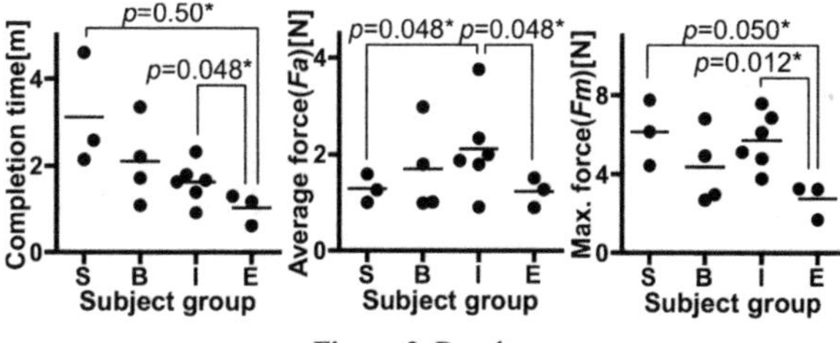

Figure 3. Results.

nasal walls, and c) Movement of forceps outside the endoscope's visual field, causing abrasion of the mucosa. Inexperienced physicians tended to be unaware of intranasal damage being caused by instrument-mucosal contact; Group I was particularly inept, corroborating a survey on laparoscopic cholecystectomy[4] revealing that 90% of injuries occur in a surgeon's first 30 cases.

The low *Fa* in Group S matched that in Group E, but Group S produced poor results. Thus, it was determined that low *Fm* and *Fa* are not predictors of good GP. Subjective assessment by experts combined with feedback of *Fm* and *Fa* has the potential to increase patient safety.

4. Conclusions

We confirmed that *Fa* and *Fm* applied to the patient model are effective and objective measures of surgical skill assessment in ESS through the analysis of GP. Force has a clinical implication not provided by *T*. More experienced subjects naturally required shorter *T*. In contrast, *Fa* increased and *Fm* did not improve with experience, except among experts. These results imply that young surgeons pay less attention to force applied to patients or tissues, potentially leading to unexpected bleeding during surgery and poor prognosis caused by unnecessary pressure on tissues. Force is not predictable from video records and must be measured for proper assessment.

The small deviations in *T*, *Fa*, and *Fm* among experts suggest that an optimal task technique exists. Analysis of expert techniques and development of training that enables trainees to acquire this expertise is essential for safe and swift introduction of newly developed surgical procedures such as minimally invasive surgery.

Future work should include analysis of torque data, the study of learning curve in conseccutive GP tasks, and assessment of ethmoidectomy.

Acknowledgements

This study was supported in part by the 2005 Industrial Technology Research Grant Program of the New Energy and Industrial Technology Development Organization (NEDO) of Japan.

References

[1] S. Payandeh, A.J. Lomax, J. Dill, C.L. Mackenzie, C.G.L. Cao, On Defining Metrics for Assessing Laparoscopic Surgical Skills in a Virtual Training Environment, *Stud Health Technol Inform* **85** (2002), 334-340.

[2] J. Rosen, B. Hannaford, C.G. Richards, M.N. Sinanan, Markov Modeling of Minimally Invasive Surgery Based on Tool/Tissue Interaction and Force/Torque Signatures for Evaluating Surgical Skills, *IEEE Trans on Biomed Eng* **48**-5(2001), 579-591.

[3] J. Yamashita, K. Yokoyama, O. Morikawa, M. Kitajima, T. Kumagai, Questionnaire Survey on Validity of AIST Incisive Nasal Model in ESS Training, *Oto-Rhino-Laryngology, Tokyo* **49** (2006) (in press, in Japanese).

[4] V.C. Gibbs, A.D. Auerbach, Learning Curves for New Procedures - the Case of Laparoscopic Cholecystectomy, In: *Making Health Care Safer, Evidence Report/Technology Assessment No.43*, Agency for Healthcare Research and Quality (2001), 213-220.

Medicine Meets Virtual Reality 15
J.D. Westwood et al. (Eds.)
IOS Press, 2007

A Proposal of Speculative Operation on Distributed System for FEM-based Ablation Simulator

Naoto KUME [a] Yoshihiro KURODA [b] Megumi NAKAO [c] Tomohiro KURODA [d]
Keisuke NAGASE [d] Hiroyuki YOSHIHARA [d] and Masaru KOMORI [e]

[a] *Kyoto University Hospital, JSPS Research Fellow*
[b] *Graduate School of Engineering Science, Osaka University*
[c] *Graduate School of Information Science, Nara Institute of Science and Technology*
[d] *Kyoto University Hospital*
[e] *Department of Medicine, Shiga University of Medical Science*

Abstract. This study aims to provide physics-based force feedback system on distributed system for simulating invasive operation such as ablation. conventional PC-based VR surgical simulators with haptic interaction are hard to provide sufficient computational resources for the simulation of physics-based soft tissue fracture. For proper presentation of force feedback as real operations, physics-based simulation is inevitable. At the same time finite element method requires huge computational complexites. In this paper, the authors propose server-side speculative operation method on application layer for hiding the calculation latencies. The proposed method would achieve the response acceleration without the decomposition of conventional simulation process. The theoritical estimates of speculation parameters are mentioned.

Keywords. Speculation, PC-Cluster, FEM, Ablation

Introduction

Various VR-based surgical simulators were provided for teaching force sense in operation. Physics-based modeling is quite important for rendering the similar sensation of the real operation. However, conventional simulators can not present the force sense of soft tissue fracture due to the computational complexities of physics-based model. This study aims to provide an ablation training simulator supporting haptic feedback. From a view point of physics, ablation is a combined operation of soft tissue deformation and fracture. So far, this study constructed FEM-based ablation model [1]. Soft tissue deformation is simulated by conventional FEM-based method [2]. The model defines the threshold of continuous deformation as shearing stress. After the determination of rupture, the model processes the reconstruction of inverse stiffness matrix. Because the matrix reconstruction requires huge computational resources, the model had not achieved simulation in real-time on PC-based system. Currently, distributed massive simulation system such as PC cluster is usable for high performance VR applications [3]. Therefore, the model is conducted to install on a PC cluster.

1. Application Level Speculation

Distributed system faces on several delays such as communication delay and calculation delay. Calculation delay including the matrix reconstruction is the most critical part on the ablation model for real-time response. Therefore, hiding reconstruction delay which is required in fracture process is desired. General use of PC cluster employs parallel processing of a simulation loop. In contrast, this paper proposes application level speculative operation of matrix reconstruction on server-side simulation. The proposed method manages every server-side processing unit as a simulator. User interface is handled on client-side system. Physics-based massive simulation is managed by server-side system. Fig. 1 illustrates the server-side system which consists of front-end and back-end system. The prediction of stress distribution generates several speculation orders of matrix construction. Stiffness matrix is reconstructed beforehand by predicted parameters, and the matrix is replied immediately to the simulation request generated by user's manipulation. The method theoretically requires the number of processing units as same as the number of the predicted stress distribution patterns. Therefore, the speculation system employs pattern reduction parameters which are based on the prediction depth and pattern priority. The number of the fracture pattern which should be prepared in advance is reduced by depth which assumes continuous manipulation. Pattern priority for the prediction of the fracture elements is defined by stress distribution which assumes varied manipulation on direction. Both parameters are adjusted to the employed simulation model and computational resources.

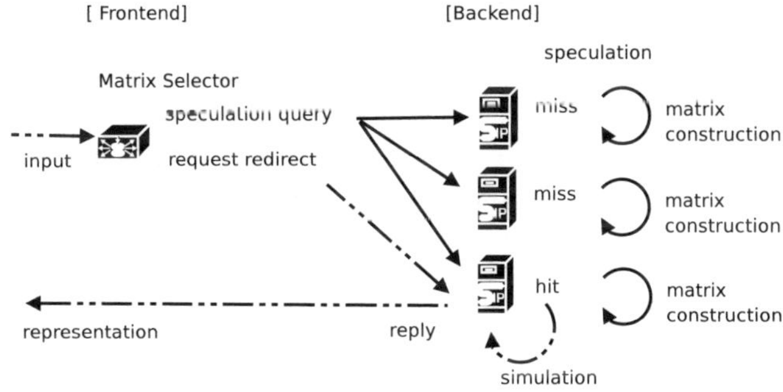

Figure 1. Server-side speculation and response

2. Estimation

Performance measurement of server response time was performed. Performance of the proposed method was analyzed on the conventional ablation model. Server response time was approx 9 msec including the communication delay and the memory loading delay of stiffness matrix. The result of estimation was that the response to user takes 11.6 msec including visualization in the best performance. The relation between the number of required processing unit and the reduction parameters is illustrated in Fig. 2. The relation between the parameters and the available size of soft tissue model are mapped on each line.

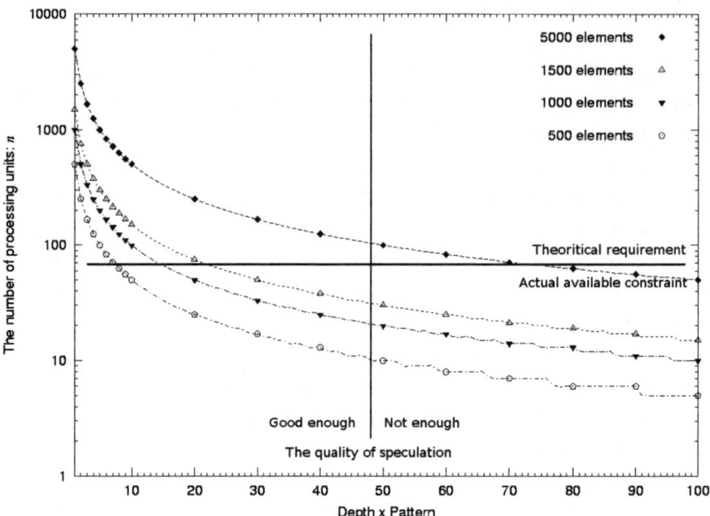

Figure 2. Relation between the number of required processing unit and the reduction parameters

3. Conclusion

This study aims to provide an ablation training simulator which presents the haptic sensation of soft tissue rupture. This paper proposed an acceleration method of server-side response for haptic interaction on distributed system. Application level speculative operation would provide quick response with physics-based massive simulation. The result of estimation indicated that the response from server to client is settle in real-time while the speculation hits. The proposed method will be implemented in the future.

Acknowledgements

This research was partly supported by Grant-in-Aid for JSPS Fellows and Grant-in-Aid for Scientific Research(S) (16100001) from the Japan Society for the Promotion of Science, supported by Grant-in-Aid (H18-Medicine-General-032) from the Ministry of Health, Labour and Welfare, Japan, and supported by Grant-in-Aid for Young Scientists (A) (17680008) and Exploratory Research (18659148) from The Ministry of Education, Culture, Sports, Science and Technology, Japan.

References

[1]   N. Kume, et.al.: FEM-based Soft Tissue Destruction Model for Ablation Simulator, *MMVR13*, Long Beach, 2005, 263–269.
[2]   K. Hirota and T. Kaneko: Haptic representation of elastic objects, *Presence* **10**(5) 2001, 525–536.
[3]   B. Raffin, et.al.: PC clusters for virtual reality, *IEEE Virtual Reality Conference*, 2006, 215–222.

Medicine Meets Virtual Reality 15
J.D. Westwood et al. (Eds.)
IOS Press, 2007

Tissue Resection using Delayed Updates in a Tetrahedral Mesh

Kishalay KUNDU [a] and Marc OLANO [a]

[a] *Department of Computer Science, University of Maryland Baltimore County*

Abstract. In open surgery simulations, cuts like incisions and resections introduce irreversible changes to underlying geometry. In such circumstances, updating tetrahedral meshes for sophisticated physical modeling methods like finite elements becomes computationally intensive.

We present an algorithm that does not need to update every time there is an incision. It allows multiple incisions and only performs subdivision after resection. We will show that this leads to lesser subdivisions and increases the interactivity of the simulation.

Keywords. geometric model, surgical simulation, cuts

Introduction

Computer based simulation of surgeries provide safe and repeatable environments for surgeons and residents to hone their skills. One of the chief challenges of surgical simulation is accurate representation of deformable organs. Many existing simulations focus on minimally invasive procedures which avoid the need to cut or limit the types of cuts.

Simulating cuts is a difficult process in *open surgery* simulation because they change the underlying data. Simulation systems that use physics-based deformation methods like mass-spring or finite elements (FEM) are particularly vulnerable to this. Cuts force introduction of new nodes and recomputations of the stiffness matrix, which makes the system slow and non-interactive.

Many FEM-based simulations model deformable organs as a mesh of tetrahedra. Bielser [1] describes a geometric data structure that preserves state information for a tetrahedra-based FEM model. In their system, a tetrahedron being cut by a line tool exists in one of twenty-four states, based on the status of their cuts. Nienhuys and van der Stappen [3] describe a cutting algorithm that constantly deforms tetrahedra so that the cut-trajectory aligns with the tetrahedra face or edge. This method is reduces the need to introduce new nodes but can produce many degenerate tetrahedra.

Newer methods like XFEM, work around the node-growth problem by enriching nodal shape functions instead of introducing new nodes [4]. We present a geometric model that preserves cut information. We assume that our cuts are piecewise-planar (3D) instead of piecewise-linear (2D). Planar cuts do not trigger tetrahedral subdivision unless resection occurs, that is, a part of the mesh is completely severed from the rest. This reduces the rate of element-growth.

1. Methods and Tools

We have implemented a novel geometric data-structure where every tetrahedron maintains its state information including the number and position of cuts. The top level mesh maintains an overall information of the state of the mesh, like the number and state of non-contiguous cuts.

The mesh is divided into an octree-based hierarchical structure to improve the speed of collision detection. The top-level mesh maintains a set of cuts, each of which may be comprised of several polygons. A new cut is defined when a new incision occurs, or when an old cut changes trajectory and is no longer on its previous plane. Logical cut information is maintained by tetrahedra. Visual and haptic feedback are derived from these logical cuts.

Resection does not occur when a tetrahedron is cut through but only when a portion of the mesh is completely severed from the rest. When this happens, multiple cuts are merged and the affected tetrahedra are subdivided along the cut plane.

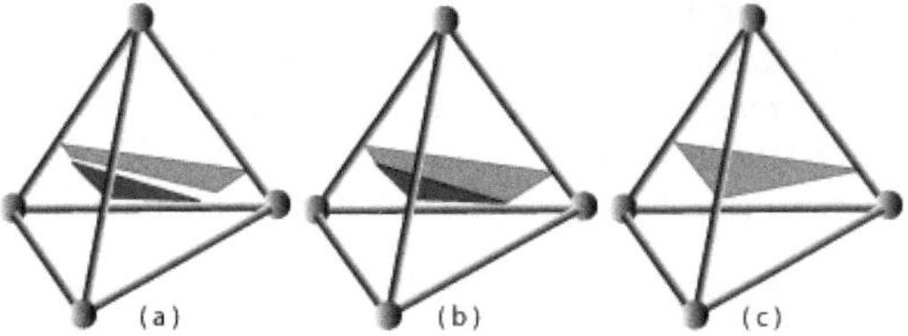

Figure 1. Merging cuts. Two separate cuts become one cut plane before subdivision

Figure 1 shows how two cuts can potentially merge into a single cut. It is to be noted that at the end of state (Figure 1c,) subdivision occurs only if the rest of the top-level cut causes resection. Our method leads to potentially fewer degenerate tetrahedra and thus provides stability to the overall system.

Bielser [1] proposed a state-machine-based tetrahedral cutting algorithm that maintains state information about tetrahedra and performs subdivision based on state changes. We have modified the concept to include multiple cuts and delayed subdivision based on mesh state instead of tetrahedron state.

2. Results

Figure 2 shows the various stages of cutting a tetrahedral mesh. Figure 2a shows the wireframe image of a tetrahedralmesh that is partially cut. While Bielser's method prompts tetrahedral subdivision at this stage, we suspend subdivision till later. Figure 2b shows our cut architecture's capacity to store multiple cuts. The bottom-right tetrahedron has been completely resected, yet remains intact.

Figure 2c shows complete mesh resection and tetrahedral subdivision. Figure 2d shows a partially cut mesh that is textured using a 3D texture map. Our lazy subdivision results in significantly lower tetrahedral subdivision for multiple cut procedures.

Our collision detection algorithm performed interactively at a rate of 28 fps with a mesh model of 1024 tetrahedra. We were able to sustain a maximum of 4 cuts, each of which spanned more than a quarter of the mesh, for the above model at a frame rate of 15 fps.

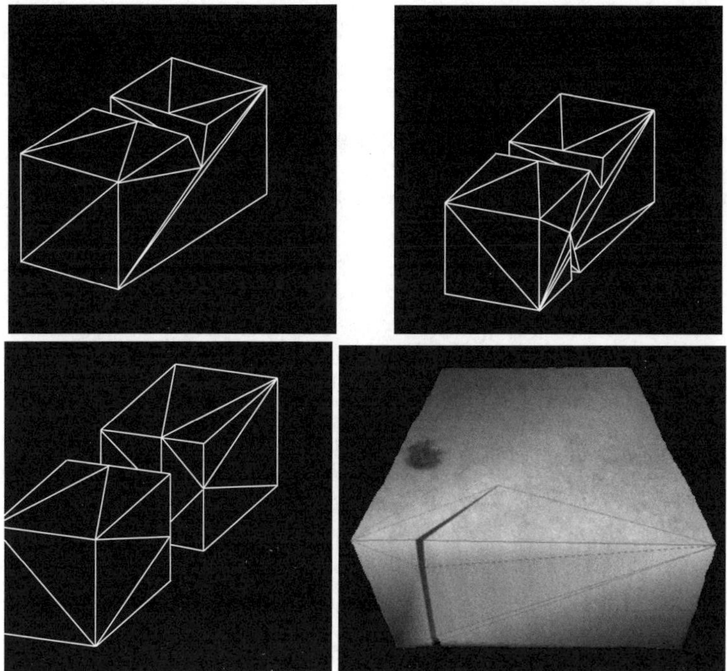

Figure 2. a. Single partial cut in mesh, b. Multiple partial cut, c. Resection and subdivision, d. 3D-texture mapped volume

3. Conclusion

We have designed and implemented a data-structure to reduce overall tetrahedral subdivision in open surgery simulations. This in turn, makes our system more robust and scalable. We do not restrict our cuts to be 2-dimensional. They may be planar in nature. We also allow multiple cuts to exist in the model. Subdivision only occurs in the event of resection.

In addition, our scheme is a logical fit with XFEM-based tissue modeling methods. We hope that these methods alleviate some of problems that traditional mesh-based models have had with cuts in open surgery surgical simulation.

References

[1] D. Bielser, *A framework for open surgery simulation*, Ph.D. thesis, Swiss Federal Institute of Technology, ETH, Zurich, 2003.

[2] N. Moës, J. Dolbow and T. Belytschko, A finite element method for crack growth without remeshing, *International Journal for Numerical Methods in Engineering*, **46**(1999), 131–150.

[3] H-W. Nienhuys and A.F. van der Stappen, Supporting cuts and finte element deformation in interactive surgery simulation, Technical Report, Universiteit Utrecht, 2001.

[4] L.M. Vigneron, J.G. Verly and S.K. Warfield, Modelling surgical cuts, retractions and resections via extended finite method, *Proceedings of the $7^t h$ International Conference on Medical Image Computing and Computer-Assisted Intervention (MICCAI)*, 311–318, 2004.

Medicine Meets Virtual Reality 15
J.D. Westwood et al. (Eds.)
IOS Press, 2007

Organ Exclusion Simulation with Multi-finger Haptic Interaction for Open Surgery Simulator

Yoshihiro KURODA[a], Makoto HIRAI[b], Megumi NAKAO[c],
Toshihiko SATO[d], Tomohiro KURODA[e], Keisuke NAGASE[e],
Hiroyuki YOSHIHARA[e]

[a]*Graduate School of Engineering Science, Osaka University, Japan*
[b]*Production Systems Research Laboratory, Kobe Steel, Ltd., Japan*
[c]*Graduate School of Information Science, NAIST, Japan*
[d]*Institute for Frontier Medical Sciences, Kyoto University, Japan*
[e]*Department of Medical Informatics, Kyoto University Hospital, Japan*

Abstract. Exclusion is a surgical manipulation of pushing aside organ in open surgery. Recently, training opportunity of surgeon is decreasing due to animal protection and patient's rights. In this study, we propose an organ exclusion training simulator with multi-finger haptic device and stress visualization. The method was applied to a medical application of exclusion which is an important manipulation to make a hidden tissue visible or to enlarge workspace. The system equips FEM-based soft tissue deformation and multi-finger haptic device. Real-time simulation was achieved with a prototype system. Experimental results of training trial suggested the effectiveness of the system and stress visualization for exclusion training. Results of subjective evaluation by surgeons were highly positive as to realism of manipulation and usefulness of the simulator.

Keywords. Multi-finger Interaction, Stress visualization, Force Feedback, Surgical Simulation

1. Introduction

In conventional surgical training, surgeons cannot avoid training their skills with real patients, because training with rubber models and animals does not have enough realism. In addition, less and less training opportunity is a problem, because animal is forbidden to be sacrificed just for training in some countries. So far, virtual reality based surgical simulator has been intensively studied and some simulators are commercially available [1]. Previous simulators give an opportunity to know surgical procedures and how to use an endoscopic instrument (e.g. endoscopic forceps), or provide training environment with a surgical tool (e.g. knife, needle). However, no training simulator of organ exclusion, which is a surgical manipulation of pushing aside organ to make a hidden object visible or to enlarge workspace as shown in Fig.1, has been developed. Improper manipulation causes fatal damage of soft tissue. This paper proposes an exclusion training simulator which provides interactive environment with multi-finger haptic display and interactive visualization of stress distribution.

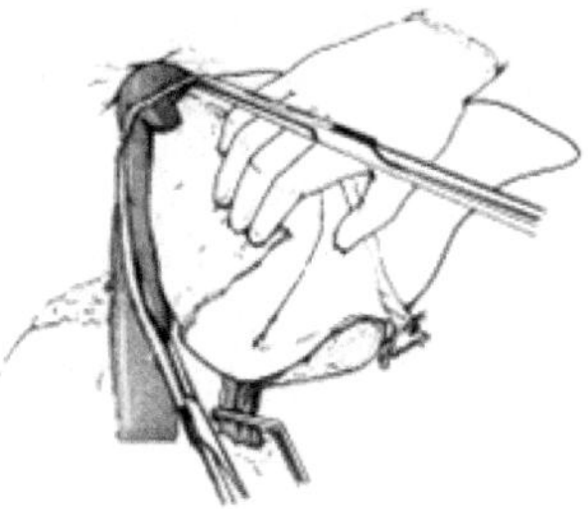

Figure 1. Liver exclusion. A vessel behind a liver is visible by exclusion with fingers.

2. Exclusion simulation with multi-finger haptic interaction

2.1. Requirements

Exclusion is conducted with multiple fingers. Hence, exclusion training system should allow interactive manipulation with realistic force sensation on each finger. If stress exceeds a limit, soft tissue is destructed and loses its function. Because exclusion includes tissue deformation, a manipulation without stress concentration is an essential skill. Information of stress distribution will be helpful for understanding a nature of the relationship between manipulation and its effect. Information can be displayed in various manners like visual, haptic and audio display. However, visual display gives easy understanding of spatial distributed information.
Therefore, requirements for exclusion training system can be defined as follows.
- Visual display of accurate and interactive soft tissue deformation based on physics
- Haptic display of accurate reaction force
- Visual display of stress distribution based on physics
- Free and multi-finger haptic interaction with elastic object

2.2. Multi-finger interaction environment

Fig.2 illustrates interaction method of multiple fingers with an elastic object. The method considers passive contact which is arisen by other finger's action to the object. In exclusion simulation, both active and passive contacts between a finger and an object must be considered and accurate deformation and reaction are calculated.

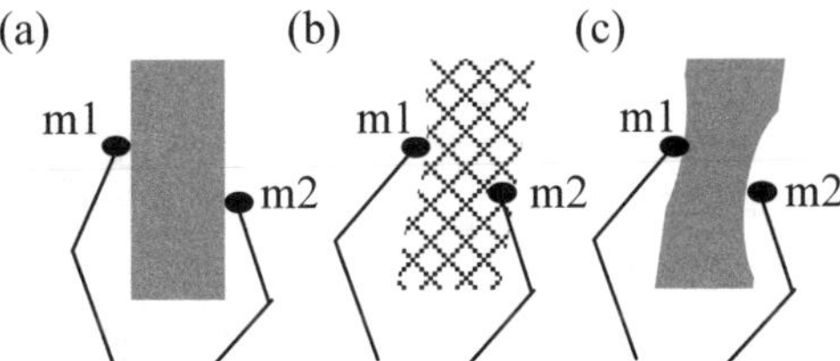

Figure 2. Temporary deformation based multi-finger interaction method with an elastic object. (a) Initial state. (b) Temporary state. An object is deformed by a manipulator (m1). Other manipulator (m2) invades into the object. (c) Simulation result. Contact by both manipulators is treated.

Interactive simulation system with haptic display requires high update rate of reaction force (more than 300 Hz or higher [2]). In surgical simulation, finite element method (FEM) has been recognized as one of the most accurate methods. The real-time simulation of non-linear elastic deformation is hard with current CPU power. Thus, FEM with linear elasticity is employed for soft tissue deformation in the system. Hirota proposed a method of real-time calculation of reaction force with finite element model [3]. Forces on finger contact node are calculated as following equations.

$$f = Ku \ , \ L = K^{-1} \qquad (1)$$

where f, u are force and displacement of nodes, respectively. K is stiffness matrix.
If multiple fingers touch with node i,j and applied forces can be assumed zero except contact nodes, forces on node i,j are calculated as follows.

$$\begin{pmatrix} * \\ u_i \\ u_j \\ * \end{pmatrix} = \begin{pmatrix} * & \cdots & \cdots & * \\ \vdots & L_{ii} & L_{ij} & \vdots \\ \vdots & L_{ji} & L_{jj} & \vdots \\ * & \cdots & \cdots & * \end{pmatrix} \begin{pmatrix} * \\ f_i \\ f_j \\ * \end{pmatrix} \qquad (2) \qquad \begin{pmatrix} f_i \\ f_j \end{pmatrix} = \begin{pmatrix} L_{ii} & L_{ij} \\ L_{ji} & L_{jj} \end{pmatrix}^{-1} \begin{pmatrix} u_i \\ u_j \end{pmatrix} \qquad (3)$$

Here, inverse matrix L can be computed in pre-processing. For haptic rendering, Equation (3) must be solved in 3^n patterns, where n is number of contact fingers [3,4].

3. Experiments and results

3.1. Prototype system

Many haptic devices have been developed. However, PHANToM cannot display force to more than two fingers [5]. SPIDAR8 has narrow workspace and restricts finger's manipulation. CyberForce^{TM}[1] is a typical exoskeleton-type haptic device, which allows free and multi-finger manipulation with force feedback. The system consists of PC (Intel Xeon 2.6GHz x 2, 1GB memory, RADEON9600 256MB graphic board), display and CyberForce system (CyberForce, CyberGrasp, CyberGlove) as shown in Fig.3. Position data is updated at 100Hz. Although high stiffness requires high refresh rate, interaction with low stiffness like soft tissue can be realized at around 100 Hz. MVL (Medical Virtual reality Library) is used for simulation modules [6].

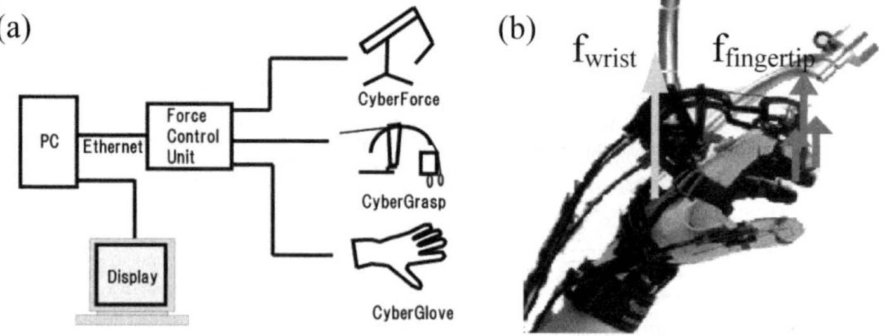

Figure 3. System configuration and haptic device. (a) System configuration (b) Multi-finger haptic device CyberForce. Forces can be displayed to each finger and a wrist.

CyberForce has only 1DOF for force display on fingertip. Reaction force is simply projected to tangential direction of a finger. On the other hand, with this device, no force is conveyed to a wrist because of its mechanism. The authors simulate internal force of wrist, which is arisen by applied force on fingertips. Sum of finger forces is output to the wrist as shown in Equation 4. The force is equivalent to real wrist force, when fingertips do not move fast and a hand can be regarded as a rigid body.

$$f_{fingertip} = f_i \cos\theta \quad , \quad f_{wrist} = \sum_i^5 f_i \ (i=1,2,3,4,5) \qquad (4)$$

3.2. Simulation results

Table 1 shows calculation time for reaction force and deformation of the model (820-noded object). Time for reaction forces with four fingers was less than 10msec, which is update time required for 100Hz refresh rate. It is sufficient for exclusion simulation, because exclusion with simultaneous contact of five fingers is not common. Figure 4 shows a simulation example of multi-finger haptic interaction with soft tissue models and results of stress visualization. Figure 5 shows stress concentration in the case, where an object has several parts of different stiffness. The object is modeled as a lung, which has a harder part in the bronchus and Pulmonary-artery.

Table 1. Calculation time for reaction force and deformation

Number of contact fingers	1	2	3	4	5
Reaction force	0.20	0.63	2.36	8.18	29.7
Deformation	1.32	1.95	4.41	12.29	32.36

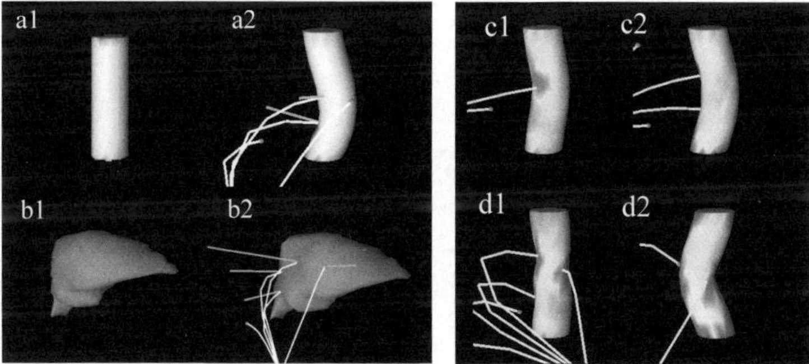

Figure 4. Exclusion simulation. (a1, 2) vessel (b1, 2) liver exclusion. Stress distribution by different finger numbers (c1,2) and by different manipulation (d1,2).

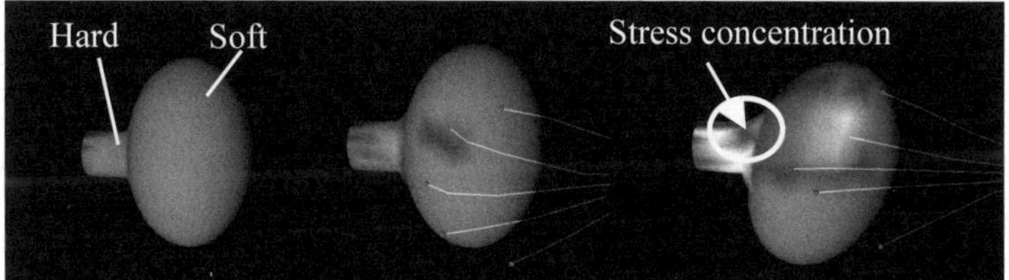

Figure 5. Stress concentration occurred in a simplified lung situation

3.3. Experiments for examining training effect

The effectiveness of a prototype system for exclusion training was examined. Figure 6 shows two environments of the experiment (object A and B). Object A has 0.3MPa Young Modulus in whole body, and object B has 0.1MPa and 1.0MPa Young Modulus in soft and hard regions, respectively. 0.4 Poisson's ratio is set to both objects. A task was to push aside a target object to make a hidden line visible for one second. 13 volunteers performed 30minutes training in every successive 5days. Stress visualization was provided to group1 (7 persons) and not to group2 (6 persons). A subject was told that he/she tried performing a task with less max stress value. In each day, 3 minutes training and a test was performed without stress visualization.

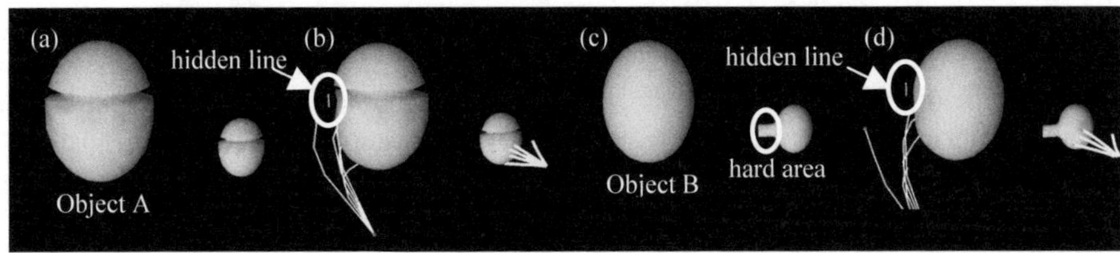

Figure 6. Two environments of training trial. Left side is a front view and right side is a side view in each figure. To make a hidden line visible by pushing is a task.

Figure 7 shows results of the experiment. In both groups, max stress converges in the case of both objects. No clear difference was found in fourth and fifth day. However, less max forces were found in first three days, except second day in the case of object B. The results suggested efficient training was conducted with stress distribution.

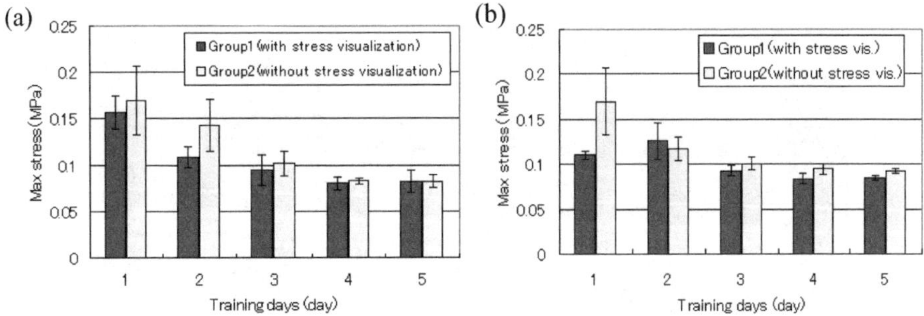

Figure 7. Result of exclusion training with object A (a) and B (b)

3.4. Subjective Evaluation by surgeons

Fig. 8 shows a view of the developed system. Three skilled surgeons participated in subjective evaluation of developed exclusion simulator. The system configuration was described in subsection 3.1. Answer was obtained 5 point scale (-2,-1,0,+1,+2) with a questionnaire. Questions and average scores were as follows.

1.   The system provides haptic sensation of organ. (average score: +1.3)
2.   The system is useful for training of organ exclusion. (average score: +1.7)
3.   Stress visualization is beneficial. (average score: +1.7)

Results of the questionnaire showed high evaluation of the developed system in effectiveness for training by surgeons with some room for improvement. Following free comments were obtained.

- The organ gives three-dimensional existence and stiffness is similar with real liver
- Manipulation is not perfectly supported, because organ can be touched only with fingertips.
- Considerably effective. Perfectly suit for OSCE (Objective Structured Clinical Examination) of medical student and training of residents

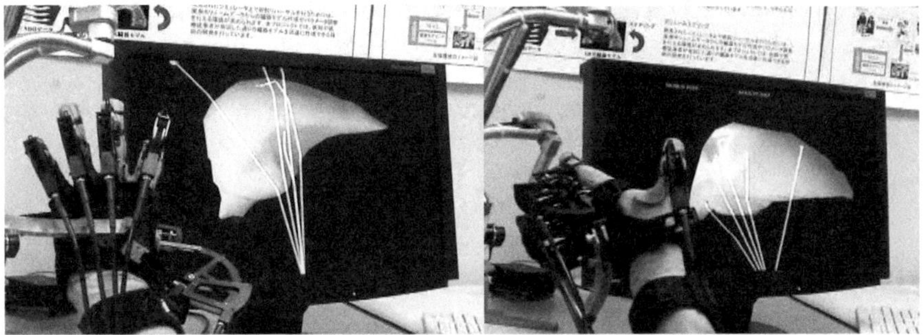

Figure 8. Developed system. Liver is excluded with pinching. Color corresponding to stress value is overlaid on the liver in right image.

4. Conclusion

This paper proposed an organ exclusion training simulator with multi-finger haptic device with stress visualization. The experimental results and subjective evaluation by surgeons suggested effectiveness of the developed system. As a future work, collision of middle phalanx and palm with virtual organ will be implemented. In addition, perceptual features in multi-finger haptic interaction should be studied.

Acknowledgement

This research was partly supported by Grant-in-Aid (S:16100001, A:18680043, E:18659148) and (H18-Medicine-General-032) from JSPS and the Ministry of Health, Labour and Welfare, Japan, and Nakajima fund and Kurata fund, Japan.

References

[1] Immersion, www.immersion.com
[2] Burdea, G., and Coiffet, P., "Virtual Reality Technology", Wiley Interscience, 2003.
[3] Hirota, K., and Kaneko, T., "Haptic Representation of Elastic Objects", MIT Presence, 10(5), pp.525-536, 2001.
[4] Zilles, C.B., and Salisbury, J.K., "A ConstraintBased God-Object Method For Haptic Display", in Proc. of IEE/RSJ International Conference on Intelligent Robots and Systems, Vol.3, pp.146-151, 1995.
[5] SensAble, www.sensable.com
[6] Kuroda, Y., Nakao, M., Kuroda, T., Oyama, H., and Yoshihara, H., "MVL: Medical VR Simulation Library", Proc. of 13th Medicine Meets Virtual Reality Conference, pp.273-276, 2005.

Medicine Meets Virtual Reality 15
J.D. Westwood et al. (Eds.)
IOS Press, 2007

Semi-automatic Development of Optimized Surgical Simulator with Surgical Manuals

Yoshihiro KURODA[a], Tadamasa TAKEMURA[b], Naoto KUME[c],
Kazuya OKAMOTO[d], Kenta HORI[e], Megumi NAKAO[f],
Tomohiro KURODA[b] and Hiroyuki YOSHIHARA[b]

[a]*Graduate School of Engineering Science, Osaka University, Japan*
[b]*Dep.t of Medical Informatics, Kyoto Univ. Hosp.,* [c]*JSPS Research Fellow, Japan*
[d]*Graduate School of Informatics, Kyoto University, Japan*
[e]*Department of Radiology, Gunma Prefectural College of Health Sciences, Japan*
[f]*Graduate School of Information Science, NAIST, Japan*

Abstract. Recently, simulation platform and libraries are provided from several research groups. However, development of VR-based surgical simulator takes much effort not only for implementing simulation modules but also for setting surgical environment and choosing simulation modules. Surgical manual describes knowledge of manipulations in surgical procedure. In this study, language processing is used to extract anatomical objects and surgical manipulations in a scene from surgical manual. In addition, benchmark and LOD control of simulation modules optimize the simulation. We propose a framework of semi-automatic development of optimized simulator with surgical manuals. In the framework, SVM based machine learning is adapted in extracting surgical information and XML file was made. Simulation programs were crated from XML file using a simulation library in different system configurations.

Keywords. Simulator development, Language processing, Optimization

1. Introduction

So far, a lot of studies have been done for simulation of soft tissue characteristics, modeling of surgical manipulations, skill transfer, skill analysis, development of specific simulators, and so on. Thanks to these efforts, simulation technologies are highly advanced. Recently, several research groups provide simulation libraries or open-source software for standardization and supporting development of surgical simulators [1, 2, 3, 4]. However, for simulating a surgical procedure, medical doctors and engineers have to spend much time to describe surgical environment, scenarios and successful criteria of manipulation. In order to record or analyze surgeon's skill using virtual environment, various surgical situations must be defined only for the purpose. On the other hand, surgical manuals have been written for describing surgical situations and scenarios with sophisticated manner from the dawn of medicine and can be used as knowledge source of surgical simulators. In this study, semi-automatic development of surgical simulator with knowledge in surgical manuals by machine learning based language processing is proposed. Simulation is optimized with considering system configuration.

2. Background

Typical virtual reality based surgical simulator consists of physics simulation engine, visual and haptic interface. A simulator provides an environment which allows interactive surgical manipulation with virtual organs with visual and haptic feedback. VR environment in the simulator represents physical object and phenomena. A surgical procedure has several major surgical scenes. In a scene, anatomical objects are located in three-dimensional environment and surgical manipulation is conducted to the objects. Hence, anatomical objects and conducted manipulations are key information to construct a virtual surgery environment.

Surgery manuals have been written for giving information about what and how to do in a surgical scene. Common knowledge is omitted in the manual, although key information such as target anatomical objects and conducted manipulations are described. Although J.Bacon et al. focused on definition of markup language and modeling of surgical scenarios [5], extraction of surgical scene from surgical manuals is never treated. No previous study has tried extracting key information of constructing a surgical scene from surgery manual.

SVM (Support vector machine) is a powerful learning methodology, which was proposed by Vapnik [6]. The method is powerful in classification in language processing by abstract understanding of sentences and not by strict understanding of a sentence structure. SVM learns plenty of words in a document as training data to determine hyper plane which divides a space. Then, SVM classifies a new document by examining where the document is plotted in a space.

Soft tissue modeling is one of the most important issues in surgical simulation. Mass-spring model, Finite Element (FE) Model and many other models have been proposed and applied to applications. Because each model has advantages and disadvantages from the aspect of computational requirement and functional possibility, a suitable model is chosen for each application. Cutting and ablating manipulations are destructive manipulations. In this case, structure of tissue model changes and it becomes more complicated. Cutting and ablating are also different from the aspect of determination of destruction place [7, 8]. For example, cutting model can define destruction place easily by defining a separating plane, which divides object structure as if knife passes through it [7]. However, ablation model has to consider physical stress to determine destruction place [8]. Accuracy and interactivity are trade-off, because physics-based simulation requires high computational resource. It is important that simulation modules are switched if a processor cannot achieve real-time computation. Computational power of a computer and requirements of simulation modules are key factors for it.

Developing simulation modules takes much effort for developers, because technical background of VR-based surgical simulation ranges extremely wide (computer graphics, physics, haptics, real-time simulation, and so on). Recently, open source and simulation libraries are provided by several research groups [1, 2, 3, 4]. Thus, such simulation modules can be used for efficient and high quality development of a simulator. It is important for simulation modules to provide module's information which enables communication between scenario extraction modules and simulation modules.

3. A framework for semi-automatic development of optimized surgical simulation

3.1. Concept & design

Fig.1 (a) shows an overview of a whole procedure of developing optimized VR simulator with surgical manuals. Fig.1 (b) shows data flow in each step. Knowledge of surgical manuals is extracted by language processing and represented once with Surgical Simulation Markup Language (SSML), which is an eXtended Markup Language (XML). Although J.Bacon et al. focused on describing surgical scenarios [5], the authors focus on extraction of surgical environment from surgical manuals and optimization of surgical simulator. SSML represents a surgical procedure, which consists of target organs, surgical manipulations, initial state of the scene, a goal of the manipulation, and pitfalls to be taken care of. Language processing is applied for extracting scene components. Simulation program, which is written with APIs of simulation modules, is produced from SSML and system configuration. Rendering methods (surface or volume rendering) of organ models and the accuracy and functionality of surgical manipulation (mass-spring or FEM, destructive or non-destructive) are chosen. GUI based authoring tool supports correcting SSML and editing of simulation setting.

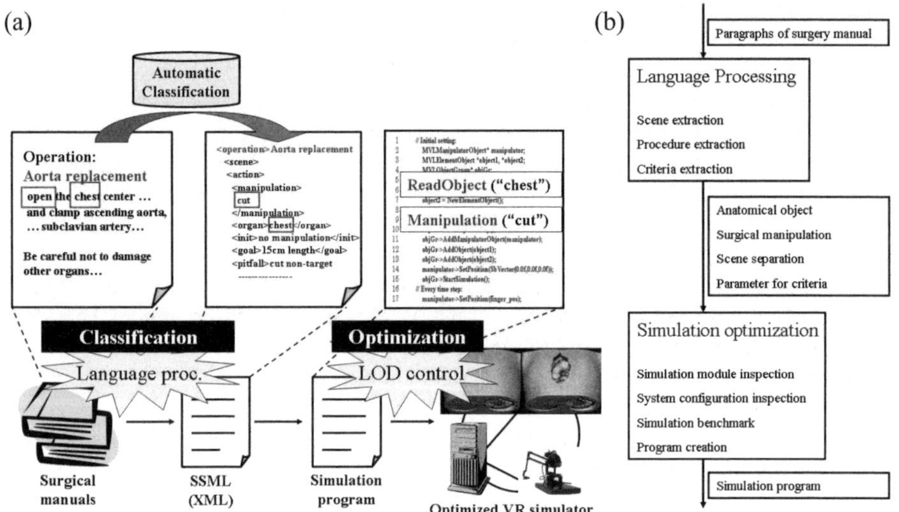

Figure 1. (a) An overview of a framework of developing optimized VR simulator with surgical manuals. (b) Data flow in the framework.

3.2. Methodology

Fig.2 (a) shows an example of SSML. SSML represents a surgical procedure, which consists of target organs, surgical manipulations, initial state of the scene, a goal of the manipulation, and pitfalls to be taken care of. Fig.2 (b) and (c) show representative surgical manipulations and anatomical objects, respectively.
This study focuses especially on extraction of surgical environment, which includes related anatomical objects and surgical manipulation in a situation, because physical

environment and phenomena are most basic and important factors in surgery. Related objects are target organ and other tissues accessed by surgeon in approaching the target. Cutting, suturing, palpating and other surgical manipulations are conducted to the tissues. SVM will be a powerful tool for finding a key object and a key manipulation. Hence, anatomical objects and manipulations are extracted from a surgical manual using SVM.

SVM has three steps in this study. In first step, SVM sets axis from all nouns and verbs appeared in the text. In second step, SVM learns from training data and defines a hyper plane. A point plotted on the space represents frequency of appearance of a word in a text. If fifty anatomies and seven manipulations exist, support vector space has fifty seven dimensions. Points are plotted on multi-dimensional space. In the teacher data, classification of a text is given in advance. A point of the data is marked. After all points from teacher data are plotted, SVM defines a separating plane, which classifies space. In third step, SVM classifies a point plotted from input text into axis of surgical manipulation and anatomical object by examining the point's location in a space divided by hyper plane. SVM determines a key anatomical object and manipulation in input text.

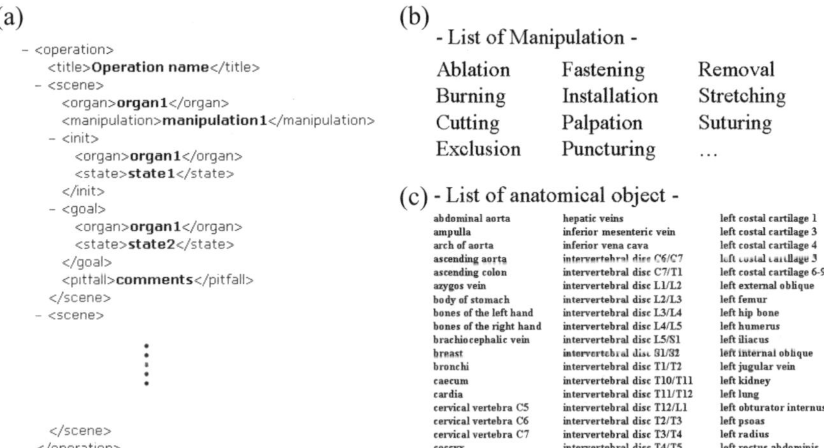

Figure 2. SSML describes surgical scenes in surgical operation. (a) Typical format of SSML (b) A part of surgical manipulations (c) a part of anatomical objects

Soft tissue model is chosen as it runs real-time for interactive manipulation with expense of its accuracy or its freedom of representation. Simulation benchmark is necessary for choosing simulation modules for each computational resource.

The system loads a SSML file and output a simulation program by decoding a structure of SSML. Fig.3 shows an example of SSML file and produced simulation program using MVL simulation library [4]. If the number of CPU is more than one and CPU power is higher than 1GHz in each processor, interactive simulation was enabled. Otherwise, interactive simulation is disabled and animation is created with given parameters.

4. Results and discussions

400 examples with cutting breast were input as training data of SVM. In an experiment, simulators with correct situations were automatically developed in 25 out of 42 example cases (60%). About 200 anatomical objects were prepared. The simulation program was successfully created from documents about Thoracoabdominalaorta approaching. Fig.3 shows created SSML file and simulation results by created simulation programs. Fig.3 (b1) shows initial state of first scene in the operation. Cutting manipulation of breast is available in the first scene. Fig.3 (b2) shows surgical scene after breast cutting. Lung hides internal body. Exclusion manipulation of lung is available in the second scene. Fig.3 (b3) shows surgical scene after lung exclusion. Aorta in the center of a body is visible. In a computer with dual CPU (2.6GHz), interactive simulation was available. In a computer with one CPU, animation was shown.

(a)   (b1)

```
- <operation>
    <title>Thoracoabdominalaorta approaching</title>
  - <scene>
      <organ>breast</organ>
      <manipulation>cutting</manipulation>
      <init />
    - <goal>
        <organ>breast</organ>
        <state>cut</state>
      </goal>
      <pitfall>tearing</pitfall>
    </scene>
  - <scene>
      <organ>lung</organ>
      <manipulation>exclusion</manipulation>
    - <init>
        <organ>breast</organ>
        <state>cut</state>
      </init>
    - <goal>
        <organ>aorta</organ>
        <state>visible</state>
      </goal>
      <pitfall>stress concentration</pitfall>
    </scene>
  </operation>
```

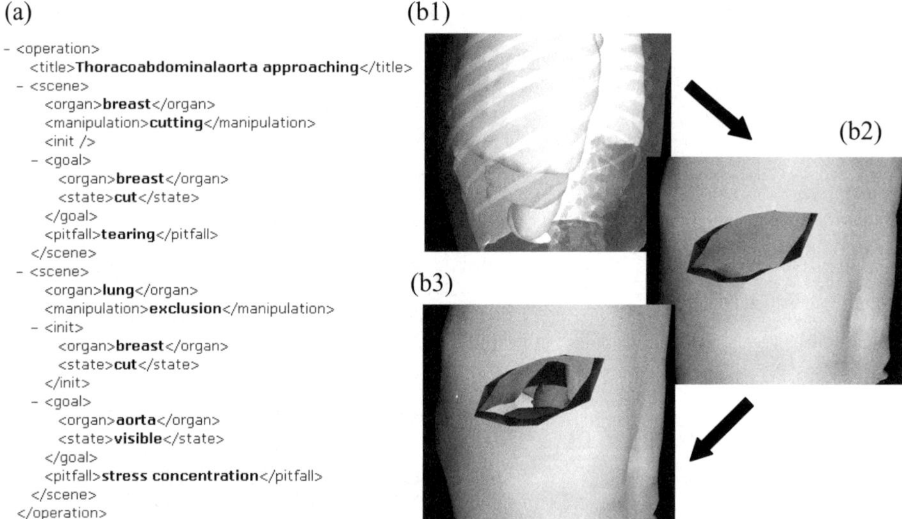

Figure 3. Result of simulation development from surgical documents. (a) SSML data (b) Simulation scenes.

Extraction of surgical scene by language processing will be improved by using ontology of anatomical objects and surgical manipulations. Construction of ontology is a future work. Extraction of pitfalls, which are hidden or not easily recognized danger or difficulty, will be helpful for training simulator. In the current implementation, control of accuracy and function of surgical manipulation is not possible. As a future work of system creation, advanced control of availability of surgical manipulation will be done.

5. Conclusion

This paper proposed semi-automatic development framework of optimized surgical simulation with surgical manuals. Results of experiments showed 60% correct extraction of surgical scene in a specific operation. The simulation program was successfully created from surgical documents. Improvement of scene extraction, progress of simulation control, and construction of simulators with various surgical procedures are future works.

Acknowledgement

This research was partly supported by Grant-in-Aid for Scientific Research (S) (16100001) from JSPS, Grant-in-Aid (H18-Medicine-General-032) from the Ministry of Health, Labour and Welfare, Japan, Grant-in-Aid for Young Scientists (A) (18680043) and Exploratory Research (18659148) from The Ministry of Education, Culture, Sports, Science and Technology, Japan, and Kurata Fund, Japan.

References

[1] K. Montgomery, C. Bruyns, J. Brown, S. Sorkin, F. Mazzella, G. Thonier, A. Tellier, B. Lerman and A. Menon, "Spring: A General Framework for Collaborative, Realtime Surgical Simulation", Proc. of Medicine Meets Virtual Reality 2002, 296-303, 2002.

[2] M. Cavusoglu, T. Goktekin and F. Tendick, "GiPSi: A Framework for Open Source/Open Architecture Software Development for Organ Level Surgical Simulation", IEEE Transaction on Information Technology in Biomedicine, Vol.10, No.2, pp.312-322, 2006

[3] S. Cotin, et al., SOFA, "Collaborative Development of an Open Framework for Medical Simulation", http://sourcesup.cru.fr/docman/view.php/98/201/SOFA.pdf

[4] Y. Kuroda, M. Nakao, T. Kuroda, H. Oyama and H. Yoshihara, "MVL: Medical VR Simulation Library", Proceedings of 13th Medicine Meets Virtual Reality Conference, pp.273-276, 2005.

[5] J. Bacon et al., "The Surgical Simulation and Training Markup Language (SSTML): An XML-based Language for Medical Simulation", Proc. of MMVR14, pp.37-42, 2006.

[6] V. Vapnik, "Statistical Learning Theory", Wiley, 1998.

[7] M. Nakao, T. Kuroda, H. Oyama, M. Komori, T. Matsuda and T. Takahashi, "Planning and Training of Minimally Invasive Surgery by Integrating Soft Tissue Cuts with Surgical Views Reproduction", Computer Assisted Radiology and Surgery (CARS), pp. 13-18, 2002.

[8] N. Kume, M. Nakao, T. Kuroda, H. Yoshihar and M. Komori, "FEM-Based Soft Tissue Destruction Model for Ablation Simulator", Proc. Medicine Meets Virtual Reality 13 (MMVR13), pp. 263-269, 2005.

Medicine Meets Virtual Reality 15
J.D. Westwood et al. (Eds.)
IOS Press, 2007

Avatars Alive!
The Integration of Physiology Models and Computer Generated Avatars in a Multiplayer Online Simulation

Laura KUSUMOTO, MS[a], Wm. LeRoy HEINRICHS, MD, PhD[b], Parvati DEV, PhD[b],
and Patricia YOUNGBLOOD, PhD[b]

[a] Forterra Systems, Inc
[b] Stanford University Medical Media and Information Technologies (SUMMIT)

Abstract. In a mass casualty incident, injured and at-risk patients will pass through a continuum of care from many different providers acting as a team in a clinical environment. As presented at MMVR 14 [Kaufman, et al 2006], formative evaluations have shown that simulation practice is nearly as good as, and in some cases better than, live exercises for stimulating learners to integrate their procedural knowledge in new circumstances through experiential practice. However, to date, multiplayer game technologies have given limited physiological fidelity to their characters, thus limiting the realism and complexity of the scenarios that can be practiced by medical professionals. This paper describes the status of a follow-on program to merge medical and gaming technologies so that computer generated, but human-controlled, avatars used in a simulated, mass casualty training environment will exhibit realistic life signs. This advance introduces a new level of medical fidelity to simulated mass casualty scenarios that can represent thousands of injuries. The program is identifying the critical instructional challenges and related system engineering issues associated with the incorporation of multiple state-of-the-art physiological models into the computer generated synthetic representation of patients. The work is a collaboration between Forterra Systems and the SUMMIT group of Stanford University Medical School, and is sponsored by the US Army Medical Command's Telemedicine and Advanced Technologies Research Center (TATRC).

Keywords. Physiology models, game technology, avatars, mass casualty response.

Introduction

This research and development program is developing a general application program interface (API) between Forterra Systems' massively multiplayer simulation technology, the Online Interactive Virtual Environment (OLIVE), and two specific physiological models. To provide context for the design of the API, we are developing curricula for training medical personnel, in which the physiology models will drive the medical states of multiple avatars in a virtual environment that simulates the mass casualty scenarios.

The program extends the curriculum for response to mass casualty incidents beyond the performance of triage, in which victims first reaching the hospital are quickly examined and sorted into categories of urgency. Using the same classifications as the START triage system adopted by Stanford Hospital, mass casualty patients are classified as Immediate, Delayed, Minor, or Deceased. In the simulation, the virtual patients then enter into the care of the emergency department, where they are transported to the appropriate treatment area, examined and diagnosed, and treated and monitored as appropriate.

As emergency department physicians and nurses, the audience for this curriculum is well versed in the treatment of patients, but dealing with a mass casualty disaster requires handling more patients simultaneously, often within unfamiliar roles and responsibilities prescribed by the hospital's disaster action plan. Sound medical judgment is required for success, but the quality of teamwork and resource management can be equally critical for delivering care to a large number of patients.

For the simulation of a mass casualty incident to seem realistic to medical professionals, it must provide a way for the trainees to treat virtual patients and for the patients to respond to their care. How the medical team members perform should impact their virtual patients. The technology must calculate and reflect medical outcomes in a sufficiently believable fashion to support learning from medical mistakes as well as triumphs. It is for this reason that integration with medical models is being undertaken.

1. Selecting Physiology Models

Before physiology models can be integrated with the game technology, it is important to understand what they must represent. Requirements for the models were determined in this program by designing of a series of medical scenarios that will stimulate the learning objectives of the curricula. For each type of simulated disaster , a specific set of patient cases was designed. For example, for simulating a dirty bomb attack on a public building, a mixture of injury profiles was designed to cause the hospital triage team to decide upon a variety of classifications, and then to stimulate the emergency department treatment areas with sufficient number and variety of cases to surface their need to work as a team and manage critical resources such as beds and blood supplies. Example cases include men and women of varying ages and conditions, receiving such injuries as lacerations, compound fractures, pneumothorax, major pelvic trauma, bruising, head injury, and liver lacerations. Each patient case describes the patient overall (gender, age, preexisting medical conditions), injuries caused by the disaster, the diagnoses and treatments that an expert team might make, and the responses the patient will show if properly treated in time, or not.

With sets of cases for a dirty bomb and sarin exposure in hand, the project team then surveyed physiological models available from universities and commercial sources, and identified two basic types for further investigation, namely rule-based models and mathematical models. We found that these types of model can provide an adequate representation of the patient's physiology and state, in more or less detail. The key difference between rule-based and mathematical models is in how the medical scenarios that play out over time are programmed. Rule-based medical models provide a great deal of flexibility but require detailed description of each possible interplay between the parameters of a scenario. Mathematical modeling provides a powerful, abstract representation of the physiology with parameters that respond to any stimuli, but they can be more difficult to extend to handle aspects of physiology not covered by the representation. To study these and other differences between models, we have chosen to integrate one of each type into this program, and we will use both in trials with representatives of the user community this year.

2. Visualizing Physiology Models

The design challenges inherent in visualizing the output of the medical models in a multiplayer virtual environment include:

- Determining the optimal presentation of avatar symptoms and medical treatments (e.g., spoken word, text, images, representations on the 3D avatar)
- Managing the computational load of multiple physiological models within a computationally demanding, 3D online virtual environment, and
- Optimizing the interactions between medical models, human control, and artificial intelligence (AI) control in determination of avatar state and behaviors.

To meet these challenges, tradeoffs must be made between the most "realistic" presentation, the computational impact of a particular style of presentation, and whether the presentation is sufficient for meeting learning objectives. For example, examining the patients' pupil response is very important, but adding that detail to the avatars and providing a close-up camera to make avatar pupils visible would be expensive. We have decided that we will not model the patients' pupil response on the 3D avatars in this phase of the project, but instead, when a physician elects to examine the pupil, an illustration will be displayed showing the state of the pupil as determined in the medical model. On the other hand, bleeding and bruising cannot be relegated to pictures that are separate from the avatar that is laying on the bed, so bleeding and bruising will be depicted on the 3D avatar.

Acknowledgements

The authors would like to acknowledge the work of Arnold Hendrick, Senior Product Designer at Forterra Systems, on the functional design of this application, and Dr. Phillip M. Harter MD and Eric A.Weiss MD for their contributions as subject matter experts in emergency department responses to mass casualties.

References

M. Kaufman; W.L. Heinrichs; P.Youngblood, Training of Medical First Responders for CBRNE Events Using Multiplayer Game Technology, Presentation at MMVR 14, January 24-27, 2006.

Medicine Meets Virtual Reality 15
J.D. Westwood et al. (Eds.)
IOS Press, 2007

Evaluation of a Simulation-based Program for Medic Cognitive Skills Training

Fuji LAI, Eileen B. ENTIN, Tad BRUNYE, Jason SIDMAN, Elliot E. ENTIN
Aptima, Inc., Woburn, MA
Email: fujilai@aptima.com

Abstract. Simulation-based training is a promising instructional approach for training military and civilian first responders. In addition to training in relevant taskwork skills, there is increasing need for first responder training in cognitively-based skills such as situation assessment and decision making. The First Responder Simulation Training (FIRST) program trains cognitive skills using complex and degraded situations. The program is comprised of five detailed scenarios, evaluation instruments, debriefing guidelines for each scenario, a multimedia tutorial that explains how to use the evaluation and debriefing instruments, and a detailed scenario guide for administering the scenarios. We conducted an evaluation of the FIRST program to assess its training utility and usability. The program was well-received by both instructors and participants. Instructors noted the importance of training cognitive skills and found the instructor materials valuable for teaching them how to administer a simulation-based training program. Participants found the scenarios realistic and challenging, and noted that such simulation-based training would be a valuable supplement to medic curricula

Keywords. Simulation, training, cognitive skills, medical first responder

1. Background

Simulation-based training is rapidly gaining widespread acceptance across the military and civilian medical first response domains as an effective medium for learning taskwork skills in an innovative, engaging, and relevant manner. However, in addition to training critical taskwork skills, there is a need to train first responders in recognizing, evaluating, and appropriately responding to novel, complex, and dynamic contextual influences. The present effort leverages relevant research in cognitive skills training to develop the First Responder Simulation-based Training (FIRST) program. The program uses mannequin-based simulator technology to address the identified need for targeted training by focusing on four cognitive skills: communication, situation awareness, prioritization, and resource management. These skills are fundamental to successful performance in emergency medical situations. For example, situation assessment involves the monitoring for and recognition of meaningful cues, causes of events, and patterns in the patient and the environment. Without this skill, emergency first responders may introduce unnecessary risk, for example, by not recognizing an increasingly severe contextual or medical situation.

The FIRST program is comprised of a multimedia tutorial, instructor's guide, five detailed scenarios, and a set of evaluation and debriefing instruments. The multimedia tutorial educates instructors on the cognitive skills being trained and the proper use of the evaluation and debriefing instruments. The instructor's guide complements the tutorial by providing both general and detailed guidance for running scenario-based training, including mannequin settings, required props, and actors needed for supporting roles such as dispatchers, bystanders, or on-line medical control (OLMC). Evaluation materials include both instructor-observer and student-observer instruments, and the debriefing instrument provides semi-structured guidelines for promoting useful and dynamic debriefing sessions.

Each of the five scenarios exercises particular cognitive skills by manipulating the occurrence of critical events. For instance, the obstetrics scenario places medics into a simulated situation involving the transfer of a pre-eclamptic expectant mother from a rural to urban medical facility. The patient's condition progressively worsens en route and the medics are placed in a situation which requires prioritization of team and medical facility resources, and communication with the receiving hospital and OLMC. As a scenario is carried out, the instructors use observer-based evaluation instruments to record trainee performance in response to changing scenario demands. These instruments provide a basis for recording trainee performance within the temporal and critical-event response framework. The obstetrics scenario, for instance, calls for communication with OLMC for valium dosing and administration permissions, prioritizing patient safety by diverting mid-route to a tertiary facility, and communicating with receiving staff. Using the evaluation instrument, the instructor can monitor and record actions as they are associated with critical scenario events (e.g., seizing mother), and link these actions to the post-scenario debriefing.

Each of the FIRST scenarios is designed to be executed by a team of two or three medics. Like the obstetrics scenario above, each scenario places the participating medics into evolving complex situations in which they must deal not only with the patient(s), but with interpersonal dynamics between themselves, patient relatives, bystanders, and hospital staff. That is, while all of the scenarios necessitate the application of medical procedures (e.g., intubation), these procedures are conducted within rich contexts designed to evoke and reinforce specific cognitive skills. During training, unfolding scenarios can be observed by any number of non-participating students. A student-observer form is used to focus attention on the trainees' cognitively-based performance, and provide a medium for recording thoughts to be later integrated with the debriefing session. In this manner, non-participating students become active participants and can benefit from observational learning opportunities.

2. Methods

We evaluated FIRST at a community college that trains first responders. Three instructors at the college and twelve emergency medical responders participated. Each instructor viewed the multimedia tutorial to familiarize themselves with the cognitive skills being trained, the program goals, and the evaluation and feedback materials.

The evaluation involved running each scenario twice, using two different teams and instructors. During each run two medics participated in the scenarios and two others acted as student observers. The instructor conducted an introductory briefing that familiarized the medics with the features of the simulator to be used. Then, the scenario was performed while the instructors and students used their respective evaluation and observation instruments. Following each scenario a debriefing session was held, during which the instructor discussed scenario events within the framework of the debriefing guide, highlighting behaviors indicative of the cognitive skills in the context of critical scenario events. Finally, participants completed a survey, the results of which are detailed below.

3. Results

The participating EMS instructors were enthusiastic about the training, including both the scenarios themselves and the debriefing materials. They praised the concept of training cognitive skills. All instructors agreed that the multimedia tutorial was time efficient and effective for understanding how the materials should be used, and elucidating the relationships between the cognitive skills, scenarios, evaluation instruments, and debriefing materials.

Overall, survey results indicated that participants found the five scenarios to be realistic (mean score = 4.1 on a 5-point scale), and the training program as a whole to be helpful for training cognitive skills (mean score = 4.7). Ten of the 12 participants identified at least one cognitive skill into which they felt they gained new insight, with communication being the most frequently cited. Furthermore, participants indicated that the scenarios helped them learn how to work with their teammates (mean = 4.6).

Furthermore, participants found that observing others in a scenario was a useful learning tool (mean = 4.7). Several participants remarked that the experience of being involved in a scenario and observing a scenario were quite different, and emphasized the utility of observational learning through the modeling of peer behavior. All participants said they would participate in similar training exercises again (mean=5.0) and would recommend such training to others (mean=5.0). Finally, participants felt that the FIRST program is appropriate at any point in a trainee's career development.

4. Discussion

The FIRST program is an off-the-shelf training program for medical first responders. The program is modular, portable, affordable, extensible across simulator platforms, targets cognitive skills, and can be administered without an expert trainer or simulation expert. The program has been evaluated for usefulness and usability and has been well-received by both instructors and scenario participants.

Simulators have the potential to enhance medic training but their widespread use has been hindered by limited availability of curricula infrastructure and expertise needed to run such programs. The FIRST program meets those needs and represents a step towards extending the integration of simulation-based training into existing medic curricula to ultimately result in improved patient care.

Acknowledgements

This work was supported by U.S. Army Medical Research and Materiel Command, Contract DAMD17-03-C-0059.

Medicine Meets Virtual Reality 15
J.D. Westwood et al. (Eds.)
IOS Press, 2007

Human Factors Engineering for Designing the Next in Medicine

Fuji LAI, *Aptima, Inc., Woburn, MA*
Email: fujilai@aptima.com

Abstract. Good design of emerging medical technology in an increasingly complex clinical and technological environment requires an understanding of the context of use, workload, and environment as well as appreciation for ease of use, fit into clinical workflow, and the need for user feedback in the design process. This is where human factors engineering can come into play for good design. Human factors engineering involves the application of principles about human behaviors, abilities, and limitations to the design of tools, devices, environments, and training in order to optimize human performance and safety. The human factors engineering process should be an integral part of the emerging technology development process and needs to be included upfront. This can help ensure that the new product is safe, functional, natural to use, seamlessly integrated into existing clinical workflow, and embraced by users to be incorporated into practice for maximum benefit to patient safety and healthcare quality.

Keywords. Human factors, ergonomics, design, performance, patient safety

1. Background

Good design of emerging medical technology in an increasingly complex clinical and technological environment requires an understanding of the context of use, workload, and environment as well as appreciation for ease of use, fit into clinical workflow, and the need for user feedback in the design process to ensure adoption of the new technology into actual practice. This is where human factors engineering can come into play for good design and ultimate impact of the product on patient safety and healthcare quality.

Human factors engineering involves the application of scientific principles about human behaviors, abilities, and limitations to the design of tools, systems, environments, and training in order to optimize human performance and safety. This is accomplished by gaining, in a targeted setting, a thorough understanding of human sensory-motor capabilities, anthropometry, ergonomics, cognitive processes, decisionmaking abilities, teamwork issues, training, and social and organizational issues.

2. Approach

The user-centered design philosophy is that the purpose of the system is to serve the users and that the system design should be driven by users and work environments instead of being driven by the technology. In applying human factors to the medical domain, the ultimate goal is a safe, functional and usable medical system design that addresses the user need and is natural to use and easily incorporated into practice.

With the accelerated pace of technology development, clinical environments are fast becoming highly complicated. In such environments it is important to understand the multiple facets of the impact that a new technology will potentially have. There needs to be an understanding of all the layers of how the technology is going to be used, who the users are, the physical and spatial environment, social and team interactions, organizational environment, as well as the safety and regulatory environment. Hence a fundamental need in the design of any new medical technology is to analyze the clinical environment from a systems perspective to understand the workflow and human-technology interactions. This is a system, rather than a single user, perspective in order to "let the system do no harm." This approach seeks to create the conditions and build the systems that help the clinician do the right thing in complex and stressful situations. In other words, a good system design promotes successful outcomes, and the more intuitive and transparent the design, the better.

The human factors design process first brings together all the stakeholders including engineers, clinicians, and users, to understand the task and work environment using techniques such as user interviews and observations to contextualize the user need and characterize the problem at hand. These requirements are then translated into a concept. Detailed design then takes place and prototypes can be constructed. The system design process is an iterative spiral development process (Figure 1). This means that there is ongoing evaluation by representative users and folding back in of their feedback in order to refine the concept and design at each stage. Such an approach increases the ultimate fit of the technology to the user and work environment.

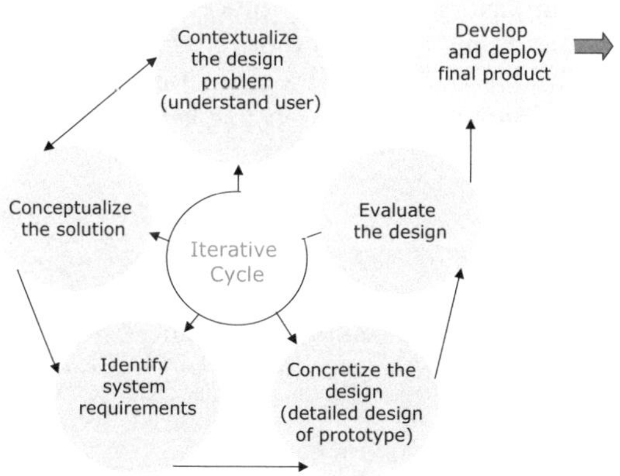

Figure 1. Human factors design process

Throughout the development process national and international human factors and healthcare quality guidelines need to be taken into account. These include standards set forth by the Association for the Advancement of Medical Instrumentation (AAMI) and the American National Standards Institute (ANSI) [1] and recognized by the Food and Drug Administration [2]. It should be emphasized that human factors needs to be introduced into the technology design process at the earliest stage possible. Involvement would occur ideally while still at the concept stage, possible at pre-Investigational Device Exemption (IDE) or IDE stage, but should be prior to 510(k) or Premarket Approval (PMA) stage.

3. Benefits

Consideration of human factors in development of new medical technologies can help ensure products are safe, natural to use, require less training, more seamlessly integrated into the clinical workflow, and are ultimately adopted into actual use. From a cost effectiveness standpoint benefits may include reduced need for customer support and also fewer product liability issues. Systems that include upfront the human factors design considerations can also obviate the need for potentially costly design changes later on due to safety, functionality, usability or integration issues.

Furthermore good design is becoming even more crucial in easing the relationship between users and revolutionary, unfamiliar new technologies. Also, with the current trend towards an aging population requiring more home healthcare delivery and in-home use of medical technology by the consumer-patient, thoughtful design which helps the technology seem more accessible and less daunting to the user will become even more pivotal for technology adoption.

4. Conclusions

There is a critical need for human factors in the design of emerging medical technology. The human factors engineering process should be an integral part of the development process and needs to be incorporated upfront. This can help realize the next generation of medical technology that is safe, effective, easy to use, and embraced by users for maximum benefit to patient safety and healthcare quality.

References

[1] AAMI/ANSI HE74-2001, *Human factors design process for medical devices*. Association for the Advancement of Medical Instrumentation, Arlington, VA, 2001.
[2] FDA, *Medical device use-safety: Incorporating Human Factors Engineering into risk management*. Food and Drug Administration, US Dept of Health and Human Services, Washington, DC, 2000.

Medicine Meets Virtual Reality 15
J.D. Westwood et al. (Eds.)
IOS Press, 2007

In-vivo Validation of a Stent Implantation Numerical Model

Denis LAROCHE [a,1], Sebastien DELORME [a], Todd ANDERSON [b]
and Robert DIRADDO [a]
[a] *Industrial Materials Institute, Boucherville, QC, Canada*
[b] *University of Calgary, AB, Canada*

Abstract. A large deformation finite element model for the patient-specific prediction of stent implantation is presented as a potential tool to assist clinicians. The intervention simulation includes the complete stent deployment under balloon inflation and deflation in the artery. This paper describes the proposed model and presents an in-vivo validation of the model using pre- and post-intervention data from a patient who underwent stent implantation. Predicted cross-section areas at different artery positions are compared to post-intervention measurements. This work demonstrated the model's potential to become a relevant tool for predicting the arterial response to the intervention.

Keywords. Finite elements, model, angioplasty, stent, multi-body contact.

Introduction

Percutaneous Transluminal Coronary Angioplasty (PTCA) is the most common intervention for the treatment of a stenosed artery. In most cases, a stent is deployed and permanently implanted to prevent elastic recoil of the artery. The intervention strategy, including balloon type selection, device positioning and inflation pressure, is typically determined by angiographic images, patient clinical information and clinician's experience. The most frequent complication of angioplasty, restenosis, is an excessive repair reaction of the arterial wall related to its mechanical damage during the intervention: 1) overstretch injury of the arterial wall and 2) denudation of the endothelium (the cell monolayer that lines the interior part of the arterial wall) due to contact with the device. The specific contribution of both types of injury to restenosis is still debated [1],[2]. Whether because of patients comeback after 6 months for target vessel revascularization or because of the use of expensive drug-eluting stents, it is generally recognized that restenosis increases by 25 to 30% the total cost of this intervention.

The success of angioplasty depends on a balance between two conflicting objectives: 1) maximizing the final deformation of the artery and 2) minimizing the mechanical damage to the arterial wall. Few research groups have attempted to simulate angioplasty with numerical or analytical models and predict its outcome. Angioplasty simulation, combined with current artery imaging technique such as

---

[1] Corresponding Author : Denis Laroche, Industrial Materials Institute, 75 de Mortagne, Boucherville, QC, Canada, J4B 6Y4; E-mail : denis.laroche@cnrc-nrc.gc.ca

intravascular ultrasound (IVUS), has the potential to become a clinical tool to assist in the selection of an appropriate intervention strategy for a specific patient. This could be done by virtually testing various strategies.

In this work, a finite element model for simulating the device/artery behavior during stent implantation is presented [3-5]. The goal of this numerical tool is to assist clinicians in the selection of appropriate intervention strategy for a specific patient by predicting the artery response to a given intervention using IVUS imaging data. Pre- and post-intervention images of a coronary artery that underwent direct stenting are used to validate the model's ability to correctly predict the instantaneous artery reopening.

1. Experiments

Direct stenting was performed in the mid-LAD of a 54 year old female. A 3x12mm Taxus stent (Boston Scientific) was deployed at balloon inflation pressure of 18 atm. Digital intravascular ultrasound (IVUS) pullback images were obtained with 40MHz catheter (Atlantis SR Pro, Boston Scientific) at a pull-back speed of 0.5 mm/sec, 7 minutes before stenting and again 8 minutes after stenting. Equally spaced images (one per cardiac cycle) were selected and imported into the Amira software (Mercury Computer Systems, Chelmsford, MA) as a 120x120x136 voxel field. The average cardiac cycle rate over the whole sequence was measured from observation of the images. The lumen and media-adventitia borders were manually segmented. Interpolation between image frames was used to compensate for shadow artifacts. Figure 1 shows the artery segment geometry including two bifurcations. The initial stent position is also illustrated. Proximal and distal cross-sections are located at 15% from the stent ends, while the center cross-section is at the center of the stent.

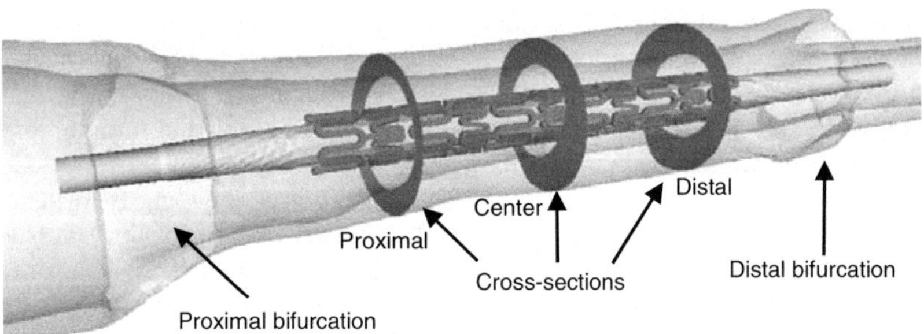

Figure 1: Artery segment showing bifurcations, stent and positions of cross-section cross-sections.

Lumen cross-section areas from pre- and post-intervention data were computed. Figure 2 gives the lumen area distribution along the targeted segment. It shows a lumen reopening to a uniform cross-section area of 6 mm, with a narrower section at the center of the stent.

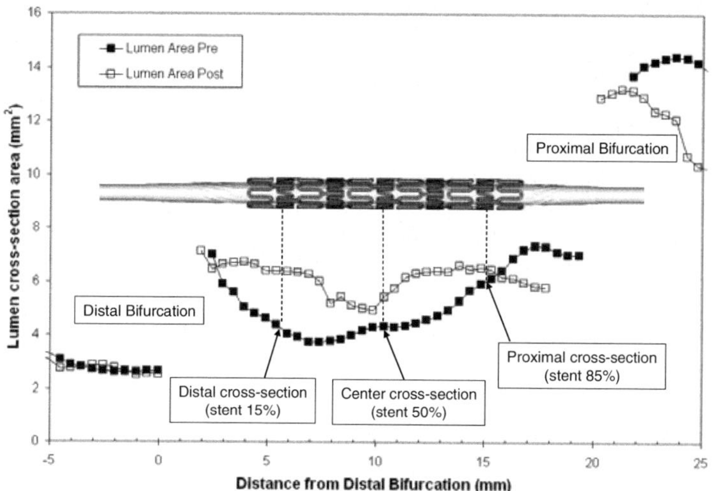

Figure 2: Cross-section area of the lumen along the artery segment.

2. Angioplasty Model

A large deformation finite element modeling software is used to solve balloon/stent/artery interactions that occur during balloon/stent deployment into the stenosed artery [3-5]. It predicts the resulting artery lumen reopening, including stress and strain distribution in the arterial wall, for a specific balloon/stent and inflation pressure. A multi-body contact algorithm developed for implicit finite element computation is used to predict friction between the balloon, the stent and the arterial wall. A continuous algorithm detects collisions between virtual nodes and surfaces moving with large displacement steps, fully respecting the non-penetration constraint. Once contact is detected, it is handled with an augmented Lagrange algorithm that computes slip and friction forces. The technique is stable for large displacement increments and is therefore applicable to finite deformation analysis.

2.1. Device Model

In this work a 3x12mm Taxus stent was used. It is mounted on a 13-mm long balloon having a diameter of 3.0 mm. The balloon is pre-folded and wrapped with a 3-ply configuration. Since it is a thin structure, the balloon is modeled with triangular membrane elements. The geometry of its wrapped shape is constructed by mapping the coordinates of the nodes of the deployed balloon onto the wrapped configuration, as described in [3]. The mechanical properties of the polymeric balloon are given by the Ogden hyperelastic constitutive equation, as proposed in [4]. The strain energy W of the Ogden model with 2 terms is given by Equation 1 where λ_1, λ_2 and λ_3 are the stretch ratios in the three principal directions, μ and α are the model constants.

$$W = \sum_{i=1}^{2} \frac{\mu_i}{\alpha_i}\left(\lambda_1^{\alpha_i} + \lambda_2^{\alpha_i} + \lambda_3^{\alpha_i} - 3\right) \tag{1}$$

Table 1 gives the constants used for the balloon.

Term	μ	α
1	154.	0.2
2	13.	12.

Table 1: Ogden model constants used for the angioplasty balloon.

High resolution digital micrographs of the crimped stent mounted on its balloon were used to measure the stent geometry. The stent was meshed using incompressible 8-node hexahedral elements. The stainless steel behavior is modeled with a hyperelastic neo-Hookean constitutive model. A Young's Modulus of 3 GPa is used to represent the work-hardening of the material in the plastic range. Therefore, the model predicts a realistic stress level at high strain while it significantly under-estimates the initial modulus. Figure 3 shows the finite element mesh of the stent (18684 nodes) mounted on the wrapped balloon (7200 nodes).

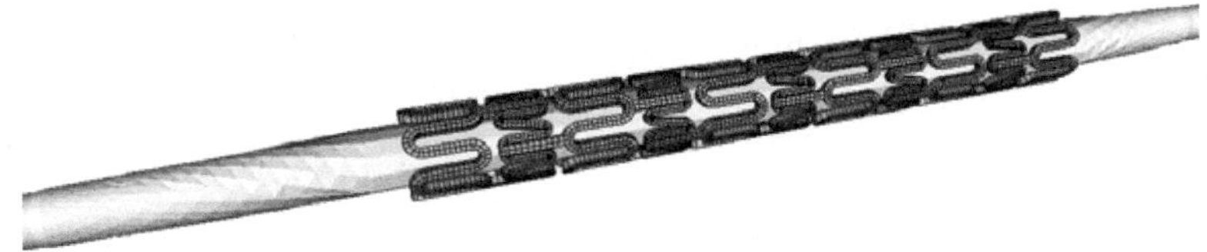

Figure 3: Finite element mesh of the stent mounted on the wrapped balloon.

2.2. Artery Model

The pre-intervention IVUS sequence was used to build the finite element mesh of a 52-mm long artery segment. An initial surface mesh was created using the marching cube algorithm. From this surface mesh, a tetrahedral mesh was then produced using the advancing front method. The mesh was edited to avoid tetrahedrons with a large aspect ratio, in order to prevent ill-conditioning of the finite element problem. The second IVUS sequence was used for validation purposes (see Section 3). The artery is modeled with the neo-Hookean hyperelastic constitutive model with a homogeneous shear modulus of 0.04 MPa, as suggested in [6]. This model can predict the elastic deformation but cannot accuratery predict the visco-plastic behaviour at high deformation level.

3. In-vivo Validation

A finite element simulation of the device deployment was performed. The nodes at the proximal end of the artery and balloon meshes were fixed in all directions. The nodes at the distal end of the artery and balloon meshes were fixed in the transverse plane. The pressure inside the balloon was progressively increased up to a pressure of 18 atm. At this pressure, the nodes on the stent mesh were fixed. The balloon was then gradually deflated. Figure 4 shows the predicted stent and artery deformation during the balloon inflation. The simulation predicts an almost uniform stent deployment along its length. Its final shape is slightly bended axially due to the initial artery shape and to the stiffness of the arterial wall. The simulation predicted a maximum artery deformation of 50%, located at the mid section of the stent.

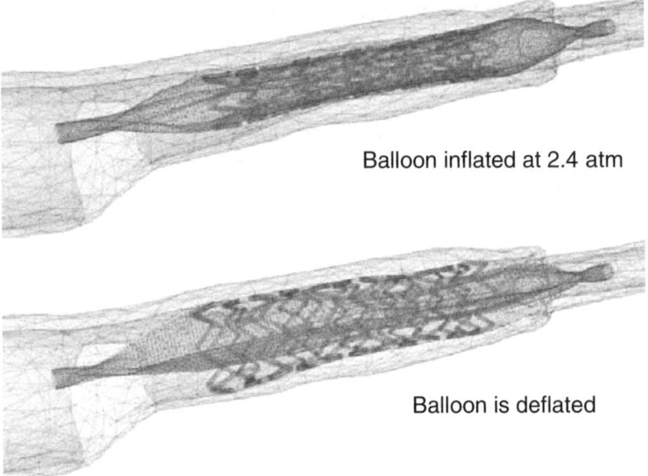

Figure 4: Simulation results of device deployment into the artery, showing predicted deformation at a balloon pressure of 2.4 atm, as well as after balloon deflation.

For comparison purposes, the predicted artery shape was aligned with the post-intervention images using the position and orientation of the bifurcations. Images extracted at proximal, center and distal positions were segmented and the lumen border was identified on each image. Figure 5 shows predicted and measured cross-sections of the artery.

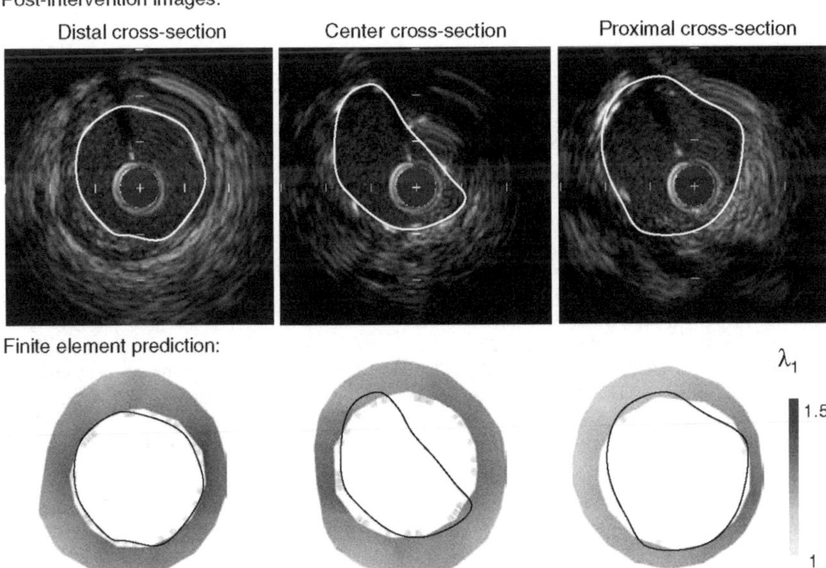

Figure 5: Measured (top) and predicted (bottom) artery shape on three cross-sections. Grey-scale shows the predicted distribution of stretch ratio in the principal direction (λ_1).

The comparison of numerical results of lumen cross-sections with post-intervention data shows that the model correctly predicted the final lumen shape at both extremities of the stent. However it overestimated the lumen area at the mid-length of the stent. This may be due in part to the use of homogeneous mechanical properties for the arterial wall, instead of a layer-specific model that could include a stiffer atheromatous plaque.

An over-prediction of the artery deformation was also expected because the elastic recoil of the stent was not modeled. This could be improved by using an elasto-plastic constitutive model for the stent. As observed in Figure 2, the reopening is more pronounced for the distal cross-section. This was well predicted by the numerical model.

4. Conclusion

In this work a finite element model for predicting patient-specific stent implantation was presented. The model can predict the complete deployment of a stent through the inflation and deflation of a pre-wrapped balloon. Artery/stent/balloon interactions are predicted, including friction and slip. An in-vivo validation using pre- and post-intervention IVUS images from a patient who underwent direct stenting of its mid-LAD artery was presented. The results showed good agreement between predicted and measured artery post-intervention shape. It also highlighted the need for an appropriate elasto-plastic constitutive model for the stent, and a layer-specific model for the artery. Future work will include appropriate constitutive models for the artery and the stent in order to better predict the elastic recoil and the final artery shape.

References

[1]   Clowes AW, Clowes MM, Fingerle J, Reidy MA. Kinetics of cellular proliferation after arterial injury. V. Role of acute distension in the induction of smooth muscle proliferation. *Lab Invest* 1989; **60**:360-364.

[2]   Fingerle J, Au YP, Clowes AW, Reidy MA. Intimal lesion formation in rat carotid arteries after endothelial denudation in absence of medial injury. *Arteriosclerosis* 1990 **10**:1082-1087.

[3]   Laroche, D., Delorme, S., Anderson, T. DiRaddo, R. Computer Prediction of Friction in Balloon Angioplasty and Stent Implantation. *Biomedical Simulation: 3rd Int. Symp, ISBMS*, Zurich, Switzerland 2006: 1-8.

[4]   Laroche, D., Delorme, S., Anderson, T., Buithieu, J., DiRaddo, R. Computer Prediction of Balloon Angioplasty from Artery Imaging, *Medicine Meets Virtual Reality 14, J.D. Westwood et al. (Eds), Technology and Informatics* 2006; **119**: 293-298.

[5]   Delorme S, Laroche D, DiRaddo R, Buithieu J. Modeling polymer balloons for angioplasty: from fabrication to deployment. *Proc Annual Technical Conference (ANTEC), SPE*, Chicago, IL, 2004.

[6]   Holzapfel, G.A., Stadler, M., Schulze-Bauer, C.A.J.: A layer-specific three-dimensional model for the simulation of balloon angioplasty using magnetic resonance imaging and mechanical testing, *Ann. Biomed. Eng.*, 2002; **30**: 753-767

Medicine Meets Virtual Reality 15
J.D. Westwood et al. (Eds.)
IOS Press, 2007

Progressive Update Approach to Real-time Cutting of Finite Element Models in Surgical Simulation

Bryan LEE [a,b,1], Dan C. POPESCU [a] and Sébastien OURSELIN [a]

[a] *BioMedIA Lab, Autonomous System Laboratory, CSIRO ICT Centre, Australia*
[b] *School of Electrical and Information Engineering, University of Sydney, Australia*

Abstract. We present an extension of our work on topology modification and deformation for Finite Element Models, in which the inverse stiffness matrix is updated rather than recomputed entirely. Previously we integrated condensation to allow for realistic interaction with larger models. We improve on this by redistributing computational load to increase the system's real-time response. Removing a tetrahedron only requires data associated with the nodes of that tetrahedron, and the surface nodes, to be updated, in order to drive the simulation. However, the update procedure itself needs the entire data structure to be updated. The equations used to update the inverse stiffness matrix are split up such that calculations are only performed for the affected nodes. Data regions corresponding to the surface nodes necessary for deformation calculations are computed immediately, whilst remaining regions can be computed as required, resulting in up to a ten-fold improvement in system response times.

Keywords. Surgical Simulation, Finite Element Method, Topology Modification, Cutting, Condensation, Real-time, Haptics

Introduction

Finite Element Methods (FEM) based on linear models are suitable for certain surgical simulation procedures as they are accurate for small displacements and efficient for real-time interaction [1]. Quasi-static schemes benefit from the precomputation of the stiffness matrix K. Furthermore, the precomputation of K^{-1} allows for considerable savings in computational complexity, to provide realistic haptic feedback. Integrating topology modification, such as cutting, requires K^{-1} to be updated. As this inverse matrix is not sparse, updating it at real-time haptic rates (300 to over 1000 Hz) is challenging.

In [2] we presented an efficient method of updating K^{-1}, without computing the full inversion of the modified K matrix. We extended this approach to integrate condensation [3], permitting larger meshes in the order of 7,500 nodes and 40,000 tetrahedra to be simulated. To permit real-time deformations, surface node data is kept in memory for fast access, whilst the data of internal nodes is stored on disk. While this enabled

---

[1] Correspondence to: Bryan C. Lee, CSIRO ICT Centre, Macquarie University, Locked Bag 17, North Ryde, NSW, 1670, Australia. Tel.: +612 9325 3267; Fax: +612 9325 3101; E-mail: BryanC.Lee@csiro.au.

the simulation of larger models, I/O and other overhead meant computation times were slower than the original method.

1. Method

We propose to improve the system's real-time response for topology modifications by redistributing the computational load required to make a cut. Using condensation, only the surface nodes are required for haptic and visual feedback of deformations. Following this idea, removing a tetrahedron only requires data associated with the nodes of that tetrahedron, and the surface nodes, to be updated.

While the entire inverse matrix is required to be updated after each cut to maintain integrity of the models, only data associated with the surface nodes has to be updated immediately. As the ratio of the number of surface nodes compared to the total number of nodes is quite small, computational requirements are reduced significantly, resulting in faster system response times. The remaining matrix data can then be updated in the background, at a later time, when spare cpu cycles are available.

2. Mathematical Model

The equations used to update K^{-1} are split up such that calculations are only performed for the affected nodes. This is achieved by selecting smaller regions of K^{-1}, corresponding to the surface nodes that require immediate calculation (see Fig. 1).

From [2], the final equations for our topology modification algorithm are:

$$A = I - U_i G_i K^{-1} G_i^T U_i^T \tag{1}$$

$$M = K^{-1} G_i^T U_i^T R^T \Lambda^{-1} R U_i G_i K^{-1} = W^T \Lambda^{-1} W \tag{2}$$

where $W = R U_i G_i K^{-1}$. G_i is a 0's and 1's "globalisation" matrix, and multiplications with this matrix only require the extraction of the corresponding rows and columns. A is 6×6, symmetric, and can be decomposed as $A = R^T \Lambda R$ with Λ the diagonal matrix of the eigenvalues, and R a rotation matrix formed with the eigenvectors of A. U_i is a precomputed 6×12 matrix, and only the 6×6 rotation matrix R and the 6×6 diagonal matrix Λ need to be computed in real-time.

From these equations we notice that with U_i precomputed, apart from the calculation of R and Λ, and subsequently A, the only information from K^{-1} to be extracted is the $12 \times 3n$ sub-matrix corresponding to tetrahedron i, where n is the number of nodes. As this sub-matrix contains non-surface node data, it will have to be accessed from disk.

Similar to the modification integrating condensation in [3], the update matrix M is then calculated by multiplication in blocks, but the full $3n \times 3n$ matrix does not have to be calculated. Only the rows (or columns, depending on convention selected) corresponding to the new set of surface nodes are required to be updated immediately. Remaining rows (or columns) are progressively updated using spare cpu cycles during less computationally intensive simulation times.

3. Results

As the ratio of surface nodes to total number of nodes can be as low as 10%, it was found that utilising the progressive update approach can reduce the real-time computational load by up to 90%. Less critical data regions are processed later, as required, to eventually update the entire stiffness matrix, but timings on these calculations depend heavily on the subsequent interactions.

Better results would be expected if the haptic and visual modules were separated into individual threads and run on a multi-processor machine. This progressive update approach would furthermore benefit from a third thread dedicated to the cutting component. This thread would perform cutting calculations immediately, as well as computing the progressive updates in the background.

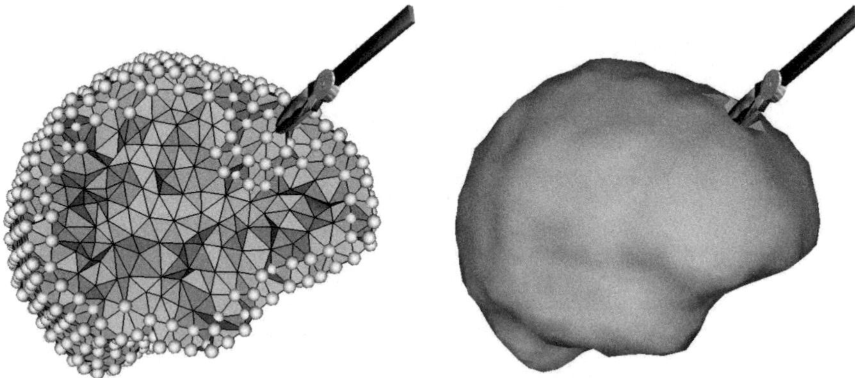

Figure 1. Topology modification with model of a brain. Left: Cross-section to highlight different nodal regions. Data corresponding to nodes marked with a sphere is updated immediately. These nodes are selected to be those near surface nodes or the local cut area. Data corresponding to remaining nodes is updated only as required. Right: Model after topology modification.

4. Conclusion

We have improved a topology modification technique by identifying and computing local updates to the inverse stiffness matrix. Data regions necessary for deformation calculations are computed immediately, whilst remaining regions can be computed as required, resulting in up to a ten-fold improvement in system response times within the framework of our surgical simulator.

References

[1]   M. Bro-Nielsen and S. Cotin; *Real-time Volumetric Deformable Models for Surgery Simulation using Finite Elements and Condensation*, Computer Graphics Forum, vol.15, no.3, pp.57–66, 1996.

[2]   D. C. Popescu, B. Joshi and S. Ourselin; *Real-time topology modification for Finite Element models with haptic feedback*, In Proceedings of The 11th International Conference on Computer Analysis of Images and Patterns, Springer, LNCS vol.3691, pp.846–853, 2005.

[3]   B. Lee, D. C. Popescu, B. Joshi and S. Ourselin; *Efficient topology modification and deformation for finite element models using condensation*, Stud Health Technol Inform (MMVR 14), vol.119, pp.299–304, 2006.

Medicine Meets Virtual Reality 15
J.D. Westwood et al. (Eds.)
IOS Press, 2007

Towards an Immersive Virtual Environment for Medical Team Training

Chang Ha LEE [a,1], Alan LIU [a], Sofia DEL CASTILLO [a], Mark BOWYER [a],
Dale ALVERSON [b], Gilbert MUNIZ [a] and Thomas P. CAUDELL [c]

[a] *The National Capital Area Medical Simulation Center*
[b] *School of Medicine, University of New Mexico*
[c] *Department of Electrical and Computer Engineering, University of New Mexico*

Abstract. Many computer based medical simulators focus on individual skills training. However, medical care is frequently rendered by teams. In addition, the conditions under which care is provided can be a crucial factor in training. For example, mass-casualty events can involve the management and triage of large numbers of victims under austere environments. Learning to care for the injured warfighter during combat requires realistic simulation of battlefield conditions. Current simulation systems do not adequately address team training requirements within lifelike environments. This paper describes our work toward the development of an immersive virtual environment that meets these needs.

Keywords. Immersive virtual environment, medical training, CAVE, display wall

Introduction

Traditional methods of medical team training include apprenticeship, rehearsals, and role playing. As medical interns, physicians not only improve their technical skills, but learn the roles and responsibilities of the medical team when treating patients. First responders improve team coordination through repeated exercise and rehearsals. Elaborate scenarios involving many volunteers acting as casualties permit multiple levels of the healthcare system to practice and coordinate their efforts, and to identify weaknesses in operational procedure.

These approaches have several shortcomings. Interns can receive different experiences due to variations in institutional culture. Re-learning may be required when they graduate to become full practitioners. Rehearsals and role playing can require elaborate preparation prior to the event. Realism can be limited. For example, it can be difficult to realistically recreate the kind of damage caused by weapons of mass destruction. Feedback is available only after the event. There is also limited ability to re-run portions of a scenario if errors or weaknesses are identified.

Virtual environments are gaining prominence as simulators for medical team training. They can increase the realism of the training scenario. It has been demonstrated that

---

[1] Corresponding Author: Chang Ha Lee, The National Capital Area Medical Simulation Center, Bethesda, MD, USA; E-mail: clee@simcen.usuhs.mil.

individuals trained in sterile classroom settings perform poorly when placed in significantly different surroundings [1]. Immersive environments can generate conditions that
are difficult or impossible to recreate, such as a mass-casualty event, or a combat zone.
They can also be paused in mid-training, and portions repeated to incorporate changes
in procedure or to improve team response. Wiederhold and Wiederhold [2] developed
a virtual environment for training combat medics, and to provide stress inoculation as
a means of preventing or reducing the severity of post traumatic stress disorder. Their
system uses game-like environment to help trainees to control fear and anxiety in combat situations. Johnston and Whatley [3] have developed an interactive virtual training
system for civilian and military health care practitioners. The system emphasizes experiential learning, and mirrors the complexities and conflicting demands of an operational
healthcare facility. Alverson *et al.* [4] developed an immersive virtual environment for
network-based medical team training. Their system allows trainees to interact over the
network to treat virtual patients with an evolving epidural hematoma following a ve-
hicular accident. Their system facilitates group and collaborative learning. Individuals
that are otherwise geographically separated are brought together within the same virtual space. Kaufman *et al.* [5,6] developed an virtual environment for training medical
first response in CBRNE (Chemical, Biological, Radiological, Nuclear and Explosive)
events. Multiple trainees can collaborate each other and interact with live actors over the
network.

While these methods are an improvement over traditional techniques, the level of
immersion is still limited. Trainees generally interact with the virtual environment via
computer monitors or head-mounted displays. The former provides very little immersive
effect, while the latter can be cumbersome. In both cases, trainees generally do not interact directly with team members. In fact, direct visual contact with each other can be
impossible with head-mounted displays.

This paper describes our work toward the development of an immersive virtual environment for medical team training. Our system is based on the CAVE [7], a fully immersive display modality that can accommodate teams of individuals. Unlike head-mounted
displays, team members can interact with each other in a natural fashion. In addition,
equipment and other gear, such as protective clothing, can be carried within the environment, thus improving realism.

1. Methods

1.1. Hardware Components

A CAVE-like system is used to display our immersive environment. A CAVE consists
of 3 walls upon which stereoscopic images are displayed. An observer standing in the
enclosed space perceives the illusion of being immersed in a 3D environment.

To accommodate larger teams, the adjacent walls in our implementation are angled
at 135°. Figure 1 shows our screen setup. Stereoscopic images are displayed using a
paired DLP projectors. Passive stereo projection is used. Users wear lightweight polarized glasses to view the scene. To handle very complex scenes and interactive frame-
rates, a scalable hardware configuration is adopted. Each projector is driven by an Alien-
ware Aurora ALX computer, with dual nVidia 7800 GPUs in an SLI configuration. A

total of six display computers and six projectors are used for three screens. Additional improvements in display resolution and rendering capability can be obtained by tiling the display to increase the number of rendering computers used. Figure 2 shows the rendering/projection hardware for one screen. Our system also accommodates a 5.1 channel sound system for acoustic presence.

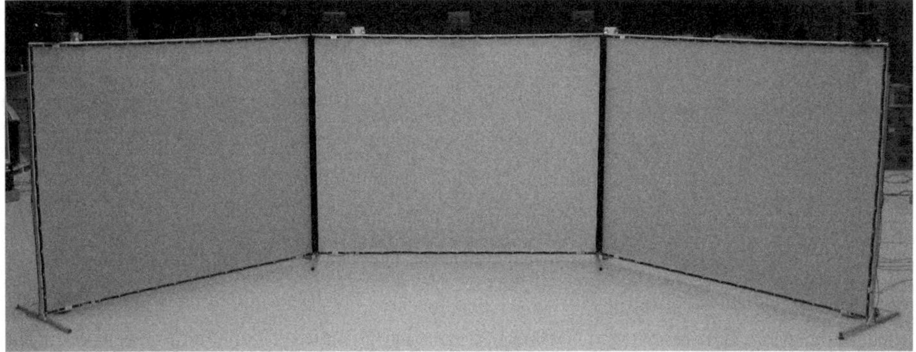

Figure 1. Screen setup.

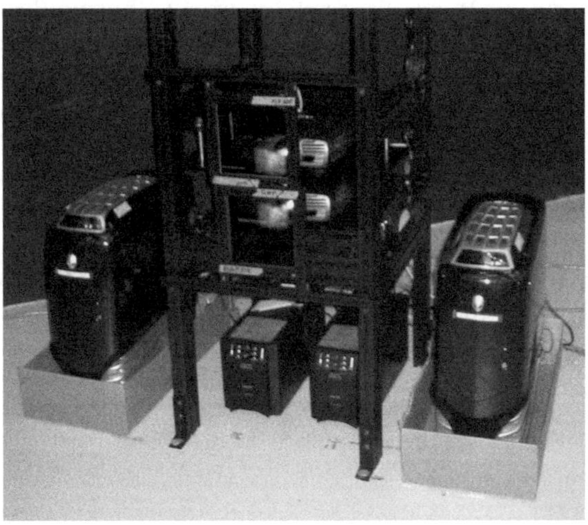

Figure 2. Projectors with polarized filters for stereoscopic display.

1.2. Rendering

Rendering software generates images for display. The software takes a 3D model of the virtual environment, then generates the virtual scene with appropriate lighting and texture models. Visual effects, such as smoke, and fire are incorporated. Animated elements, such as virtual characters and vehicles, are added for greater realism.

We have adopted Flatland [8] as our rendering platform. Flatland is an immersive 3D environment that permits multiple networked individuals to interact, explore, examine, and manipulate objects in real-time. Flatland was originally designed for use with tracked head-mounted displays. We have adapted the code to run with our CAVE display system.

The use of multiple rendering computers requires the images to be synchronized. Synchronization across all computers is essential for maintaining the illusion of immersion. Even subtle variations in rendering speed between computers can cause unacceptable image jitter for the observer. Two forms of synchronization are required: event synchronization and frame synchronization. Changes in the virtual environment require event synchronization. The movement of virtual characters, smoke, and flame effects must be synchronized across displays. Flatland incorporates mechanisms for event synchronization. In our application, Each display computer runs its own instantiation of Flatland. Events within each instantiation is synchronized across the network so that all events occur at the same time across all instantiations.

In addition to synchronizing events within the virtual world, successive frames for each display must be displayed synchronously. Failure to accomplish this results in unacceptable jitter between images on each screen, and even between images for each eye. We have developed a network frame synchronization algorithm that reduces jitter down to visually imperceptible levels. Our method consists of a server and n rendering clients ($n = 6$ in the current implementation), and takes advantage of the double buffering mechanism in the graphics display pipeline. The server drives the locomotion and scenario events. For each frame, the server sends locomotion parameters and events to the rendering clients r_i ($0 \leq i < n$). The renderers generate the scene and write to the back buffer, then wait for a synchronization packet from the server. When the server sends this packet, all renders swap display buffers simultaneously. To compensate for variations in hardware performance, the server adaptively changes frame rates to ensure all rendering clients are ready to swap buffers before they receive the synchronization packet. While intended to eliminate minor variations in rendering speed across different machines, we have found that the algorithm is sufficiently robust that it successfully synchronizes computers with widely differing CPU and graphics capabilities. Our tests used three rendering computers. One had dual nVidia 7800 GPUs in an SLI configuration, another had an nVidia 6800 GT, and the final computer used a 3D Labs 6100 Wildcat. These three machines represent three generations of graphics hardware. When tested, rendering was synchronized within 50 frames after initialization, and the entire configuration ran at a consistent 18 frames per second.

1.3. 3D Modeling and Rendering

Mass-casualty and combat scenarios require realistic environmental effects, such as smoke, fire, and explosions. We have implemented a fire model using a sprite-based particle system with animated textures [9]. Sprites are instantiated, moved about, and removed based on the parameters such as initial position, velocity, and decay time. Animated textures are displayed on each sprite to simulate the appearance of a fire. This way, we can simulate realistic effects with fewer particles, which results in the performance enhancement. A smoke model has been implemented in a similar fashion.

Comprehensive training requires the development of a suite of scenarios and virtual environments. We have streamlined scenario development by developing a bridge between 3D modeling tools, such as 3D Studio Max and Flatland. 3D environmental models are created in 3D Studio Max, then exported to Flatland. Plug-ins were developed for 3D Studio Max for our smoke and fire models. Information such as the position, direction and intensity of these effects are then used for rendering within the immersive environment. The Cal3D library [10] is used for rendering skeleton based animations. Human characters, vehicles, and other animated objects are modeled by using 3D Studio Max, and exported in Cal3D file format for display in Flatland.

2. Results

Figure 1 shows our screen setup and synchronized rendering results. The wide angle of screens provides a spacious effective area for large teams. Our system provides synchronized rendering across screens. The fire and smoke effects shown in Figures 3 and 4(a) give more realistic presence in mass-casualty or battlefield scenarios. Figure 4(b) shows animated characters.

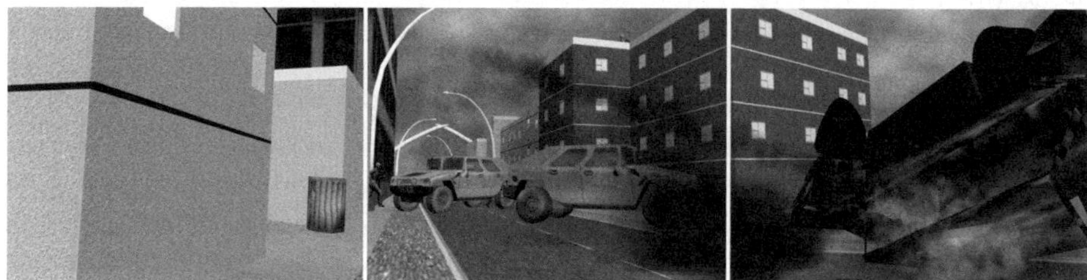

Figure 3. Synchronized rendering across three screens.

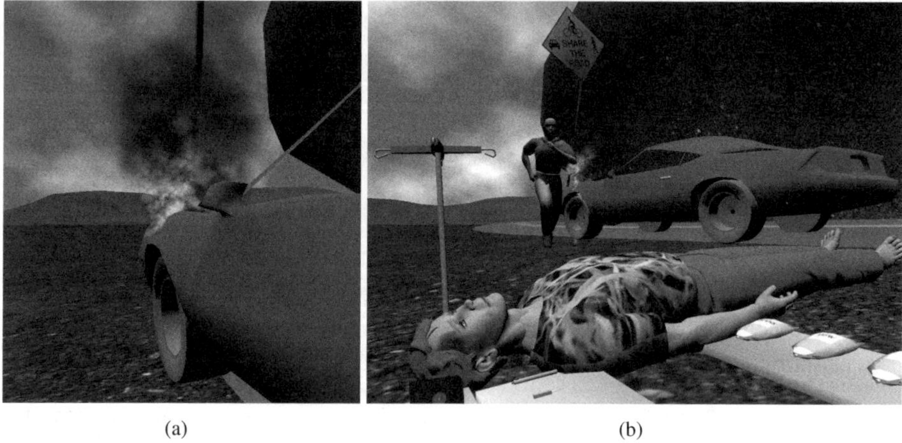

(a)   (b)

Figure 4. (a) The fire and smoke model adds realism, and (b) an animated running man modeled by using 3D Studio Max is plugged in Flatland.

3. Discussion and Conclusion

We are currently developing an immersive virtual environment for medical team training. A CAVE-like display is used to physically accommodate team members. Our approach differs from systems using computer monitors and head-mounted displays in that all members of the team are in physical proximity, yet are still able to interact within a virtual space. A scalable, network-based rendering approach permits highly complex scenes to be rendered in real-time with minimal temporal mismatch between displays. We have also developed a framework for 3D model development that simplifies the transfer of scenarios between the 3D modeling tool and the immersive environment. Work is currently underway to develop educational case content that will use our immersive environment.

Acknowledgments

This work is supported by the US Army Medical Research Acquisition Activity, Contract W81XWH-04-1-087. The views, opinions and/or findings contained in this report are those of the authors, and should not be construed as the official positions, policies, or decisions of the US Army unless so designated by other documentation.

References

[1] M.W. Scerbo, Weireter L.J., Bliss J.P., Schmidt E.A., and Hanner H. An examination of surgical skill performance under combat conditions using a mannequin-based simulator in a virtual environment. In *NATO RTO Human Factors in Medicine, St. Pete Beach, FL*, 2005.

[2] M. D. Wiederhold and B. K. Wiederhold. Training combat medics using VR. In *Proceedings of CyberTherapy*, 2004.

[3] C. L. Johnston and D. Whatley. Pulse!! - a virtual learning space project. *Studies in health technology and informatics (MMVR14)*, 119:240–242, 2006.

[4] D.C. Alverson, S.M. Saiki Jr, T.P. Caudell, K.L. Summers, Panaiotis, A. Sherstyuk, D. Nickles, J. Holten, T. Goldsmith, S. Stevens, S. Mennin, S. Kalishman, J. Mines, L. Serna, S. Mitchell, M. Lindberg, J. Jacobs, C. Nakatsu, S. Lozanoff, D.S. Wax, L. Saland, J. Norenberg, G. Shuster, M. Keep, R. Baker, R. Stewart, K. Kihmm, M. Bowyer, A. Liu, G. Muniz, R. Coulter, C. Maris, and D. Wilks. Distributed immersive virtual reality simulation development for medical education. *Journal of the Association of International Medical Science Educators*, 15:19–30, 2005.

[5] Matt Kaufman. Team training of medical first responders for CBRNE events using multiplayer game technology. In *Proceedings of Medicine Meets Virtual Reality*, 2006. http://www.forterrainc.com.

[6] M. Kaufman, P. Dev, and P. Youngblood. Application of multiplayer game technology to team based training of medical first responders. In *The Interservice/Industry Training, Simulation & Education Conference (I/ITSEC)*, 2005.

[7] C. Cruz-Neira, D. J. Sandin, and T. A. DeFanti. Surround-screen projection-based virtual reality: The design and implementation of the CAVE. In *Proceedings of ACM SIGGRAPH*, pages 135–142, 1993.

[8] T.P. Caudell, K.L. Summers, J. Holten, T. Hakamata, M. Mowafi, J. Jacobs, B.K. Lozanoff, S. Lozanoff, D. Wilks, M.F. Keep, S. Saiki, and D. Alverson. Virtual patient simulator for distributed collaborative medical education. *The Anatomical Record (Part B: New Anat.)*, 270B:23–29, January 2003.

[9] H. Nguyen. Fire in the vulcan demo. In R. Fernando, editor, *GPU Gems*, chapter 6, pages 87–105. Addison Wesley, 2004.

[10] Cal3D – 3D character animation library. http://cal3d.sourceforge.net/.

Medicine Meets Virtual Reality 15
J.D. Westwood et al. (Eds.)
IOS Press, 2007

Haptic Rendering of Device and Patient Impedances in Catheter-Based Simulation

Christopher LEE
Medical Simulation Corporation

Abstract. The complexity of devices used for endovascular interventions has grown rapidly in the last decade. While older simulations render simpler devices such as wires, catheters, stents, and balloons, current simulations need to haptically render the dynamics of devices which may not feel passive. This paper describes the control strategy for the SimSuite® haptic platform and some of its mechanical characteristics.

Keywords. Haptic, impedance, catheter, endovascular, simulation, control

1. Introduction

Simulation has become a powerful tool for endovascular intervention training. Haptic transparency is a key factor in the sense of immersion in catheter-based simulation [1]. Haptic rendering must include both the feedback from the patient anatomy and from the medical devices themselves. The dynamics of these devices have become increasingly intricate. For example, the patent foramen ovale (PFO) closure devices [2] have 'binders' that straddle the atrial septum. As these are deployed at the septum, the delivery catheter pops forward in a spring-like manner. In the case of abdominal aortic aneurysm (AAA) interventions, wires threaded through one insertion point must be seen moving out another. This is one of several cases where as many as four wires and catheters can be inserted through each of several points. The SimSuite simulator has been designed to accept up to five exchangeable catheters and wires simultaneously through each of two insertion points (see Figure 1).

In this paper, section two briefly describes some mechanical characteristics pertinent to wire and catheter control. Section three presents a combined passive and active haptic rendering strategy based on impedance control [3] and the computational platform used in the SimSuite medical simulator.

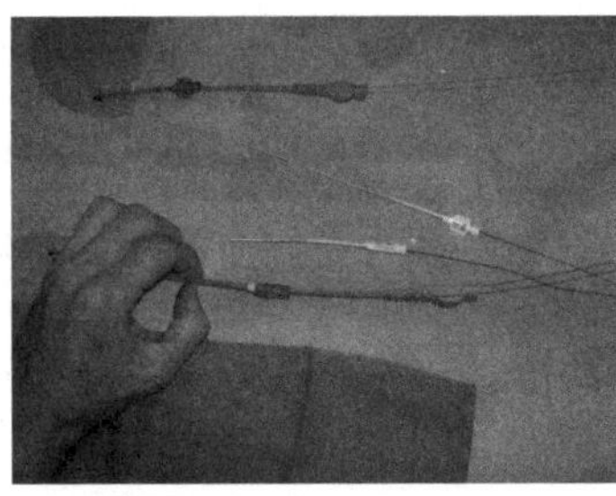

Figure 1. Dual access points hosting up to 5 wires or catheters each

2. Mechanical characteristics

Several haptic rendering hardware implementations have been proposed. In the passive implementation, minimal mechanical impedance from the simulator allows excellent free feel, but complex non-passive device and anatomy haptics cannot be rendered.

In the active implementation (e.g. [3]), the wires and catheters are driven by very small motors, allowing a greater range of haptic rendering. The active implementation is more difficult to control due to the drive train dynamics. It requires an effective control methodology and high fidelity sensing to subdue mechanical artifacts.

The SimSuite system incorporates both passive and active implementations, depending on the type of haptic feedback required. For the actively controlled catheters and wires, force sensors are attached at the contact point between the catheter/wire and the simulator hardware to measure translational force. The force sensors have a range of ± 2.5 N, with an A/D resolution of 0.000076 N. Catheter position is measured using encoders with an accuracy of 0.004mm for translation and 0.5 degrees for rotation. The high position accuracy is necessary for the stability of the impedance control loop.

3. Control strategy

The control strategy is force-based impedance control [4]. An inner loop controls the force felt by the user, while an outer impedance loop calculates desired forces based on the impedance of the virtual environment, comprised of both the patient anatomy and the dynamics of the devices. Figure 2 shows this architecture. The dedicated Haptic Interface Computer (HIC) runs a real time operating system (RTOS) at a hard 500 Hz refresh rate on a Pentium III processor with 16 bit A/D and D/A cards, as well as 24 bit position decoding. The main simulation computer runs other functionality of the simulator, such as fluoroscopic and EKG screens, vascular and pharmacological models, catheter navigation, case flow, and other modalities.

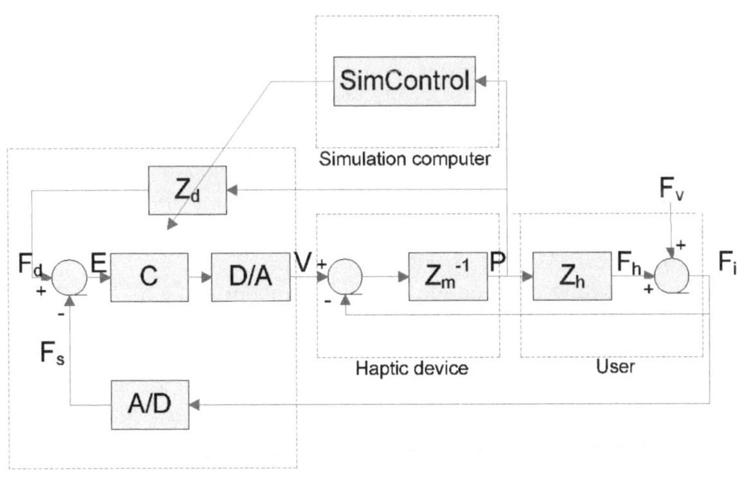

Figure 2. Block diagram for the haptic interface

In Figure 2, the user's hand impedance is Zh, which relates the positions and rotations, P, to the hand forces, *Fh*. The voluntary component of user-applied forces is *Fv*. The interaction forces between user and device are Fi. The haptic device dynamics are Zm, and the desired impedance to be felt by the user is Zd, which incorporates device and vessel dynamics. The components of Zd are triggered on and off by the simulation computer that contains the patient vascular model and device types. The feel of Zd is tunable in real-time during simulations by clinicians. The force controller, C, is driven by the error, E, between the measured interaction force, Fs, and the desired force, Fd. C determines the voltage, V, sent to the motors to control the catheter/wire motions.

In order to quantify haptic interface performance, a useful metric is the total impedance tracking bandwidth [5]. The total impedance of the simulator, Zt, is the relationship between the measured interaction force, Fi, and the position, P. Ideally, this would be Zd. Zt can be calculated using standard block diagram derivation from Figure 2. Assuming, as a simplification, perfect A/D and D/A conversion, we find:

$$F_i = \frac{Z_h C}{Z_m + Z_h(C+1)} Z_d P = Z_t P$$

$$\{C \to \infty\} \Rightarrow \{Z_t \to Z_d\}$$

Hence, large gains in C drive the total impedance of the system to Zd. Although human sensitivity in the fingers extends beyond 300 Hz [6], the bandwidth of human-induced motion is closer to 8 Hz. To achieve good performance up to 8 Hz, large gains in C must be stably achieved. The design technique for C generally follows [7].

4. Conclusions

The SimSuite haptic interface combines passive and active mechanical implementations. Whereas the passive implementation yields superior free feel, the active implementation allows for the rendering of complex device and anatomy dynamics. The control strategy is implemented on a RTOS running at 500 Hz. The device has been successfully implemented in numerous full case simulations including carotid, coronary, PFO, and others. It has received positive feedback for its haptic fidelity in a wide range of clinical cases.

References

[1] J. Korndorffer et al. "Haptic Interfaces: Do They matter?", *MMVR 14*, Jan 2006.

[2] Bernhard Meier, MD, "PC-Trial: Patent Foramen Ovale and Cryptogenic Embolism", Retrieved July 13, 2006, from http://www.clinicaltrials.gov

[3] T. Moix, D. Ilic, H. Bleuler. "A Haptic Device for Guide Wire in Interventional Radiology Procedures", *MMVR 14*, Jan. 2006.

[4] C. D. Lee, D. A. Lawrence, and L. Y. Pao. " Modeling of a 5-DOF Haptic Interface for Multivariable Force Control Design," *Proc. IFAC Conf. Mechatronic Systems*, Berkeley, CA, pp. 559-565, Dec. 2002.

[5] S.J. Bolanowski, G.A. Gescheider, R.T. Verrillo, and C.M. Checkosky. "Four Channels Mediate the Mechanical Aspects of Touch," *J. Acoust. Soc. Am.*, Vol. 84, No. 5, pp. 1680-1694, 1988.

[6] C. D. Lee, D. A. Lawrence, L. Y. Pao. "A High-Bandwidth Force-Controlled Haptic Interface", *Proc. 9th Annual Symposium on haptic Interfaces for Virtual Environment and Teleoperator Systems"*, held at the Int. Mech. Engr. Cong. and Expo., Orlando, FL, November 2000

Medicine Meets Virtual Reality 15
J.D. Westwood et al. (Eds.)
IOS Press, 2007

Collaborative Virtual Desktop as decision support system for surgical planning

Pascal LE MER and Dominique PAVY
France Telecom Div R&D – 2 av. Pierre Marzin – 22307 Lannion Cedex – France

Abstract. Today, diagnosis of cancer and therapeutic choice imply strongly structured meeting between specialized practitioners. These complex and not standardized meetings are generally located at a same place and need a heavy preparation-time. In this context, we assume that efficient collaborative tools could help to reduce decision time and improve reliability of the chosen treatments. The paper presents an activity analysis and the first outcomes of a participatory design method involving end users.

Keywords. GUI 3D, Collaborative Decision Support System, Surgical planning.

Introduction

Today, diagnosis of cancer and therapeutic choice imply strongly structured meeting between specialized practitioners. These complex and not standardized meetings are generally located at a same place and need a heavy preparation-time in order to take the best decision as promptly as possible with the available part of the medical history.

However, a lot of reasons such as delocalised skill centres, home constraints or busy schedules, don't allow practitioners to attend all the meeting they could be expected for. Thereof, several overview studies [1] or technical experiments [2] underline the potentiality of collaborative tools to reduce decision time and improve reliability of the chosen treatments. Indeed looking for the most experienced second opinion is crucial in decision making activity. But despite striking needs, a large deployment of distance collaborative tools didn't really yet occurred in medical communities, even though tremendous tools are easy to implement and exist since several years. From our point of view, this situation could be partly explained by unsuitability of the available tools as well as a lack of network infrastructures to share efficiently medical histories.

In the European project Odysseus (Eureka 3184) INRIA, IRCAD and France Telecom R&D investigate how to design a Collaborative Decision Support Systems (CDSS) for surgical planning. And the project priorities are focused on adequacy of the CDSS with both activity and infrastructure aspects.

We present here ergonomic requirements pointed out from several analysis. Then we explain how we assume that 3D and more generally Virtual Reality techniques could contribute to overcome unsuitability of existing collaborative tools. And finally, we describe a first prototype of Graphic User Interface (GUI) designed to contribute to an iterative participatory design method [3] involving end users.

1. Activity analysis and requirements

Decision making is not a lonesome activity. Practitioners we have interviewed in several hospitals are requested each day if not several times a week for medical opinions. The majority of these opinions are asked in order to talk about a complex situation or to reach a consensus in the close practitioners' circle. And whether they are inside or outside the hospital, they are used to talking by phone. In the specific context of cancer treatment, structured meetings are generally organised in the majority of the French and European hospitals. The aim of these meetings is to provide a reliable diagnosis and follow therapeutic choices along the treatments.

Odysseus focuses on this last specific use case activity. Indeed, we assume there is a strong need of distance collaboration before, during and after these meeting. Before the meetings, practitioners need to prepare relevant elements of the medical histories with a team physically dissipated. During the meeting skill centres could be delocalised as well. And after a meeting practitioners could need to call for details about a treatment or a surgical operation.

In order to determine delocalised activity requirements, we first investigated co-localised ones. Features we have observed are the following: number of the attendees, length of the meeting, time dedicated to each patient, non-usual attendees number for each meeting, time dedicated to remind each patient history, content of the medical history, collaboration steps and rhythm of a meeting. Thus, we determined following requirements:

- Minimize efforts to memorize the medical histories
- Minimize the time of diagnosis and therapeutic choices for each patient data
- Capability to alternate between face to face communication and examination of medical histories
- Maintain the confidentiality of several medicals information
- Ensure the connectivity to the Hospital Information System (HIS)
- Be compatible with all the office, pictures and 3D data formats of the HIS
- Allows a connectivity with practitioners outside of the HIS

Seeing that these requirements depend strongly on the efficiency and the acceptability the user interface, we decided to focus our efforts on the Graphic User Interface (GUI) design. And especially we decided to explore the potentiality of 3D to improve the efficiency and the acceptability of collaborative tools.

2. Iterative participatory design method

It is very difficult to obtain from practitioners expected functionalities for such a system. The main reason comes from the difficulty for everybody of projecting himself onto other way of working. And today only co-localised decision meeting exist. Therefore, we assume that using a CDSS might imply not easy to anticipate changes in the way of working. Above all, these difficulties increase when it is a non-usual 3D interface.

In order to introduce progressively a CDSS in such an activity without changing the way of working, it is mandatory to keep in eyes to fit with the original activity. Therefore we have designed a first prototype bound to initialize an iterative participatory design method [3] involving end users.

3.   Argonaute: a prototype of Collaborative Virtual Desktop for decision making

Our main idea is to integrate a windowing system upon a 3D collaborative platform. This approach appeared few years ago with new desktop such as Task Gallery [4] or more recently Looking Glass (http://www.sun.com/software/looking_glass/), but only for lonesome activity. Therefore we tried to make evolve the windows paradigm [5] used for twenty years, to take into account collaborative decision requirements.

Our windowing manager allows sharing medical contents such as DICOM pictures and office data format. In a near future a 3D planning application will be integrated too. Several techniques such as control gestures are integrated in the GUI in order to improve the efficiency of interactions with windows and automatically contribute to reduce the decision time for each medical history. Hereunder two snapshots of the GUI (figure 1) show a public view and a private view.

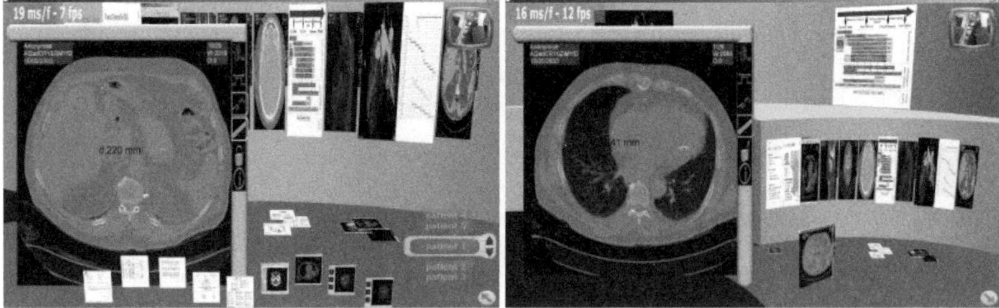

Figure 1: CDSS user interface – Left image: public space; Right image: private space

A public view allows a shared space organization of data for each patient history in order to aids practitioner to remind rapidly previous diagnosis and decisions. A private view allows simultaneously, manipulating confidential data and attend to the collaborative. A dynamic organization of attendees' videos allows an alternation between face to face communication and examination of medical histories as well.

4.   Conclusion

We have designed a 3D collaborative virtual desktop dedicated to surgical decision activity. The system integrates the main functionalities required to start an iterative participatory design process involving end users. Moreover we hope this 3D CDSS could also be used by practitioners to explain a chosen therapy to citizen-patients and in a general way constitute a breakthrough in surgery planning.

References

[1] Quintero J. M. and al., "Medical decision-making and collaborative reasoning", Proceeding of Bioinformatics and Bioengineering Conference, pp 161-165, November 2001.
[2] Le Mer P. and al., "Argonaute 3D: a real- time cooperative medical planning software on DSL network", Proceeding of MMVR12, pp 203-209, Newport Beach, California, USA, January 2004.
[3] Muller M. and Kuhn S. Special Issue on Participatory Design, CACM 36:6 pp 24-28, June, 1993.
[4] Robertson G. and al. "The Task Gallery: A 3D Window Manager". Proceeding of CHI. pp. 494-501, 2000.
[5] Myers B. "A taxonomy of window manager user interfaces". IEEE Computer Graphics and Applications, 8(5):65–84, September/October 1988.

Medicine Meets Virtual Reality 15
J.D. Westwood et al. (Eds.)
IOS Press, 2007

Low Cost Eye Surgery Simulator with Skill Assessment Component

Rainer LEUSCHKE [a], Anuja BHANDARI [b], Brian SIRES [b] and
Blake HANNAFORD [a]

[a] *Department of Electrical Engineering*
[b] *Department of Ophthalmology*
University of Washington, Seattle, WA 98195-2500, USA
e-mail: [rainer\bhandari\blake]@u.washington.edu

Abstract. Ophthalmic surgeons require years of training and continuous practice to successfully manipulate the delicate tissues of the human eye. Development of the fine motor skills is a crucial component of this training. Virtual eye surgery simulators have come on the market in recent years leveraging the advantages of virtual procedures. However adoption is limited by the high initial investment and availability of models. Our approach consists of a low cost hybrid approach that employs a standard porcine model for cataract training and a platform that is instrumented to record interaction forces and video. In a preliminary study we have recorded procedure data for a small number of experts which shows good signal-to-noise ratio suitable for development of objective skill assessment models.

Keywords. Surgical Training, Skill Assessment

Introduction

The human eye is one of the most delicate structures in the human body. Ophthalmic surgeons need years of training and continuous practice to carefully and successfully manipulate the tissues. Tool motions and forces used in these procedures are extremely small. Development of the fine motor skills is therefore an important component of resident training and generally consists of wetlab practice on cadaveric eyes and assisting experts with surgery in live cases in the operating room.

For wetlab practice a cadaveric eye is mounted in a Styrofoam training prop. The ex-vivo specimens are used to practice various common intraocular surgical procedures such as cataract removal, glaucoma and retinal surgery [1]. In a simulated wetlab procedure the resident in training can carry out several complete procedures in a short time frame and practice critical steps without risk to a patient. However in order to obtain performance feedback for the resident, a skilled surgeon has to observe and evaluate the practice session [2]. Due to the workload demands on expert surgeons and high cost of their time, residents currently go through only one supervised and 5 to 10 unsupervised wetlab sessions. The residents are quickly transitioned into the OR working live cases. The expert surgeon will perform most of the procedure at first and assign increasingly larger and more difficult parts of the procedure to the resident. With this approach, the resident will practice critical steps in the procedure for only a few brief periods per patient once basic skills are fully mastered.

Virtual eye surgery simulators such as the EYESI® from VRmagic GmbH have come on the market in recent years leveraging the advantages of simulated procedures [3,4]. Due to the virtual nature of the model, they are well suited to simulate standard procedures as well as unexpected and rare circumstances. Performance assessment is feasible since the state of the model is known. These simulators currently do not provide tactile feedback for tissue interaction [5,6,7,8,9]. This component is critical in developing the motor skills necessary to successfully handle the extremely delicate tissues of the human eye.

With availability of high fidelity data of surgeon/tool and tool/tissue interaction, objective skill assessment for surgical applications has recently been subject to intense study. Integrative and averaged metrics have been employed to this goal [10,11]. More recently approaches using stochastic tools such as Markov models have been employed to capture the dynamic nature of the surgical task. [12,13,14,15,16]

The goal of this project is to improve the understanding of the biomechanical properties of the human eye, eye socket and surgical tools, leading to the development of objective surgical skill assessment methodology and improved training tools for ophthalmic surgeons. Current trends in medical training indicate that simulator based certification for surgical procedures may become more common. The device proposed here lends itself to training and certification of proficient surgeons for new procedures and materials. In the initial phase of this project, we developed, built and tested a surgical platform for data collection during cataract procedures on porcine and human ex-vivo eyeballs and collected preliminary data.

1. Methods

1.1. Simulator platform

We developed a novel device to measure, record and evaluate surgical tool/tissue interaction data for eye surgery. A cup supporting an ex-vivo human or porcine eye is placed on top of a 6-axis force/torque sensor (Nano 17 from ATI Industrial Automation). The cup is available in several sizes to allow a somewhat customizable fit to the specimen size. Because the force/torque sensor is easily damaged by exposure to fluids, the cup and supporting structure are shaped to allow fluids from the surgical site to drain to the base without pooling or contacting the sensor. An internal channel in the platform connects the fluid catch basin with a hose barb, where external drain tubing can be attached. A Styrofoam head prop representing patient anatomy is mounted to the platform. The head prop is mechanically isolated from the sensor to allow the surgeon to use it for support as is commonly done in real surgery.

With its placement directly below the specimen, the 6-axis sensor allows us to track direction and magnitude of resulting forces and torques applied to the specimen throughout the procedure. Placing the sensor on the specimen enables the use of unmodified surgical tools as well as standard handpieces used with phacoemusification machines.

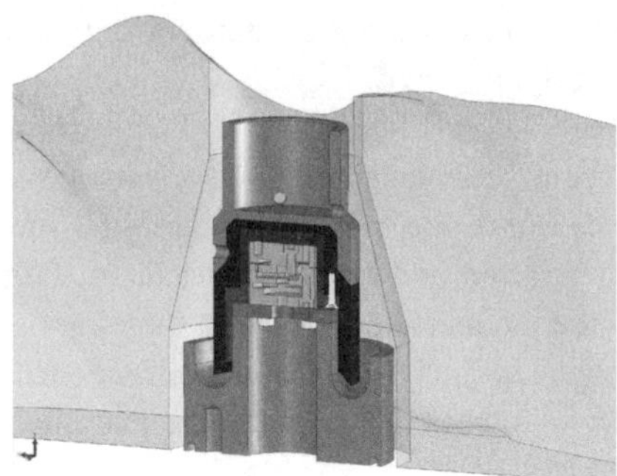

Figure 1. CAD rendering of sensor support with drainage system and specimen cup.

1.2. Specimen Suspension and Pressure Regulation

Preliminary testing with the platform revealed that the porcine eyes obtained from Sierra for Medical Science Inc. made it difficult to place the specimen in the cup with satisfactory consistency and biomechanical realism of the suspension. Several methods of attachment of the eye were considered and tested. Method 1 is a simple velcro lining of the bottom of the cup to increase friction between specimen and cup. Method 2 consists of fixation with a needle transversely penetrating the specimen, holding the eyeball more rigidly to the cup. Method 3 is a 10mm pin penetrating the globe from the back. The pin is attached to rubber bands that suspend the pin flexibly to the inner circumference of the cup. These methods were tested with cup sizes of 22, 25 and 28mm inner diameter.

The specimens we obtained varied in intraocular pressure mainly due to decreased and variable vitreous volume. To improve specimen consistency and maintain intraocular pressure throughout the procedure we implemented a simple pressure regulator based on a gravity feed of saline solution to a needle that penetrates the posterior segment from the side. With this placement of the needle port, the workspace of the surgeon was not affected and correct pressure could be maintained continuously. Normal intraocular pressure (18mmHg) was obtained with reservoir fluid level at 25cm above the cornea.

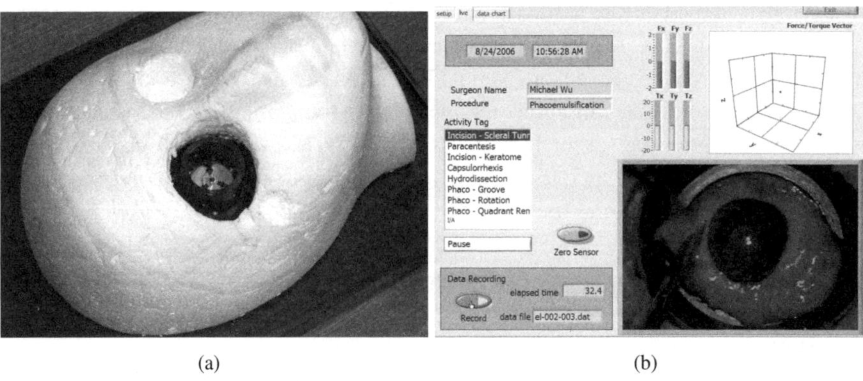

(a)   (b)

Figure 2. Device with Styrofoam prop, cup and suspended pin (a) graphical user interface (b)

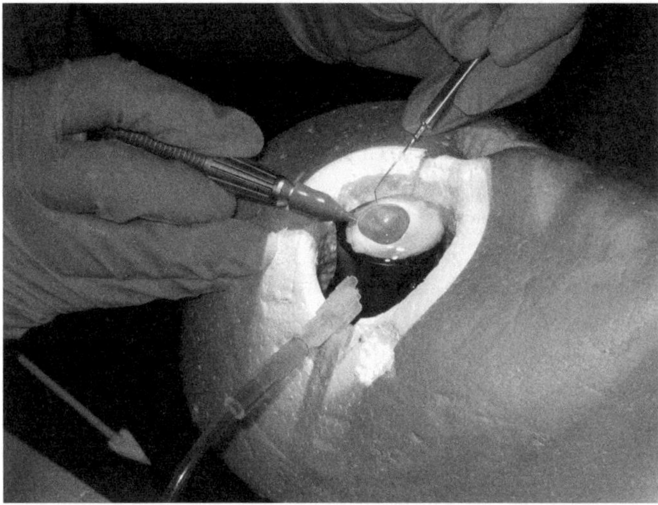

Figure 3. Test procedure performed on a porcine specimen

1.3. Data and Video Acquisition

The sensor data is acquired and recorded using a National Instrument data acquisition card and a Labview program. Force/torque data is recorded at 100Hz. The software provides a simple user interface that allows the surgeon or a nurse to record data and view results with little or no training. To aid with development of the skill assessment component the recorded data can be tagged manually to identify data corresponding to distinct procedural steps during a phacoemulsification procedure. Tags are displayed in a list and the user simply selects the appropriate item. The Labview program also displays and records live video from the microscope camera to facilitate off line evaluation and model validation.

2. Results

The cornea size of 6 porcine eyes was measured. The cornea is slightly elliptical and the average length of the major axis was measured at 15.1mm with a standard deviation of 1.2mm. For evaluation of the suspension, the eyes were reformed using the pressure regulator. Fit was tested for cups of 21, 25 and 28mm inner diameter and found to be best for the 25mm cup. The suspension methods for the eye were evaluated for realism of suspension, expected consistency and sensitivity to eyeball size. Method 1 (velcro) resulted in moderately realistic suspension; consistency of the method and sensitivity to changes in specimen size were poor. Method 2 (transverse needle) resulted in consistent, size insensitive, but very unrealistic rigid suspension of the eyeball. Method 3 (suspended pin) showed good consistency and size insensitivity with very good physiological accuracy of the suspension. This method was selected for further experiments.

To date, multiple procedures performed by two experts were recorded during phacoemulsification procedures on porcine eyes (see Figure 3 and 4). The collected data displays a high signal to noise ratio with peak forces during phacoemulsification recorded at around 0.7 N. Similar values were recorded by Charles et al. with a tool-based measurement [17]. The data shows well defined periods of activity corresponding to the typical steps of the procedure and the manually assigned tags. Video of the procedure was recorded simultaneously. Average procedure completion time of the procedure was 838s ($\sigma = 141s$), completion time for the phaco sections was 235s ($\sigma = 40s$).

3. Conclusion and Future Work

A novel device for training in eye surgery has been proposed. Much like traditional wet-lab work, residents train on porcine models. The collection of force and torque data provides the means to develop a better understanding of the interaction of tissue and surgical tools in this discipline. The data will also be used to develop statistical models for assessing resident skill objectively. Primarily aimed at improving the training experience of surgical residents, this approach lends itself to broad adaptation due to its relatively low complexity and cost.

We are in the process of collecting data from procedures by more experts as well as less experienced residents and are evaluating the feasibility of using artificial eyes with our device.

Acknowledgments

The authors would like to acknowledge support from Department of Ophthalmology, Bucy Chair Memorial Funds and University of Washington Technology Gap Innovation Funds. The authors would also like to thank Dr. Michael Wu.

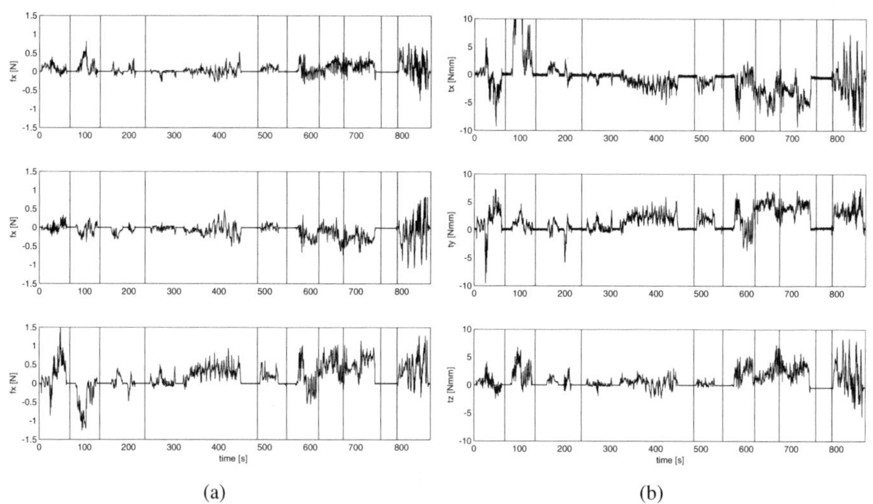

(a)   (b)

Figure 4. Sample of recorded forces (a) and torques (b)

References

[1]   T.D. Lenart, C.A. McCannel, K.H. Baratz, and D.M. Robertson. A contact lens as an artificial cornea for improved visualization during practice surgery on cadaver eyes. *Archives of Ophthalmology*, 121(1):16–19, January 2003.

[2]   S.L. Cremers, J.B. Ciolino, Z.A. Ferrufino-Ponce, and B.A. Henderson. Objective assessment of skills in intraocular surgery (OASIS). *Ophthalmology*, 112(7):1236–1241, July 2005.

[3]   M. Colvard and S. Charles. How to be a virtually perfect surgeon. *Review of Ophthalmology*, January 2005.

[4]   C.G. Laurell, P. Söderberg, L. Nordh, E Skarman, and P. Nordqvist. Computer-simulated phacoemulsification. *Ophthalmology*, 111(4):693–698, April 2004.

[5]   Y. Cai, C.K. Chui, Y. Wang, Z. Wang, and J.H. Anderson. Parametric eyeball model for interactive simulation of ophthalmologic surgery. *Lecture Notes in Computer Science*, 2208:465, January 2001.

[6]   I.W. Hunter, L.A. Jones, M.A. Sagar, S.R. Lafontaine, and P.J. Hunter. Ophthalmic microsurgical robot and associated virtual environment. *Comput Biol Med*, 25(2):173–182, March 1995.

[7]   P.J. Berkelman, L.L. Whitcomb, R.H. Taylor, and P. Jensen. A miniature instrument tip force sensor for robot/human cooperative microsurgical manipulation with enhanced force feedback. *Lecture Notes in Computer Science*, 1935:897–906, February 2000.

[8]   R. Kumar, P. Berkelman, P. Gupta, A. Barnes, P.S. Jensen, L.L. Whitcomb, and R.H. Taylor. Preliminary experiments in cooperative human/robot force control for robot assisted microsurgical manipulation. In *IEEE Intl. Conference on Robotics and Automation, ICRA 2000*, pages 610–617, 2000.

[9]   M.A. Schill, S.F. Gibson, H.J. Bender, and R. Männer. Biomechanical simulation of the vitreous humor in the eye using an enhanced chainmail algorithm. *Lecture Notes in Computer Science*, 1496:679, January 1998.

[10] L. Verner, D. Oleynikov, S. Holtmann, and L. Zhukov. Measurements of level of surgical expertise using flight path analysis from Da Vinci^{TM} robotic surgical system. In *Studies in Health Technology and Informatics - Medicine Meets Virtual Reality*, volume 94, pages 373–378. IOS Press, January 2003.

[11] L. Moody, C. Barber, and T.N. Arvanitis. Objectice surgical performance evaluation on haptic feedback. In *Studies in Health Technology and Informatics - Medicine Meets Virtual Reality*, volume 85, pages 304–310. IOS Press, January 2002.

[12] T.M. Kowalewski, J. Rosen, L. Chang, M. Sinanan, and B. Hannaford. Optimization of a vector quantization codebook for objective evaluation of surgical skill. In *Proc. Medicine Meets Virtual Reality 12*, pages 174–179, January 2004.

[13] T. Mackel, J. Rosen, and C. Pugh. Data mining of the E-pelvis simulator database A quest for a generalized algorithm for objectively assessing medical skill. In *Proceedings of Medicine Meets Virtual Reality*, pages 355–360, Long Beach, CA, January 2006.

[14] J. Rosen, J.D. Brown, M. Barreca, L. Chang, B. Hannaford, and M. Sinanan. The blue DRAGON - A system for monitoring the kinematics and dynamics of endoscopic tools in minimally invasive surgery for objective laparoscopic skill assessment. *Studies in Health Technology and Informatics - Medicine Meets VirtualReality*, 85:412–418, January 2002.

[15] J. Rosen, J.D. Brown, L. Chang, M. Sinanan, and B. Hannaford. Generalized approach for modeling minimally invasive surgery as a stochastic process using a discrete markov model. *IEEE Transactions on Biomedical Engineering*, 53(3):399–413, March 2006.

[16] C. Richards, J. Rosen, B. Hannaford, M. MacFarlane, C. Pellegrini, and M. Sinanan. Skills evaluation in minimally invasive surgery using force/torque signatures. *Surgical Endoscopy*, 14(9):791–798, 2000.

[17] S. Charles and R. Williams. Measurement of hand dynamics in a microsurgery environment: Preliminary data in the design of a bimanual telemicro-operation test bed. In *Proceedings of the NASA Conference on Space Telerobotics*, volume 1, pages 109–118, 1989.

Medicine Meets Virtual Reality 15
J.D. Westwood et al. (Eds.)
IOS Press, 2007

Computer Simulation of Corticospinal Activity during Transcranial Electrical Stimulation in Neurosurgery

Daliang Leon LI[1,3], H. Louis JOURNEE[4], Arjen van HULZEN[4],
William T. RATH[1,2], Robert J. SCLABASSI[1,2,3], and Mingui SUN[1,2,3]
*Laboratory for Computational Neuroscience, Depts. of [1]Neurosurgery,
[2]Bioengineering, and [3]Electrical Engineering, University of Pittsburgh,
Pittsburgh, PA 15261*
[4]*Dept. of Neurosurgery, University of Groningen, The Netherlands*

Abstract. Transcranial Electrical Stimulation (TES) is an important procedure in intraoperative motor monitoring. When neurosurgery is performed at certain difficult locations within the central nervous system (CNS), TES evaluates CNS functions during surgical manipulations to prevent post-operative complications. In TES, electrical stimulation is provided to the motor cortex through electrodes placed on the scalp, generating action potentials which travel through the nervous system. Despite widespread use, the sites of activation (AP generation) within the brain are not well understood. We have integrated computational and neurophysiologic models including a 3D volume conduction head model computed using the finite element method, a realistic corticospinal tract (CST) model, and a geometry-specific axon activation model for the CST to predict the sites of activation along the CST as a function of electrode placement and stimulation voltage, which have been verified by epidural recordings. We then develop a simple meshing and rendering algorithm to display the activating function along the CST. We have found that the AP generation appears closely linked to regions of high CST curvature. Our model and rendering algorithm provide a window to visualize the effects of TES in the brain.

Keywords. Activation Function, Computer Simulation, Corticospinal Tract, Finite Element Analysis, Nerve Tract Rendering, Transcranial Electrical Stimulation

1. Introduction

1.1. Background

Transcranial electrical stimulation (TES) is often performed during neurological surgery for the resection of tumors in certain difficult locations in the central nervous system (CNS), such as intramedullary spinal cord tumors and intrinsic brain stem tumors. In TES, electrical stimulation is provided to the motor cortex through electrodes placed on the scalp of an anesthetized patient, generating action potentials (APs), in a process known as activation, through the stimulation of neurons in the brain.

Clinical neurophysiologists can then monitor the descending volleys along the central motor pathways ([1], [2]). If abnormality is detected, corrective actions can be taken.

Although TES has been widely utilized, its exact mechanisms inside the brain with respect to various tissues and structures are not clearly understood. Localizing the sites of action potential generation under electrical stimulation improves the understanding of TES and allows for more effective optimization of TES parameters such as voltage, impedance, and electrode geometry. The critical problem yet to be solved is how to predict the locations of action potential generation, or sites of activation, given an external stimulus in a complex geometric domain such as the human head. We present a 3D finite element model of TES, consisting of a 3D model of the human head and the corticospinal tract (CST). Our modeling technique has produced a powerful computational tool to determine the sites of activation during TES as a function of stimulation parameters. We then use a simple rendering algorithm to display these distributions along the CST, providing a tool to better visualize the effects of TES.

1.2. Descending Volleys (D waves)

Presently, experimental research has suggested that TES activates neurons in the corticospinal tract ([1], [3]). The evoked volleys, or D-waves then descend through the CST to the spinal cord, where they can be recorded through epidural electrodes inserted in the spinal cord. As stimulation voltage increases, D-wave latencies decrease in discrete jumps, resulting from deeper neuronal activations at higher voltages. These latencies result from the propagation time required for a descending volley to travel through the CST before reaching the recording electrodes.

1.3. Model of Axon Activation – Activating Function

The most widely accepted nerve activation micromodel has been provided in [4], where it is suggested that a nerve axon under an external electric field is activated when the second derivative of the external potential along the direction of an axon, defined as the activating function, exceeds a certain threshold value.

1.4. Unifying Model

In this paper, we combine a finite element macromodel with the nerve activation micromodel to compute the sites of activation during TES. First, we utilize a finite element model [5] of the human head to compute the potential and current distribution in the brain resulting from TES. We then add a realistic model of the CST constructed using diffusion tensor imaging (DTI), and calculate the activating function along the corticospinal tract to localize TES-elicited neuron activation. D-wave latencies between any two sites are estimated using the distance between the sites and the conduction velocity of corticospinal fibers, and then compared with experimental latency data. Our model is the first to integrate computational and neurophysiologic models including a volume conduction head model computed using the finite element method, a realistic CST model constructed through image processing of DTI data, and a geometry-specific microscopic axon activation model for the CST.

2. Methods

For the computational study of TES, the head may be viewed as a volume conductor [6] with different conductivities for different regions. We have chosen to approximate the head as a 3D, four-layer spherical model, consisting of the scalp, skull, cerebral spinal fluid (CSF), and brain. In this volume conduction system, the voltage-current relationship obeys the law of electrostatics. It is well known that this relationship is governed by the Poisson's Equation. Since electrical stimulation occurs through electrodes on the scalp and the resulting signal is several orders of magnitude stronger than the spontaneous brain waves, we can assume that no current sources exist within the simulation domain. Then, within this domain,

$$\nabla \cdot (\sigma \nabla \varphi) = 0 \tag{1}$$

where φ is the electric potential (a scalar), ∇ is the gradient operator (a vector), and σ is the conductivity value. In the general case, σ is a tensor describing the anisotropy of the volume conductor. In our case, for simplicity, we assume that it is a scalar constant within each of the four tissue types. To further reduce complexity in computation, we use four concentric spheres in our model of the head, with one sphere for each of layer. The simulation domain also contains two 2cm diameter cylindrical stimulation electrodes on the scalp (Figure 1a).

The diameter of the brain in our model is 13cm, and the CST, skull, and scalp layer widths are 0.7, 0.4, and 0.5cm respectively. The conductivities of the brain and CSF are 0.15S/m [7] and 1.8S/m [8] respectively, while the skull and scalp conductivities are determined by the scalp:skull:brain conductivity ratio of 1:1/15:1 [7]. DC voltages are used in our model to simulate the electrical activity inside the brain. We also assume that tissue conductivities do not have any dielectric components. The assumption of DC voltages does not cause loss of generality because the simulation result is considered to be instantaneous and can be scaled according to arbitrary input voltage values and polarities. The positive and negative electrodes are assigned Dirichlet boundary conditions of 100V and 0V, respectively, again without loss of generality since Laplace's equation is linear. Thus, the specific solution to Eq. (1) can be generalized. All other segments on the outer boundary (scalp) are assigned the Neumann condition $\nabla \varphi = 0$ based on the physical constraint that no current can escape from the scalp and flow into the air. The model is solved numerically for the potential and electric field distribution using the finite element method (FEM).

We create a model of the CST through Diffusion Tensor Imaging (DTI), which employs fiber tracking algorithms to locate nerve tracts within the brain. We use the methods in [9] and manually adjusted the seed fiber region of interest and fractional anisotropy threshold value on the DT-MRI slices of a patient with no known lesions near the CST to obtain the course of the CST from the corona radiate to the brain stem, shown in Figure 1a. We assume that the nerve tracts have the same conductivity as the rest of the brain layer, since this conductivity value arises from the bulk measurements of brain tissue [7], and thus we may ignore the thickness of the CST and consider it to be a continuous curve (zero thickness) connecting the cortex to the brainstem. This assumption greatly simplifies finite element modeling because, then, we do not create a separate complex subdomain for the CST, reducing computational complexity. The

CST curve is smoothed using spline interpolation and is included inside the model during meshing to increase the accuracy of the solution near the CST curve.

The potential φ along the CST is sampled at 1mm intervals, in accordance with the approximate distance between nodes of Ranvier, and then the difference between successive elements is computed twice to estimate the activating function

$$A(l) = \Delta^2 \varphi / \Delta l^2 \ [\text{V/cm}^2] \tag{2}$$

where l is the length along the CST from the motor cortex. The first difference quotient $\Delta \varphi / \Delta l$ gives the electric field strength along the tract.

3. Results

The potential, activating function, and curvature along the CST is shown in Figure 2b for the C3-C4 configuration, where the symbols are standard notations in electrophysiology for electrode locations. The potential along the length of the CST only spans approximately 0.5V, consistent with earlier simulation results showing the shielding effect of the poorly conductive skull [5]. As stimulation is applied, membrane potentials increase towards its excitation threshold at the rate proportional to its activating function magnitude, causing the action potentials to be first initiated at locations with larger activation function values [4]. We assume that the activating function threshold along the CST is constant, reasonable given that the CST fibers in the range modeled are of similar diameter. Thus, local peaks in the activating function curves represent sites of activation. However, peaks which are too close together will only elicit one action potential, due to an axon's refractory period. Regions of activations, D1 (near the motor cortex), and D2 (near the brain stem), are labeled in Figure 2, with a distance of approximately 5-6 cm between them. Each region encompasses local peaks which are too close together to elicit separate activations. Since the activating function peaks of D1 are higher than those of D2, D1 will activate first, and then followed by D2 as stimulation voltage is increased. Assuming a constant conduction velocity of 60m/s, the latency of D2 will be between 0.8 and 1ms less than that of D1.

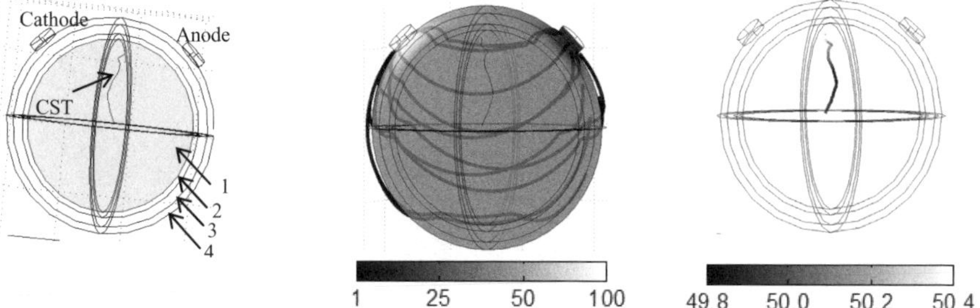

Figure 1: Left: Simulation domain. Center: Potential distribution (V) and electric field lines in the head (central sagittal slice) using 100V stimulation voltage. Right: Potential distribution along the CST for C3-C4 configuration. 1: brain, 2: CSF, 3: skull, 4: scalp.

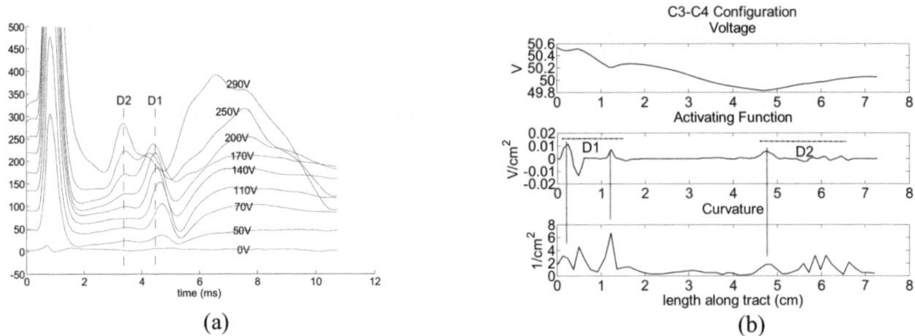

Figure 2: (a): D waves from epidural recordings. (b): Potential, activating function, and curvature along the CST for stimulation from C3-C4 electrodes using stimulation voltage 100V. Length is measured in cm from the motor cortex. D1 and D2 are predicted D wave activation sites.

Patch graphics, consisting of connected polygons, are employed to better visualize the activating function. A desired section of the tract is discretized to obtain p equally spaced coordinates. A polygonal "layer" is constructed using an n vertex regular polygon around each coordinate. This layer is then rotated such that it faces the direction of the tract, or that the unit vector perpendicular to the face of the polygonal layer is in the same direction as the Jacobian of the tract curve. In this way, the "smoothness" of the tract is better preserved. Successive layers are connected using $2n$ triangular faces to create a meshed representation of the tract, as shown in Figure 3a with $p=3$ layers and $n=6$. As n increases, the polygonal layer approximates a circular disk and the mesh takes on the appearance of a smooth tube — the desired rendering appearance of the CST. The mesh is colored using the activating function, evaluated along the vertices of each layer, and then linearly interpolated on all faces to create a smooth, rendered tract. The activating function along the D1 region (0-2cm) and D2 region (5-7cm) regions of the CST is rendered in Figure 3b and c respectively using $p = 80$ and $n = 40$. The effect of curvature on activation is clearly visible.

Epidural recordings from single pulse TES is used to verify our simulation results. A single pulse waveform of 100μs is applied at C3 anode and C4 cathode, consistent with our simulation model. D waves were recoded using epidural electrodes and then amplified and filtered. (Figure 2a) The latency of stimulation between D1 and D2 is approximately 1.1ms, matching and validating the latency calculations from our model.

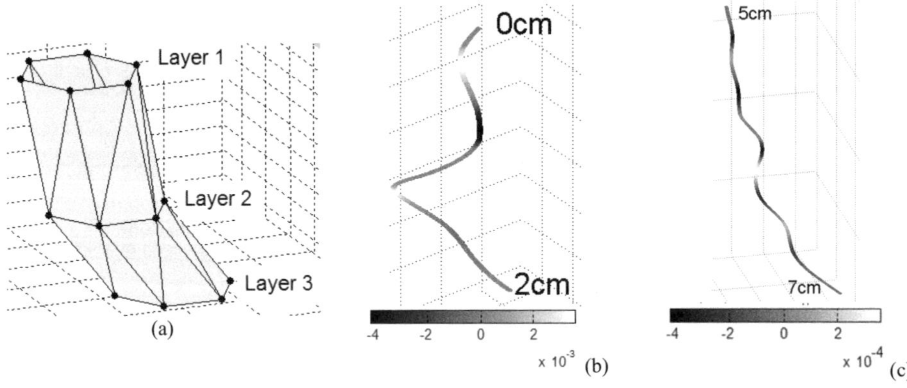

Figure 3: (a): 3 layered patch graphics model of a nerve tract. (b): Activating function (V/cm^2) along the 0-2cm region (D1 region) of the CST in the C3-C4 configuration. (c): Same for 5-7cm (D2 region).

4. Discussion

We have presented a computational approach to the study of transcranial electrical stimulation (TES) for neurosurgical monitoring. Finite element models of the human head and corticospinal tract (CST) have been developed and utilized to perform realistic computer simulation. This computational approach allows us to compute the potential and electric field distributions inside the head and predicts the regions of TES-elicited action potential generation, providing the neurophysiologists with a unique window to observe the electrical and neural activity in the brain from TES. Our simulation results have specifically shown two CST activation sites for the C3-C4 electrode configuration modeled. Graphically rendering the activating function along the CST has provided a method to visualize the clear effect of curvature on activation. The computed latencies between the two sites quantitatively match the TES data measured in the operating room.

Our rendering algorithm uses simple polygons and procedures to provide a fast and simple way to graphically display data along nerve bundles. Our computational methods described in this paper can be modified and extended to modeling electrical stimulation of both the central and peripheral nervous systems in other clinical and research studies.

References

[1] Rothwell J and et al., "Transcranial electrical stimulation of the motor cortex in man: further evidence for the site of activation." *J Physiol*. 1994;481.1:243-250.

[2] Journee HL, Polak HE, de Kleuver M, Langeloo DD, Postma AA. "Improved neuromonitoring during spinal surgery using double-train transcranial electrical stimulation." *Med Biol Eng Computing* 2004 Jan;42(1):110-113.

[3] Burke D, Hicks RG, Stephen JP, "Corticospinal volleys evoked by anodal and cathodal stimulation of the human motor cortex." *Journal of Neurophysiology*. 1990;425:283-299.

[4] Rattay F, "Analysis of models for external stimulation of axons." *IEEE Trans Biomed Eng*. 1986;33:974–977

[5] Li DL, Rath WT, Journee HL, Sclabassi RJ, Sun M, "Finite Element Analysis of Transcranial Electrical Stimulation for Intraoperative Monitoring," in *Proc.IEEE 31st Northeast Bioengineering Conference*, April, 2005, pp. 96-97.

[6] Malmivuo J and Plonsey R, *Bioelectromagnetism*, Oxford; New York: Oxford University Press, 1995, pp. 133-147

[7] Oostendorp TF, Delbeke J, Stegeman DF, "The conductivity of the human skull: results of in vivo and in vitro measurements, *IEEE Trans Biomed Eng*, Nov 2000, 47:11, p1487-1492

[8] Baumann SB, Wozny DR, Kelly SK, Meno FM, "The electrical conductivity of human cerebrospinal fluid at body temperature," *IEEE Trans Biomed Eng*, March 1997, 44:3, p220-223

[9] Kamada K and et al., "Functional Identification of the Primary Motor Area by Corticospinal Tractography." Neurosurgery. 56(1) *Operative Neurosurgery Supplement* 1:98-109, January 2005

Medicine Meets Virtual Reality 15
J.D. Westwood et al. (Eds.)
IOS Press, 2007

An Overview of 3D Video Transmission and Display Technologies for Telemedicine Applications

Qiang Liu [a], Robert J. Sclabassi [a], Amin Kassam [a], Feng Zhu [b], Ron Machessault [c], Gary Gilbert [c] and Mingui Sun [a]

[a]*Department of Neurological Surgery, University of Pittsburgh, Pittsburgh, PA*
[b]*Shenyang Institute of Automation, Chinese Academy of Sciences, Shenyang, Liaoning Province, China, 110016*
[c]*Telemedicine and Advanced Technology Research Center (TATRC), US Army Medical Research & Material Command (USAMRMC), Fort Detric, Frederick MD 21702*

Abstract. Digital 3D visualization provides a fundamental platform to render both the real world and computer generated objects in a highly comprehensive form. It has a number of significant applications in telemedicine, such as telesurgery, patient monitoring and remote surgeon training. Towards utilizing the 3D visualization technologies for these applications, we present an overview of state-of-the-art 3D display devices and discuss related data transmission technologies to support the remote 3D display.

Keywords. 3D video transmission, 3D display, telemedicine

Introduction

In this paper, we present an overview of the current state-of-the-art three-dimensional (3D) visualization technologies and discuss their potential applications to the rapidly growing field of telemedicine. Here, 3D visualization is defined as a means to provide more geometrical information about objects in space than 2D displays. The relevant technologies, including 3D display devices, 3D data modeling and rendering, and 3D data transmission, have been developed over the past three decades. Thanks to these technologies, many medical applications, such as computerized training, surgical planning, and image-guided surgery, are ready to embrace new advancements and improvements in information processing and decision making. We will concentrate on the telemedicine applications where 3D imaging data are remotely displayed. Two key technologies, 3D display devices and 3D data transmission, are discussed. We will first review two major categories of 3D display methods: autostereoscopic and volumetric. A number of cutting-edge products that are not yet widely marketed will be compared. Then, we will discuss several 3D image/video transmission techniques focusing on image coding methods that reduce required bandwidth.

1. 3D Display Devices

1.1. Autostereoscopic displays

The original idea of 3D display can be traced back to Leonardo da Vinci who suggested two paintings, one for each eye, to be displayed simultaneously for capturing true reality [1]. This may be the earliest concept of stereoscopic display. Following this concept, a variety of 3D display devices have been invented, including stereoscopes, anaglyph glasses, polaroid glasses and shutter glasses. While these traditional devices are still being utilized, new state-of-the-art devices that display two or multiple images simultaneously and require no glasses are being developed. These new devices are often referred to as autostereoscopic displays and are designed based on the following two principles: 1) interleaving a pair of or multiple pairs of images and displaying them on a single screen, and 2) directing the ray emitted light from each image pixel to the corresponding eye.

There are two dominant techniques in autostereoscopic display: 1) barrier parallax and 2) lenticular arrays. The concept of barrier parallax, as illustrated in Fig. 1, is simply to block the path of a light ray from reaching the "wrong" eye.

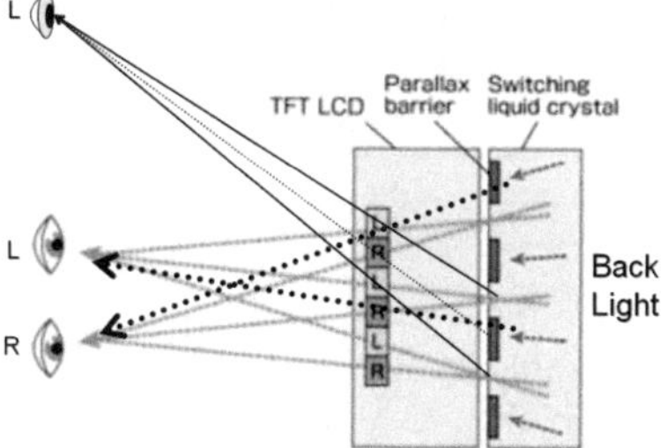

Figure 1. Autostereoscopic display based on barrier parallax (courtesy of Sharp Inc.).

This type of design contains three essential components, a back light for illumination, interleaved pixels (column-wise) for the left and the right eyes, and parallax barriers that can be switched on and off (e.g. by changing the polarization of the back light). The important variables of this design include the distance d_1 between the barrier plane and the pixel plane, the distance d_2 from the eye to the barrier plane, the pixel width w, the separation s between the eyes and the refractive index n of the LCD. A simplified relation between these variables is given by $d_2 = \frac{d_1 \cdot s}{w \cdot n}$, upon which the viewing distance can be determined. This relation also indicates an important limitation of this technique in that the user must adjust his/her position to observe the 3D effect. However, as seen from Fig. 1 the barrier parallax allows multiple viewing positions, implying that multiple users may perceive the 3D effect simultaneously.

The lenticular array techniques employ a micro-sized prism coupled to each pixel column to convey the light rays to the corresponding eyes. Figure 2 shows a typical product of SeeReal Technologies Inc.. that displays a pair of column-interleaved images. Like the barrier parallax technique, in this design a pre-defined viewing position is assumed. The most important advantage of the lenticular array technique is that the light rays from the pixels that are switched on are focused onto the user's retina, therefore providing superior luminance and contrast. The

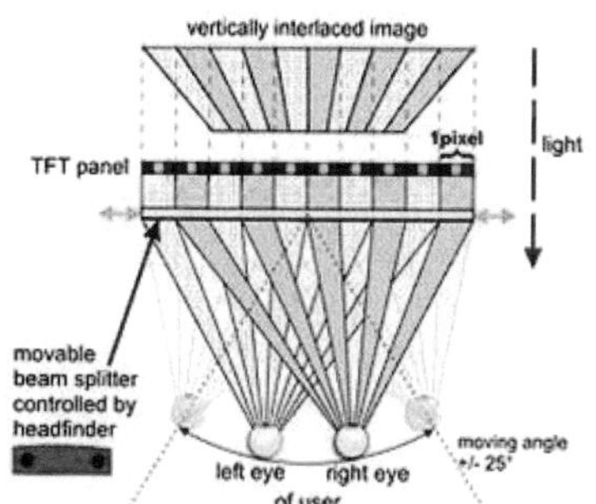

Figure 2. Autostereoscopic display based on lenticular array (courtesy of SeeReal Technologies Inc.).

weakness, however, is that the user is restricted to a certain position. To maximize the 3D display effect, a device called headfinder is designed which consists of a pair of cameras and a set of image processing routines to track the position of the user's eyes and adjust the position of the lenticular array accordingly. The current display system equipped with this device can only translate the lenticular array in the horizontal direction, allowing a change of viewing angle within $\pm 25^o$, but supporting a single

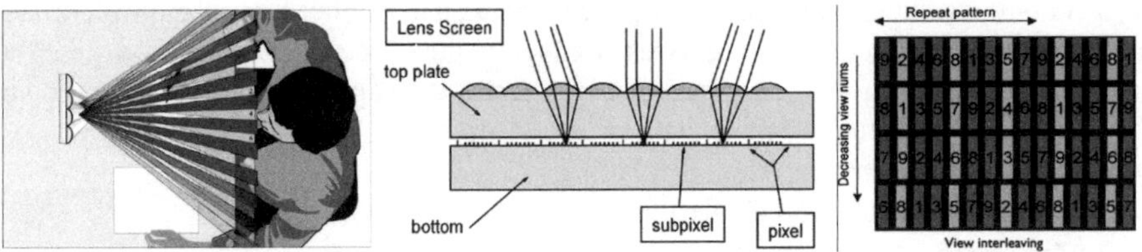

Figure 3. Autostereoscopic display based on lenticular array that accommodates multiple users (courtesy of Philips Inc.).

user. A more advanced technique that can accommodate multiple users has been investigated by Philips Inc. Up to 9 views can be interleaved into one image for display. Each pixel in the display is composed of 9 sub-pixels, which represent the 9 views separately. Therefore, this design requires the display to possess high horizontal resolution. The interleaving pattern is shown in the right panel of Fig. 3, where each cell represents a subpixel. A pixel is coupled by a micro-lens that directs the light ray from the subpixel to a specific direction as shown in the middle panel. Therefore, this technique provides 3D display to either multiple users at fixed viewing positions or a single user with a flexible or changing viewing position. Both of these lenticular array based techniques in general have higher complexity than the barrier parallax based designs, and thus a much higher cost. However, the images delivered by the lenticular array based displays are of better quality, while the barrier parallax displays are more oriented towards consumer products.

1.2. Volumetric displays

Stereoscopic displays, although providing 3D perception, do not render volumetric images in space. Therefore, some important 3D cues, such as motion parallax, are not available with the stereoscopic devices. Volumetric display devices however, recreate volumetric images and are thus referred to as "true" 3D displays. Currently, there are three major technologies realizing volumetric display: holography, solid-state volume and swept volume. We will only describe the latter two here, as holography has been a traditional display

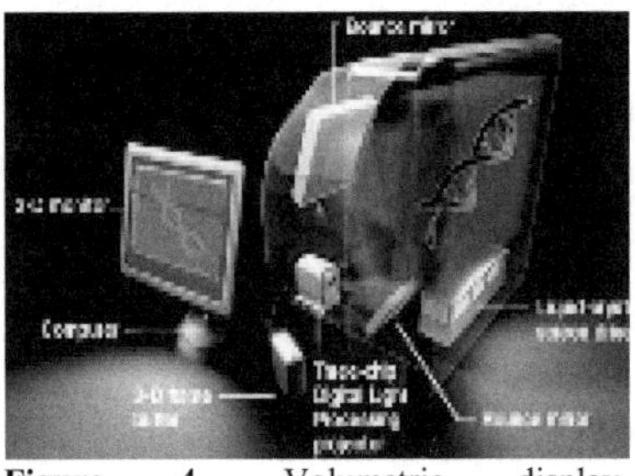

Figure 4. Volumetric display incorporating 20 LCDs (courtesy of LightSpace Technologies Inc.).

method. A solid-state volumetric monitor (developed by LightSpace Technologies Inc.) incorporates 20 LCDs, each about 5mm from the next. The images are displayed at 1200 frames per second at 60 Hz refresh rate. The current technology supports a resolution of 1024x748x608 voxels, where the last dimension denotes the resolution of depth. This is achieved by applying an "anti-aliasing" technique that exploits human perception: if two pixels with the same intensity are displayed on two aligned transparent panels, one pixel with twice the intensity located in the halfway between the two panels is perceived. Therefore, by manipulating the pixel intensities on the 20 LCD panels, human eyes can "interpolate" the voxels along the z-direction.

Swept volume displays, such as the Actuality System's Perspecta, implement a half transparent, quickly rotating screen in a volume. During the rotation, more than 200 images are projected onto the screen and each held for a certain amount of time (e.g. 100 μ s). At a sufficient speed, for instance, 15 revolutions per second, a smooth, solid 3D image is rendered, taking advantage of the persistence of the human visual system. The visual quality, in terms of the delivered 3D cues, is superb. However, limitations do apply, such as a smaller display size (currently up to 25cm in diameter), requiring a careful mechanical balance, and a lower color resolution. The swept volumetric display is being tested on the CT and MRI scans and demonstrating outstanding performance significantly better than the 2D displays [2].

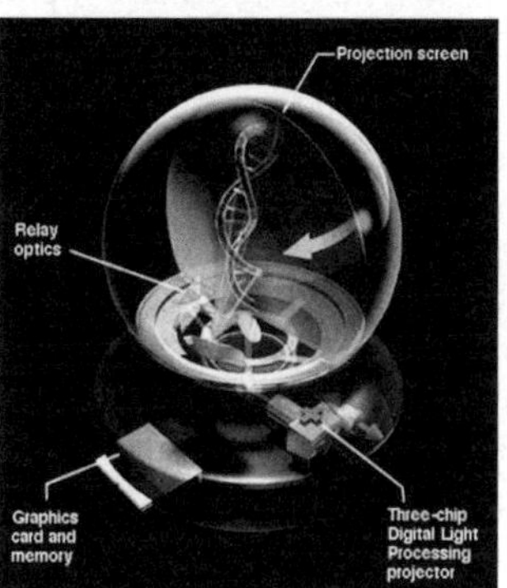

Figure 5. Swept volume display (courtesy of Actuality Systems Inc.).

2. 3D Data Transmission

Transmission of 3D imaging data is an active research field due to the typical mismatch between massive 3D data and limited network bandwidth. Depending on the data type, which includes volumetric data (e.g. MRI and CT), 3D surface data, stereoscopic video and free viewpoint video, the coding schemes for the data transmission are different.

In general, both lossy and lossless coding methods are needed to compress volumetric medical data. The popular 2D image coding schemes such as SPIHT [3] can be extended to 3D image coding. An important feature for the coding of volumetric data is that in most cases the visualization can be performed prior to the completion of the entire data transmission. This is due to the fact the user will only view a small portion of the 3D volume at a time. Therefore, it is necessary for the coding scheme to allow a scalable data stream. The latest standard for the compression of medical images is JPEG2000, which support a number of functions, such as interactive visualization across the Internet and the wavelet-based scalable coding. Some recent research [4] has extended JPEG2000 to coding volumetric data, emphasizing on the demand-driven visualization that allows the user to rapidly retrieve the specified anatomical contents. We believe that this strategy can be used to design a realistic medical volumetric data transmission system for remote display.

The spherical mapping method encodes a 3D surface whose shape can be approximated by a sphere. This spherical surface is then represented by a mesh with scalable density (higher density leads to less distortion of the

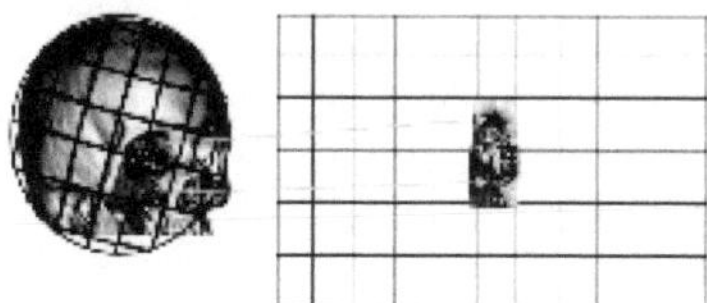

Figure 6. Spherical surface mapping coding: the texture on each mesh grid can be mapped onto a 2D image.

mapping). The texture on each mesh grid can be mapped onto a 2D image with equal-area projection, by associating the mesh vertices with the pixels, as shown in Fig. 6.

The texture map, i.e. the 2D image with the surface texture, can be coded with regular image/video codecs.

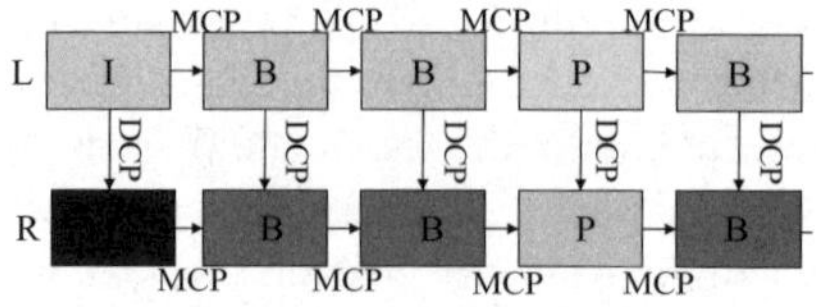

Figure 7. MPEG stereo coding profile.

The stereo video coding can be implemented using both a standardized scheme, i.e. the MPEG-2 or MPEG-4 stereo profile, and a disparity map based scheme. The standardized scheme carries out video compression based on two main strategies (see Fig. 7) by decorrelating the stereoscopic video frame pair, called disparity compensated prediction (DCP), and by decorrelating in the temporal domain, i.e. motion compensated prediction (MCP), as in the case of the regular mono-view video. The disparity map based scheme utilizes a mono-view video with an associated depth map (in gray level) to represent a stereo video. Both techniques can achieve significant compression, while the latter may support more interactivity by adapting the depth map to the user's viewing position [5]. This type of coding is supported by layered coding scheme such as MPEG-4 AFX [6]. A simplified layered 3D video transmission system is highlighted in Fig. 8.

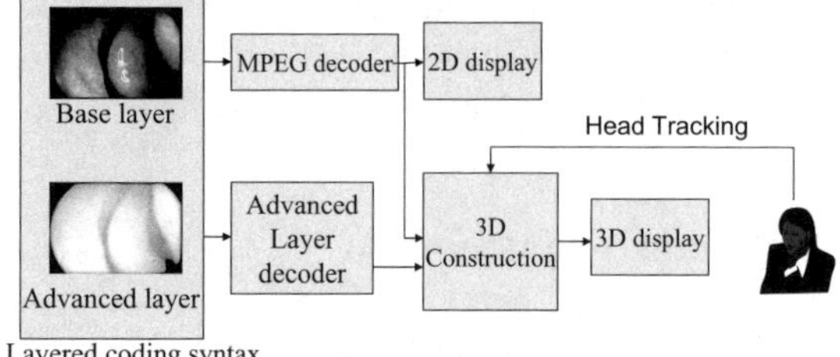

Figure 8. Layered coding/transmission system.

Another coding scheme that aims at rendering an arbitrary perspective view of an object, often referred to as the free viewpoint coding technique, extends the stereo coding schemes by deploying multiple cameras or video sources. When these video are acquired at appropriate positions, in terms of complete coverage of a scene with low redundancy, a 2D image of the scene from any specified view point can be generated by combining the views from the correlated cameras [7].

3. Telemedicine applications

3D visualization technology promises many telemedicine or medical telepresence applications. A short list includes education and consultation over distance, telesurgery, especially image-guided robotic surgery, pre-, intra-, or post-operative

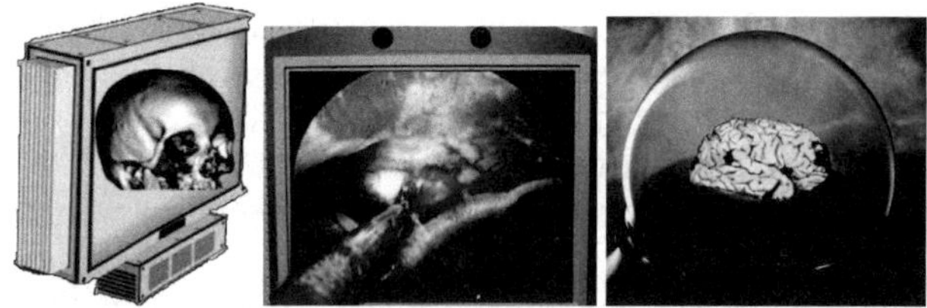

Figure 9. Potential medical applications of 3D visualization. From left to right: preoperative data displayed on solid-state volumetric monitor for training and surgery planning applications; stereoscopic endoscopic surgery visualized on autostereoscopic monitor; physiological data fused with brain MRI volume and displayed with swept volumetric device.

monitoring of patients, and tele-rehabilitation. More specifically, we provide several examples here to highlight these important applications. 1) Preoperative data such as

MRI and CT can be rendered with volumetric displays, which will better serve surgery planning and training purposes by presenting real 3D anatomy; 2) Many minimally invasive surgeries, which utilize stereoscopic surgical video, will benefit from the autostereoscopic displays since the conventional head-mounted-devices are cumbersome in prolonged surgical procedures; 3) Neurophysiological data, which can be fused with the volumetric data (e.g. with FreeSurfer), can be rendered with volumetric displays to visualize the functional activities of the brain, facilitating intra-operative monitoring during high-risk surgical manipulations; And 4) for monitoring patients or caring for elderly people, multiple cameras can be utilized to cover the entire visible space, and the volumetric rendering, especially the swept volume, techniques can be utilized to render the subject's position and activity. All these potential applications can be performed through computer networks, which will inevitably employ the 3D data transmission technologies reviewed previously. It can be seen that such coding schemes are complementary to each other when considering the operational fields, data modality, transmission bandwidth, quality constraints, and costs. Although 3D data coding and transmission are still under active research, the available techniques are ready to be exploited in numerous 3D telemedicine applications.

4. Conclusion

We have presented a review of state-of-the-art 3D display technologies, including autostereoscopic and volumetric devices. Although some of these technologies are not yet commercialized, they promise a wide variety of medical and telemedical applications. In addition, 3D data coding and transmission techniques, including volumetric data coding, stereoscopic video coding, and free viewpoint video coding, have also provided important tools to support these applications. Together, these technologies have great potential to create a significant impact on future medical practices.

Acknowledgement

This work was supported in part by NIH Grants NS/MH38494 and EB002309; Telemedicine and Advanced Technology Research Center, US Army Medical Research and Materiel Command; and Computational Diagnostics, Inc.

References

[1] I. Sexton and P. Surman, "Stereoscopic and autostereoscopic display systems," *IEEE Signal Processing Magazine*, Vol. 16, No. 3, pp. 85-99, May 1999.
[2] Available:http://www.actuality-systems.com/site/content/medical_imaging.html/.
[3] A. Said and W. A. Pearlman, "A new fast and efficient image codec based on set partitioning in hierarchical trees," *IEEE Trans. Circuits Syst. Video Technol.*, Vol. 6, No. 3, pp. 243–250, Jun. 1996.
[4] K. Krishnan, M. Marcellin, A. Bilgin and M. S. Nadar, "Efficient transmission of compressed data for remote volume visualization," *IEEE Trans. Medical Imaging*, Vol. 25, No. 9, pp. 1189-1199, Sep. 2006.
[5] A. Smolic and P. Kauff, "Interactive 3-D video representation and coding technologies," *Proceedings of the IEEE*, Vol. 93, No. 1, pp. 98-110, Jan. 2005.
[6] "Text of ISO/IEC 14 496-16:2003/FDAM4," Int. Standards Org./Int. Electrotech. Comm. (ISO/IEC), ISO/IEC JTC1/SC29/WG11, Doc. N5397, Dec. 2002.
[7] EyeVision [Online]. Available: http://www.pvi-inc.com/eyevision/.

Medicine Meets Virtual Reality 15
J.D. Westwood et al. (Eds.)
IOS Press, 2007

Real-Time Image Mosaicing for Medical Applications

Kevin E. LOEWKE [a], David B. CAMARILLO [a], Christopher A. JOBST [b], and
J. Kenneth SALISBURY [a,b,c]

[a] *Department of Mechanical Engineering, Stanford University*
[b] *Department of Computer Science, Stanford University*
[c] *Department of Surgery, Stanford University*

Abstract. In this paper we describe the development of a robotically-assisted image mosaicing system for medical applications. The processing occurs in real-time due to a fast initial image alignment provided by robotic position sensing. Near-field imaging, defined by relatively large camera motion, requires translations as well as pan and tilt orientations to be measured. To capture these measurements we use 5-d.o.f. sensing along with a hand-eye calibration to account for sensor offset. This sensor-based approach speeds up the mosaicing, eliminates cumulative errors, and readily handles arbitrary camera motions. Our results have produced visually satisfactory mosaics on a dental model but can be extended to other medical images.

Keywords. Mosaic, image mosaicing, real-time, medical robotics

Introduction

Tissue biopsy, the removal of tissue and subsequent laboratory examination, results in a lengthy disconnect between diagnosis and treatment of many diseases. Recently, the development of micro-endoscopes has allowed for tissue structures to be observed *in vivo*. These optical biopsies [1] are moving toward unifying diagnosis and treatment within the same procedure. The application of micro-endoscopes for this purpose, however, is inherently limited by the tunnel-vision effect of their small field-of-view. In order to improve physician confidence during optical biopsies, it will be necessary to visualize tissue at micron-scale cellular resolution across centimeter-sized fields-of-view for greater tissue coverage. One approach is to apply image mosaicing techniques to stitch multiple images together and widen the field-of-view. These "optical biopsy mosaics" can provide macro scale views of tissue structures while retaining micro-architectural detail.

Recent efforts in mosaicing microscopic images from an *in vivo* video sequence have shown promise, but required post-processing [2]. In this paper we describe an approach for achieving real-time performance by integrating robotic technologies, which have proven to be useful in the surgical suite for sensing, processing, and actuation [3]. Specifically, we describe a new method for real-time image mosaicing that incorporates robotic position sensing into the mosaicing software to provide the algorithms with a fast initial estimate of the relative geometric motion among images. This is a useful alternative to image processing techniques that are often slow, require large image overlap, have trouble with homogeneous images (such as biological cells), and impose restrictions on camera motion.

1. Image Mosaicing Background

Image mosaicing is an active field of research in computer vision and has found applications in several areas such as panorama imaging, mapping, tele-operation, and virtual travel. Traditionally, a mosaic is created by stitching two or more overlapping images together to create a single larger image through a process involving registration, warping, re-sampling, and blending. The central step, image registration, is used to precisely align the images and can be achieved through a combination of different techniques [4].

Due to the computational demands of image registration, mosaicing in real-time can be a challenging task. Prior efforts using optical flow achieved processing times ranging from 10-20 frames/second [5], but required significant image overlap and simple camera motions. Other efforts such as *VideoBrush* [6] and *Panoramic Viewfinder* [7] handled arbitrary camera motions, but were designed as real-time previews for the consumer and required post-processing to accurately align the images.

There have been very few efforts aimed at using position sensing to speed up the mosaicing process. While this idea has surfaced in medical imaging, these efforts used motorized microscope stages and were limited to left/right camera translations only [8] [9]. In this paper we use five degree-of-freedom robotic position sensing for the initial image alignment, and the Levenberg-Marquardt iterative nonlinear least-squares routine [10] for the secondary alignment. This readily handles arbitrary camera motions and allows the images to be mosaiced in real-time.

2. Experimental Setup

The experiments presented in this paper were performed using a Phantom Premium 1.5 robot [11]. The robot has optical encoders that are used to determine the five degree-of-freedom position and orientation of the end-effector. The end-effector is a Sony miniature CCD camera mounted on a stylus. The robot is not actuated, and thus the user engages the device manually via the stylus to scan a region of interest while watching the corresponding image mosaic develop. Metal pins near the camera help the user maintain focus by keeping at least one pin in contact with the scene. This bench-top setup was used to simulate an endoscope with position sensing for proof-of-concept.

Individual still images are captured by a Euresys PCI frame grabber. Image processing takes place on a 2.79 GHz Pentium 4 processor using the Intel OpenCV library.

3. System Framework

In this section we present a framework for developing our real-time, robotically-assisted image mosaicing system. Specifically, we discuss how to integrate knowledge from the fields of projective geometry, camera calibration, sensor-based robot kinematics, hand-eye calibration, and image mosaicing algorithms. While some of the assumptions are specific to our particular application, this general approach can be followed for other image mosaicing systems that use multiple degree-of-freedom position sensing.

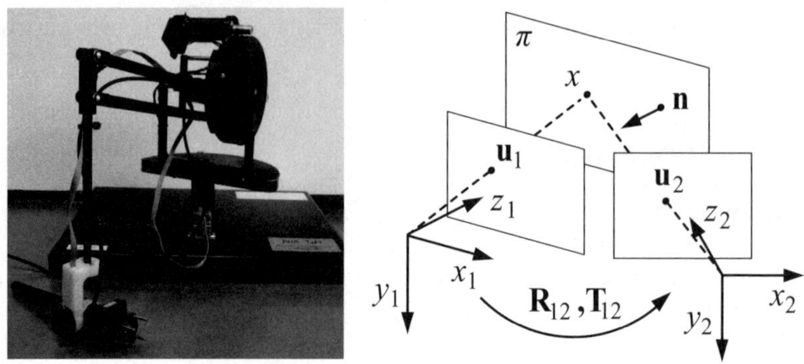

Figure 1. Left: experimental setup from Section 2. Right: diagram of projective geometry from Section 3.1.

3.1. Projective Geometry

We begin by assuming that the camera is taking pictures of a planar scene in 3D space, which is a reasonable assumption for certain tissue structures that may be observed *in vivo*. The camera is allowed any arbitrary movement with respect to the scene as long as it stays in focus and there are no major artifacts that would cause motion parallax.

Using homogeneous coordinates, a world point $\mathbf{x} = (x, y, z, 1)$ gets mapped to an image point $\mathbf{u} = (u, v, 1)$ through perspective projection and rigid transformation,

$$\mathbf{u} = \begin{bmatrix} \mathbf{K} & \mathbf{0} \end{bmatrix} \begin{bmatrix} \mathbf{R} & \mathbf{T} \\ \mathbf{0}^T & 1 \end{bmatrix} \mathbf{x}, \tag{1}$$

where $\mathbf{R}$ and $\mathbf{T}$ are the 3×3 rotation matrix and 3×1 translation vector of the camera frame with respect to the world coordinate system. The 3×3 projection matrix $\mathbf{K}$ is often called the intrinsic calibration matrix, with horizontal focal length f_x, vertical focal length f_y, skew parameter s, and image principle point (c_x, c_y).

Next we consider two different projections $\mathbf{u}_1$ and $\mathbf{u}_2$ of a point $\mathbf{x}$ on plane π. The plane can be represented by a general plane equation $\mathbf{n} \cdot (x, y, z) + d = 0$, where $\mathbf{n}$ is a unit normal extending from the image plane towards the first view and d is the distance between them. If we orient the world coordinate system with the first view, the relationship between the two views can be written as $\mathbf{u}_2 = \mathbf{Hu}_1$, where $\mathbf{H}$ is a 3×3 homography matrix [12] defined up to a scale factor,

$$\mathbf{H} = \mathbf{K} \left(\mathbf{R}_{12} + \mathbf{T}_{12} \frac{\mathbf{n}^T}{d} \right) \mathbf{K}^{-1}. \tag{2}$$

3.2. Camera Calibration

In order to determine the homography between image pairs, we need an accurate measurement of the intrinsic camera parameters. We determined parameters of $f_x = 934$, $f_y = 928$, $s = 0$, and $(c_x, c_y) = (289, 291)$, with roughly $1 - 3\%$ error. This relatively large error is a result of calibrating at sub-millimeter scales. The camera calibration also provided radial and tangential lens distortion coefficients that were used to un-warp each image before processing. In addition, the images were cropped from 640×480 pixels to 480×360 pixels to remove blurred edges caused by the large focal length at near-field.

3.3. Robot Kinematics

In near-field imaging, camera translations $\mathbf{T}$ are often on the same scale as the imaging distance d. If we cannot use the assumption that $|\mathbf{T}| \ll d$, it becomes important to measure camera translation in addition to orientation. We therefore use the Phantom forward kinematics to measure the rotation and translation of the point where the 3 gimbal axes intersect. Stylus roll is ignored since it does not affect the camera motion. With these measurements, we can calculate the transformation required in (2) as

$$\begin{bmatrix} \mathbf{R}_{1j} & \mathbf{T}_{1j} \\ \mathbf{0}^T & 1 \end{bmatrix} = \begin{bmatrix} \mathbf{R}_1 & \mathbf{T}_1 \\ \mathbf{0}^T & 1 \end{bmatrix}^{-1} \begin{bmatrix} \mathbf{R}_j & \mathbf{T}_j \\ \mathbf{0}^T & 1 \end{bmatrix}, \tag{3}$$

where $\mathbf{R}_1$ and $\mathbf{T}_1$ are the rotation and translation of the first view and $\mathbf{R}_j$ and $\mathbf{T}_j$ are the rotation and translation of all subsequent views as seen by the robot's reference frame.

3.4. Hand-Eye Calibration

The transformations in (3) refer to the robot end-effector. The transformations in (2), however, refer to the camera optical center. We therefore need to determine the rigid transformation between the end-effector and the camera's optical center, which is the same for all views. This hand-eye (or eye-in-hand) transformation is denoted as a 4×4 transformation matrix $\mathbf{X}$ composed of a rotation $\mathbf{R}_{he}$ and translation $\mathbf{T}_{he}$. Hand-eye calibration arises in many applications including medical imaging [13], and becomes critical for near-field imaging where the assumption $|\mathbf{T}_{he}| \ll d$ is no longer valid.

To determine $\mathbf{X}$ we define two poses $\mathbf{C}_1 = \mathbf{A}_1\mathbf{X}$ and $\mathbf{C}_2 = \mathbf{A}_2\mathbf{X}$, where $\mathbf{C}$ refers to the camera and $\mathbf{A}$ refers to the robot. Hand-eye calibration is most easily solved during camera calibration, where $\mathbf{A}$ is measured using the robot kinematics and $\mathbf{C}$ is determined using the calibration routine. Denoting $\mathbf{C}_{12} = \mathbf{C}_1^{-1}\mathbf{C}_2$ and $\mathbf{A}_{12} = \mathbf{A}_1^{-1}\mathbf{A}_2$, we obtain the hand-eye equation $\mathbf{A}_{12}\mathbf{X} = \mathbf{X}\mathbf{C}_{12}$. Further details on how to solve this equation are deferred to [14]. The resulting hand-eye transformation can be used to augment (3) which is in turn used in (2) to find $\mathbf{H}$.

3.5. Image Mosaicing Algorithms

At this point we have established how to estimate the homography between two images using position sensing. The resulting matrix $\mathbf{H}$, however, will have errors and certainly will not have pixel-level accuracy. The final step is to integrate mosaicing algorithms to accurately align the images. We implement a variation of the Levenberg-Marquardt (LM) iterative nonlinear routine to minimize the discrepancy in pixel intensities [10].

The LM algorithm requires an initial estimate of the homography in order to find a locally optimal solution, making it an ideal candidate for integrating our position sensing. The initial estimate is often obtained using optical flow, feature detection, or correlation-based techniques in the spatial or frequency domain. By replacing these methods with the robotic position sensing, we very quickly obtain an accurate estimate of the homography that requires relatively few iterations of the LM algorithm for optimization. In addition, the position sensing is robust since it will always provide an estimate that is near the locally optimal solution regardless of the camera motion or image homogeneity.

An additional advantage of position sensing is that it eliminates cumulative error. That is, if each new image is aligned to the previous image, alignment errors will propagate through the image chain [15], becoming most prominent when the path closes a loop or traces back upon itself. The position sensing eliminates this effect, since our initial alignment is always defined relative to a global reference frame. Each new image is then aligned to the entire image mosaic, rather than the previous image. To ensure accurate results, we perform seam blending on the mosaic before each new image is added.

4. Results

Figure 2 shows two image mosaics of a dental model. The mosaics are composed of roughly 25 (left) and 70 (right) images, and were created in real-time at a rate of just over 1 image/second. Although this is a 3D model, the scenes are roughly planar when viewed from a few millimeters away. The black dotted lines represent the size and location of the first image. In the larger mosaic, the user moved the camera in a clockwise circle and back through the middle to show that cumulative errors have been eliminated.

Experimentally, we found that alignment errors can sometimes occur due to the camera motion (blurred images, loss of focus). These situations, however, can be handled by taking a second pass over the misaligned areas. Being able to fix any arbitrary portion of the mosaic in real-time is a useful advantage of having an initial global position estimate.

5. Discussion

We have presented a real-time, robotically-assisted image mosaicing system designed for near-field medical imaging. We have shown that position sensing is useful for reducing the processing load, eliminating cumulative errors, and handling arbitrary camera motions. The next step in this project is to use a micro-endoscope for very close-field medical imaging. The main challenge associated with this is that the position sensing from the Phantom will be relatively less accurate. We therefore plan to explore the use of other sensors with increased sensitivity, such as MEMS accelerometers. Another technique would be to use the homography determined by the mosaicing as feedback to improve the position estimates. A crucial challenge associated with medical imaging is patient (or tissue) motion during camera scans. We plan to address this issue through additional sensors or alternative processing techniques on existing sensor data.

Acknowledgements

This work was supported by an NSF Graduate Research Fellowship and a Stanford Bio-X Graduate Fellowship. The authors would like to thank Sean Walker for helpful discussions and assistance with the software platform.

References

[1] R. DaCosta, B. Wilson, N. Marcon, Optical Techniques for the Endoscopic Detection of Dysplastic Colonic Lesions, Current Opinion in Gastroenterology, vol. 21(1), pp. 70-79, 2005.

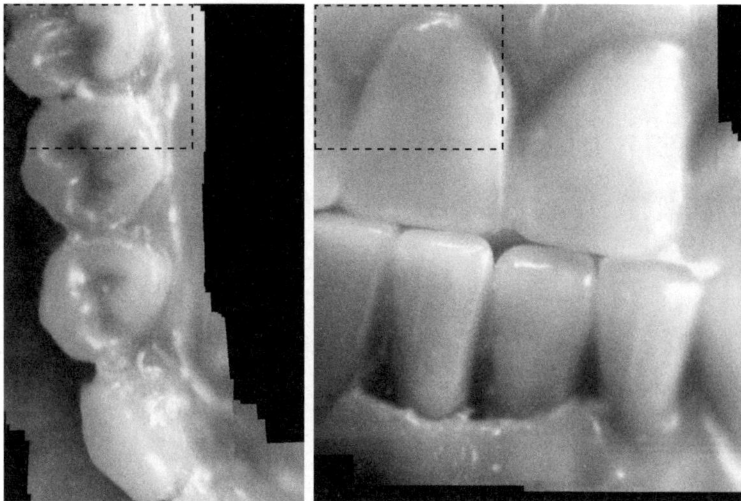

Figure 2. Two image mosaics of a dental model, composed of roughly 25 (left) and 70 (right) images. The mosaics were created in real-time at just over 1 image/second. Individual images are size 480 × 360 pixels.

[2]   T. Vercauteren, A. Perchant, X. Pennec, N. Ayache, Mosaicing of Confocal Microscopic In Vivo Soft Tissue Video Sequences, Proceedings of MICCAI'05, Palm Springs, CA, October 26-29, 2005.

[3]   D. Camarillo, T. Krummel, K. Salisbury, Robotic Technology in Surgery: Past, Present and Future, American Journal of Surgery, vol. 188(4A Suppl), pp. 2-15, 2004.

[4]   L. Brown, A Survey of Image Registration Techniques, ACM Computing Surveys, vol. 24(4), pp. 325-376, December 1992.

[5]   J. Hoshino, M. Kourogi, Fast Panoramic Image Mosaicing Using One-Dimensional Flow Estimation, Real-Time Imaging, vol. 8(2), pp. 95-103, April 2002.

[6]   H.S. Sawhney, R. Kumar, G. Gendel, J. Bergen, D. Dixon, V. Paragano, VideoBrush^{TM}: Experiences with Consumer Video Mosaicing, Proceedings of WACV'98, pp. 56-62, October 1998.

[7]   P. Baudisch, D. Tan, D. Steedly, E. Rudolph, M. Uyttendaele, C. Pal, R. Szeliski, Panoramic Viewfinder: Providing a Real-Time Preview to Help Users Avoid Flaws in Panoramic Pictures, Processings of OZCHI'05, Canberra, Australia, November 2005.

[8]   S.K. Chow , H. Hakozaki, D.L. Price, N.A.B. MacLean, T. Deerinck, J. Bouwer, M.E. Martone, S. Peltier, M.H. Ellisman, Automated Microscopy System for Mosaic Acquisition and Processing, Journal of Microscopy, vol. 222(2), pp. 76-84, May 2006.

[9]   V. Rankov, R.J. Locke, R.J. Edens, P.R. Barber, B. Vojnovic, An Algorithm for Image Stitching and Blending, Proceedings of SPIE Volume 5701, Three-Dimensional and Multidimensional Microscopy: Image Acquisition and Processing XII, pp. 190-199, March 2005.

[10]   R. Szeliski, Video Mosaics for Virtual Environments, IEEE Computer Graphics and Applications, vol. 16(2), pp. 22-30, March 1996.

[11]   Sensable Technologies website, Available at http://www.sensable.com/

[12]   O.D. Faugeras, F. Lustman, Motion and Structure from Motion in a Piecewise Planar Environment, International Journal of Pattern Recognition and Artificial Intelligence, vol. 2, pp. 485-508, 1988.

[13]   F. Vogt, S. Krüger, J. Schmidt, D. Paulus, H. Niemann, W. Hohenberger, C.H. Schick, Light Fields for Minimal Invasive Surgery Using an Endoscope Positioning Robot, Methods of Information in Medicine, vol. 43(4), pp. 403-408, 2004.

[14]   R. Tsai, R.K. Lenz, A new Technique for Fully Autonomous and Efficient 3D Robotics Hand/Eye Calibration, IEEE Transactions on Robotics and Automaion, vol. 5(3), June 1989.

[15]   S.D. Fleischer, S.M. Rock, R.L. Burton, Global Position Determination and Vehicle Path Estimation from a Vision Sensor for Real-Time Video Mosaicking and Navigation, Proceedings of OCEANS '97, Halifax, Nova Scotia, October 1997.

Medicine Meets Virtual Reality 15
J.D. Westwood et al. (Eds.)
IOS Press, 2007

Magnetically Levitated Nano-Robots: An Application to Visualization of Nerve Cells Injuries[1]

Mingji LOU and Edmond JONCKHEERE
Dept. of Electrical Engineering—Systems, University of Southern California
Los Angeles, CA 90089-2563 {mlou, jonckhee}@usc.edu

Abstract. This paper proposes a swarm of magnetically levitated nano-robots with high sensitivity nano-sensors as a mean to detect chemical sources, specifically the chemical signals released by injured nervous cells. In the aftermath of the process, further observation by these nano-robots would be used to monitor the healing process and assess the amount of regeneration, if any, or even the repair, of the injured nervous cells.

Keywords. Nano-Robots, Nerve Cells Injuries, Magnetic Levitation

Introduction

Traditionally, clinicians and researchers have incorporated surface Electromyography (sEMG) as a diagnostic tool to take out much of the guesswork in the assessment of muscle and even Central Nervous System (CNS) functions [1]. One problem is that the noninvasive sEMG electrodes collect the nervous signals only indirectly and corrupt them with noise. As such, sEMG signals are sometimes very difficult to analyze. Here we propose nano-robots with the properties of high sensitivity and tiny size as the best candidates to be used as direct nervous chemical signature detectors.

The neuro-chemical signatures of primary interest here are Nitric Oxide (NO) and Calcium ions (Ca^{2+}) since they are related to the mechanisms of numerous brain injury phenomena [2] and nerve cell functions [3]. Other chemical signals can also be utilized for detection of CNS injuries, though.

From the perspective of fabrication, nanowire (NW) or nanotube (NT) modified with receptors or ligands for specific detection have been extended in many directions. NO and calcium ions nano-sensors have been discovered and fabricated by different methods such as those reported in [4] and [5].

Following Requicha [6], communication and coordination for a swarm of nano-robots would be function-limited. Signal output channel would be ten times larger than the sensor itself. Clearly, a novel method to alleviate the above bottlenecks in the sensing applications of nano-robots is an emerging research issue. In this paper, a system-level scheme is proposed to magnetically levitate the nano-robots so that imaging their position provides sensor output. The swarm of magnetically levitated nano-robots is controlled to detect the injured spinal nerve cells, which are releasing

---

[1] © M. Lou and E. Jonckheere.

NO or Ca^{2+} in this case. This technology can be identified under the acronym SPIMALs™, **SPI**nal **I**njury **IMA**ging by **MA**gnetically **L**evitated **s**ensors.

1. Methodology

The nano-robots in this project are fabricated by coating the NO and Ca^{2+} nano-sensors with magnetic material such as Fe_2O_3 or Neodymium. The nano-robots are magnetically levitated and guided. Soft X-Ray microscopy is used to visualize the position of the swarm. A feedback control from the image to the magnetic levitation recursively clusters the nano-robots around the injury area. The system-level scheme of the magnetic levitation is shown in Figure 1.

1.1. Magnetic Levitation

To levitate the nano-particles in 3D, 3 pairs of solenoids are placed along the x, y, z axes in Euler space. The fields generated by the electromagnets can be modified by adjusting the current through the coil of these solenoids. Soft X-ray microscopy with, to date, a spatial resolution of 43 nm [7] is used to monitor the current 3D position of the nano-robots and provides the signal output from the nano-sensor robots. Hall Effect sensors [8] are used to observe the distribution of the magnetic field in space. The coordinate of the local NO or Ca^{2+} density center is obtained in the Digital Signal Processing (DSP) module by anglicizing the distribution of the nano-robots and the output signal from their sensors. Then this coordinate is inputted as the reference to the controller. To move the physical center of the swarm of nano-robots to the local dense center, the controller calculates the desired magnetic field and compares it with the current magnetic field observed by the Hall Effect sensors. Finally the control decision is transferred to electrical current format (and/or the related position of solenoids if necessary) and synchronized by the external crystal.

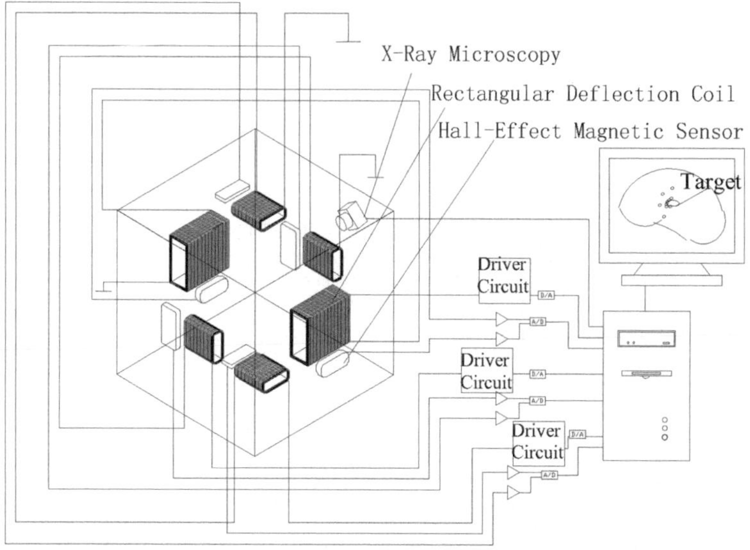

Figure 1: System-level architecture of the magnetic levitation concept

1.2. Detecting the NO or Ca^{2+} Signal Source by the Swarm of Nano-robots

The scenario in this section is as follows: a swarm of nano-robots is released in the CSF around the area where injured spinal nervous branches release NO or Ca^{2+} to their neighbors. The mission for the suspended nano-robots is to try to find the diffusion center of the above chemical signal, which, probably at the same time, is the position of the injured cells.

To achieve this mission, the swarm of nano-robots needs to have proper distribution to cover the potential injury area when they are injected at the beginning. Then, the sensor in the robot begins to work and detect the local chemical concentration. The X-ray device observes the physical center of the swarm of nano-robots, and the local highest chemical concentration. With a highly efficient controller, the outside magnetic field moves the physical center to the chemical center. At the same time, the distribution area of the swarm is decreased, and the X-ray microscopy zooms. By repeating the above process, the nano-robots finally cluster around the signal source.

1.3. Stabilization of the swarm

Initially, the nano-robots are charged so as to repel one another and arrange themselves in a volume that covers the chemical diffusion areas. This self-organizing process imparts sub-stability of the robots relative to each other, which would attract one another by van der Waals forces and magnetic forces under normal conditions. At time goes on, this spatial volume should be decreased by bleeding off the charges and magnetic confinement as the physical center becomes closer and closer to the chemical center.

Further prospects

In the aftermath of the process, further observation by these nano-robots would be applied to monitor the healing process and assess the amount of regeneration, if any or even the repair, of the injured nervous cell. This research is still under progress.

References:

[1] E. A. Jonckheere, P. Lohsoonthorn, and V. Mahajan, ``ChiroSensor---An array of non-invasive sEMG electrodes," The 13th Annual Medicine Meets Virtual Reality (MMVR 13) Conference, Long Beach, CA, 2005; IOS Press (Edited by J. D. Westwood et al), Technology and Informatics 111, Amsterdam/Berlin/Oxford/Tokyo/Washington, DC, ISBN 1 58603 498 7, 2005, pp. 234-236.

[2] B.Stefano, Y. Coumon, T. V. Bilfinger, I. D. Welters, P. Cadet (2000) "Basal nitric oxide limits immune, nervous and cardiovascular excitation: human endothelia express a mu opiate receptor." Progress in Neurobiology 60, 513-530.

[3] P. G. Kostyuk, A. N. Verkhratsky, "Calcium Signaling in the Nervous System" , 1996.

[4] Cui et al., "Nanowire nanosensors for highly sensitive and selective detection of biological and chemical species", Science, Vol. 293, pp. 1289-1292, 17 August 2001;

[5] http://www.wpiinc.com/WPI_Web/Biosensing/NewISONO.html

[6] Requicha, "Nanorobots, NEMS and Nanoassembly", Proc. IEEE, November 2003, Sec. II;

[7] Center for X-ray Optics (CXRO), Berkeley Lab. http://www-cxro.lbl.gov/microscopy

[8] Shrivastava, "Introduction to Quantum Hall Effect", Nova Science Publishers, Inc, New York, 2002.

Medicine Meets Virtual Reality 15
J.D. Westwood et al. (Eds.)
IOS Press, 2007

313

Telesurgery Via Unmanned Aerial Vehicle (UAV) with a Field Deployable Surgical Robot

Mitchell J.H. Lum[*], Jacob Rosen[*], Hawkeye King[*], Diana C.W. Friedman[*], Gina Donlin[*], Ganesh Sankaranarayanan[*], Brett Harnett[+], Lynn Huffman[+], Charles Doarn[+], Timothy Broderick[+], Blake Hannaford[*]

[*]*University of Washington, Seattle, WA, USA*
[+]*University of Cincinnati, Cincinnati, OH, USA*

Abstract: Robotically assisted surgery stands to further revolutionize the medical field and provide patients with more effective healthcare. Most robotically assisted surgeries are teleoperated from the surgeon console to the patient where both ends of the system are located in the operating room. The challenge of surgical teleoperation across a long distance was already demonstrated through a wired communication network in 2001. New development has shifted towards deploying a surgical robot system in mobile settings and/or extreme environments such as the battlefield or natural disaster areas with surgeons operating wirelessly. As a collaborator in the HAPs/MRT (High Altitude Platform/Mobile Robotic Telesurgery) project, The University of Washington surgical robot was deployed in the desert of Simi Valley, CA for telesurgery experiments on an inanimate model via wireless communication through an Unmanned Aerial Vehicle (UAV). The surgical tasks were performed telerobotically with a maximum time delay between the surgeon's console (master) and the surgical robot (slave) of 20 ms for the robotic control signals and 200 ms for the video stream. This was our first experiment in the area of Mobile Robotic Telesurgery (MRT). The creation and initial testing of a deployable surgical robot system will facilitate growth in this area eventually leading to future systems saving human lives in disaster areas, on the battlefield or in other remote environments.

1. Introduction

Just as minimally invasive techniques revolutionized the way many surgical interventions are performed, robot-assisted surgery stands to further revolutionize the medical field and provide patients with more effective healthcare. In most robot-assisted cases the surgeon is present in the operating room with the patient. However, surgical robotic systems teleoperate from the surgeon console to the patient; this can occur in either the same room or across the world. The challenge of surgical teleoperation across long distances was most prominently solved using standard means of telecommunication in a transatlantic experiment [1]. The challenge is now to deploy a surgical robotic system in a mobile setting or extreme environment and to control it through an unconventional data link such as an Unmanned Aerial Vehicle (UAV). This has implications for battlefield trauma, disaster response and rural or remote telesurgery.

2. Methods

Research systems rarely leave the operating room or lab environment in which they were conceived. Deployment introduced problems rarely faced by researchers, including environmental concerns such as dust and high temperatures, and durability concerns such as shock absorption and packing. As a collaborator in the HAPs/MRT (High Altitude Platforms/Mobile Robotic Telesurgery) project, The University of Washington surgical robot system [2] was deployed in the desert of Simi Valley, CA for telesurgery experiments on an inanimate model.

Deploying the surgical robot system into an outdoor desert environment exposed the mechanisms, electronics and computer hardware to dusty winds and hot temperatures. To protect the surgical manipulators' motor packs (actuators, brakes, encoders and electrical wiring), 3-piece covers were designed and produced. The covers featured ventilation holes and a mounting point for a PC fan to cool the actuators in the desert heat. Clean power is not a primary concern in a hospital or lab, but in the field this was an important consideration. In order to prevent damage due to generators spikes two 1200W line regulators from APC were used. The ability to safely transport all the equipment to the remote site was also very important. Custom foam lined cases were designed to hold the surgical manipulators, surgical tools and master console devices (Phantom Omnis). The majority of the electronic components, including the control computer, power supplies, Maxon brushless motor amplifiers and USB2.0 interface device, were mounted inside two SKB Industrial Roto-Shock Rack cases. These cases have shock isolation between the plastic hard-shell exterior an internal frame.

In order to transport the system a Chevy Express cargo van was filled with approximately 700 kg of equipment. This included cases containing the two surgical manipulators, the SKB shock isolated cases, a custom made portable OR table, the surgeon console, tools, and back-up equipment.

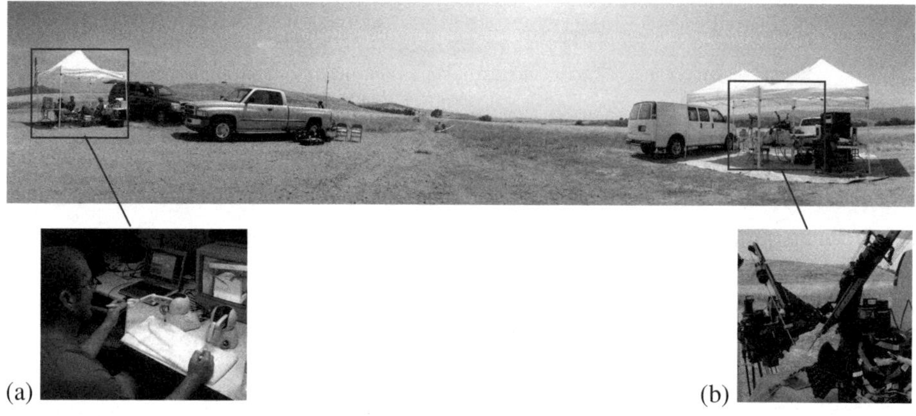

(a)   (b)

Figure 1. The surgical robotic system deployment in Simi Valley, CA. (a) The surgical Console (Master) (b) The surgical robot (slave)

The surgical manipulators were set up in one tent and the surgical console was set up in a second tent 100m away. Because of the UAV's range, the surgeons site and operation site could have been separated by a distance of up to 2km, but a closer distance was chosen for convenience in testing and debugging. Two surgeons interacted with inanimate objects that simulated internal organs; a modality commonly used to train surgeons. The surgeons performed gross manipulation tasks via a wireless communication link through Aerovironment's PUMA UAV. The radio link onboard the PUMA provided a TCP/IP Internet-style link between the two sites. The video signal was encoded using MPEG-2 transmitted at 800 kbps by a Hai560 hardware codec provided by HaiVision Inc. of Montreal, Canada.

3. Results

The experiment demonstrated telesurgery via wireless communication with limited bandwidth and variable time delays. A maximum time delay of 20 ms for robot control signals and 200 ms for video stream were observed. During the three days of field deployment, both kinematic data from the surgeons' commands and data characterizing the network traffic were collected. The two surgeons were able to perform the telemanipulation protocol through the wireless link. This experiment demonstrates the feasibility of performing telesurgery through wireless communication in remote environments.

Kinematic control signals were going to be sent to the manipulators at a 1kHz rate, and video signals sent to the surgeon using 2MB/s bandwidth. However, packet loss became a major problem (80% loss) during the initial testing at full bandwidth. When the overall bandwidth was scaled back packet loss was reduced to between 3%-15%. For the majority of the task experiments robot control signals were sent at 100 Hz and video bandwidth was 800kB/s. The surgeons noted increased pixilation in the video stream but did not feel it affected their task performance.

4. Conclusions

This was our first experiment in the emerging area of Mobile Robotic Telesurgery (MRT). Beyond the obvious environmental concerns, the experiments highlighted the need for minimal bandwidth, bandwidth scaling, a stable network and the support personnel to maintain a reliable communication link. It also demonstrated that under minimal or low visual feedback and network time delay, surgeons are still able to perform surgical tasks. When deploying in the field it is necessary to plan for all contingencies by bringing spare parts and tools; something the military has known for years. The creation and initial testing of a deployable surgical robot system will facilitate growth in this area and eventually lead to future systems which will save human lives in isolated or extreme environments.

References

1.   J. Marescaux. "Transatlantic robot-assisted telesurgery." *Nature*, 413, Sept. 27. 2001
2.   M.J.H. Lum, et al. "Multidisciplinary approach for developing a new minimally invasive surgical robot system." *In Proc. of the 2006 BioRob Conference*, Pisa, Italy, February 2006.

Acknowledgments

The HAPs/MRT project was supported by the US Army, Medical Research and Material Command grant number W81XWH-05-2-0080. We would also like to thank our collaborators from AeroVironment and HaiVision.

Medicine Meets Virtual Reality 15
J.D. Westwood et al. (Eds.)
IOS Press, 2007

Application of Hidden Markov Modeling to Objective Medical Skill Evaluation

Thomas MACKEL [1], Jacob ROSEN [1,2], Ph.D., Carla PUGH [3], M.D., Ph.D.
*[1] Department of Electrical Engineering, [2] Department of Surgery,
University of Washington, Seattle, WA, USA*
[3] Department of Surgery, Northwestern University, Chicago, IL, USA
E-mail:{tmackel ,rosen}@u.washington.edu drpugh@northwestern.edu
Biorobotics Lab URL : http://brl.ee.washington.edu

Abstract: The methodology for assessing medical skills is gradually shifting from subjective scoring of an expert which may be a variably biased opinion using vague criteria towards a more objective quantitative analysis. A methodology using Hidden Markov Modeling (HMM) and Markov Models (MM) were used to analyze database acquired the E-Pelvis (physical simulator) during a pelvic exam. The focus is on the method of selection of HMM parameters. K-Means is used to choose the alphabet size. Successful classification rates of 62% are observed with the HMM as opposed to 92% with the MM. Moreover, the MM provide an insight into the nature of the process while identifying typical sequences that are unique to each level of expertise, where the HM, given their nature as a black box model, do not.

1. Introduction

Currently, many accepted methods of training rely on the subjective analysis of performance by an expert. The methodology for assessing surgical skill as a subset of surgical ability is gradually shifting from subjective scoring of an expert which may be a variably biased opinion using vague criteria towards a more objective quantitative analysis. The ultimate aim is therefore to develop a modality independent methodology for objectively assessing medical competency. The methodology may be incorporated into a simulator, surgical robot, or performance tracking device during a real procedure and provide objective and unbiased assessment based on quantitative data resulting from the physical interaction between the physician and modality used to measure competency.

Markov Modeling (MM) and Hidden Markov Modeling (HMM) are effective methods for deconstructing and understanding speech data. An analogy between spoken language and medical procedure [1] is used to apply these methods towards objective surgical skill analysis. An effective method of evaluation using MM was developed [2]. In our previous work, MM was found to successfully classify 82 subjects into two classes (expert and novice) with a 92% success rate [3]. Another study used MM to classify 30 subjects (25 residents and 5 attending surgeons – 5 subjects form each year of residency) using MIS step and animal model. The coloration factor an objective assessment (MM) and subjective assessment (expert video evaluation) was 87.5% [4]. Significant differences between surgeons in different levels of residency were found: 1) Magnitude of applied Forces/Torques; 2) Types of tool/tissue interactions; 3) time intervals spent in each tool/tissue interaction [5]. Evidence was obtained which supported the idea that a major portion of laparoscopic surgical capabilities is acquired between the first and third years of residency training.

The difference between MM and HMM is a subtle but important one. In MM, observed data is converted into model states, hence the model states directly reflect the physical reality of the process being modeled. In HMM, the states of the model do not directly reflect the physical reality. Instead, the model states represent an underlying *hidden* stochastic process that, similar to reality, could produce the observed data. Can HMM classify subjects more correctly than MM? This study uses HMM to classify a dataset that was previously classified using MM.

2. Method

Two HMM models were defined based on data of 15 expert subjects and 15 novice subjects performing a pelvic exam with the E-Pelvis physical simulator [6-8]. These are the same data that were used as the training set in the previous MM study [2]. Data of subjects that were not included in training the HMM are scored against the two trained models by finding the probability for the most likely observation sequences with each model. The subject is classified as a member of the class for which the probability is highest.

3. Results

The number of states in the model is chosen by creating 29 different models, each with a different number of states ranging from 2 to 30. The 4-state model classified the training data most correctly with the best error margin, and therefore we chose to work with this 4-state model during the rest of the reported data analysis. The data was quantized to N clusters using K-Means clustering. Nine clusters (N=9) were selected as a trade-off between computational concerns and distortion. For N>9, to gain more improvement in distortion would require significant loss of silhouette as compared to N<=9 (see Figure 1). The clusters correspond to observations in the HMM.

Successful classification occurred for 62% of subjects over all trials. Experts were classified correctly 64% of the time, and novices correctly 59% of the time. During the selection of the number of states to use, all subjects tended to score closer to novice as the number of model states was increased. This result is not superior to the previous MM work, but HMM may have other merits.

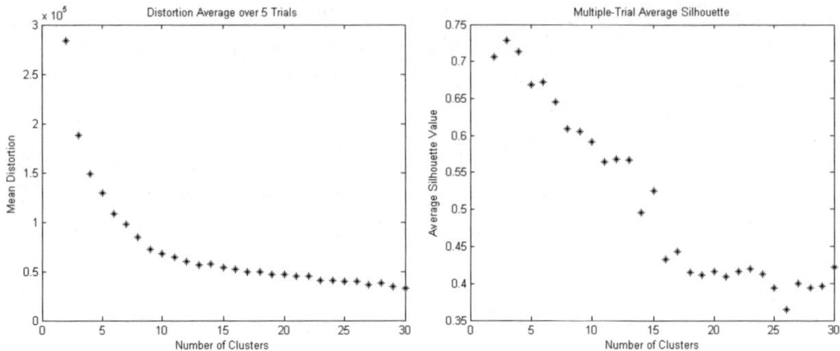

Figure 1: Clustering analysis of the e- pelvis database: Plots of distortion (left) and silhouette/distortion ratio (right) for selecting the optimal number of clusters

4. Conclusions

HHM and MM ware used to classify students and expert performing a pelvic exam utilizing a database collected by the e-pelvis simulator. The results indicates that the MM classified the students and experts with a success rate 92% where as the HMM classification had 62% success rate for the same database. Moreover, the MM provide an insight into the nature of the process while identifying typical sequences that are unique to each level of expertise, where the HM, given their nature as a black box model, do not.

References

[1]   Rosen J., Chang L., Brown J., Hannaford B., Sinanan M., Satava R. Minimally Invasive Surgery Task Decomposition – Etymology of Endoscopic Suturing. Studies in Health Technology and Informatics, vol. 94, pp. 295-201, IOS Press, Fairfax, VA 2003.

[2]   Rosen J., Brown J., Chang L., Sinanan M., Hannaford B. Generalized Approach for modeling Minimally Invasive Surgery as a Stochastic Process Using a Discrete Markov Model. IEEE Transactions on Biomedical Engineering, vol. 53, pp. 399-413, March 2006.

[3]   Mackel T., Rosen J., Pugh C. Data Mining of the E-Pelvis Simulator Database: A Quest for a Generalized Algorithm Capable of Assessing Medical Skill. Studies in Health Technology and Informatics, vol. 119, pp. 355-360, IOS Press, Fairfax, VA 2003.

[4]   Rosen, J., Hannaford B., Richards C., Sinanan M. Markov Modeling of Minimally Invasive Surgery Based on Tool/Tissue Interaction and Force/Torque Signatures for Evaluating Surgical Skills. IEEE Transactions on Biomedical Engineering, vol. 48, pp. 579-591, 2001.

[5]   Rosen, J., Solazzo M., Hannaford B., Sinanan M. Objective Evaluation of Laparoscopic Surgical Skills Using Hidden Markov Models Based on Haptic Information and Tool/Tissue Interactions. American College of Surgeons Annual Meeting, Washington State Chapter, Lake Chelan, WA, 2000.

[6]   Pugh C., Srivastava S., Shavelson R., Walker D., Cotner T., Scarloss B., et al. The effect of simulator use on learning and self-assessment: the case of Stanford University's E-Pelvis simulator. Studies in Health Technology and Informatics, vol. 81, pp 396-400, IOS Press, Fairfax, VA 2001.

[7]   Pugh C., Rosen J. Qualitative and quantitative analysis of pressure sensor data acquired by the E-Pelvis simulator during simulated pelvic examinations. Studies in Health Informatics and Technology, vol. 85, pp. 376-379, IOS Press, Fairfax, VA 2001.

[8]   Pugh C., Youngblood P. Free in PMC, Development and validation of assessment measures for a newly developed physical examination simulator. J Am Med Inform Assoc. 2002. 2002 Sep-Oct; 9(5):448-60.

[9]   Rabiner, L. A Tutorial on Hidden Markov Models and Selected Applications in Speech Recognition. Proceedings of the IEEE, vol. 77, no. 2, Feb 1989.

Medicine Meets Virtual Reality 15
J.D. Westwood et al. (Eds.)
IOS Press, 2007

Manual registration of ultrasound with CT/Planning data for hepatic surgery

Mathias Markert[1], Stefan Weber, Tim C. Lueth
MIMED • Micro Technology & Medical Device Engineering • TU München • Germany

Abstract. In this article an approach for assistance for soft tissue surgery through instrument navigation is presented. It can sufficiently be integrated into the clinical workflow. The presented methods are part of an assistance system for open liver surgery and supports surgeons during tumor resections or living donor liver transplantation. To combine preoperative CT data with intraoperative ultrasound images, the registration process is directly controlled by the surgeon through a 6D mouse (space ball). This simple yet effective approach overcomes existing limitations of automatic algorithms relying on stable image features within both ultrasound and CT images. As a first result, the described surgery assistance system was successfully applied in clinical routine.

Keywords: hepatic surgery, instrument navigation, images registration

1. Introduction

Instrument navigation and its application is a relatively novel to the area of soft tissue surgery. Known methods from hard tissue surgery (Dental-, ENT-, Neuro surgery and Orthopedics) can not directly transferred as the intraoperative shape, position and volume of soft tissue differs significantly from its preoperative shape. Stable algorithms for registering ultrasound with CT/MR images automatically based on vessel tree models have been demonstrated [1, 2], but lack stability and clinical applicability. In this article a method is described to register intraoperative and navigated ultrasound images with an existing preoperative planning model by means of a manually controlled process. The approach is being integrated in an already developed assistant system for open liver surgery [3].

2. Material

The assistance system consists of a Tablet-PC (PaceBlade TetraLight20 – Centrino, 1.5 GHz). It is controlled via touch screen. An additional input device is a 6D mouse (3Dconnexion Spaceball 5000), which is primarily used for alignment of the 3D planning model. The system contains integrates an intraoperative navigated ultrasound transducer (Terason by Teratech). Alternatively, any other external ultrasound system can be connected via standard video interface. An optical position measurement system (Vicra by NDI) is used to obtain the spatial position and orientation of the ultrasound

---

[1] Corresponding Author: Department Micro Technology and Medical Device Engineering, TU München, Boltzmannstr. 15, 85748 Garching, Germany; E-Mail: mathias.markert@tum.de

transducer. All components are fixed at a moveable stand (Fig. 1) but can also be mounted at the operation table. For application within the situs, sterile drapes are applied. On opposite sides of visual display of the system both the 3D preoperative planning model and the actual ultrasound image are shown. The planning model contains the boundary of the liver, possible tumors and existing vascular structures. The intraoperative ultrasound is available in B-mode, Doppler and Power-Doppler with full adjustable ultrasound properties.

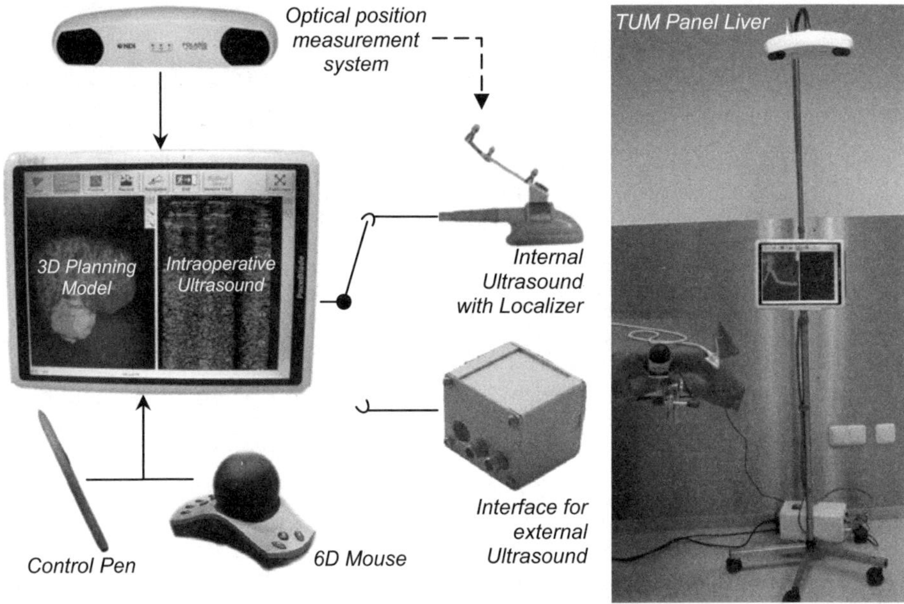

Figure 1: The assistance system comprises of a Tablet-PC, connected with a position measurement system and an ultrasound device (internal and external). It is controlled by a control pen and a 6D mouse (© MiMed 2006).

3. Methods

After the surgeon has loaded the preoperative digital planning data into the system, an alignment of the 3D planning model according to the personal visual perspective onto the situs is possible. By manipulating the 6D mouse rotation, translation and zooming of the 3D model is available. Thereafter, the surgeon explores the liver with the ultrasound transducer to perceive additional intraoperative imaging information. An analysis of the anatomical structure of the liver and a comparison of the relative position of vessels and tumors in the ultrasound image will be conducted. Using the parallel display of preoperative planning data and intraoperative ultrasound a thorough understanding of the actual clinical situation is at hand. Registration of preoperative CT with intraoperative ultrasound images is a prerequisite of displaying one image modality virtually within the other at the correct spatial position. Therefore the spatial position and orientation of the ultrasound transducer is measured by the optical position measurement system. Initially the location of the first ultrasound image relative to the 3D planning model has to be defined. Thus the surgeon manually registers the ultrasound images with the preoperative 3D model (Figure 2) using the 6D mouse to align the ultrasound image within the planning model. The surgeon applies his expert knowledge about the anatomical structure of vascular, parenchyma and tumor structures visible in the ultrasound image. Only relative position and orientation need to be set by the manual registration process.

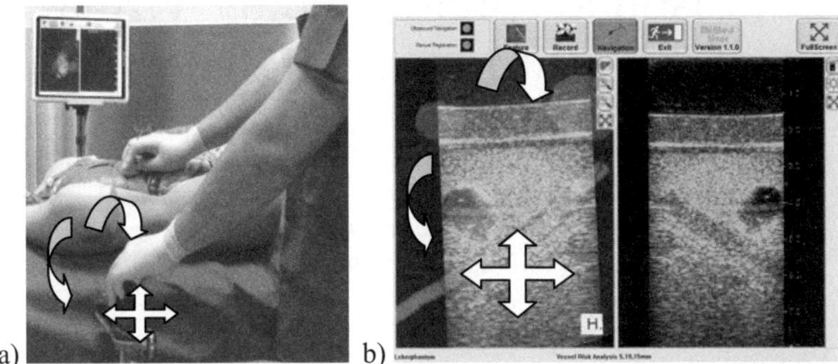

a)   b)

Figure 2: During manual registration the surgeon aligns the ultrasound image according the visible anatomical structure with the 6D mouse (a). Thus the position and orientation of the ultrasound image within the planning model is defined (© MiMed 2006).

Afterwards the preoperative planning data is registered with the intraoperative situation. The ultrasound images are displayed at the correct spatial location according to the 3D planning model. Thus the surgeon is able to check changes in size and position of structures and can transfer the preoperative information to the intraoperative situation.

4. Results

In this article an assistance system for liver surgery was presented. It was evaluated in a number of clinical interventions. The system is easily integrated into the clinical workflow. Because of the immediate visual feedback the usage of the 6D mouse is very intuitive and can be learned very fast. The manual registration of the preoperative and intraoperative data allows navigation to be applied in soft tissue surgery. This step is performed by the surgeon without support of an assistant. This provides an easy solution for intraoperative navigation without need for automatic registration methods. Thus, it is shown that is possible to develop an assistant system for soft tissue surgery. It is planned to re-evaluate the whole system in clinical routine. The goal of ongoing development is the integration of instrument navigation specifically for hepato-biliary surgery.

References

[1]   Lange, T.; Eulenstein, S.; Hünerbein, M.; Lamecker, H.; Schlag, P.M: Augmenting Intraoperative 3D Ultrasound with preoperative Models for Navigation in Liver Surgery in C. Barilloot, D.R. Haynor and P. Hellier (Eds.): MICCAI 2004, LNCS 3217, pp.535-541, 2004

[2]   Penney, G.; Blackall, J.; Hamady, M.; Sabharwal, T., Adam, A.; Hawkes, D.J.: Registration of freehand 3D ultrasound and magnetic resonance liver images. Medical Image Analysis (8) 2004, pp. 81-91

[3]   Markert M., Weber S., Kleemann M., Bruch H.P., Lüth T.C.: (2006): Comparison of fundamental requirements for soft tissue navigation with a novel assistance system for open liver surgery, 20th International Congress and Exhibition for Computer Assisted Radiology and Surgery 2006, Osaka, Japan 28th June – 1st July, 2006

Medicine Meets Virtual Reality 15
J.D. Westwood et al. (Eds.)
IOS Press, 2007

2D Ultrasound Augmented by Virtual Tools for Guidance of Interventional Procedures

John Moore [a,1], Gerard Guiraudon [a,b,c], Doug Jones [b,c], Nick Hill [a,c],
Andrew Wiles [a,c], Dan Bainbridge [b,c], Chris Wedlake [a] and Terry Peters [a,b,c]

[a] *Robarts Research Institute, London, Ontario, Canada*
[b] *CSTAR, London, Ontario, Canada*
[c] *University of Western Ontario, London, Ontario, Canada*

Abstract.
Many intracardiac procedures can currently be performed on the heart only after it has been arrested, and the patient has been placed on cardio-pulmonary bypass. We have developed a new method for operating on multiple targets inside the beating heart, and describe a procedure for accessing them under virtual-reality (VR)-assisted image guidance that combines real-time ultrasound with a virtual model of tools, and the surgical environment acquired from pre-operative images. This paper presents preliminary results aimed at assessing the operator's ability to accurately position and staple an artificial valve to a "valve orifice" within a cardiac phantom when guidance is performed via ultrasound alone, and with US augmented by the VR environment.

Keywords. image-guided surgery, virtual reality, cardiac surgery

1. Introduction

"Surgery is a side-effect of therapy". This rather provocative statement underlines the fact that most complications that are associated with "surgical" procedures, relate not to the therapy itself, but to the process of approaching the target to be treated. In order to reduce patient trauma, many conventional surgical procedures are being replaced by minimally invasive approaches. If most therapies could be achieved without the need for significant surgery to access the site of disease, procedure time would be shortened, patient trauma and side effects minimized, and health costs correspondingly reduced.

While cardiac surgery has relied for 50 years on cardiopulmonary bypass technology, new technologies are now available to transform the "old" open-heart approaches into target-specific interventions with fewer invasive side effects. Conventional open-heart surgery provides unobstructed direct vision and access to the target. However, direct access and vision comes with the high price of side effects including general anaesthesia, cardiopulmonary bypass, aortic cross-clamping, cardiotomy, cardiac arrest, myocardial preservation and permanent neurological damage (an occasional side-effect of cardiopulmonary bypass surgery). The surgical

---

[1] Corresponding Author: John Moore, Robarts Research Institute, 100 Perth Drive, London ON, N6A 5K8, Canada. E-mail: jmoore@imaging.robarts.ca

delivery of the treatment is a side effect responsible for most of the morbidity and mortality associated with the intervention. Catheter-based interventions separate access (via the vascular system) from visualization (using X-ray or ultrasound imaging, and when feasible, electrophysiological recording/ablation). Their use is associated with fewer side effects and positive outcomes. Unfortunately the open-heart approach is still routinely employed for most intracardiac targets like valves, septal defects, and aneurysms.

Recently, we embarked on a project to modernize procedures inside the beating heart using new surgical technologies and support of image-guidance via pre-operative imaging and intraoperative 2D Ultrasound (echo-cardiography) to substitute for direct vision. Our goal was to provide a system with a safe cardiac port access that augmented the traditional ultrasound approach with virtual reality to substitute for the absence of direct vision, while at the same time delivering quality therapy to the target. As an example of our goals, we describe our methodology with respect to the implantation of a mitral valve. Validation, both laboratory-based and clinical is being reported elsewhere.

2. Materials and Methods

2.1. The Universal cardiac Introducer

The first task was to design a device that could provide safe heart port access, which could accommodate up to four tools, instruments or devices, access all cardiac cavities and intracardiac targets, and which could be removed at the end of the intervention. This device, the Universal Cardiac Introducer® (UCI) [1] (Fig. 1) has been tested in animal studies to demonstrate feasibility for endocardial atrial fibrillation surgery, and mitral valve replacement. The UCI is designed as an "air lock" between the cardiac cavity containing blood, and the atmosphere. It comprises an insertion cuff, which is attached to the heart port access, and which in turn is connected to the introductory chamber. This chamber can be affixed to the heart via a mini-thoracotomy, can accommodate bulky devices and has 3 or 4 sleeves that allow the introduction of the tools or

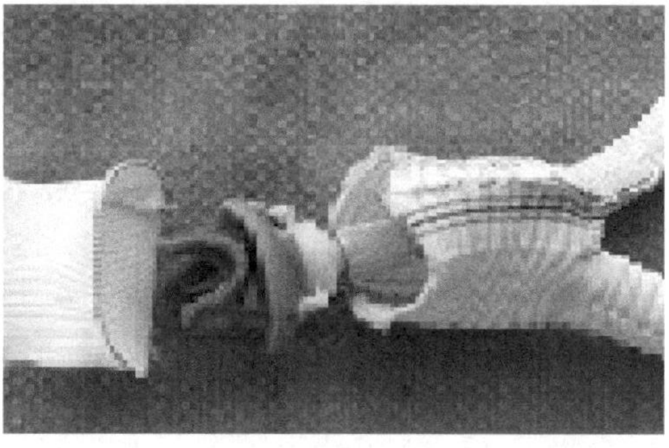

Figure 1. Universal Cardiac Introducer (UCI) showing its components including the three arms to accommodate instruments, along with an artificial mitral valve and holder

holders. The introductory chamber is "loaded" with the device and tools before being connected to the cuff. For mitral valve implantation, the sleeves of the introductory chamber accommodate the valve holder, a pressure line and a "clip applier". The introducer is safe and versatile and does not compromise the manipulation of tools.

2.2. Image-guidance using Ultrasound: Limitations

Echocardiographic guidance uses technology that is readily available in the cardiac operating room. Cardiac ultrasound systems are available in several forms including trans-esophogeal echography (TEE), and intra-cardiac echography (ICE). A limited number of 3D systems are also available, but the transducers are large, image acquisition is restricted to trans-thoracic views, and the 3D dynamic data are not readily available to the user.

In order to demonstrate both the feasibility of the intracadiac procedure using the UCI, and to highlight the limitations of using US alone as a navigation tool, we employed a TEE system to navigate a bioprosthetic mitral valve into the left ventricular inflow tract of a pig. In this study, a full sternotomy was employed to provide ready access to the site with epicardial ultrasound employed as an adjunct visualization modality. When we felt that the valve was appropriately positioned, a 3D transthoracic US probe was used to acquire an image of the left ventricular base from the epicardial surface. Once the valve was in place, it was fastened to the valve annulus using a laparoscopic clip applier introduced via the UCI. Doppler US was then used to assess the quality of valve placement.

Our initial experience in valve placement through the left atrium into the mitral valve orifice relied on ultrasound image guidance alone, and emphasized the significant limitations imposed by the low quality 2D images. The US images were often difficult to interpret due to lack of anatomical context, and required cautious trial-and-error manipulation of the valve based upon the imperfect US images. In these tests, the final positioning of the valve was performed using a large dynamic 3D ultrasound transducer placed on the epicardium. Such devices are very bulky and have a small field of view, and access to the target may be compromised. Tools and targets are poorly perceived in both 2D and 3D images. From our initial experience, we conclude that the use of 2D TEE guidance has significant limitations when used as the sole imaging modality. Estimation of orientation of tools and their motion is virtually impossible to assess since the 2D cross section image does not provide the necessary context of the 3D cardiac anatomy. As demonstrated below, this limitation can be addressed by augmenting the 2D dynamic cardiac US with virtual models of the surgical instruments and target. This approach offers the advantage of real time 3D imaging while employing only standard 2D US modalities.

In spite of the limitations discussed above, the Doppler capability of ultrasound imaging is ideal for assessing the quality of the intervention based on blood-flow measurements. Residual flow around the valve seat, inappropriate flow through the valve, or incomplete Atrial Septal Defect repair, can be readily identified through aberrant flow patterns.

2.3. Cardiac Intervention Phantom and tracking Devices

Our preliminary studies were performed using a custom-built heart phantom. This phantom (Fig. 2) is similar in concept to that described by Rettmann et al [2]. Three plates (two horizontal, one vertical, approximately 7cm x 12cm) hold PVA cryogel membranes [3] that can represent various cardiac walls and chambers.

To ascertain the position of an ultrasound image in space relative to the patient the transducer must be tracked relative to some coordinate system. The US modalities generally used in cardiac surgery create images via a transducer placed in the esophagus, (TEE), or in the heart chamber itself (ICE): Since line-of-sight

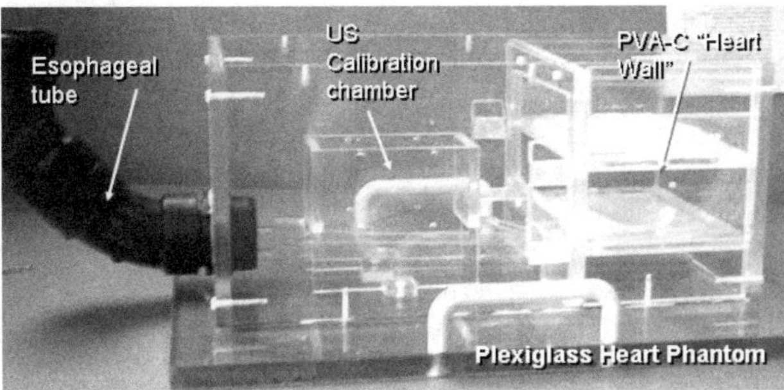

Figure 2. The cardiac intervention phantom showing esophageal tube, US calibration chamber and heart tissue membranes.

is not available in these cases, magnetic tracking must be used. To this end, we track both the ultrasound and instruments using the NDI Aurora® system, which identifies the position and orientation of miniature 6 Degree-of-freedom (DOF) sensors (not commercially available at this time), fixed to the transducer and tools.

Three tracked objects are needed for the mitral valve implantation procedure, one for tracking the US transducer, and another for tracking the valve insertion tool, and a third for determining the position and orientation of the stapler or "clip fixation device".

3. Experimental Methodology

We examined the accuracy with which an experienced cardiac surgeon could guide the valve prosthesis, place it accurately over the aperture, and staple it in place using a laparoscopic clip. This process was performed first under 2D US guidance alone, and then with US complemented by the virtual representation of all tools. The target in this case was a hole in a pliable PVA-C membrane that could move freely under pressure from the valve and tool as the valve was being positioned. The virtual environment included a CT scan of the cardiac phantom with the membrane. However, since in practice the virtual (pre-op) model may not be precisely registered with the target (because of registration errors, motion etc), we deliberately misaligned the target aperture by several mm from its virtual representation. This emphasized the fact that the pre-operative virtual model is there to give context to the US image rather that for accurate final guidance to the target. The virtual environment nevertheless contained an accurate representation of the tracked manipulation tool and valve, robustly registered with respect to the ultrasound transducer.

A 4-7.5MHz 2D TEE ultrasound probe was used to visualize the instruments and target. A virtual target was also placed within the volume by interactively aligning it with the edges of the actual aperture as seen in the 2D US images. We emphasize that even though the target is represented in the pre-operative images, because of the pliability of the artificial membrane material, the target as seen in the pre-operative scans is unlikely to be precisely registered with the actual target. This is also a realistic representation of what will happen in practice in a real heart. Virtual representations of both instruments, along with live images acquired from the video stream of the US system were mapped into the virtual visualization environment.

When manipulating the valve, the US image depicts the sonic reflections from the intersection plane of the holder or the valve, and while certain characteristics of the tool may be appreciated, it is extremely difficult to determine exactly where the tool is and what its relationship is to the target. The position of the target may be determined by interpreting the US image as it is swept across the valve. However, when the US image is complemented by a virtual representation of the tool, navigation of the valve towards the target becomes trivial. Once the valve is in place superimposing the target, it is a relatively simple matter to introduce the clip fastener, place the staple head at several points around the valve flange, and staple it to the membrane as demonstrated by Fig. 3.

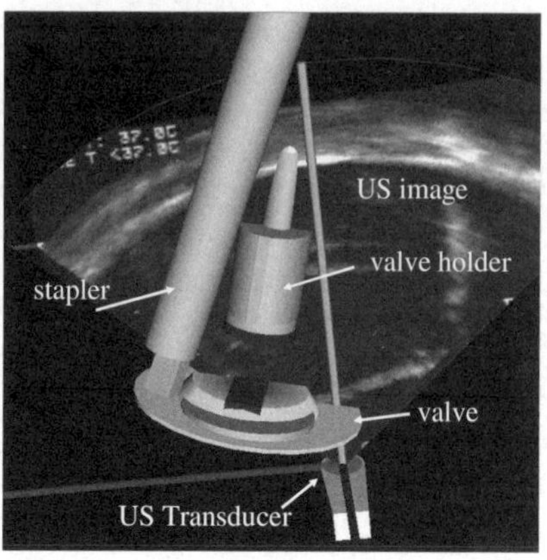

Figure 3. Virtual environment showing valve, valve holder, stapler, ultrasound transducer and US image.

4. Results

Three attempts were made to place the valve in a free-hand manner in the aperture under both 2D US guidance alone, and US/VR. The results were visualized using an endoscope directed at the target.

The results of using the 2D ultrasound alone to position the valve were consistent with those from our previous experience, i.e. that parts of the valve circumference could be identified but that the image was contaminated with artifacts. Positioning that seemed appropriate using US alone, was often

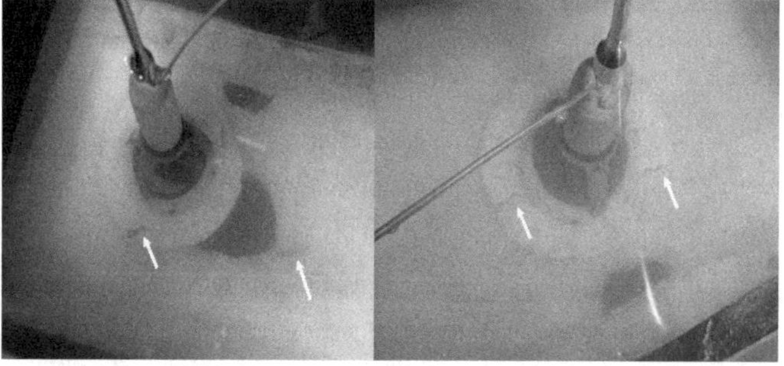

Figure 4. a) Poorly placed and stapled valve placed under US only navigation (left), while b) the image on the right shows the correct positioning and stapling achieved under US/VR guidance. Arrows indicate the staples in both cases.

several mm off target, both in translation and angulation (Fig 4a). When the valve placement was complemented by the VR environment, the operator found it was much easier to place the valve close to the final target initially, and that the refinement of the positioning could then be carried out using the 2D US. Typically the valve seating was much closer to the ideal under these conditions. Perhaps the most helpful characteristic of the virtual environment was its ability to visualize the entire 3D valve and insertion tool and to appreciate its orientation with respect to the plane of the target – information that is not immediately evident in the US-only approach.

At the time of writing, the placement and fixation task had been performed several times with US guidance alone, and with VR assistance. In all cases the US-guidance attempt was unsuccessful in properly placing the valve on the aperture, or achieving a patent fastening of the valve to the membrane (Fig 4a). However, with VR/US guidance, the success rate has been 100% (Fig 4b).

5. Conclusions and Future Work

This project is still in its infancy, and a great deal of additional work remains to be done. However this early series of experiments has convinced us that the use of the VR environment can be a key element to enhance the performance of off-pump, beating, intracardiac surgery. When using US guidance alone to position the stapler and fix the valve to the underlying membrane, the procedure proved to be complex and largely unsuccessful. However, when the same task was attempted using VR and US, the same task became trivial. Enhanced with US imaging for final positioning, the combination provides both the elements of visualization of the target, planning optimal routes to the target, and the guidance for directing therapeutic interventions. The phantom allows evaluation of the surgical approach as well as training of the team. Future developments will need to incorporate dynamic motion and flow to the phantom and then to refine the imaging to be useful for intracardiac surgery. While we used a laparoscopic "stapler" to fasten the valve in place, there are other fixation technologies that need to be explored as well. We also note that it would be ideal to employ dynamic 3D US within this environment, however this facility is not generally available and so we must achieve a similar effect by complementing the 2D US images with the 3D virtual environment.

Last but not least, we must design tools and devices that deliver the required treatment to the target, while being compatible with standard imaging and tracking systems.

Acknowledgements

We wish to acknowledge funding for this work that has been provided by the Ontario Research and Development Challenge Fund; the Ontario Innovation Trust; the Canadian Foundation for Innovation; the Canadian Institutes for Health Research, and the National Science and Engineering Research Council. We would like to thank Louis Estey for assistance with tool design, and Dr. David Gobbi, Dr. Mark Wachowiack, Xishi Huang, and Dr. Hualiang Zhong for useful discussions

References

[1]   Guiraudon G.M., "Universal Cardiac Introducer," US Patent 20050137609, 2005.
[2]   M. E. Rettmann, D. R. Holmes, III, Y. Su, B. M. Cameron, J. J. Camp, D. L. Packer, and R. A. Robb, "An integrated system for real-time image guided cardiac catheter ablation," *Studies in Health Technology & Informatics. 119:455-60,* 2006.
[3]   K. J. M. Surry, H. J. B. Austin, A. Fenster, and T. M. Peters, "Poly(vinyl alcohol) cryogel phantoms for use in ultrasound and MR imaging," *Physics in Medicine and Biology,* vol. 49, no. 24, pp. 5529-5546, Dec.2004.

Medicine Meets Virtual Reality 15
J.D. Westwood et al. (Eds.)
IOS Press, 2007

Smooth Haptic Interaction from Discontinuous Simulation Data

Jesper MOSEGAARD[a,b,1], Bo Søndergaard CARSTENSEN[c],
Allan RASMUSSON[c], Thomas Sangild SØRENSEN[c]
[a]*Institute of Information and Media Studies, University of Aarhus, Denmark*
[b]*Department of Computer Science, University of Aarhus, Denmark*
[c]*Centre for Advanced Visualisation and Interaction, University of Aarhus, Denmark*

Abstract. When a physical simulation that relies on haptic interaction is temporarily paused due to e.g. visualization, noticeable discontinuities are introduced in the interaction as well as the haptic-feedback. The source of this problem is a discrepancy between the notion of time in the simulation and in the real world. In this paper we analyze the general problem of executing simulation steps that each represent a constant amount of simulation time but are distributed non-uniformly in real world time. We have devised a solution that realigns the two notions of time, hereby insuring smooth interaction data and haptic feedback.

Keywords. Haptic rendering, noise-filtering, discontinuous simulation, GPU acceleration, surgical simulation

Introduction

In this paper we deal with a specific problem within the field of haptic-rendering, namely to achieve smooth haptic interaction from simulation-data that is sampled non-uniformly over time. The problem occurs specifically in GPU (graphics processing unit) based simulations where execution of several simulation steps for each visualization step is common [1,2]. The problem arises since the simulation is briefly suspended during each visualization step. The user continues to move the interaction device however, and when the simulation resumes, the position of the virtual instrument, as seen from the simulation timeline, will appear to have moved extraordinarily (or discontinuously) since the previous simulation step. This introduces noise and "jumps" in the interaction with the simulated tissue as well as in the haptic feedback. In Figure 1, graphs based on measurements demonstrate this undesired effect. The problem is clearly exhibited in the relatively large perturbations (solid line) in interaction *a)* and haptic-feedback *b)*. Notice how the errors from Figure 1 *a)* are more distinct in Figure 1 *b)* since the physical simulation collects perturbations as additional energy whereby oscillations occur. As humans are very sensitive to even the smallest discontinuities in the haptic rendering, this is an important problem to solve.

A naive "solution" would be to try and smooth the haptic forces through a filter. This is not a viable solution unfortunately, since a substantial amount of smoothing

---

[1] Corresponding Author: Jesper Mosegaard, Institute of Information and Media Studies, Helsingforsgade 14, 8200 Aarhus N, Denmark; E-mail mosegard@daimi.au.dk

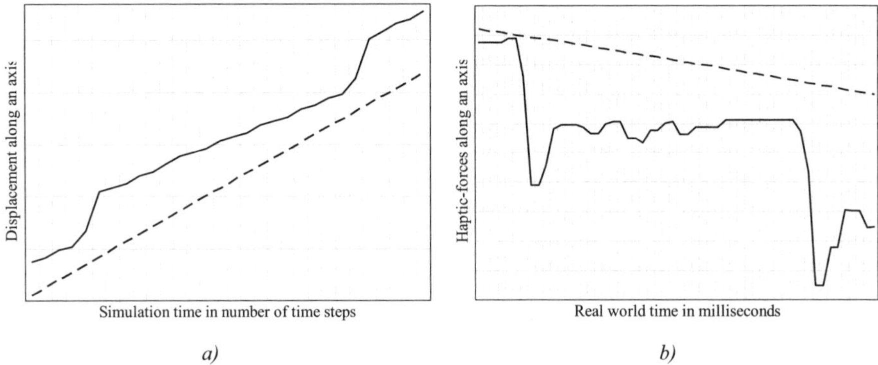

Figure 1. An interaction-device is moved with constant velocity (programmed) along an axis in the GPU-based simulator. The solid graphs are based on measurements of *a)* motion of interaction in simulation time and *b)* haptic-feedback in real world time. Delays in the execution of simulation-steps are clearly seen as noise and "jumps" in the two graphs. The dotted graphs are based on measurements of the simulator using the proposed mapping (Figure 3) to correct *a)* the motion of interaction in simulation time and the proposed inverse-mapping (Figure 4) to correct *b)* the haptic-feedback in real-world time. Notice how the dotted graphs are very close to the theoretically optimal linear graph of constant velocity.

would be required, which again seriously dampens the desired haptic changes that should be felt when manipulating the simulated tissue. In this paper we analyze the problem and present a method to solve the actual problem rather than repairing its symptoms.

This specific problem has not previously been described in the field of haptic-rendering, although other related subjects of interpolation and extrapolation, to achieve a sufficient update rate of more than 500hz, has been dealt with in e.g. [3,4].

1. The GPU-based surgical simulator

We observed the behavior described in the introduction in GPU-based simulators, which effectively utilize the large amount of computational power in consumer-level programmable graphics processing units for the computation of tissue deformation. On the GPU, several simulation-steps can be performed for each visualization-step due to much faster computation of each simulation step compared to a CPU implementation [1,2]. The large number of simulation-steps per second ensures a fast, responsive, and stabile simulation. To obtain the highest quality of haptic feedback, forces are collected after each simulation step. In [2] a Geforce 7800 GTX is reported to sustain a simulation rate (and consequently a haptic feedback rate) of 450 Hz for a system of 20.270 particles (of 18 springs each) with two haptic-devices. This system was used to simulate surgical procedures on congenital heart defects. A visualization of 137.490 faces is executed at 30 Hz. This corresponds to 15 simulations-steps for each visualization step. The non-uniform distribution of simulation-steps not only arises from these pauses during visualization, but also from internal resource priorities on the GPU. That is, even a pure sequence of simulation steps may not arrive at regular intervals.

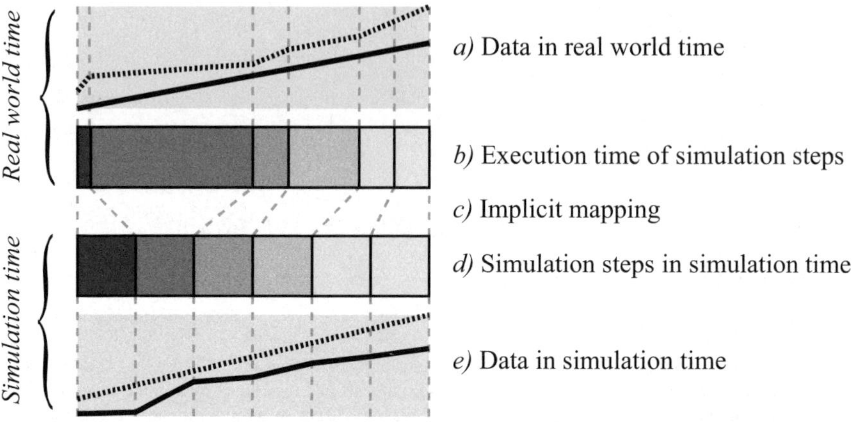

Figure 2. This figure illustrates the errors introduced when directly applying data from real world time in simulation time (and visa versa). The dotted graph is linear in simulation time, while the solid graph is linear in real world time. The mapping between the two notions of time *c)* is applied through the relationship between constant sized simulation-steps as seen from the simulation *d)* and the non-regular execution times as seen from real world time *b)*.

2. Analysis

In a computer simulation we have two notions of time; real world time and simulation time. The real world time is the time as measured by the internal clock of a computer and experienced by the user. The simulation time is the time "measured" by the numerical simulation of some phenomenon. The surgical simulation we consider, uses a discretized notion of simulation-time where each simulation-step increments the simulation-time by a *constant* factor. We analyze the problems arising when the simulation-steps are non-uniformly distributed in real world time but uniformly distributed along the simulation time-line. These issues become clear when specific actions in the real world manipulate the simulated object (and visa versa), specifically during interaction with simulated tissue and the corresponding haptic feedback.

To illustrate, consider directly using interaction data sampled at the beginning of each simulation step (in real world time) as input to the simulation. The interaction data would not be sampled at constant intervals due to run-time variation as mentioned previously. However, in the simulation the sampled data is assumed to represent interaction sampled in regular intervals. This transformation on interaction data is illustrated in Figure 2. The reader should follow the transformation of the fat line from real world time (Figure 2 *a)*) to simulation time (Figure 2 *e)*), where the fat line has become severely distorted. The same problem affects information calculated by the simulation but applied in the real world, such as haptic forces. This is illustrated by the transformation of the dotted fat line in simulation time (Figure 2 *e)*) to real world time (Figure 2 *a)*). Our solution to both problems is to introduce a mapping from both real world time to simulation time, as well as simulation time to real world time.

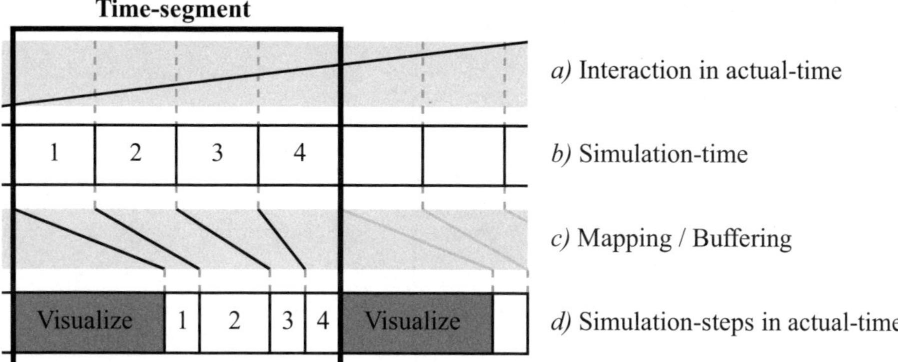

Figure 3. Consider a time-segment of one visualization-step and four simulation-steps. *a)* shows the interaction-data in real world time. *b)* shows the division of the time-segment into four equal parts, each corresponding to one of the four simulation steps. *c)* shows the mapping from execution time of simulations steps in d) and the corresponding division of the time-segment in *b)*. For each simulation step 1-4 in *d)* the mapping in *c)* provides the actual time *a)* at which to retrieve interaction-data from.

We can now see why the above identified issues are rarely problematic in conventional CPU-based simulators (See [5] for a good introduction). In many such simulators a simulation-step is always followed directly by a visualization step, thereby introducing the same delay of visualization for each simulation-step. Interaction can consequently be delivered directly to the simulation and haptic-forces can be retrieved directly.

3. Method

Without loss of generality we now further explore the case of the GPU-based simulator, in which the visualization step was the largest source of delay. A visualization-step and a set of simulation steps (up until the next visualization step) will be named a *time-segment*, see Figure 3. We assume that the execution time of a time-segment is constant – or slowly changing. The calculation of the execution time is based on a weighted average of several successive time-segments. We propose to construct a mapping (Figure 3 *c)*) from real world time to simulation time as follows. First, let us consider how the execution of simulation steps should have been distributed, in real world time, across a time-segment to reflect the constant sized time-step in the simulation. Since each time-step in the simulation is constant, the execution of simulation steps should also be uniformly distributed across a time-segment. By splitting a time-segment equally into a number of time slots, one for each simulation-step, we consequently know the point of time, in real world time, that the simulation-step corresponds to. Figure 3 *b)* can be said to show both this division into time slots, as well as the time-steps as seen in simulation-time. The actual execution time of a simulation step (Figure 3 *d)*) cannot be changed though. Instead we retrieve the correct interaction prior to the execution of a simulation step. We have chosen a time-segment such that a large delay (the visualization) is in the beginning of the time-segment (Figure 3 *d)*). This means that interaction-data is available before it is required in the simulation. We consequently buffer that incoming interaction-data until the corresponding simulation-step is ready to be executed. When the simulation-step is

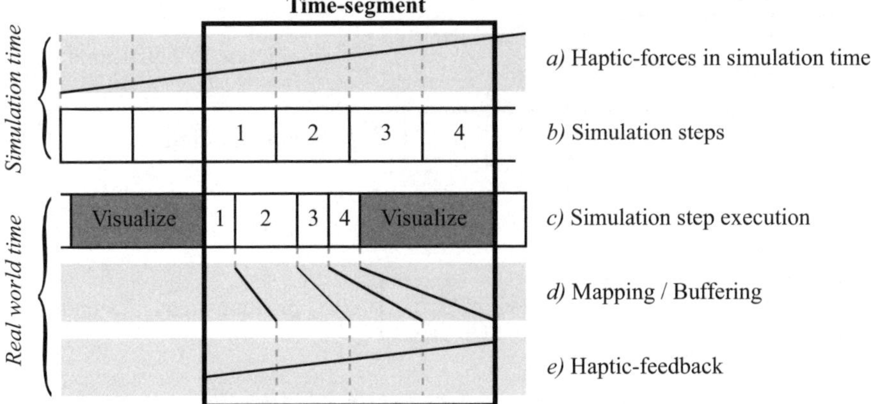

Figure 4. This figure represent the inverse mapping of Figure 3, now going from simulation time to real world time. The haptic-force in *a)*, calculated in simulation time *b)*, are mapped *d)* to real world time through a uniform distribution the simulation-steps *c)* in a time-segment. The result is that haptic-forces calculated in simulation-time *a)* are mapped correctly to real world time *e)*.

about to be executed, it retrieves the buffered interaction data according to its assigned time slot in the time-segment, see Figure 3 *c)*. The buffer is constructed of sampled interaction values and supports linear interpolation of these values when data is retrieved from the buffer.

Although the interaction is now correctly aligned, the haptic-forces calculated after each simulation step, should not be directly applied to the haptic hardware. As discussed in the previous section, we must apply the inverse mapping to the calculated forces to transfer data from simulation-time to real world time. Refer again to Figure 2, and follow the fat dotted line (which could represent haptic-forces) in simulation time to real world time, and notice the severe perturbations if the inverse mapping is not applied. We consequently buffer the resulting haptic-forces, distribute the forces equally across a time-segment, and send them on to the haptic-hardware at regular intervals, see Figure 4.

Although the presented solution was specific to a scenario with one relatively long visualization step and a series of non-regular simulation steps, the method is generally applicable. The only demand is that a cycle of repeating execution times can be found. The buffering of data from either interaction or haptics must be large enough for the access of data in the buffer never to catch up with the buffered content.

4. Results and Discussion

The result of applying the proposed method is that interaction data from the haptic-device arrives at the simulation-step at correct simulation-time, delayed maximally with one visualization-step. Haptic-forces are recorded after each step of the simulation, and are realigned with real world time, delayed maximally one further visualization step. Since the interaction was already delayed one visualization step, the haptic-feedback is delayed two visualization steps compared to the interaction that caused it. In the example from [2] a visualization-step is executed in 11.1 ms. Hence, this delay in interaction is barely noticeable. The results of applying the proposed scheme can be inspected in Figure 1 *a)* (the dotted line). The results on the quality of haptic-feedback can be inspected in Figure 1 *b)* (the dotted line). The results in both cases are actual measured values from the GPU-based surgical simulator [1], and are very close to the theoretical optimal linear line.

In our solution we have assumed that the execution time of each time-segment is constant or slowly changing since this is used to define the "length of time" to divide by the number of simulation steps. We have also assumed that a cycle of repeating execution times is present. In the case of the GPU accelerated simulator these assumption hold.

Practically all simulators are based on differential equations, and consequently solved by numerical integrators. The issues identified in this paper originate from the fact that the time-step was constant. There exist numerical integrators that support varying time-step lengths from one simulation step to the next. Those are most often used to actively guarantee a given precision of approximation though, and not as a *reaction* to expected run durations. The problem with this solution is that the time-step length directly influences the stability of the numerical integration. This is a critical drawback in a real-time simulation and hence not a viable solution.

The proposed scheme solves the problems of constant length time-steps, hereby maintaining the stability of the simulation.

Acknowledgments

We kindly acknowledge the funding we received from the Danish Research Council's Program Committee on IT-Research (grant #2059-03-0004) and The Danish Heart Foundation (grant #05-10-B359-A657-22265).

References

[1] J. Mosegaard, T.S. Sørensen. GPU accelerated surgical simulators for Complex Morphology. In proceedings: IEEE Virtual Reality (IEEE VR), Bonn, Germany, 2005; 147-53.

[2] T.S. Sørensen, J. Mosegaard. Haptic Feedback for the GPU-based Surgical Simulator. 14th Medicine Meets Virtual Reality 2006. Stud Health Technol Inform; 119:523-8.

[3] F. Mazzella, K. Montgomery, J. C. Latombe. The Forcegrid: A Buffer Structure for Haptic Interaction with Virtual Elastic Objects. ICRA 2002:939-46.

[4] G. Picinbono, J-C. Lombardo, H. Delingette, N. Ayache. Improving realism of a surgery simulator: linear anisotropic elasticity, complex interactions and force extrapolation. Journal of Visualisation and Computer Animation, 13(3):147-67.

[5] A. Liu, F. Tendick, K. Cleary and C. R. Kaufmann. A survey of surgical simulation: applications, technology, and education. Presence: Teleoperators and Virtual Environments. 2003;12(6):599–614.

Medicine Meets Virtual Reality 15
J.D. Westwood et al. (Eds.)
IOS Press, 2007

Cybertherapy
New applications for discomfort reductions

Surgical Care Unit of Heart, Neonatology Care Unit, Transplant Kidney Care Unit, Delivery Room-Cesarean Surgery and ambulatory surgery, 27 case reports

°José Luis MOSSO, ¹Skip RIZZO, ²Brenda WIEDERHOLD, ³Verónica LARA , ³Jesús FLORES, ³Edmundo ESPIRITUSANTO, *Arturo MINOR, **Amador SANTANDER, ***Omar AVILA, °Osvaldo BALICE, •Benjamin BENAVIDES

*°Clínica de Especialidades A. Pisanty del ISSSTE, ¹Southerm University, CA, USA, ²The Virtual Reality Medical Center, San Diego, CA, USA, ³Hospital de Ginecología y Obstetricia, Tlatelolco, IMSS, *Centro de Investigación y de Estudios Avanzados del IPN, **Hospital General CMNR, IMSS,***Hosp. Fdo. Quiroz G. ISSSTE, •Hospital General y Regional No. 25 del IMSS*

Email: quele01@yahoo.com, bwiederhold@vrphobia.com, arizzo@usc.edu

Abstract. We demonstrate the feasibility of virtual reality scenarios to reduce discomfort in patients during ambulatory and obstetric surgeries and patients hospitalized in postoperative care units from Cardiac, nephrology, and neonatology unirs. 27 patients have been participated in this preliminary reports from 3 public hospitals from Mexico city in 2006. The VR scenarios were developed in the Virtual Reality Medical Center of San Diego CA, USA, and the HMD is from the Southern University of los Angeles, CA, USA. The majority of patients demonstrated comfort with virtual scenarios during surgical procedures or hospitalization. In ambulatory surgeries the reduction of medication dosage was real. We present the first applications in surgery, obstetrics and care units. The preliminary results must be supported in the future with more number of cases and statistical results; however we can predict the usefulness because we have found reduction of medication in ambulatory surgeries. Explore new applications in different areas in medicine is a challenge of Virtual Reality.

Key words. Cybertherapy, ambulatory surgery, obstetric, unit cares, neonatology.

Introduction

Recent studies have suggested that Virtual Reality (VR) can be effectively used to produce analgesic relief in patients undergoing painful or uncomfortable medical procedures by way of distracting attention away from the perception of pain. We will report data from exploratory investigations of the VR analgesic experiences of 18 patients hospitalized in a Surgical Unit for Heart Care, two pregnant women who underwent natural labor and cesarean surgery and a case of a patient hospitalized in a kidney transplant care unit where VR was applied to promote positive emotion behavior. We will also briefly report some early tests of a VR HMD used to promote neurological stimulation in a nursing infant in the neonatology care unit and 3 cases of patients underwent short surgeries.

1 Methodology

Patients from four public health institutions in Mexico City, participated in this project from March-July, 2006. The VR pain distraction software (Enchanted Forest and Icy Cool World) was developed at the Virtual Reality Medical Center of San Diego,

California, USA. The 18 heart patients (avg. age = 60.5) underwent coronary vessels revascularizations or cardiac valve replacements and experienced the VR scenarios 24-48 hours post surgery for approximately 30 minutes, Figure 1. The pregnant women were 40 weeks pregnant, this was their first delivery and they used the VR scenarios for 5 hours. The kidney transplant patient was a 14-year old teenager who was emotionally depressed after a fistula complication required an extended hospital stay. The nursing infant (age = 2 months and 23 days) was hospitalized in the Neonatal Care Unit following a gastrointestinal surgery of bowel resection and end to end colo-colo-anasthomosis, Figure 2. In general surgery, 3 adult patients had an extensive underarm lipoma, umbilicus hernia and in the last patient various cysts lesions, they didn´t present pain during surgery. The medication employed to local infiltration in the surgical region were, 20 cc of lydocaine 1-2%, 8 cc of bicarbonate, 4 cc of buphibacayne, and 2 cc of epinephrine. Relaxation medication were phentanil 75 mgr.and mydazolam 1 mgr in 1 of 3 patients.

2 Results

The cardiac patients reported higher well-being while using VR on the pain scale employed (HMD VR=7.25 vs. No VR=3.12). Their metabolic, homodynamic and gasometry responses are not important because all rates are in normal levels such as: Increase of glycemie of 109 to 155; increase of blood pressure of 123.5/72.25 to 132.62/72.5 mmHg. In myocardium conduction disorders, normal catecholamine's production may produce arrhythmias (one patient presence cardiac arrhythmias). Regarding the two pregnant patients, one of them underwent natural labor Figure 3, and the other had to undergo a cesarean surgery Figure 4. In the natural labor case, the response without epidural block in the pain scale was 1 without HMD VR and 5 with HMD VR. Following an epidural block, the ratings were: without HMD VR=3 and with HMD VR=10. VR scenarios distract pregnancy. The teenager following a kidney transplant reported an increase on the well-being scale of 1 to 9 after using the HMD VR. His HR decreased from 115 to 106 per minute during VR use due to well-being, while his breath rate was the same, at 28 per minute. The nursing infant who had undergone gastrointestinal surgery showed normal metabolic response, an increase in his heart rate (128 to 133), a decrease in breath rate (31 to 15 per minute) and a decrease in arterial oxygen saturation (98% to 91%) following presentation of the HMD delivered stimuli. During surgery, medication phentanyl, mydazolam medications were reduced 75 % of the amounts. No pain presented in the 3 patients during surgery, the scale pain before surgery was 8, during 9, after 10.

3 Preliminary Conclusions

Our initial observations from these cases suggest that the HMD VR scenarios were useful for decreasing the experience of pain in patients following surgical procedures. When using HMD VR following such significant cardiac surgical procedures, we suggest a constant heart measure with close attention to the electrocardiogram due to the possible occurrence of heart arrhythmias. In obstetrics, the virtual scenarios were reported to be useful when the mother and the fetus had no complications before or during labor. Many hospitals don't use epidural block, in these cases we recommend the HMD also. In our patient following a kidney transplant, the virtual navigation was useful in improving his emotional state and during surgical cleanings. In the case of the infant, we recognize that presenting imagery via a VR HMD is a rather speculative procedure. However, future research might explore this with small displays as a form of neurological stimulation that might be helpful during extended stays on neonatology care units. Finally, in some cases it may be helpful for the VR navigation to run in a "forced-flythrough" mode to reduce patient arm activity that could interfere with treatment. Special thanks to Prof. Brenda of The Virtual Reality Medical Center for the virtual scenarios we used in the present project and for Prof. Skip Rizzo for the HMD. We present the first results in the worldwide in patients in unit cares, obstetrics and ambulatory surgery. In surgery, is important to recognize the decreasing of medication doses of phentanyl and mydazolam 75 % of their doses. An experience of infiltration of medication in the surgical area is important to avoid pain during surgery. The virtual scenarios in surgery are a complementary treatment to reduce surgical discomfort.

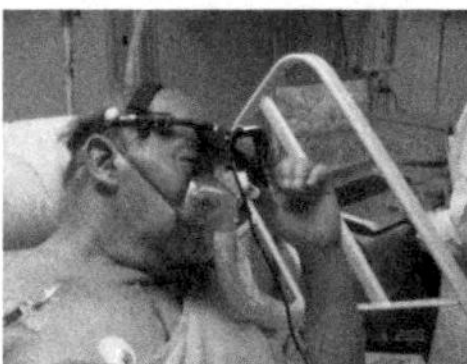

Figure 1
Patient within 24 hrs. after cardiac surgery in Heart Unit Care. National Medical Center la Raza of the IMSS.

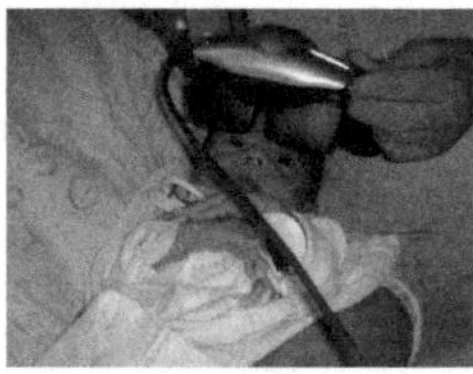

Figure 2
Patient of 2 months and 23 days, hospitalized in a neonatology unit care. Fernado Quiroz Hospital. ISSSTE.

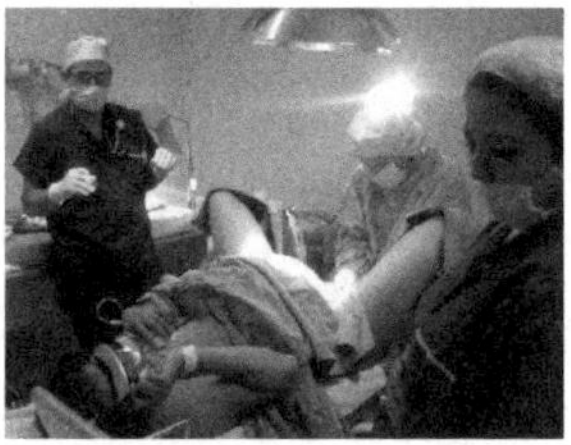

Figure 3
Patient in delivery room with epidural block. Gynecology and Obstetric Hospital, Tlatelolco Unit of the IMSS.

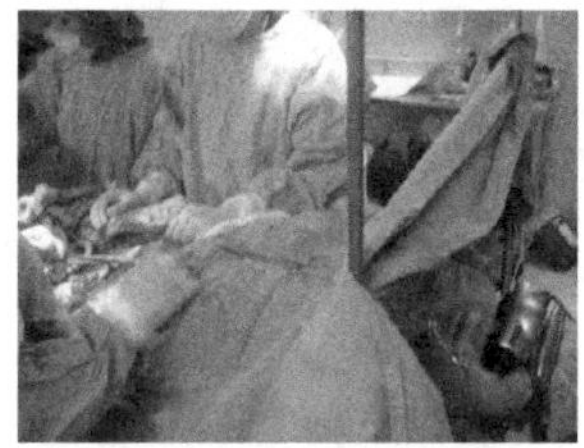

Figure 4
Patient during cesarean surgery with epidural block. Gynecology and Obs-Tetric Tlatelolco Hospital, IMSS.

References

[1]   New applications of virtual reality: Surgical cleaning in infected, extensive and Soft tissues, cervical conization with diathermia loop, and upper gastrointestinal Procedures in MMVR 13, Long Beach CA, USA, 2006.

[2]   Rizzo, A.A. (1994). Virtual Reality applications for the cognitive rehabilitation of Persons with traumatic head injuries. In Murphy, H.J. (ed.), *Proceedings of the 2nd International Conference on Virtual Reality and Persons With Disabilities.* CSUN: Northridge.

[3]   Rizzo, A.A. , Buckwalter, J.G., & Neumann, U. (1997). Virtual reality and cognitive rehabilitation: A brief review of the future. The Journal of head Rehabilit. 12(6),1-1 -15.

Medicine Meets Virtual Reality 15
J.D. Westwood et al. (Eds.)
IOS Press, 2007

Applications of Computer Assisted Surgery and Medical Robotics at the ISSSTE, México: Preliminary Results

[0]José Luis MOSSO, [1]Mauricio POHL, [1]Juan Ramon JIMENEZ, [1]Raquel VALDES, [1]Oscar YAÑEZ, [1]Veronica MEDINA, [2]Fernando ARAMBULA, [2]Miguel Angel PADILLA, [2]Jorge MARQUEZ, [2]Alfonso GASTELUM, [3]Alejo MOSSO, [3]Juan FRAUSTO

[0]Clínica de Especialidades A. Pisanty del ISSSTE, [1]Universidad Autónoma Metropolitana, campus Iztapalapa, [2]Universidad Nacional Autónoma de México, CCADET, [3]Instituto Tecnológico y de Estudios Superiores de Monterrey, campus Cuernavaca
Email: quele01@yahoo.com

Abstract. We present the first results of four projects of a second phase of a Mexican Project Computer Assisted Surgery and Medical Robotics, supported by the Mexican Science and Technology National Council (*Consejo Nacional de Ciencia y Tecnología*) under grant SALUD-2002-C01-8181. The projects are being developed by three universities (UNAM, UAM, ITESM) and the goal of this project is to integrate a laboratory in a Hospital of the ISSSTE to give service to surgeons or clinicians of Endoscopic surgeons, urologist, gastrointestinal endoscopist and neurosurgeons.

Key words. Simulation, Robotics, neuronavigatoion, virtual endoscopy.

Introduction

We present technological preliminary advancements from the second of three stages (three years) of 4 projects developed at Mexican universities and a national medical center of the ISSSTE (*Instituto de Seguridad y Servicios Sociales de los Trabajadores del Estado*) comprising a neuronavegator, a system for TURP surgery, a gastrointestinal endoscopic simulator and a robot for laparoscopic surgery.

1. Methodology

Neurosurgery planning system. Researchers at Universidad Autónoma Metropolitana, Iztapalapa are developing a system to support neurosurgery planning. The system allows the fusion of anatomical information, obtained through three-dimensional (3D) reconstructions from Computer Tomography (CT) or Magnetic Resonance images (or MRI), with functional EEG maps. The main goal is to estimate the location of epileptogenic foci by solving the inverse problem from EEG scalp recordings. The inverse solutions are computed for each voxel in the real anatomic model, thus increasing precision and assuring protection of critical zones of the brain in the pre-operatory phase. Potential users of this surgery planning system may include neurologists, internship physicians, pediatricians and radiologists [1], [2], [3].

The *prostatic simulator for TURP surgery* and the *virtual endoscope* are under development by researchers of the CCADET from the *Universidad Nacional Autónoma de México* (UNAM); the first project comprises a graphic model of the prostate, using a mesh with virtual springs and masses, the proximity of a surgical tool is detected with a collision detection algorithm, and from this information the mesh is deformed, displacing the nodes in contact with the tool. Tissue resection is simulated by removing nodes and updating the mesh [4]. The second system, a *virtual endoscopy system* comprises: (1) a computer model of the high gastro-intestinal system, built from the color cryo-anatomical images of the *Visible Human Project* [5]., (2) a virtual endoscope and (3) an electro-mechanical interface (under development) to navigate through the computer model and to simulate endoscopical procedures. The model is characterized by simulated physical collapsing of the esophagus, typical lens distortion (barrel) and illumination as in real endoscopes. Dynamical behavior was added to the tissue walls, using a two-layer mesh, and a simplified collision algorithm using distances fields in 3D. Dynamical behavior includes persitaltic waves along the esophagus, and simulation of insuflation thru the endoscope, using a physics-based approach called *Smoothed Particle Hydrodynamic* [6]. *The laparascopic surgery robot* consists in the technological development of the final efector that will hold laparoscopic surgical instruments that perform sutures, and manipulation of other surgical instruments. The final efector is also being adapted to a *Fanuc* industrial robot.

2. Results

Neurosurgery planning system. A graphical user interface was made using QT (a development tool of programming that uses libraries of Borland C++) and the graphical handling of the data is made through VTK (Visualization ToolKit) (Figure 1).

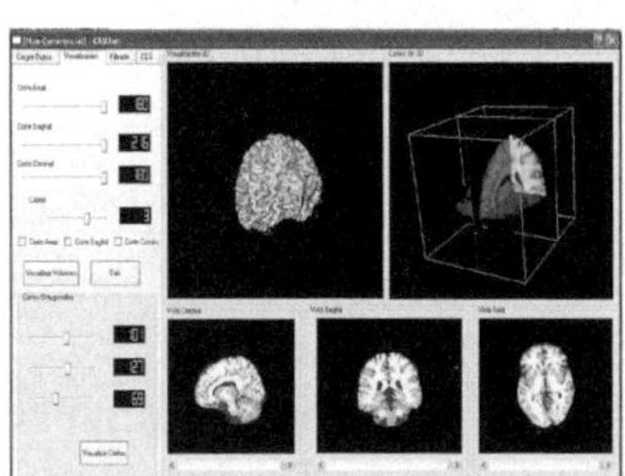

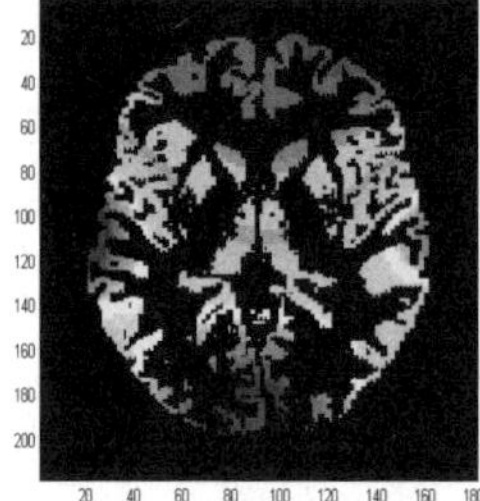

Figure 1. GUI of the neurosurgery system   **Figure 2.** Synthetic MR slice planning system

We have obtained the inverse problem solution according to the standardized minimum norm method, taking 8197 voxels of gray matter as the space solution (Figure 2). The 3D rendering of the inverse solution projected over the anatomical model is shown in Figure 3, for two simulated sources.

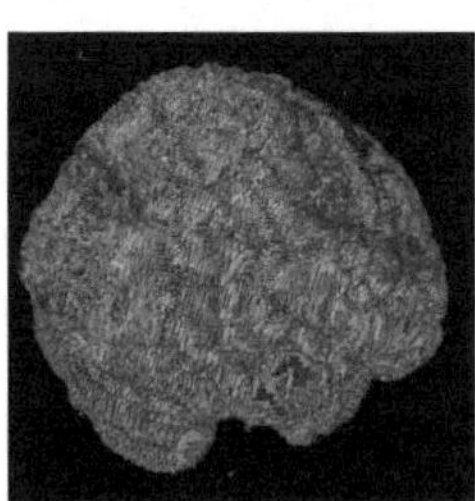

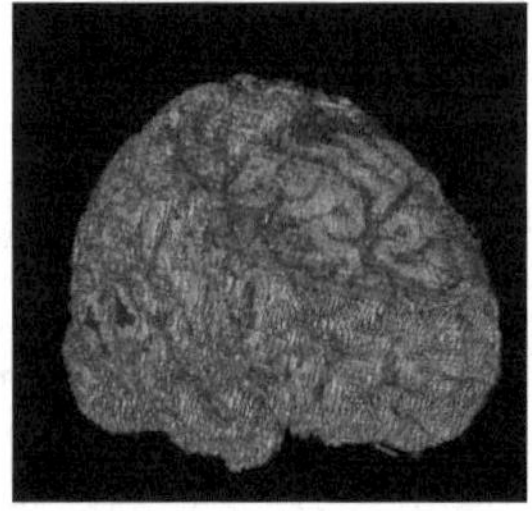

Figure 3. 3D rendering of the inverse solution projected over the anatomical model

The graphical model, (*prostate simulator*) shown in Figure 4, allows to simulate deformations and tissue resection in an approximated form, with a video rate of 8 frames per second. In the *virtual endoscopy system, a* video rate of 4 frames per second was attained with the much larger and complex endoscopy model, adding in this case a Radeon 1900X graphics accelarator; the endoscopical navigation (Figure 5) includes optical distortion, color mapping from real video endoscopies, small light source illumination and dynamical behavior.

3. Conclusions

The following tasks are to be completed. *Neuronavigator.* The next step will be to integrate the realistic head model (such as BEM) on the definition of the lead matrix, in order to enhance source location and resolution. Other than LORETA there are other iterative and enhanced methods for inverse solutions, that we will be integrating shortly into our planning system. *The prostate simulator* will increase in realistic behavior, by including new collision detection algorithms, and by identifying mechanical constants optimal for the mesh, as well as by optimizing calculations and speed, while increasing visual quality. *The virtual endoscope* requires development of haptic hardware, undergoing at present several tests in order to interact with the virtual model (fig. 5), information from video endoscopies and radiograph videos will be used to obtain several parameters for a realistic dynamical response and to visualize special pathological conditions. *Robot.* A robotic arm is under development for laparoscopic and surgical tasks such as suturing, and grasping, the robot is at present at the integration stage with a five degree of freedom robot and an efector mechanism to hold endoscopic instrumentation.

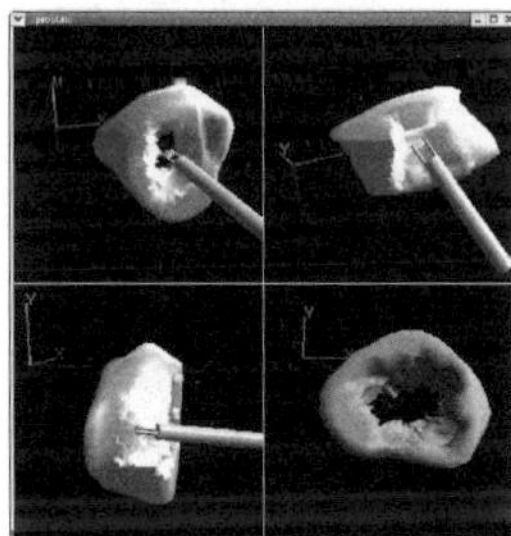
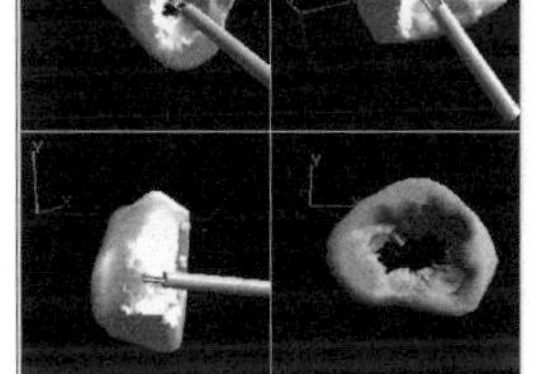

Figure 4. Prostate model and simulated TURP   **Figure 5.** Simulated endoscopy of virtual model.

References

[1]   Peters, T. M., 2000. *Image-guided surgery.* SPIE Medical Imaging Handbook, 2, Cap. 3, SPIE Press, 2000.

[2]   Jiménez, J.R., Medina, V., Yáñez, O. 2003. *Nonparametric MRI segmentation using mean shift and edge confidence maps.*   Proccedings of SPIE, 5032, 2003, 1433-1441.

[3]   Kim, P.E., Singh, M., 2003. *Functional magnetic resonance imaging for brain mapping in neurosurgery.* Neurosurgery Focus, 15, No.1, Article 1, 2003, 1-7.

[4]   MA Padilla Castañeda, F. Arambula Cosío. The deformable model of the prostate for TURP surgery simulation. Computer graphics, 2004, 28, 767-777

[5]   Gastelum A, Mosso JL and Marquez J, "A Computer Representation of the Upper Gastrointestinal System", *28th Annual International Conference of the IEEE Engineering in Medicine and Biology Society,* New York, USA, August 30 – September 3, 2006.

[6]   Gastelum A. and Marquez J. "Modelling Interactions with a Computer Representation of the Upper Gastrointestinal System" *IVCNZ'06 (Vision Computing New Zealand 2006) Conference,* Great Barrier Island, New Zealand, Nov 27-29, 2006.

Medicine Meets Virtual Reality 15
J.D. Westwood et al. (Eds.)
IOS Press, 2007

Development of an Interactive Module to Enhance and Understand Cavity Navigation

Andrés A. NAVARRO NEWBALL [a], Franco ROVIELLO [b], Domenico
PRATTICHIZZO [b], Francisco J. HERRERA [a], Cesar A. MARIN [a]

[a] *Pontificia Universidad Javeriana, Cr 103# 12C -50 Cali –Colombia*
[b] *Università degli Studi di Siena, Italy*

Abstract. The Interactive Module for Cavity Navigation (IMCA) was created in
order to enhance the Web Environment for Surgical Skills Training in
Otolaryngology (WESST – OT); later, it was found that it could be used as an
independent module which allowed the practice of path navigation in any medical
cavity, and its potential use with patients was evidenced. This paper describes the
making of IMCA and the potential use of genetic algorithms in path generation.

1. Introduction

WESST-OT was presented in previous works [1, 2]; it was then stated that it needed
some enhancements such as the support and evaluation of cavity navigation. IMCA
was created and aimed to enhance WESST – OT; this paper describes the architecture
and technologies used for IMCA's development. First, it describes the tools and
methods used; then it shows the results obtained and; finally, it provides a discussion.
This work has been possible thanks to the Coimbra Group Scholarship, the Università
degli Studi di Siena, Colciencias, the Pontificia Universidad Javeriana and the ICESI
University.

2. Tools and Methods

The first version of IMCA was approached through rapid prototyping using a modular
and object-oriented software methodology, this allowed focusing on computer graphics
and genetic algorithms techniques; it was implemented with the DirectX technology
and the .X file format, contrasting with the original WESST-OT's Java3D
implementation. Here, path generation mechanisms were compared and a validation
questionnaire was applied to health specialists and patients [3]; additionally, IMCA
was tested in the following situations: 1) IMCA displaying a generic cavity; 2) IMCA
displaying a reconstructed stomach that was obtained from a CT scan machine and
converted from the DICOM format to the .X format and; 3) IMCA displaying a
reconstructed head that was obtained from a CT scan machine and converted from the
DICOM format to the .X format.

3. Results

IMCA is capable of displaying any 3D anatomical cavity represented in the DirectX's .X format, allowing internal movements with full degrees of freedom through the use of the mouse, the keyboard and the joystick. Fig. 1a shows IMCA's architecture; at present, the *3D reconstruction module* is under development and, image reconstruction and export to the .X format are done using third party tools [4, 5]; at this point, the *pre processing module* is used to generate bounding boxes [6] that allow the identification of a path point inside the cavity; the *cavity navigation engine* allows 3D displacement inside the cavity; additionally, the *path generation module* can be used to suggest a path either using an automatic technique based upon genetic algorithms or mathematical averages or, using the path proposed by an expert; finally, after navigation, the *evaluation module* can be used to objectively evaluate the path followed by a user. Fig. 1b shows a stomach where critical points have been displayed; here, the red spheres are critical points that should not be touched, the green spheres are objective points that should be touched and the blue spheres represent a suggested path. Fig. 1c shows IMCA displaying a reconstructed head.

"Genetic algorithms are a methodology for searching through the space of solution possibilities, using the concept of evolution. By constructing individual chromosomes that consist of possible solutions in the search space, genetic algorithms determine the fitness (F) of an individual based on an objective function" [8]; they have been used for trajectories before [9]; In IMCA, the chromosome takes into account factors like distance to a wall of the anatomical cavity (W), distance to a critical point (C) and, distance to an objective point (O); additionally, the genetic algorithm is applied once for each bounding box; also, coefficients for the objective function Eq. (1) were empirically obtained. Fig. 1b displays a path generated using 20 generations of 30 chromosomes. Fig. 2a shows a path generated using mathematical averages; averages are calculated by finding the middle point inside a bounding box (Fig. 2b). Fig. 2c shows a path from a human expert that got 4.93 out of 5 after being evaluated according to the genetic algorithm's path.

$$F = 10 \times W + 2 \times C + 100 \times O \tag{1}$$

Surgical simulation educational potential has been evident for some years [10]; also, the potential use of IMCA for patients' education [3] and the use of WESST-OT in surgical training [1] were evidenced in previous works; moreover, 9 of 10 interviewed doctors considered that IMCA enhanced WESST-OT realism and functionality.

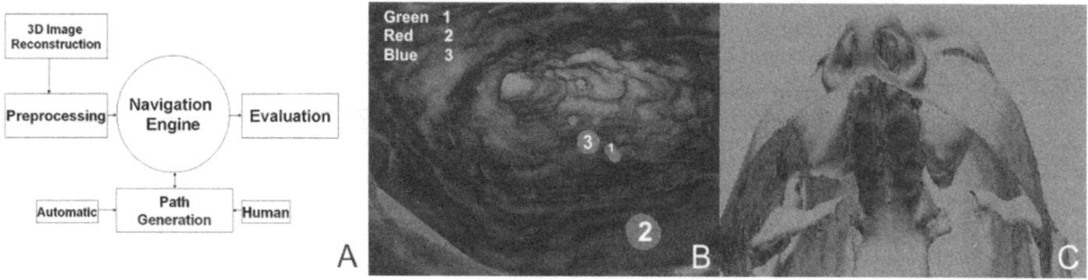

Figure 1. a) Architecture; b) stomach and genetic path; c) reconstructed head.

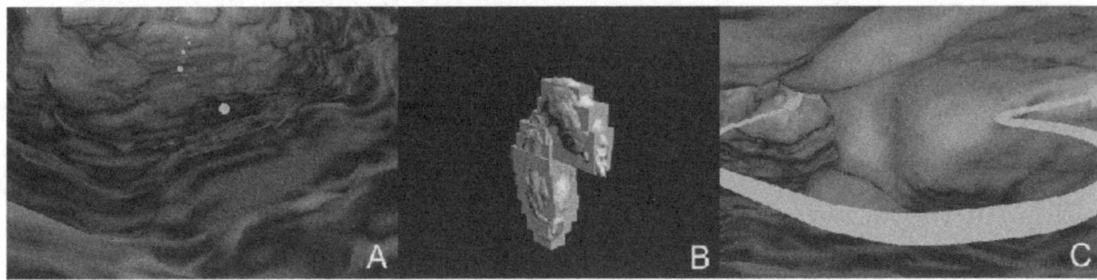

Figure 2. a) Average path; b) stomach and bounding boxes; c) human path

4. Discussion

Validations show that IMCA can be used independently and that it can enhance patients´ and surgeons´ experience; additionally, IMCA can enhance the WESST - OT simulator. On the other hand, critical and objective points shown can be enhanced to represent polyps, cancer, vessels or other tissues. It is recommended that the 3D reconstruction module is fully implemented; however, rapid prototyping was useful to know the advantages and disadvantages of IMCA and the techniques used. At the same time, techniques used provide an objective path evaluation mechanism.

Genetic algorithms have great potential, tests done show a rapid convergence using a few generations for small populations in order to find a path; comparing them with other techniques, it has been found that they can be more useful when avoiding critical points or approaching objective points; also, genetic algorithms can be used to identify more than one path; meanwhile; the mathematical averages technique is better when no critical or objective points are defined; however, path navigation is influenced by the quality of the bounding box generated; in contrast, a route generated by a human expert can contain more path points without the need of bounding boxes.

5. References

[1]   AA Navarro N, CJ Hernández, JA Vélez B, LE Múnera S, GB García, CA Gamboa, AJ Reyes. Virtual Surgical Telesimulations in Otolaryngology. *Studies in Health Technology and Informatics* 111 (2005), 353-355.

[2]   A Cardona, E Mazuera, FJ Herrera, AA Navarro N, CA Gamboa, JA Vélez. Incorporación de un Módulo para la Práctica de la Habilidad de Ubicación Espacial al Simulador de Otorrinolaringología – WESST – OT. *Sistemas & Telemática* 7 (2006), 43-53.

[3]   AA Navarro, FJ Herrera, CA Marín. Using an interactive module to enhance and understand 3D cavity navigation: a patient's view. Accepted for TeleMed & eHealth London November 2006. Submitted to the Journal of Telemedicine and Telecare.

[4]   TB Software. *Rheingold3D: the 3D Polygon Modeler.* http://www.tb-software.comProducts_1.html. Last checked 1 October 2006.

[5]   Able software. *3D-DOCTOR: Vector-Based 3D Medical Modeling and Imaging Software.* http://www.ablesw.com/3d-doctor/. Last checked 1 October 2006.

[6]   JD Foley, A Van Dam, SK Feiner, JF Hughes. *Computer Graphics: Principles and Practice.* 1996.

[8]   AM Howard. Role Allocation in Human-Robot Interaction Schemes for Mission Scenario Execution. *Proceedings of the 2006 IEEE International Conference on Robotics and Automation* 2006, 3592.

[9]   JH Joon, O Kwon, JS Yeon, Park JH. Optimal Trajectory Generation of Serially-Linked Parallel Biped Robots. *Proceedings of the 2006 IEEE International Conference on Robotics and Automation* 2006, 1610 – 1615.

[10] Robb RA. The Virtualization of Medicine: A Decade of Pitfalls and Progress. *Studies in Health Technology and Informatics* 85 (2002), 1-7.

Medicine Meets Virtual Reality 15
J.D. Westwood et al. (Eds.)
IOS Press, 2007

Design Methodology for a Novel Multifunction Laparoscopic Tool: Engineering for Surgeons' Needs

Carl A. NELSON [a,b], David J. MILLER [a], Dmitry OLEYNIKOV [b]
[a] *Dept. of Mechanical Engineering, University of Nebraska-Lincoln*
[b] *Dept. of Surgery, University of Nebraska Medical Center*

Abstract. In minimally invasive surgery (MIS), the small number of incisions necessitates the insertion and removal of many different instruments to complete a given procedure. Using the technique of functional decomposition, it was found that some functions are repeated for different instruments, such as positioning and actuation of the tool's tip. Axiomatic design principles motivated a redesign of current technology to consolidate these repeated functions into a single multifunction tool. The investigators surveyed a laparoscopic surgeon to obtain functional requirements and their relative importance in MIS. These requirements were used in a Quality Function Deployment analysis to design a laparoscopic tool which combined the functionalities of multiple tools into one handheld device, and allowed the integration of the surgeon's needs into the design. This novel tool eliminates the need to remove and reinsert multiple tools during a surgical procedure and decreases the OR time, monetary cost and trauma to the patient.

Keywords. Minimally invasive surgery, functional decomposition, axiomatic design, quality function deployment, laparoscopic surgical tool.

1. Background

In laparoscopic surgery, a small number of functionally similar tools are used [1,2]. With a limited number of access ports, minimally invasive surgery (MIS) often requires the complete removal of one tool and reinsertion of another. This can result in increased trauma and longer patient recovery time [3].

Multifunction surgical tools [4] can diminish these problems by allowing the surgeon to change tool functions without removal and reinsertion. Soft computing techniques have been used previously in medical applications [5-8] and can be used to optimally queue the tool tips in a multifunction tool, allowing surgeons to deliver treatment of higher quality in less time, decreasing overall cost [9] and improving outcomes. The sections which follow describe the methodology used to design a novel multifunction tool for minimally invasive surgery.

2. Methods

Three principal techniques were used to arrive at the novel tool design. Functional decomposition provided insight into the problems with the current surgical paradigm. Axiomatic design provided a systematic way of finding a solution which matched the information gained through functional decomposition. Quality function deployment allowed for mathematically determining design criteria which would positively affect the functioning of the final product.

2.1. Functional Decomposition: Motivation for Redesign

Functional decomposition [10] refers to a systematic breakdown of sub-functions performed as part of a process. Following these techniques, necessary component functions involved in MIS were broken down into four main sub-tasks, which were then further subdivided, as shown in Figure 1. The resulting functional structure motivates a change in the surgical paradigm. Looking specifically at the mechanical tasks involved in MIS (the dashed region of Figure 1), one notices that the sub-functions cut, grasp, retract and dissect, typically performed by separate tools, all have common operations – tool positioning and tool actuation.

2.2. Axiomatic Design: Influence on Redesign

The "axiomatic design" approach [10,11] is based on two main concepts:

1. Maintain the independence of functional requirements.
2. Minimize the information content.

The first axiom indicates that the quantifiable design parameters (DPs), such as weight, dimensions, etc., should ideally be coupled to a single functional requirement (FR), e.g. "compactness." This allows independent tuning of the FRs, simplifying the iterative design process. In real-world design problems, this rule can never be fully satisfied, but it serves as an overall guide for the design process. The second axiom simply states that a good design satisfies the FRs using the least number of DPs. This has been referred to colloquially as the "keep it simple" strategy. Applying these axioms to the multifunction surgical tool design implies that a single component or assembly should satisfy the repeated functions indicated in Figure 1: tool positioning and actuation.

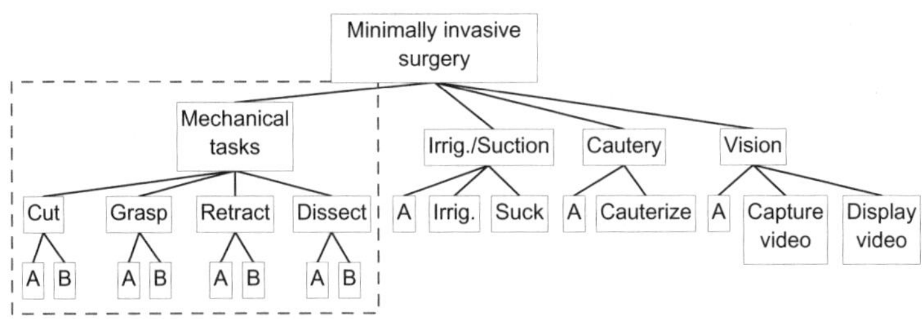

Figure 1. Decomposition of functions in MIS: A = tool positioning, and B = tool actuation.

Customer Needs	weight	length	handle size	shaft diameter	CG location	power requirement	motor size	motor speed	actuation force	material strength	material type	time between tools	Priority (1-5)	Improvement ratio	Importance	Weight
Goal (Up/Down)	D			D	D	D	D	U	D	U		D				
Features																
Cuts well									1	1	3		4	1	4	0
Grasps well									1	1	3		4	1	4	0
Retracts well									1	1	3		4	1	4	0
Dissects well									1	1	3		4	1	4	0
Operate witih 1 hand	3		9		3		1		9				5	1	5	0.1
Durable - won't break				1					1	9	3		3	1	3	0
Robust - always works right						1	3	1	1	3	1		5	1	5	0.1
Self-contained			1			3	1						4	1	4	0
Reusable											9		2	1	2	0
Quiet								3			1		2	0.9	1.8	0
Adaptable/scalable	1	1		3		3	9	1	1	1			2	2.5	5	0.1
Ergonomics																
Light	9	3	3	1			9				9		3	0.8	2.4	0
Comfortable grip	3		9		9		1			3	1		4	1.2	4.8	0.1
Easy/intuitive to use									9			3	5	1	5	0.1
Easy/fast tool change		1						9				9	4	2.5	10	0.1
Efficient use of hand motion			1						3				3	1	3	0
General																
Low power						9	3	3				1	1	1	1	0
Mobile/portable	9	1	1			1					1		3	1	3	0
Easy to sterilize		1		1							9		2	1	2	0
Efficient use of OR space		1	1			3							2	2	4	0
Integration with existing tools/tech.		3	3	9		1				1	3	1	1	1	1	0
Aesthetics	3	1	3				3				3		2	1	2	0
Low cost						1	1	1		1	3		3	0.9	2.7	0

Competitive Eval. (Σ 83, 1)

Technical Evaluation	weight	length	handle size	shaft diameter	CG location	power requirement	motor size	motor speed	actuation force	material strength	material type	time between tools	
Absolute importance	1.1	0.4	1.4	0.4	0.7	0.7	1.3	1.3	1.7	0.8	1.8	1.3	13
Relative importance (%)	8	3	11	3	5	6	10	10	13	6	14	10	100
Technical Difficulty (1-5)	3	5	4	5	4	4	3	5	4	5	5	3	
Current tools	8 oz	12 in	4 in	10 mm	0	0	0	0	5 N	50 ksi	stainless/ plastic	30 s	
Target Value	16 oz	12 in	4 in	10 mm	0	5 W	1 in	1000 rpm	5 N	50 ksi	stainless / plastic	8 s	

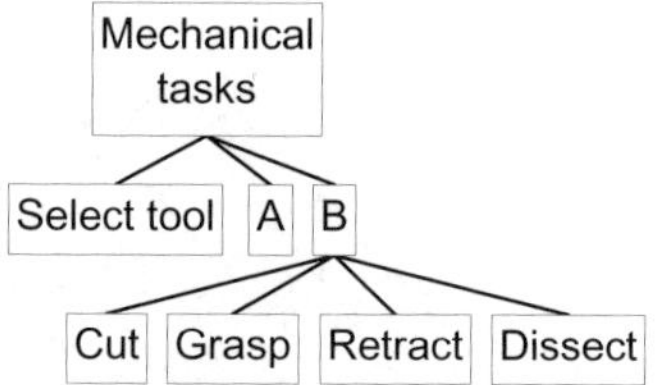

Figure 2. New functional paradigm for MIS mechanical tasks: A = tool positioning, and B = tool actuation.

2.3. Quality Function Deployment: Meeting Surgeons' Needs

Quality function deployment (QFD) [10,12] is a technique by which customer requirements are quantified and correlated to design parameters. Thus it is directly related to the FRs and DPs described by axiomatic design.

The QFD process relies on a matrix often called the "House of Quality," which quantifies the relationship between FRs and DPs. As shown in Table 1, rows of the matrix represent the FRs, and columns represent the DPs. High, medium, and low correlations between FRs and DPs are given values of 9, 3, and 1 respectively. The sparseness of the correlation matrix is a measure of how well Axiom 1 (decoupling of FRs) is adhered to for the given design. An importance value or weight is calculated for each FR based on customer ranking and the anticipated margin of improvement relative to current technology. Each row of the correlation matrix is then scaled by the corresponding weight, and the importance of each DP on enhancing product quality is calculated as the sum of the entries in its column of the weighted correlation matrix.

Using the results of the functional decomposition and axiomatic design analysis, the investigators generated 23 unique FRs for a multifunction MIS tool design. These were ranked in importance from 1-5 by a laparoscopic surgeon. A set of 12 quantifiable DPs were identified to characterize the engineering aspects of the design. A QFD matrix (Table 1) was used to correlate the FRs to the DPs, determine which DPs most influence overall quality, and competitively assess the quality of the design under consideration relative to current technology.

3. Results and Conclusions

The shaded section of Table 1 shows the outputs from the QFD analysis and the relative importance of each of the DPs with respect to overall quality. DPs with relative importance above 10% (handle size, motor size and speed, actuation force, material type, and tool-change time) were given special attention in the design since these provide the highest relative impact on customer-perceived quality. As far as axiomatic design is concerned, the QFD correlation matrix is sufficiently sparse to suggest that a reasonable amount of design iteration will result in an optimized tool. A key achievement of the design is highlighted by its functional decomposition, shown in Figure 2. The restructured functional paradigm is very streamlined, reflecting savings of time and money in the operating room.

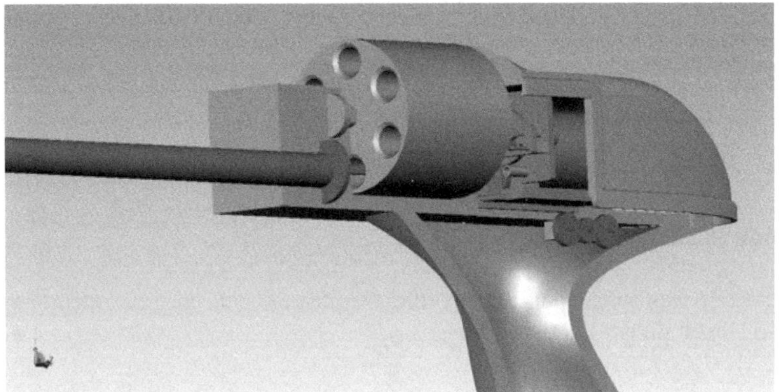

Figure 3. Laparoscopic tool design resulting from customer needs analysis.

The tool resulting from the preceding analysis is shown in Figure 3. A rotating chamber houses up to 6 instrument tips with different functions. Each tip is conveyed via electric drive through the tool shaft and then is actuated manually by input from the surgeon at the tool's handle. This strategy reduces the number of tool removals and insertions needed to perform a procedure, while still meeting the functional needs of the surgeon, decreasing OR time, cost and trauma to the patient.

This study uses the specific case of a multifunction laparoscopic tool design to illustrate how established design engineering methodologies can be applied to biomedical research problems in general. The process begins with an identification of weakness using functional decomposition. Axiomatic design then guides engineers to a candidate design. By defining needs in terms of functional requirements and numerically correlating these to quantifiable design parameters, substantial improvements in product quality are obtained and effective engineering solutions to biomedical problems are reached.

4. References

[1]   Hunter, J. G., Sackier, J. M. (eds.), 1993. *Minimally Invasive Surgery*, McGraw Hill, New York.

[2]   Soper, N. J., Swanström, L. L., Eubanks, W. S. (eds), 2005. *Mastery of Endoscopic and Laparoscopic Surgery*, Williams and Williams, Philadelphia.

[3]   Kim, V.B., Chapman, W.H.H., Albrecht, R.J., Bailey, B.M., Young, J.A., Nifong, L.W., Chitwood, W.R., 2002. "Early Experience with Telemanipulative Robot-Assisted Laparoscopic Cholecystectomy Using da Vinci," Surgical Laparoscopy, Endoscopy & Percutaneous Techniques, 12(1), pp. 33-40.

[4]   Brock, D.L., 2005, "Interchangeable Instrument," U.S. Patent No. 6,860,878. Washington, DC: U.S. Patent and Trademark Office.

[5]   "A Fuzzy Inference System for the Ordering of Laparoscopic Tools in Minimally Invasive Surgery," ASME SBC'06, Amelia Island, FL, June 21-25, 2006, ASME Paper No. BIO2006-156583.

[6]   Ross, T.J., 2004. *Fuzzy Logic with Engineering Applications*, 2nd ed., John Wiley and Sons, West Sussex, England.

[7]   Anbe, J., Tobe, T., Nakajima, H., Akasada, T., Okinaga, K., 1992. "Microcomputer-Based Automatic Regulation of Extracorporeal Circulation: A Trial for the Application of Fuzzy Inference," Artificial Organs, 16(5), pp. 532-538.

[8]   Rau, G., Becker, K., Kaufman, R., Zimmerman, H. J., 1995. "Fuzzy Logic and Control: Principal Approach and Potential Applications in Medicine," Artificial Organs, 19(1), pp. 105-112.

[9] Dexter, F., 2001.   "Maximizing Operating Room Staff Productivity," Currents, 2(3),
     www.uihealthcare.com/news/currents/vol2issue3/5operatingroom.html. Printed: 10/02/06.
[10] Dieter, G.E., 2000. *Engineering Design,* 3rd ed., McGraw-Hill, Boston.
[11] Suh, N.P., 1990. *The Principles of Design*, Oxford University Press, New York.
[12] Hauser, J.R., Clausing, D., 1988. "The House of Quality," Harvard Business Review, May-June 1988,
     pp. 63-73.

5. Acknowledgement

This research was made possible by the Nebraska Tobacco Settlement Biomedical Research Development Funds.

Medicine Meets Virtual Reality 15
J.D. Westwood et al. (Eds.)
IOS Press, 2007

349

A User-friendly Interface for Surgeons to Create Haptic Effects in Medical Simulation

Liya NI [a] David W. L. WANG [a] Adam DUBROWSKI [b] Heather CARNAHAN [b]

[a] *Dept. of Electrical & Computer Engineering, University of Waterloo, Canada*
[b] *Dept. of Surgery, University of Toronto, Canada*

Abstract. Haptics, namely the sense of touch, has been playing an important role in medical simulation. However, most medical practitioners, who are best suited to create the training environments, do not have the engineering expertise necessary for programming a haptic environment. We propose a user-friendly interface that allows surgeons to arbitrarily select regions on a 3D model of an organ, similar to "painting-by-numbers", and tune the haptic properties of each region in an intuitive way. The selected region and tuned haptic properties are recorded in a lookup table in real-time. The proposed user interface is assessed by comparing the haptic effects of a tumor on a virtual liver created by a number of surgeons.

Keywords. haptics, surgical training, user interface

Introduction

Medical simulation using virtual reality technology offers a revolutionary approach for medical training. With medical simulation, medical or nursing students can learn basic and procedural skills before touching a real patient, particularly for dextrous tasks such as laparoscopic surgery[1]. Haptics, namely the sense of touch, has been playing an important role in medical simulation[2]. However, most medical practitioners, who are best suited to create the training environments, do not have the engineering expertise necessary for programming a haptic environment. The performance of medical simulators may be suboptimal because of the gap between the medical practitioners's expectation and the designer's understanding. As an attempt to solve the above problem, we propose a user-friendly interface that allows surgeons to arbitrarily select regions on a 3D model of an organ and tune the haptic properties of each region. For example, with this interface, a surgeon can create a tumor on a liver model by selecting an area on the liver and increasing the stiffness of that area.

1. Design of Proposed User Interface

Our experimental setup includes a laptop with 2.0 GHz CPU and a PHANTOM Omni haptic device[1]. The proposed user interface consists of three components: a haptic-enabled virtual scene; a Matlab GUI; the mechanism to record the selected region and tuned haptic properties in a lookup table in real-time. The virtual scene, which contains the 3D organ model and a 3D cursor representing the Omni device position, and the Matlab GUI with slider bars, buttons, a 3D mesh plot etc., are shown in Figure 1. The

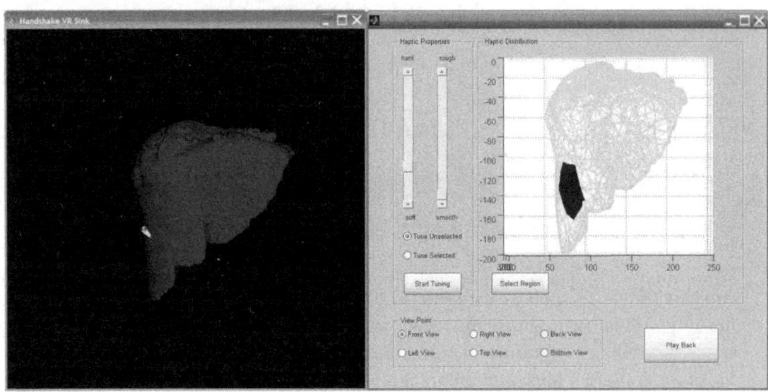

Figure 1. Virtual Scene(left) and Matlab GUI(right) of the Proposed User Interface

3D organ model exists as an IndexedFaceSet node in the VRML standard. It can be viewed from six different viewpoints: front, back, left, right, top, bottom. With a Matlab/Simulink based software called proSENSE Virtual Touch Toolbox [2], the virtual scene with the Omni device touching the 3D virtual organ can be rendered graphically and haptically.

The procedure of creating haptic effects using this interface is as follows: after the surgeon presses the "Select Region" button, each triangle that is in collision with the device end tip during the current sample period will be painted on the triangular mesh plot. These triangles are recorded and are grouped together when the surgeon presses "Finish". This is how the surgeon chooses a part of the liver to be a tumor. By pressing the "Start Tuning" button with the radio button "Tune Selected" checked, the surgeon can start tuning the haptic properties of the tumor such as stiffness and friction using the slider bars. The values of haptic parameters corresponding to the current slider bar settings are used in haptic rendering so that the surgeon feels the change in stiffness or friction immediately. The parameters are saved when the surgeon presses "Finish". The surgeon can tune the haptic properties of the unselected region in a similar way by pressing the "Start Tuning" button with the radio button "Tune Unselected" checked. In the lookup table, each group of triangles map to a set of haptic parameters. When the surgeon presses the "Play Back" button, the triangle that is currently in collision with the device will be compared to the triangles in the lookup table and the appropriate haptic properties will be retrieved from the lookup table and applied in haptic rendering. Thus the user will feel the haptic properties changing as desired when moving the device from one region to another region.

---

[1] Product of SensAble Technologies Inc., www.sensable.com.
[2] Product of Handshake VR Inc., www.handshakevr.com.

2. Surgeons' Assessments

Four surgeons at the Toronto General Hospital and Mount Sinai Hospital in Toronto were asked to create the haptic effects corresponding to a tumor on a virtual liver using the proposed interface. The four surgeons all had the experience of touching patients' livers with tumors in their surgical practice.

Since the size and location of a tumor are relatively arbitrary, we only choose the stiffness of the healthy part of liver and that of the tumor as the criteria for comparison. Figure 2 shows the stiffness tuned by different surgeons. The stiffness for the tumor is

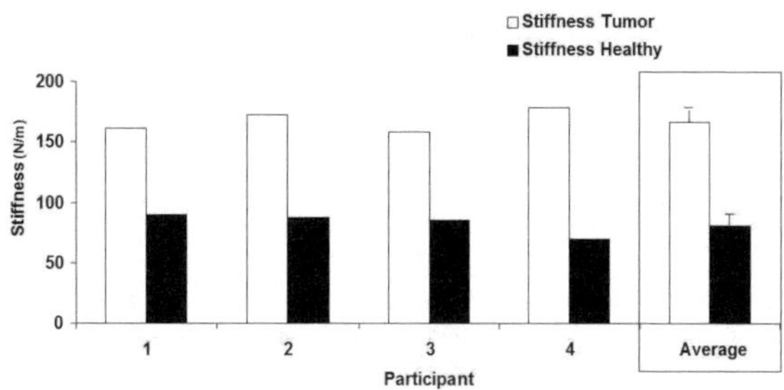

Figure 2. Comparison of Healthy Liver and Tumor Stiffness Tuned by Different Surgeons

in the range of $158.6 - 177.4 N/m$, with an average of $167.2 N/m$. The stiffness for the rest of the liver is in the range of $69.3 - 89.0 N/m$, with an average of $82.8 N/m$. The total range for stiffness tuning is $10 - 300 N/m$. Stiffness tuned by different surgeons is relatively consistent. The friction was kept at a constant low value during the tests, as we expected there would not be much difference in friction between the tumor and the rest part of the liver.

3. Conclusions

A user friendly interface for surgeons to create haptic effects in medical simulations is proposed in this paper. It is tested by four surgeons and the results show that the haptic effects created by different surgeons are relatively consistent. This user interface allows surgeons to directly input their surgical experience into the design of a virtual reality medical simulation so that the design procedure can be simplified and the performance of the simulator can be improved.

References

[1]   J. Torkington, S. G. Smith, B. I. Rees, A. Darzi: Skill transfer from virtual reality to a real laparoscopic task. *Surg Endosc.* **15**(10), (2001), 1076-1079.
[2]   P. Strom, L. Hedman, L. Sarna, A. Kjellin, T. T. Wredmark, L. Fellander-Tsai: Early exposure to haptic feedback enhances performance in surgical simulator training: a prospective randomized crossover study in surgical residents. *Surg Endosc.* **20**(9), (2006), 1383-1388.

Medicine Meets Virtual Reality 15
J.D. Westwood et al. (Eds.)
IOS Press, 2007

MODELING AND RENDERING FOR A VIRTUAL BONE SURGERY SYSTEM

Qiang Niu and Ming C. Leu
Department of Mechanical and Aerospace Engineering
University of Missouri-Rolla
Rolla, MO 65401, USA
qniu@umr.edu, mleu@umr.edu

Abstract. A virtual bone surgery system is being developed to guide a novice surgeon practicing bone surgery operations, as well as to allow an experienced orthopedic surgeon planning and rehearsing bone surgery procedures. The development of this system involves medical image processing, geometric modeling, graphics rendering, haptic rendering, and auditory rendering. It is implemented with a personal computer and a PHANToM^{TM} device capable of providing the position and orientation information of the virtual tool and generating force feedback. This paper presents the techniques we have devised for the development of this surgery simulation system.

Keywords. Virtual reality, virtual bone surgery, geometric modeling, graphic rendering, haptic rendering.

1. Introduction

To guide novice surgeons practicing bone surgery operations, as well as to allow experienced orthopedic surgeons planning and rehearsing bone surgery procedures, a virtual bone surgery system is being developed with geometric and physical models and implemented with virtual reality technologies. The development of this system consists of the following key components: medical image processing and data management for simulation preparation, geometric modeling of bones and surgical tools, physical modeling, and virtual reality rendering. The software architecture is shown in Figure 1. The developed system works as follows. It first constructs a geometric model of the bone from the processed CT (Computed Tomography) image data by applying medical data processing and management techniques established in the field. The geometric model of the bone is updated continuously during the virtual surgery process. Virtual surgical tools are represented using implicit functions, which are discretized into mesh points on the surface. A physical model is used to represent the tool-bone interaction. During the bone surgery simulation, collisions are checked between the geometric models representing the virtual tools and the bones, and the interference data is used to update the interface force and sound continuously. Virtual reality rendering is generated in real time to provide realistic visualization, force and sound feedback during the surgery simulation. Our system can provide a realistic, safe, controllable virtual reality environment allowing medical students, novice doctors and experienced surgeons to make mistakes during bone surgery practice and planning without causing serious consequences.

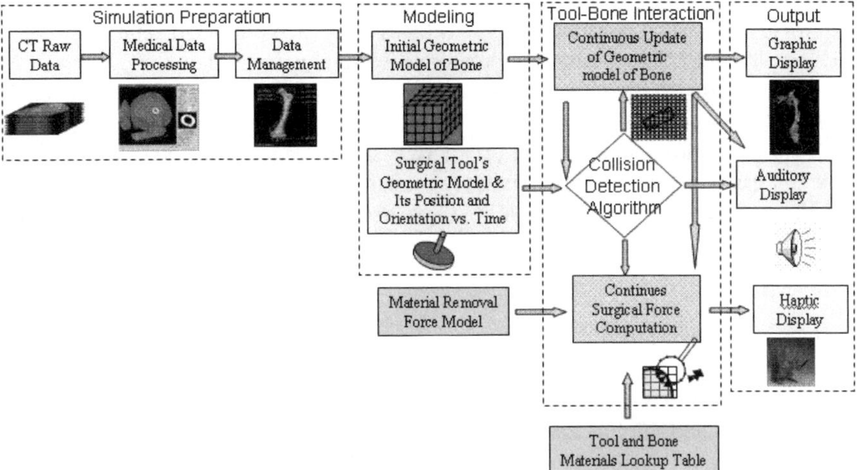

Figure 1. System architecture of our virtual bone surgery system

2. Modeling of bones

Volume modeling is used to model the geometry of a human bone from 2D image data, which is obtained from CT scans and is used as input to reconstruct 3D internal structures of the bone. CT data can show good contrast between bones and soft tissues, and they typically represent the values of some properties at various 3D locations. Image processing, region-growing segmentation, bounding volume, and quadtree techniques are applied to manage large CT scan data in order to remove irrelevant data and to organize the remaining data for improving memory efficiency and real-time performance [1]. These data are processed before the surgery simulation in order to save data processing time. A quadtree data structure is used to store and construct the bone model for the simulation.

3. Modeling of surgical tools

In order to represent different kinds of surgical tools, implicit functions are used for the representation by considering surgical tools' kind, size and geometry. The surgical tools modeled consist of cutting tools (e.g., drill, mill, saw, etc.) and non-cutting tools (e.g., guide, pin, rod, etc.), and they are virtually attached to the user's hand via the PHANToM^{TM} device. Two kinds of points, active points and passive points, are classified on the surface of the virtual tool, in order that they can be used for more accurate collision detection, force generation, and sound rendering during the tool-bone interaction.

4. Graphic, haptic and auditory rendering of tool-bone interaction

Surface rendering of the generated volume model is chosen in this research because of display quality and real-time performance requirements. The marching cube algorithm [2] is used to generate polygonal faces from the volumetric data.

During the tool-bone interaction, material removal occurs when the cutting force is greater than the penetration force limit. A multi-point collision detection algorithm and a balance-point based force calculation technique are developed for haptic rendering of bone material removal operations. An active sub-volume queue is used for model update and graphic re-rendering. Auditory rendering is also done for the bone material removal simulation in order to provide cues for the user regarding the status of the surgical operation.

5. System implementation

The overall system is implemented using C++ and VTK (Visualization Toolkit), GHOST and DirectSound as the APIs, under the MS Visual C++ environment. During simulation, a virtual surgical tool is attached to the user's hand via a PHANToM^{TM} device (a product of SensAble Technologies), which is capable of providing 6D position and orientation data of the virtual tool and generating 3D force feedback to the user. Different kinds of surgical tools can be used for different machining processes, such as drilling, milling, broaching, etc. Figure 2 shows screen shots from the medical image processing module and the simulation module of our virtual surgery system. To make the simulation system more intuitive and interactive, the overall system runs in several threads with multiple rates in parallel: a simulation thread (main working thread doing most computations), a graphic thread (working thread with a 30 Hz timer to fulfill graphic display with surface rendering), and a haptic thread (working thread with a 1kHz timer to do force rendering).

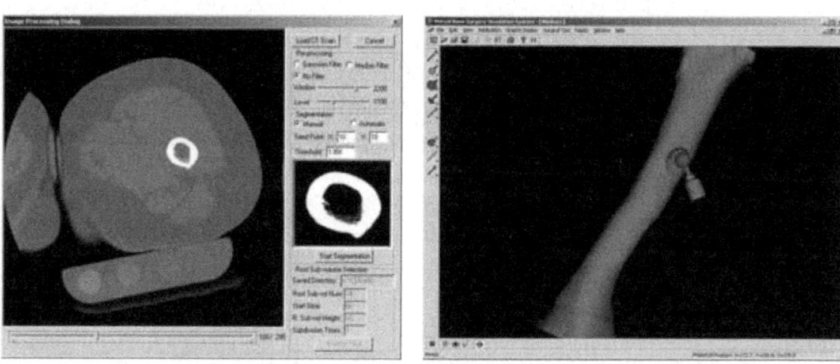

Figure 2. Screen shots from the virtual bone surgery system

References
1. Niu Q, Chi X, Leu MC. Large medical data manipulation for bone surgery simulation. Proceedings of ASME International Mechanical Engineering Congress and Exposition, Orlando, FL, 2005.
2. Lorence WE, Cline HE. Marching cubes: a high resolution 3D surface construction algorithm. Computer Graphics 21(4): 163-169.

Medicine Meets Virtual Reality 15
J.D. Westwood et al. (Eds.)
IOS Press, 2007

A Serious Gaming/Immersion Environment to Teach Clinical Cancer Genetics

Thomas M. NOSEK [a], Mark COHEN [a, b], Anne MATTHEWS [a], Klara PAPP [a], Nancy WOLF [a, b], Gregg WRENN [a], Andrew SHER [a], Kenneth COULTER [a], Jessica MARTIN [a], Georgia L. WIESNER [a, b]

[a] *Case Western Reserve University School of Medicine, Cleveland, Ohio, USA*
[b] *University Hospitals/Case Medical Center, Cleveland, Ohio, USA*

Abstract. We are creating an interactive, simulated "Cancer Genetics Tower" for the self-paced learning of Clinical Cancer Genetics by medical students (go to: http://casemed.case.edu/cancergenetics). The environment uses gaming theory to engage the students into achieving specific learning objectives. The first few levels contain virtual laboratories where students achieve the basic underpinnings of Cancer Genetics. The next levels apply these principles to clinical practice. A virtual attending physician and four virtual patients, available for questioning through virtual video conferencing, enrich each floor. The pinnacle clinical simulation challenges the learner to integrate all information and demonstrate mastery, thus "winning" the game. A pilot test of the program by 17 medical students yielded very favorable feedback; the students found the Tower a "great way to teach", it held their attention, and it made learning fun. A majority of the students preferred the Tower over other resources to learn Cancer Genetics.

Keywords. Cancer, Genetics, Serious Game, Medical Education, Simulation

Introduction

Incoming medical students, children of the computer/information age, are accustomed to an interactive learning environment that puts information at their finger tips (Information on Demand). In contrast, the traditional medical school preclinical experience is often a passive learning environment with information-packed lectures. Further, it is often difficult for new concepts in medical sciences to be integrated into traditional formats due to constraints on available lecture time. With the exponential growth of medical information, students may be better served by being exposed to basic concepts and then provided opportunities to develop their skills to gather and synthesize the most current information to solve problems. This type of learning (Information Just in Time) can be achieved in a safe, virtual environment where the student controls the pace of learning.

E-learning (web-based learning, online learning, distributed learning, computer-assisted instruction, or Internet-based learning) is defined as "the use of Internet technologies to enhance knowledge and performance" [1]. The promise of e-learning is that asynchronous, self-paced access to learning resources enhances access to the information and allows for a learner-centered educational experience that leads to the desired results. The effectiveness of e-learning has been demonstrated in a variety of higher education, government, corporate, and military environments [2.3]. Most non-healthcare e-learning resources are as good as or better than instructor-led learning when product utility, cost-effectiveness, and learner satisfaction were measured [2,4]. Learners' knowledge on standardized exams and retention were most often found to improve with e-learning. Students are typically very satisfied with e-learning, particularly because of its ease of use and accessibility. The same generalized effects were found for e-learning resources in a medical environment [5].

The newest computer-based learning resource is the "serious game". Gaming dominates the recreational time of the younger generation and has penetrated the older generations as a form of recreation and learning. Computer games create a virtual environment that the user actively engages and is captivated to master. The more difficult the game, the more students find it engaging. Through trial and error, players build a model of the underlying game based on empirical evidence collected through play. As the players refine this model, they begin to master the game world. It's a rapid cycle of hypothesis, experiment, and analysis. This is a fundamentally different form of problem-solving. Gamers treat the world as a place for creation, not consumption. Games cultivate - and exploit - possibility space better than any other medium [6]. Serious games attempt to take advantage of these features of games to achieve serious educational objectives. Barnett et al. [7] have reported the effective use of educational games to train the public health workforce. Henry [8] has demonstrated that gaming as a teaching strategy is an effective way of conveying information in a stimulating, appealing manner to adults.

Since 1998, the Office of Academic Computing at Case Western Reserve University School of Medicine has been using e-learning to provide more and varied learning resources online. This Office has collaborated with experts in cancer, genetics, and education to form the Clinical Cancer Genetics Education Group and create a web-based learning resource to teach Clinical Cancer Genetics. The group created this learning resource as a "Cancer Genetics Tower" in a serious gaming format. This paper describes the computer rendering and design of the learning environment and the results of an initial pilot of the system.

Methods

The "Cancer Genetics Tower" is available online at http://casemed.case.edu/cancergenetics. The interactive, gaming environment was created using Photoshop (to create texture maps and 2D images), Maya (to create the 3D environment), Bryce (to organize the grouped objects as .obj files), and Flash 8 Professional (to assimilate all rendered images and animations). Once the site was constructed, each file was embedded into HTML (hyper text markup language) for display on the web. To make the Tower into an interactive "gaming" environment, it was necessary to track a participant's progress through the "Tower", to determine whether or not they had accessed certain learning resources, and to assess how well they had performed on multiple choice questions. All of this information was collected and stored in a SQL database using Microsoft Intelligent Information Server (IIS), SQL Server, Visual Web Developer 2005, and .Net 2.0 Framework.

Results

The Tower is intended to be a self-paced, simulated learning environment that encourages students to achieve specific Learning Objectives (LOs) as a prerequisite for advancement to

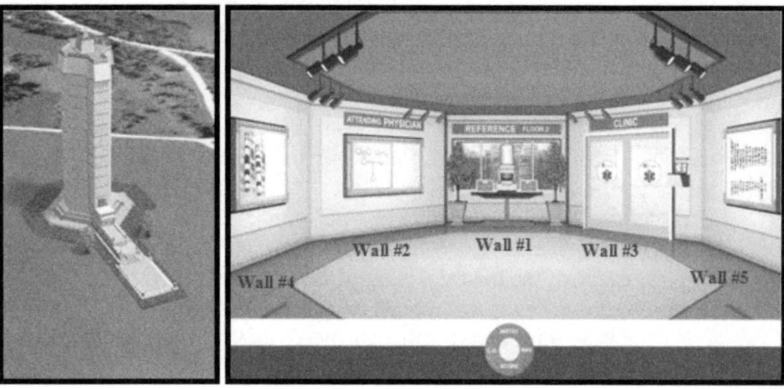

Figure 1. A screen shot of the "Cancer Genetics Tower" and a typical floor in the Tower.

"higher levels" in the learning hierarchy. Figure 1 shows a screen shot of the Tower in the left panel and a typical floor (Floor #3) of the Tower in the right panel. Wall #1 contains a Virtual Microscope, Wall #2 contains video interactions with a virtual Attending Physician, Wall #3 contains a clinic and virtual video conferencing with four virtual patients, and Walls #4 and #5 contain links to various learning resources specific to each floor.

The control circle at the bottom-center of a floor is the navigation tool for the Personal Digital Assistant (PDA) that is available on all floors of the Tower. The PDA has four tabs:

1. The LO tab provides access to the LOs specific to each floor of the Tower along with sufficient resources to enable students to achieve the LOs. This tab is the starting point for interacting with each floor of the Tower. The resources include textual and graphical material created by the authors and hot-links to web-based resources. Each LO is assigned a point value which is awarded when students demonstrate their achievement of a LO by successfully carrying out a specific activity. Activities may include navigating to a particular site in or out of the Tower, successfully playing a matching or identification game, watching a video, answering a question posed by either the Attending Physician or one of the patients, successfully gathering information from a patient and entering that data in the patient's Electronic Medical Record, etc. The Tower is a self-contained learning environment.
2. The Score tab provides each student with an indication of how many total points they have accumulated, how many points they need to achieve in order to gain access to the next higher floor in the Tower, and their score relative to other students.
3. The Notes tab provides a place to type or cut/paste information for later reference.
4. The Navigation (Nav) tab provides navigation within the Tower. Students can always freely navigate to lower floors. But to access higher floors, they must satisfy the criteria for access.

When a student clicks on the Clinic wall, they can choose to interact with one of the four virtual patients. A videoconferencing interface allows students to select a question to ask the patient. The patient can also ask the student a question. An expert answer is provided after the student enters their answer into a text field. All responses are saved in the database to follow student performance. Students can access an Electronic Medical Record (EMR) for a patient and add information to it as a result of their interactions.

The first floor of the Tower introduces students to the application, explains navigation within a room and between floors, and explains the resources in the PDA. Once the LOs for the first floor are achieved, students progress to the second floor, a reference floor which includes links to many web-based learning resources, a virtual microscope and slide collection, and the Human Ideogram linked to National Library of Medicine Human Genome resources. The third floor begins a four-floor series of basic science experiences intended to give the scientific underpinnings of Clinical Cancer Genetics. The next seven floors apply these principles to clinical practice. The pinnacle clinical simulation on the topmost floor challenges the learner to integrate all information in the application and demonstrate mastery. Mastery of the material is required to "win" the game.

The first three floors of the Tower have been completed and pilot-tested by 14 female and 3 male volunteers from the third and fourth year medical classes at Case. Feedback was solicited through an anonymous online survey. All of the students were at least slightly familiar with the field of Cancer Genetics. The 17 students were equally divided among those who were familiar, somewhat familiar, and unfamiliar with "computer gaming". The majority of the students (14) spent less than 2 hours evaluating the application. **Navigation**: Students all quickly learned how to navigate through the Tower and found navigation on a floor and between floors easy. All students liked the layout of the PDA, although some wanted more guidance on how to use this navigation tool. **Learning Activities**: The majority of students thought that the Learning Activities associated with the LOs were a good way to learn the material and fun to complete. **Scoring**: It was clear to the students how points were assigned to LOs and achieved. **Videos**: Students in general wanted transcripts of the video files available within the Tower so that they could better follow the conversations and more easily review the material. **Attending Physician and Virtual Patients**: The data in the EMR for the patients was reported by the students to be helpful. The majority of the students were able to answer the questions asked by the Attending Physician and patients from the resources and activities in the Tower. They highly rated the expert answers provided after they answered the questions. **Online Resources**: Students appreciated the links to the various online resources that helped them achieve the LOs. They found the Virtual Microscope to be particularly useful and liked the way it was integrated into learning about the virtual patients.

The overall rating of the application by the students was exceptionally positive. The quality of the Tower was rated as excellent by 10 students and good by 6. Only one student rated it as average. They all found the quality of the graphics acceptable. All students agreed that the Tower "Kept my attention and interest". Some students found the speed of downloading each floor from the web site too slow and detracted from the experience even though all had DSL or cable connections. When we asked the students, "Do you think this interactive methodology is helpful in learning cancer genetics principles and applications?", 14 answered in the affirmative and 3 in the negative. The same distribution of responses was elicited when we asked, "If the entire 'Clinical Cancer Genetics Curriculum' were available in the Tower, would you be interested in using it to learn more about cancer genetics?"

The following comments were offered by the students:

- "I was impressed with how well this program worked and how much information it contained/was linked to."
- "I enjoyed the interactive nature of the exercises. It was more interesting to go and actively find the answers to clinically relevant questions than to just sit and read a text book about cancer."

- "I liked how all the resources were available and it was interactive, including articles to read as a learning method, but some of it was just time consuming and excessive clicking back and forth to different modules. I liked the games, I liked the videos, I liked the clinical application and the ability to type in notes. I'm not sure if that makes up for the time-consumption in terms of efficiency in learning and studying. I personally might prefer to simply learn the material in the old-fashioned lecture/paper syllabus manner, and then use a program like this for application to see if I've absorbed the information."
- "I think this computer module is a great learning tool."
- "Overall a neat concept, and makes learning much more fun."
- "What an incredible program! It definitely kept my attention and made learning fun. Great job!"
- "This is a great modality and has many uses in medical education. There could be a tower of learning for absolutely everything we have to learn, and all of medical school could be made virtual! It might be interesting if other medical students were visible occupying the same virtual space that would be neat and social."
- "My aim became to achieve the learning objectives and get the 100%. I didn't really try to synthesize the information given to me."
- "I think this site is a great way to teach medical/grad students more about cancer genetics."
- "I absolutely love this learning tool, excellent structure and easy to use."

Discussion

The serious gaming movement is in its infancy and developing rapidly. In a recent article, Joel Foreman [9] interviewed four leaders of the serious gaming movement. The consensus view is that:

- Conventional instruction is dysfunctional. Today's learners/students are accustomed to learner centered curricula. Passive lectures and seminars are not part of this culture. The era of teacher centered instruction is coming to an end.
- Simulations are powerful learning environments. Computer-based games have the power of simulating an environment where the player/learner takes on a new identity and is empowered to explore the learning space to find answers to questions or to achieve the goals of the "game". Learners can have experiences in this virtual world that they just are not able to have in the "real" world.
- Computer games promise a better learning future. In good computer games, information is provided "On Demand" and "Just in time" to solve a problem, the most effective way to learn. Games are the most engaging intellectual pastime that we have invented. Features of learning resources that current cognitive sciences agree enable people to learn best are incorporated into the best computer-based games. The most important feature is frequent decision making and speed of access.

A successful learning tool requires an effective educational strategy and a cognitively efficient design to capitalize on the advantages of presenting information in multiple modalities [10]. Constructivism is a learning theory that sees knowledge as an integrated body of information where each bit of information fits into the learner's existing body of knowledge. When adopting this theory of learning, computer-based learning environments must actively engage students to interpret and reflect on the problems they are challenged to solve [11]. We adopted a constructionist approach to learning as we developed the Tower. The students' responses to the Tower suggest that the structure of our serious game is on the right track to better helping our information-age students to learn.

Grunwalk and Corsbie-Massay [10] have summarized guidelines for developing computer-based learning resources to create active learners and encourage long-term retention of newly-acquired knowledge. The feedback from the students indicate that the design of the Tower has successfully incorporated many of their guidelines, including: encouraging learners to make active choices; adopting an authentic context so that information learned can be applied to a real setting; providing feedback to learners; providing an integrated learning environment; providing an applications that is entertaining and engaging, and; providing a "virtual companion" to guide the learner.

The Tower is scheduled for completion by the summer of 2007 and will be an assigned learning resource for first year medical students matriculating in 2007. To evaluate the effectiveness of the Cancer Genetics Tower, we will compare the performance of this year's first year students (who did not have access to the Cancer Genetics Tower) on standardized multiple choice and essay examinations with the performance of next year's first year students on the same examinations.

The Cancer Genetics Tower will continue to be available to the worldwide educational community at our website and we welcome feedback from all those who access it. We believe that the time for faculty to integrate such serious gaming applications into their teaching strategies is now. This work was supported by PHS, NCI R25 CA092357-01A2.

References

[1] Ruiz, J. G., Mintzer, M. J., and Leipzig, R. M. (2006): The impact of E-learning in medical education. *Acad Med* 81, 207-12.

[2] Gibbons, A., and Fairweather, P. (2000): Computer-based instruction, pp. 410-442. In S. Tobias, and J. Fletcher (Eds): *Training & Retraining: A Handbook for Business, Industry, Government, and the Military* Macmillan Reference USA, NY.

[3] Bernard, R., Abrami, P. L., Lou, Y., and Borokhovski, E. (2004): How does distance education compare with classroom instruction? a meta-analysis of the empirical literature. *Review of Educational Research* 74, 379-439.

[4] Wentling, T., Waight, C., Gallaher, J., J., L. F., Wang, C., and Kanfer, A. (2000): E-Learning: A Review of Literature 2000. University of Illinois National Center for Supercomputer Applications, Urbana-Champaign, IL. http://learning.ncsa.uiuc.edu/papers/elearnlit.pdf

[5] Chumley-Jones, H. S., Dobbie, A., and Alford, C. L. (2002): Web-based learning: sound educational method or hype? A review of the evaluation literature. *Acad Med* 77, S86-93.

[6] Wright, W. (2006): Dream machines. *Wired Magazine* 14.

[7] Barnett, D. J., Everly, G. S., Parker, C. L., and Links, J. M. (2005): Applying educational gaming to public health workforce emergency preparedness. . *American Journal of Preventive Medicine* 28, 390-395.

[8] Henry, J. M. (1997): Gaming: A teaching strategy to enhance learning. *Journal of Continuing Nursing Education* 28, 231-234.

[9] Foreman, J. (2004): Game-based learning: How to delight and instruct in the 21st century. *Educause Review* 39, 50-66.

[10] Grunwald, T., and Corsbie-Massay, C. (2006): Guidelines for cognitively efficient multimedia learning tools: educational strategies, cognitive load, and interface design. *Acad Med* 81, 213-23.

[11] Gross, R. (1992): *Psychology: The science of mind and behavior*. Hodder and Stoughton. London.

Medicine Meets Virtual Reality 15
J.D. Westwood et al. (Eds.)
IOS Press, 2007

Surgical Scissors Extension adds the 7th axis of Force Feedback to the Freedom 6S

Marilyn J. POWERS[1], Ian P.W. SINCLAIR[1], Iman BROUWER[2], Denis LAROCHE[2]
[1] MPB Communications Inc., Montreal, QC, Canada
[2] Industrial Materials Institute, National Research Council, Boucherville, QC, Canada

Abstract. A virtual reality surgical simulator ideally allows seamless transition between the real and virtual world. In that respect, all of a surgeon's motions and tools must be simulated. Until now researchers have been limited to using a pen-like tool in six degrees-of-freedom. This paper presents the addition of haptically enabled scissors to the end effector of a 6-DOF haptic device, the Freedom 6S. The scissors are capable of pinching a maximum torque of 460 mN·m with low inertia and low back-drive friction. The device is a balanced design so that the user feels like they are holding no more than actual scissors, although with some added inertia on the load end. The system is interchangeable between the 6-DOF and 7-DOF configurations to allow switching tools quickly.

Keywords. Haptic Device, Force Feedback, Haptics, Surgical Simulation, Scissors

Introduction

Haptic interface devices deliver a sense of 'being there' to the operator of a virtual reality surgical simulator or to the operator of a master device in a teleoperated system. These devices come in a variety of degrees-of-freedom (DOF), 3-DOF, 5-DOF and 6-DOF, etc. Six-DOF devices enable the simulation of three translations and three rotations. In surgical simulation this gives the user the ability to feel torque (multiple point contact) on the end of the surgical instruments as he/she pokes and prods tissues. Enabling a grasping, pinching and cutting function provides more complete simulation of basic surgical maneuvers. Haptically enabled scissors are not new, however previous developments provide only two DOF [1]. This paper presents the specifications and performance of a detachable scissors handle to an existing 6-DOF haptic device, the Freedom 6S [2]. The resulting device provides the user with 7 degrees of force feedback and 7 degrees of positioning capability.

1. Requirements

The goal of a haptic device is to deliver forces from the virtual world to the user with maximum transparency. This requires lightweight, rigid links that permit the user to move freely in free space but also provide significant stiffness when hitting a rigid virtual object. Ideally the user should not be able to distinguish between the real world, holding their surgical instruments in this case, and the virtual world [3]. This sets up a long list of strict criteria for design. The following sections will explain those requirements.

1.1. Defining Scissor Parameters

The first criteria to define are the performance parameters. Scissors should be capable of reproducing forces typically found in a surgical procedure. Ideally these forces would be measured in-vivo on the tissues of interest. This is difficult both ethically and practically because of the hostile environment of the autoclave for sensors. Studies have been done to measure these forces in-vitro [4]. In [4], several tissues were tested giving large variability in torque requirements depending on tissue. The initial end use of our scissors is neurosurgery simulation. Therefore, much lower forces are anticipated.

To establish the ballpark range of torque needed to hold and cut a small artery, basic experiments were performed at the Industrial Materials Institute (NRC, Boucherville, QC). Teflon tubing was used to simulate the properties of an artery. Torques were applied by attaching calibrated weights at known distances from the hinge. Two types of scissors were used to measure closing torque: 14.5cm Metzembaum scissors and 10cm Lexer baby scissors. Using either scissor, 3-4N of force was required to cut the tube. The maximum peak torque is listed in Table 1.

To establish a maximum continuous torque a secure grasping test was performed using a 12.5cm mosquito hemostat and a Teflon tube. A 1N force with a lever distance of 80mm was required in order to secure the tube within the jaws of the hemostat. At this closing torque the tube would not slip even when applying an intuitively large force. The continuous torque required is listed in Table 1.

Table 1. Results of Scissor Tests

Test	Result
peak torque (4N at 9cm lever arm)	360 mN·m
continuous torque (1N at 8cm lever arm)	80 mN·m

1.2. Ergonomic Considerations

Since the scissors are the primary point of contact with the operator, ergonomics must play a key role in the design. Ergonomic considerations include the length and weight of the hand controller scissors, and the ability to achieve the same motions and grasps that a surgeon would perform using real surgical scissors.

In order to define range-of-motion parameters, we consulted with Dr. R. Del Maestro, Director of the Brain Tumor Research Centre, Montreal Neurological Institute, McGill University, Montreal, Canada. The most important factors were: how the scissors are held and the stance of the surgeon during surgery. For full range-of-motion, surgeons grasp around the scissor handles with their thumb and middle finger with the index finger resting on the hinge (Figure 1). This allows approximately 280° of rotation versus 180° if the index finger rests on the lower handle and/or the fingers are inserted in the handle loops.

With this grasp the design must allow for the operator to place his/her index finger on the hinge or center of rotation of the scissor. The handles must be the appropriate length to allow this as well. Additionally the weight and feel of the scissors must mimic that of real scissors.

The opening angle of scissors need not be larger than the maximum separation distance between the human thumb and middle finger. However, a surgeon would not use the extremes of his/her motion abilities for reasons which could include a mechanical disadvantage of the muscles at the limits or a loss of fine motor control. In examining literature on surgical cutting, it is observed that the maximum opening angle of scissors is less than 40° [5,6].

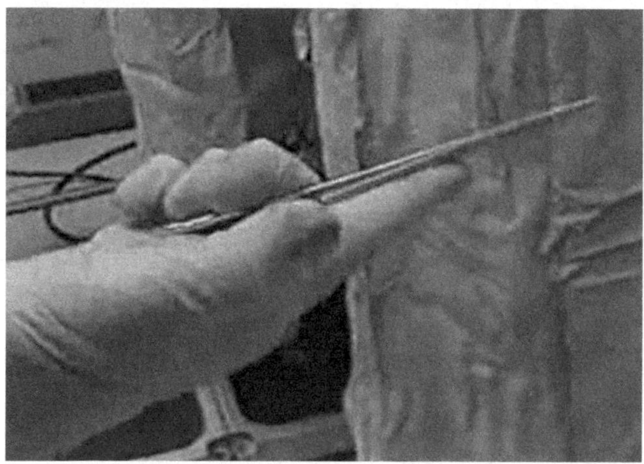

Figure 1. Recommended grip of surgical scissors for maximum rotation.

1.3. Interchangeable Tools

The seventh degree-of-freedom (DOF) need not be limited to scissors. There are many other tools used in surgery that have a similar grasping motion, such as hemostats and forceps of different kinds. As well it should be possible to convert the scissor handles back to a single handle instrument (e.g. scalpel). Therefore, one design consideration was to enable the scissor handles to be quickly changed to another type of handle.

2. Final design of the scissors

The final design is shown in Figure 2. It is shown attached to the Freedom 6S hand controller, and is appended as a seventh stage serially connected to six supporting stages. The lowest three stages are directly coupled to motors at the shoulder of the device, while the upper four stages are driven by tendons attached to a cluster of motors that are grounded to the frame of the device. The design rational has been set out in [2,7].

The scissors comprise two handles, one fixed to the roll axis and one rotating about a hinge with its axis normal to the handle roll. The handles are actually stubs with mechanical connectors, allowing for different types of handles to be attached to the device. If the movable handle is left off, a handle representing a scalpel or other single-axis instrument may be attached.

Polymeric tendons provide one of the lightest mechanisms for transferring torque from a stationary motor to a mechanism on an extended arm. The tendons are guided along the arm and the distal stage by means of pulleys mounted on low friction bearings. The scissors design required a unique set-up of idler pulleys (patent pending) to guide the tendons whilst maintaining the full range-of-motion in yaw, pitch and roll. A rotary sensor is placed on the axis of the hinge for direct angle measurement.

The design allows the index finger to rest on a flat surface, which is the top surface of the scissors pinch pulley. The final length of scissor handles was determined to be 8cm, typical of some surgical instruments but also an average 'comfort' length. The shape and size of the handle loops is similar to surgical scissors. There is one main difference between the Freedom 6S's scissors and actual surgical scissors. Surgical scissors are made of stainless steel and therefore can be made thin with a round cross section. Because of the weight considerations in a haptic device, aluminum is the material of choice. The cross section must then be larger, especially in the axis of greatest torque.

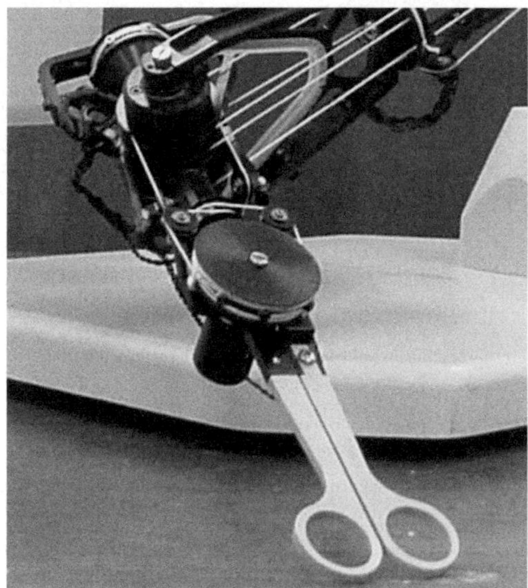

Figure 2. Scissor extension

3. Kinematics

Adding the seventh degree of freedom complicates the kinematics. Although kinematics are specific to the Freedom 6S, there are some points which are general to all machines that incorporate tendons. The pull of the tendon on joints closer to the distal stage has an effect on the torque of the lower stages. This "crosstalk" between stages is countered by a reverse torque calculated from static force and torque considerations. The effect is especially strong in the scissors, where squeezing the scissors handles against an uncompensated torque load would cause them to rotate in roll. We therefore add a counter-torque to oppose this induced roll torque.

4. Testing the Haptic Scissors

The resultant end effector including the scissor handles has an apparent mass of 40g, comparable to stainless steel surgical scissors, which are also about 40g. This light weight is possible because of the counterbalancing of the assembly. The inertia that the scissors carry when held at the hinge is estimated to be 170 g, compared to the normal 125 g inertia of the Freedom 6s.

The maximum peak force that the scissors can deliver was measured using a weigh scale (Ohaus Scout II, 400 g × 0.1 g scale). One handle of the scissors was placed on the scale, while the other was under the scale. Torque requests up to 500 mN·m were applied by instruction from a computer program; actual torque to over 460 mN·m was measured by the scale (since the software takes into account current limits in the circuits). (The displayed scale reading, say 100 g, is multiplied by gravity, 9.8 N/kg, to give 1 N; this is multiplied by the lever arm, 22 cm, to give 220 mN·m torque.)

Linearity of torque over the range of motion is also important. This can be shown by repeating the force measurements for various requested torque values. The left plot in Figure 3 shows torque linearity over a wide range of measured versus requested torque.

Position resolution is of great importance in a hand controller, since this determines in large part the ability of the device to control a robot arm in contact with a hard surface, or, equally, a virtual probe in touch with a rigid virtual surface. We placed a micrometer in a vise in such a way as to push on the end of the movable handle, while the fixed handle was held immobile in another vise. Thus we were able to compare angle measurements sensed in the hand controller to externally measured angles (Figure 3 – right). The deviation (computed from the root mean square error between the two) was 9.7 μrad.

Backdrivability of the scissors is very low, as the scissors open and close with a minimum of torque. The stiffness of the scissors, the ability to press against a virtual wall of a given stiffness without vibration, is some 11.4 mN·m/rad, exceeding the design target of 5 mN·m/rad

The addition of the scissors did not degrade the torque or workspace of the other six degrees of freedom. In fact, the newly redesigned distal center housing increased the stiffness of the roll from 0.2 to 4.4 mN·m/rad, and that of the yaw from 2.5 to 21 mN·m/rad. There is, on the other hand, some increase in roll friction on our test unit, as we have increased tension in the roll tendon. The final specifications of the Scissors attachment are listed in Table 2.

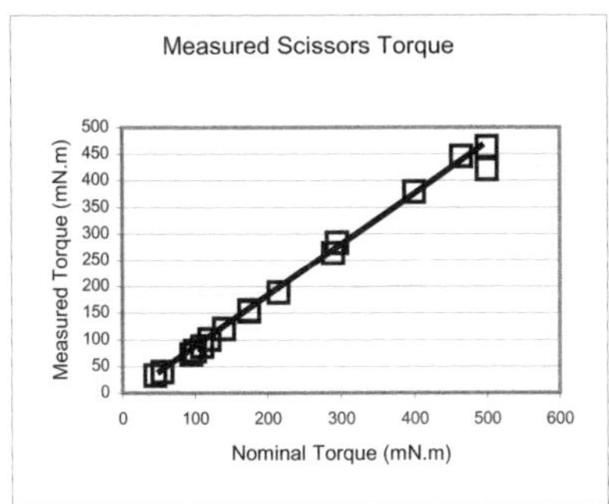

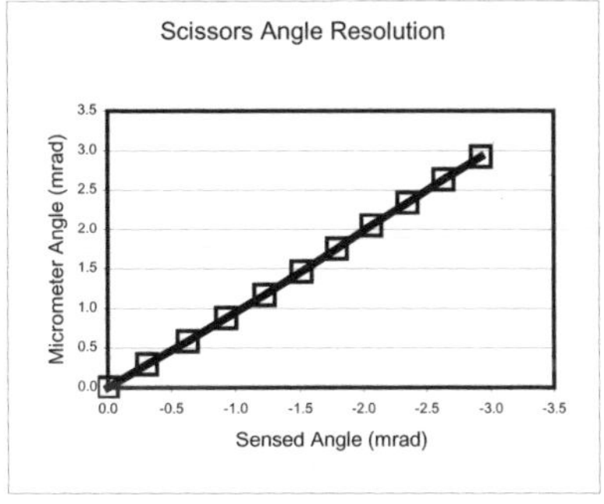

Figure 3. Sensor Angle Resolution and Torque Linearity of Scissors

Table 2. Specifications of the Haptic Scissors

Specification	Required	Achieved
Maximum torque	360 mN·m	460 mN·m
Continuous torque	80 mN·m	100 mN·m
Maximum angle	40°	40°
Position Resolution		9 μrad
Stiffness	5 N·m/rad	11.4 N·m/rad

5. Conclusions

The scissors attachment is capable of simulating a wide range of forces seen in soft tissue manipulation. The addition of scissors to a 6 DOF device provides a highly maneuverable haptic interface ideal for surgical simulation. The ability to detach the scissors and replace them with hemostats, forceps and other grasping tools responds to the surgeon requirements for adaptability and flexibility, better mirroring surgical practices.

Acknowledgements

We would like to thank Dr. Rolando Del Maestro, Director, Brain Tumour Research Centre, Montreal Neurological Institute, for his input on surgical technique. Dr. Marilyn Powers is funded through NSERC on an Industrial Research and Development Fellowship.

References

[1] Okamura, A.M., R.J. Webster III, J.T. Nolin, K.W. Johnson, H. Jafry. The haptic scissors: cutting in virtual environments. Proceedings of the 2003 IEEE International Conference on Robotics & Automation, 2003, 828-833.

[2] Demers, J.-G.S., J.M.A. Boelen, I.P.W. Sinclair. Freedom 6S force feedback hand controller. SPRO '98, 1st IFAC Workshop on Space Robotics, Montreal, Canada. October 19-22, 1998.

[3] Astley, O.R. and V. Hayward. Design constraints for haptic surgery simulation. Proceedings of the IEEE Int. Conf. on Robotics and Automation, San Francisco, CA. April 2000, 2446-2451.

[4] Greenish, S., Hayward, V., Chail, V., Okamura, A. and Steffen, T. Measurement, analysis and display of haptic signals during surgical cutting. Presence, 11:6, 2002, 626-651.

[5] Chial V.B., S. Greenish, A.M. Okamura. On the display of haptic recordings for cutting biological tissues. IEEE Proceedings of the 10th Symp. On Haptic Interfaces for Virtual Envir. & Teleoperator Systems. 2002,

[6] Mahvash, M. and Okamura, A.M. A fracture mechanics approach to haptic synthesis of tissue cutting with scissors. First Joint Eurohaptics Conference & Symposium on Haptic Interfaces for Virtual Environments & Teleoperator Systems (World Haptics), 2005, 356-362.

[7] Hayward, V., P. Gregario, O. Astley, S. Greenish, M. Doyon, L. Lessard, J. McDougall, I. Sinclair, S. Boelen, X. Chen, J.-P. Demers, J. Poulin. Freedom-7: A high fidelity seven axis haptic device with application to surgical training. ISER'97, Barcelona, Spain. June 15-18, 1997. 445-456.

Medicine Meets Virtual Reality 15
J.D. Westwood et al. (Eds.)
IOS Press, 2007

An Adaptive Framework Using Cluster-Based Hybrid Architecture for Enhancing Collaboration in Surgical Simulation

J.Qin[1], P.A.Heng[1,2], K.S.Choi[3] and Simon S.M. Ho[4]
[1] *Dept. of Computer Science & Engineering, The Chinese University of Hong Kong*
[2] *Shun Hing Institute of Advanced Engineering, The Chinese University of Hong Kong*
[3] *Department of Computing, Hong Kong Polytechnic University*
[4] *Department of Diagnostic Radiology & Organ Imaging, CUHK*

Abstract. Research on collaborative virtual surgery opens the opportunity for simulating the cooperative work during surgical operations. It is however a challenging task to design and implement a high performance collaborative surgical simulation system because of the difficulty in maintaining a high level of state consistency under limited network transmission capacity. In this paper, we present an adaptive framework using cluster-based hybrid architecture to support real-time collaboration in surgical simulation. In addition to the TCP communication protocol, the framework is also equipped with UDP for multicasting, allowing for a flexible strategy to reduce network latency. A set of techniques was proposed to assure reliable transmission on top of standard yet unreliable multicast protocols. Experimental results demonstrate that this framework can support collaborative surgical simulation with lower network latencies than traditional client-server architecture.

Keywords. Surgical Simulation, Network architecture, Reliable multicast protocol

1. Introduction

Recent years have witnessed the significant progress of computer-assisted surgical simulators to train novice surgeons and conduct rehearsals for medical procedures. While many surgical simulation systems have been developed, most of them focus on the simulation of surgical interventions involving a single user in the virtual environment. In reality, surgical operation is usually a teamwork requiring a group of medical practitioners to cooperate with each other. In this regard, collaborative architecture is a necessary component of future surgical simulators. However, it is a challenging task to design and implement a high performance collaborative surgical simulation system because of the requirement to maintain a high level of state consistency under the limitation of network transmission capacity [1]. In particular, considerable network resource is required for timely distribution of every event occurred in the virtual surgical procedures.

In this paper, we present an adaptive framework to support real-time collaboration in surgical simulation. A cluster-based hybrid network architecture is proposed to decrease network latencies using a circular topology, where the consistency of the system is maintained through an administrative server. A reliable transmission protocol supporting end-to-end principle as well as multicast approach is provided. A prototype system based on this proposed framework has been implemented. Experimental results demonstrate our framework has lower network latency than client-server architecture, meeting the requirement for state consistency in collaborative surgical simulation.

2. The Framework

2.1 Cluster-based hybrid network architecture

Network architecture supporting collaborative surgical simulation has conventionally been dominated by client-server (C-S) (Figure 1(a)) and peer-to-peer (P2P) (Figure 1 (b)) strategies [2]-[5]. Unfortunately, neither of them can sufficiently support collaborative surgical simulation. Although the C-S architecture can maintain a high level of system consistency, the network latency is relatively high because of the transmission bottleneck at the server. On the other hand, the P2P architecture can minimize the latency but consistency is not guaranteed because of the absence of a server as the arbiter. In [6], the authors proposed a multi-server architecture to avoid potential inconsistency in simulating cooperative tasks while supporting low-latency interactions. (Figure 1(c)) However, with the increase in the number of clients attached to one of the servers, network latency is still a problem. In addition, when the number of servers is large, synchronization between these servers is a time-consuming task.

Figure 1. Network architecture supporting collaborative surgical simulation. (a) Client-server (b) Peer-to-peer (c) Multi-servers (d) Our cluster-based architecture

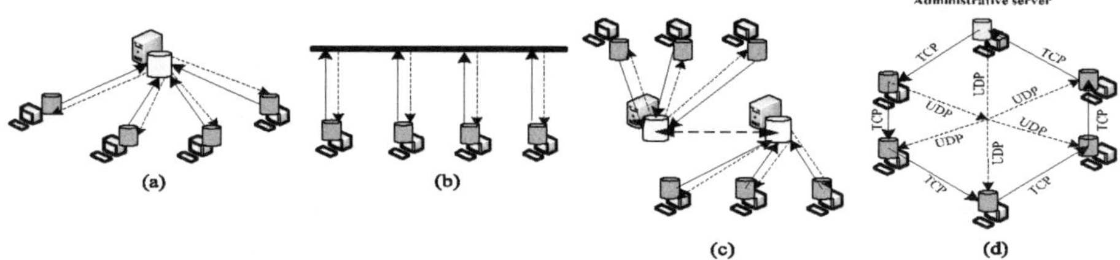

Figure 2. Pseudo code of algorithms for reliable multicast. (a) Regular reliable multicast (b) Multicast optimization based on cluster cooperation

We proposed a cluster-based hybrid architecture in which participants constitute a circular structure (Figure 1(d)). The updated information can be transmitted to the involved participants according to the topology view stored in every participant. An administrative server is assigned to manage the topology view, handling the joining and leaving requirement gracefully and informing all participants the transformation of the topology view. The proposed approach tackles the disadvantage of traditional C-S architecture by reducing the additional latency caused by the round-trip to the server as well as avoiding the transmission bottleneck at the server. Meanwhile, system consistency can be well maintained by the administrative server and a reliable transmission protocol, which will be discussed in next section.

2.2 Communication Protocol

Two communication mechanisms are provided based on the proposed cluster-based architecture. When participants transmit the updated information according to the topology view one by one, TCP protocol is used to ensure communication reliability. For some surgical simulators where computation-intensive deformable simulation and haptic rendering are involved, a multicast mechanism using UDP protocol could be adopted. Reliable message exchange on top of multicast protocols is implemented by using a number of techniques: multicast is optimized based on cluster cooperation; flow-control is handled by using sliding windows; the cluster-based collaborative algorithms is extended to facilitate distributed message acknowledgement; and the topology view is updated dynamically to prevent the blocking of message transfer due to failed instances.

2.2.1. Multicast Optimization Based on Cluster Cooperation

Reliable multicast requires all the participants involved to receive a message before the message being handled. Figure 2(a) shows the pseudo code of the basic reliable multicast algorithm where every participant transmits the received message to other participants to ensure the reliability of transmission. In our framework, cluster cooperation was utilized to simplify the algorithm based on *Distributed Message Acknowledgement*, which will be discussed in Section 2.2.3. In the algorithm, as illustrated in Figure 2(b), the function `wait()` puts a message M in the buffer and determine whether M has been received by other participants through distributed message acknowledgement. When M has been received correctly, the re-transmission operation will be omitted and substantive transmissions are avoided.

2.2.2. Flow Control Using Sliding Windows

In multicast, participants receive the messages in a random sequence due to network latencies. But in distributed surgical simulation, receiving updated information in an accurate sequence is an indispensable requirement. Sliding window technique is used in our framework to handle the flow-control problem in multicast. The principle of sliding window technique is shown schematically in Figure 3. Figure 3(a) shows the sliding window of a sender. A window of fixed width is put in the massage queue and only the messages within the window can be sent. The message blocks that have been acknowledged by all recipients are pained with a dark color. When the leftmost message in the window has been acknowledged by all the recipients, the window slides right by one or more message blocks. Correspondingly, each recipient also has a sliding

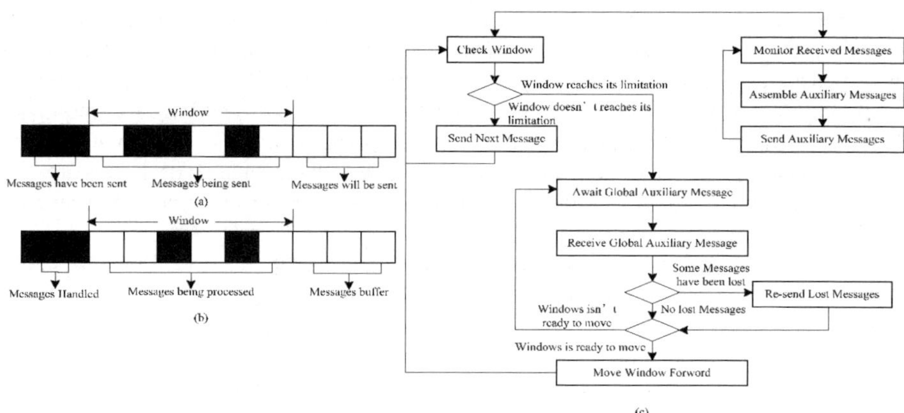

Figure 3. Flow control using sliding windows. (a) Sliding window in sender (b) sliding window in receiver (c) flow-control algorithm

window, which is illustrated in Figure 3(b). When the acknowledgment of the message with the least sequence number in the window has been received, the window slides right by one or more message blocks. Figure 3(c) shows the flow-control algorithm. The sender takes out the first massage from the queue and transmits messages until limited by the window's width W. At the same time, if the acknowledgment of the first message is not received, the send process will be blocked. The message will be re-transmitted when latency time exceeds a threshold T or an NAK message is received by the sender.

2.2.3. Distributed Message Acknowledgement

In our framework, the *Distributed Message Acknowledgment* (DMA) mechanism is used to optimize the multicast algorithm. The receiving information is encapsulated as an *Auxiliary Message*, which is resolved into two components: *Partial Auxiliary Message* (PAM) and *Global Auxiliary Message* (GAM). The administrative server is responsible for acquiring GAM by synthesizing a lot of PAMs provided by other participant. If the GAM indicates that some message has been received by all participants, the re-transmission operation will be omitted to reduce network latencies. (Figure 4)

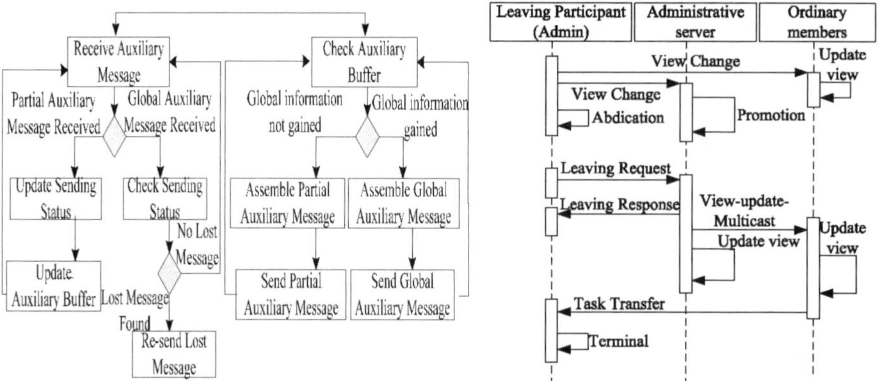

Figure 4. Distributed Message Acknowledgments   **Figure 5.** Administrative server leaving process

2.2.4 Dynamically updated topology view

Topology view of the cluster can be updated dynamically when participants join or leave. In particular, before the administrative server leaves, a new administrative server should be selected to take over its responsibility. Figure 5 shows the leaving procedure of administrative server.

2.2.5 Flexible Computational Policy

Sophisticated deformation model using in surgical simulation is a challenge for computing power and the network bandwidth. Depending on network traffic and resources, the system is adaptive by providing two computational policies: the *local-computation policy*, where deformation computation is off-loaded to individual participant; and the *global-computation policy*, where a participant with powerful computational capability handles the computation and distributes the results to other members. The bandwidth requirement for the former is low since the data transfer only involves the parameters of the computation. Provided that the network resources is adequate, the latter applicable for the situations where a high-performance machine is employed and the computing power of the other participants are limited.

3   Implementation and Results

The proposed framework has been implemented using Eclipse SDK 3.1.0. Network infrastructure and graphical rendering are respectively achieved with J2SE5.0 and OpenGL. The administrative server runs on an Intel Pentium(R) 4 computer, with 3.20GHz CPU, 1024M RAM and NVIDIA GeForce 6800 display adapter. All participants connect to the cluster through a 10Mb intranet. A comparison of the timing performance between the C-S architecture and our architecture are shown in Figure 6. In these experiments, a scalable deformation model, the force propagation model [7], is implemented to simulate some medical procedures involved in soft tissue deformation. It has a low bandwidth requirement as the information required for transfer only includes the mass points subjected to external forces and the associated force vectors. Figure 6(a) shows the timing performance when a user applies a force to 50 nodes of a virtual organ, whereas Figure 6(b) when there are five participants joining the collaborative deformation. Both experiments adopt *local-computation policy*. Obviously, the proposed cluster-based hybrid architecture can reduce the network

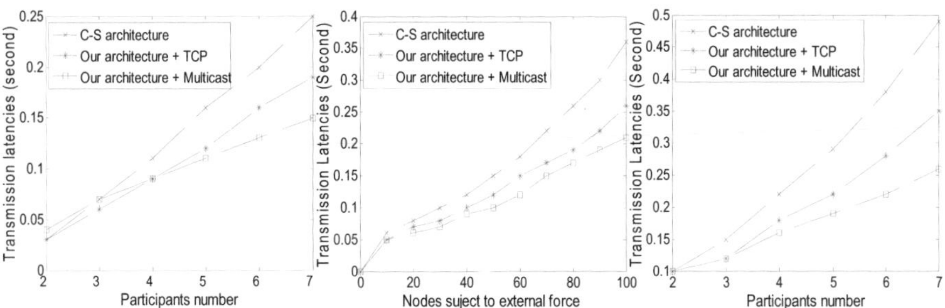

Figure 6. Timing performance of the proposed framework: local-computation policy applied for (a) 50 subjected nodes, and (b) 5 users; (c) 20 subjected nodes under the global computation policy

latency especially when the number of participants is large. The advantage is more significant when the participant number is large enough to counteract the additional overhead for the transmission reliability. Figure 6(b) shows that our architecture also avoids the transmission bottleneck occurred at the server of the C-S architecture when the number of nodes increases. Another experiment is set up to illustrate time performance of *global-computation policy* when a user applied a force to 20 nodes and force penetration depth [7] was set to 6. The results were shown in Figure 6(c). The transmission latency is greatly increased when compared to that of the *local-computation policy* (Figure 6 (a)).

4   Conclusion and Future work

In this paper, an adaptive framework for enhancing collaboration in surgical simulation is proposed. A prototype system based on this framework has been developed in our lab. Preliminary experiment results demonstrate this framework can support collaborative surgical simulation involved with sophisticated deformation models. Future work includes extending our framework to support haptically-enabled simulators and developing some clinical applications.

Acknowledgements

The work described in this paper was supported by grants from the Research Grants Council of the Hong Kong Special Administrative Region (Project no. CUHK4461/05M and PolyU 5145/05E) and CUHK Shun Hing Institute of Advanced Engineering.

References

[1]   Y.P. Chui, P.A. Heng, "Enhancing view consistency in collaborative medical visualization system using predictive-based attitude estimation", In Proceedings of the International Workshop on Medical Imaging and Augmented Reality, June 2001, IEEE Computer Society Press, pp.292-297.

[2]   K. Montgomery, C. Bruyns, J. Brown, S. Sorkin, F. Mazzella, G. Thonier, A. Tellier, B. Lerman, and A. Menon, "Spring: A General Framework for Collaborative, Real-Time Surgical Simulation", Medicine Meets Virtual Reality, Amsterdam: IOS Press, 2002.

[3]   V. Liberatore, M. C. Cavusoglu, Q. Cai, "GiPSiNet: An Open Source/Open Architecture Network Middleware for Surgical Simulations", Medicine Meets Virtual Reality 14 (MMVR 2006), 2006.

[4]   M. Oliveira, J. Mortensen, J. Jordan, A. Steed, and M. Slater, "Considerations in the Design of Virtual Environment Systems: A Case Study", Proc. Second Int'l Conf. Application and Development of Computer Games, Jan. 2003.

[5]   J. Qin, K.S. Choi, P.A. Heng, C.F. Chan and F.L. Chung, "A Distributed Simulation System for Virtual-Reality Based Medical Learning", In proceeding of World Congress on Medical Physics and Biomedical Engineering 2006.

[6]   J. Marsh, M. Glencross, S. Pettifer, and R. Hubbold, "A network architecture supporting consistent rich behavior in collaborative interactive applications", IEEE transactions on visualization and computer graphics, vol. 12, no. 3, 2006, 405-416.

[7]   K.S. Choi, H.Sun and P.A. Heng, "An efficient and scalable deformable model for virtual reality based medical applications", Artificial Intelligence in Medicine, vol.32, no.1, pp. 51-69, 2004.

Medicine Meets Virtual Reality 15
J.D. Westwood et al. (Eds.)
IOS Press, 2007

From Simulations to Automated Tutoring

Dr. Sowmya RAMACHANDRAN[a] and Dr. Barbara SORENSEN[b]
[a]Stottler Henke Associates, Inc, San Mateo, CA, USA
[b]AFRL/HEA, Mesa, AZ, USA

Abstract: Training medical personnel to maintain readiness for medical emergencies and combat-related operations is a critical problem. Distance learning solutions are required for enabling effective training while minimizing time away from the important on-the-job duties of providing quality medical care. Simulation-based training can significantly benefit learners by providing opportunities for hands on training. A simulation by itself, however, is not sufficient to enable learning. It must be accompanied by opportunities for reflection and a chance for learners to try their skills under different conditions. This means a simulation-based training course should include several scenarios. The high cost of developing and administering training scenarios renders this infeasible.

We have developed a simulation-based training framework called SimCore that incorporates intelligent, automated assessment and coaching in support of self-paced learning. This reduces the need for human facilitators. A key feature of this framework is an authoring tool that supports rapid scenario development and customization and is designed for use by subject matter experts and course developers. This brings down the cost of scenario development. The system has been designed to interface easily with third-party simulators, with minimal effort. It also includes a Flash-based simulator that can be played on a web-browser.

A beta version of SimCore is currently being distributed for evaluation.

Keywords: Simulation-based training, Intelligent Tutoring, Scenario Authoring Tool

1. Introduction

Simulation-based training can significantly benefit learners by providing them the opportunity to practice and learn from applying their skills and knowledge to realistic training scenarios [1, 2]. Traditionally, simulation-based training has meant live simulations. The logistics and cost of such simulation constrain how often they can be presented. Typically such simulations deliver one or two scenarios. With computer-based simulations, it is possible to deliver cost-effective training with the added benefit that trainees can play them anywhere, anytime. In order to support such self-paced learning, simulations must be accompanied by performance assessment and feedback. As the healthcare community starts to invest significantly in simulation-based training, it is running against the limitation of requiring hands-on instructor-led facilitation to make it effective. This is prohibitively expensive. Automated coaching and feedback reduces the need for instructor facilitation, thus making simulation-based training cost-effective and feasible.

According to Kolb [3], experiential learning is a cyclic process where a student works with a concrete situation, reflects on his experience, creates abstractions of the knowledge gained from the experience, and finally tries his new knowledge on other related situations. Simulations provide the concrete experience. Without reflection and abstraction, the experiential learning cycle would be incomplete. Typically instructors work with students to help complete the learning cycle but this makes the cost of simulation-based training considerably higher. Additionally, providing a personalized learning experience requires one-on-one instruction which can be prohibitively costly. Techniques from the field of Artificial Intelligence and Intelligent Tutoring systems can be applied to automate one-on-one personalized instruction including automated performance assessment, coaching and review. This will close the loop on the experiential learning cycle while freeing simulations from the requirement for dedicated instructors.

We are currently developing technologies for applying the concept of Intelligent Tutoring Systems (ITS) to healthcare simulations. ITSs are software tutors that are designed to provide one-on-one tutoring, much like humans [4]. As a first step in this direction, we are developing SimCore (**Sim**ulate, **Co**ach, **Re**view), a tool that adds intelligent performance assessment and coaching facilities to training simulations. Using SimCore, simulation developers can convert their simulations into automated, intelligent tutors. Freed from the need for hands-on instructor-led support, simulation systems can be used to deliver not one but a variety of scenarios, giving students the opportunity to learn by applying their newly acquired skills under varying conditions. SimCore allows for complex free-play simulations. It can be used to actively guide a student towards performing an action or a procedure, even as the simulation allows them the freedom to explore. Authoring tools are typically needed to make Intelligent Tutoring Systems a viable option [5]. SimCore includes a scenario authoring tool that can be used to rapidly customize existing scenarios or to create new ones.

2. Architecture

SimCore employs a client-server architecture with two server-side components (Figure 1): the authoring tool and the runtime server. The authoring tool enables the specification of training scenarios in abstract, high-level terms. The runtime server drives the simulation, initiates events, responds to and evaluates student actions, and provides after-action reports. The system has been designed to interface with third party simulators with minimal customization of the runtime engine or the authoring tool. A default Flash-based simulator is included with the SimCore package.

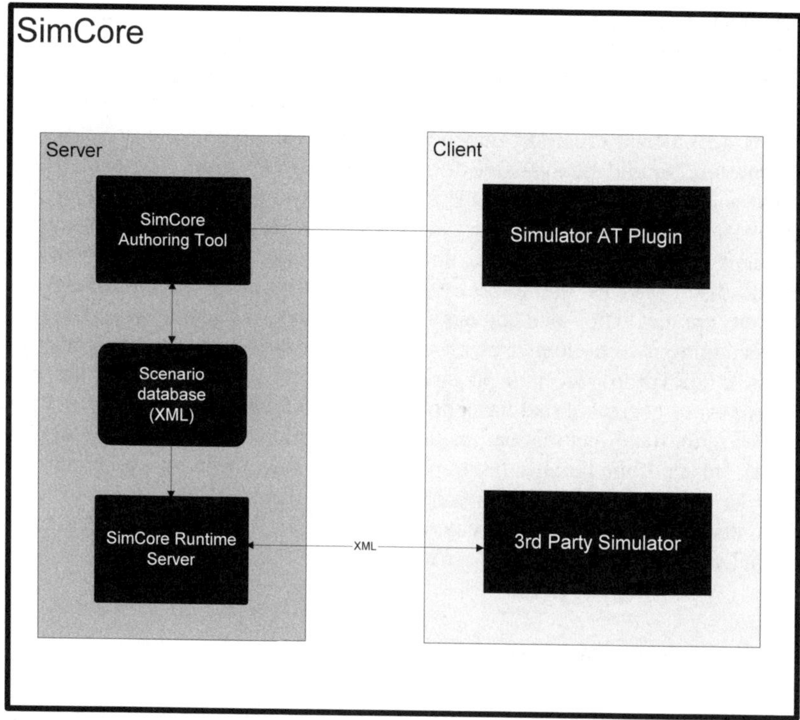

Figure 1; SimCore client-server architecture with two server-side components

The runtime server connects to a simulator via a simulator API. The simulator API must be customized to work with each specific Simulator. Communication between the runtime server and the simulator is done using XMI. In general, the simulator is responsible for maintaining the user interface for one or multiple players. The runtime server is responsible for maintaining the state of the simulated world.

3. Scenario Model

SimCore is based on a generalized, domain-independent scenario model. In the runtime server, the actions, props, etc. are represented by a set of Java Objects. These building blocks are created by the authoring tool, stored in a series of XML files, and read in by the runtime server. A scenario is composed of locations, props, NPCs (non-playing characters), and events. Locations represent the various different locations in a scenario. For example, a side of the street which is the scene of an accident can be a location. An ambulance may be a second location. Props are scenario objects in locations and can have actions performed on them. The car involved in an accident is an example of a prop. NPCs are virtual human characters in the scenario. The person hurt in the accident, as well as his companions in the car would be modeled as NPCs. Props and NPCs are associated with attributes that represent their states at any given time. For an NPC, for instance, the modeled attributes may include his/her vital signs, age, medications, allergies. The scenario model includes actions that be performed on the NPCs and Props.

Each action has a unique command name, a textual representation to display to players, a series of possible textual replies upon performing the action, a series of sub-areas on the target where the action can be performed, a set of preconditions as to when this action can be performed, and a set of effects that are executed after the action is performed. For example, "Check Blood Pressure" may be an action with the precondition that the blood pressure monitor should be available for performing this action. The action definition would also include rules specifying the simulators response when the player performs this action. A scenario also includes events. Sometimes it is necessary to change the scenario state when the player does not initiate an action. Events are the way to accomplish this. Events are a set of effects that will be performed if a set of preconditions are met. They also contain a trigger set that, if equal to true, will cause this event's preconditions to no longer be checked and the event will be made inactive. An example is a box (prop) that is supposed to explode in 30 seconds if it has not been opened. An event is created that has a precondition that checks to see if 30 seconds has passed. If so, run the effect that causes the box to explode. The inactive section of the event checks to see if the box has been opened. If so, then the event's preconditions will no longer be checked, and the box won't explode because of this event. Authoring a scenario entails instantiating the scenario model. The Runtime Server executes this model to deliver a training scenario.

4. Automated Performance Assessment and Coaching

SimCore includes an automatic performance assessment component that also guides students towards an optimal solution path. Each scenario can be associated with a solution template using the SimCore authoring tool. A solution template is a generalized procedure or protocol that is required to complete the scenario successfully. The solution template is not visible to the player; it is used behind-the-scenes to assess student performance. By a generalized procedure, we mean that the procedure can include unordered sets of actions and conditional actions. The solution template defines the actions the student should perform. The scenario author can also specify specific error rules that represent actions the student should not perform. During each scenario, the simulator software sends notification messages to the SimCore engine that describe each student action and report the values of each simulation state variable. SimCore evaluates each student action by comparing it with the solution template and the error rules contained within the scenario definition. This information is passed back to the simulation which then selects an appropriate feedback. In addition, this information is included in the after-action review. The solution template is also used by SimCore to provide just-in-time hints which are associated with the solution template during authoring.

5. Authoring tool

The authoring tool is a very important component of the SimCore framework. It enables the rapid development of training scenarios. The authoring tool has visual editors for defining the scenario model described earlier. In addition, there is a section in the authoring tool for specifying the solution templates and error rules. Hints and feedback to help coach can also be specified using these editors. Figure 2 shows the Props editor where scenario author can create Props, define their attributes, and the actions that can be performed on them.

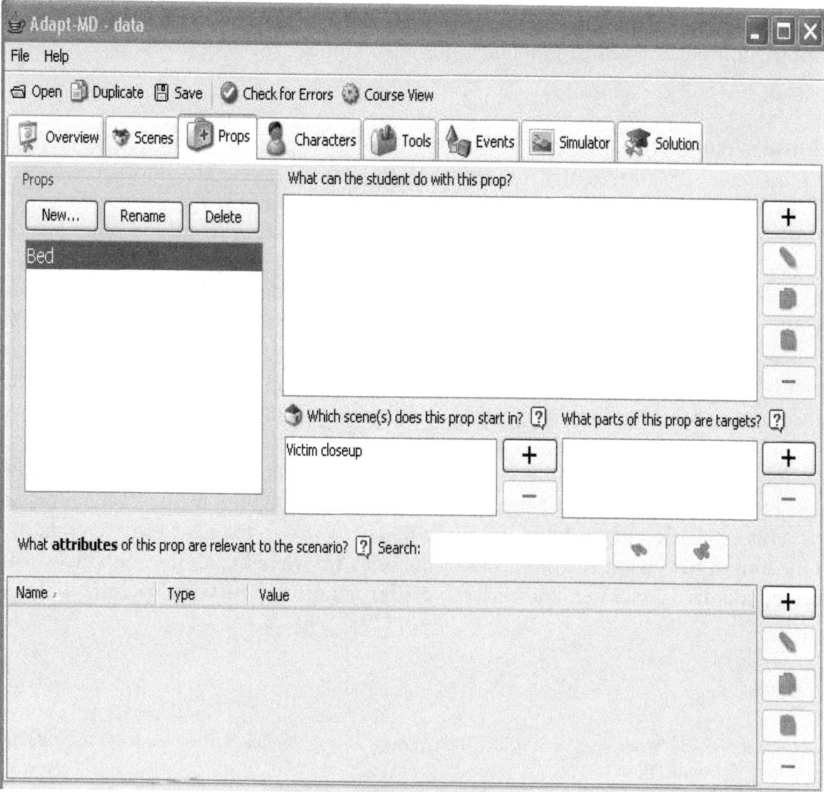

Figure 2: SimCore Authoring Tool

6. Evaluation

We developed the SimCore framework in three spirals. The software at the end of each spiral was demonstrated to experienced EMS trainers. Their suggestions have strongly influenced the design of the system. We are currently making the product available to beta testers and we will be collecting feedback from these users.

7. Related Work

A few intelligent tutoring systems have been developed for healthcare domains [6, 7]. In most such systems, the tutoring is tightly coupled with the simulation or the problem-solving interface. SimCore is based on a domain-independent scenario model and can thus be used for a broad range of domains. It is designed to be plugged into third-party simulators with minimal effort. [5] presents an in-depth discussion of authoring tools for Intelligent Tutoring Systems. The trade-off between power and usability is a central dimension that characterizes authoring tools. Our objective is to develop a tool that is usable by healthcare training experts who have little programming experience. Hence our first version of SimCore trades power for authoring simplicity. Future versions of the system will make the framework increasingly powerful while involving users in the development process to ensure that usability does not get sacrificed.

8. Future Work

SimCore beta is now available. SimCore is re-usable framework for developing low-cost, customizable simulations and training games for training EMS and other healthcare professionals. Using SimCore, subject matter experts and course developers can rapidly create simulations to test students' ability to apply their skills and decision-making capability in realistic scenarios. SimCore provides the facility to incorporate automated performance assessment and feedback, enabling organizations to create rapidly powerful, skill-application oriented self-paced training. A Flash simulator that is included as a part of the SimCore package makes the system usable by organizations that do not have a third-party simulator at their disposal.

In the near future, our primary objective to collect feedback from beta users on the system, understand how well it meets their needs, and gaps that must be addressed by future versions. Efficiency related improvements are also in the near-term agenda.

Our long-term vision for the product includes improved usability, enhanced student modeling, adaptive coaching, and reflective after-action review with Socratic dialogs.

References

[1] Schank, R. (1995), What We Learn When We Learn by Doing, *Technical Report no. 60*, Institute of Learning Sciences, Illinois.

[2] Johnson, W. B. and Norton, J.E. (1992). Modeling student performance in diagnostic tasks: A decade of evolution. In *Cognitive Approaches to Automated Instruction*. Eds. Regian, J.W and Shute, V.J. Lawrence Erlbaum Associates. 1992.

[3] Kolb, D. A. (1984) *Experiential Learning*, Englewood Cliffs, NJ.: Prentice Hall.

[4] Forbus , K. D., and Feltovich, P. J. (2001). *Smart Machines in Education*. AAAI Press.

[5] Murray, T., Blessing, S., and Ainsworth, S. (2003). *Authoring Tools for Advanced Technology Learning Environments: Toward Cost-Effective Adaptive, Interactive, and Intelligent Educational Software.* Springer.

[6] Shaw, E., Ganeshan, R., Johnson, W.L., and Millar, D (1999). Building a Case for Agent-Assisted Learning as a Catalyst for Curriculum Reform in Medical Education, In *Proceedings of the Int'l Conf. on Artificial Intelligence in Education*, July, 1999.

[7] Kizakevich, P.N., M. L. McCartney, D. B. Nissman, K. Starko, and N. Ty Smith (1998). Virtual Medical Trainer: Patient Assessment and Trauma Care Simulator. *Medicine Meets Virtual Reality - Art, Science, Technology: Healthcare (R)evolution*, J. D. Westwood, H.M. Hoffman, D. Stredney, and S.J. Weghorst, eds.,pp. 309-315, IOS Press and Ohmsha, Amsterdam.

Medicine Meets Virtual Reality 15
J.D. Westwood et al. (Eds.)
IOS Press, 2007

Haptics-Constrained Motion for Surgical Intervention [1]

Jing Ren [a,2], Huaijing Zhang [b], Rajni V. Patel [d,e] and Terry M. Peters [c]

[a] *Faculty of Engineering and Applied Science, University of Ontario Institute of Technology*
[b] *Dept. of Elect. and Comp, Qingdao Technological University*
[c] *Imaging Research Labs, Robarts Research Institute*
[d] *Canadian Surgical Technologies & Advanced Robotics (CSTAR)*
[e] *Dept. of Elect. and Comp. Engrg., Univ. of Western Ontario*

Abstract. Current open-heart procedures requiring the use of a medial sternotomy and a heart-lung machine can potentially be performed by entering the heart through the cardiac wall. A new procedure in cardiac surgery involves introducing an ablation tool through the appendage of the left atrium. This method, intended for the treatment of atrial fibrillation, septal defect repair and valve replacement, provides increased control over the ablating instrument [1]. It is believed that this procedure will ultimately be performed under robotic control and image-guidance provided by intra-cardiac ultrasound. However, the intra-cardiac guidance presents several drawbacks, such as limited field of view, temporary loss of signal, and, in some cases, difficulty with interpreting the signal. We believe that the introduction of haptic feedback into this environment will enhance the procedure by providing tactile cues to assist in the location of the surgical targets. Keywords. Artificial potential fields, haptic feedback, sigmoid functions

Keywords. Artificial potential fields, haptic feedback, Gaussian functions

1. Introduction

In minimally invasive surgery, many safety and precision issues can be addressed through the use of haptic virtual fixtures. Recent literature reveals a great diversity in the application of studies concerning haptic fixtures [1,2]. In particular, one trend involves moving virtual fixtures closer to the operating room (OR). To this extent, we have proposed the use of dynamic 3D virtual fixtures generated directly from MR data of a beating heart in order to guarantee safety and improve precision by constraining the operator's motion relative to the target surface through haptic feedback.

[1]This research was supported by the Natural Sciences and Engineering Research Council (NSERC) of Canada under grants RGPIN-1345 and RGPIN-303802, by grants from the Ontario Research & Development Challenge Fund and the Canada Foundation for Innovation awarded to Robarts and CSTAR.

[2]Correspondence to: Jing Ren, Faculty of Engineering and Applied Science, University of Ontario Institute of Technology,L1H 7K4, Tel.: 01 905 721 3111 ext. 2865; E-mail: jing.ren@uoit.ca

2. Background

Our ongoing lab work is focused on augmenting surgical guidance with haptic feedback in order to complement the intra-operative environment that is designed to guide intervention based on pre-operative MR or CT images and intra-operative ultrasound (US) images. To achieve this goal, we need to perform the following steps, which are shown in the block diagram in Figure 1

- Acquire pre-operative MR/CT images to construct a three-dimensional map
- Build a force model using MR/CT images and create a combined virtual visual/haptic model.
- Register this virtual visual/haptic model to the patient and synchronize this model to patient using the ECG as a time reference
- Acquire intra-operative US images and map them to the haptic model to provide real-time force feedback to the surgeon during the surgical procedure

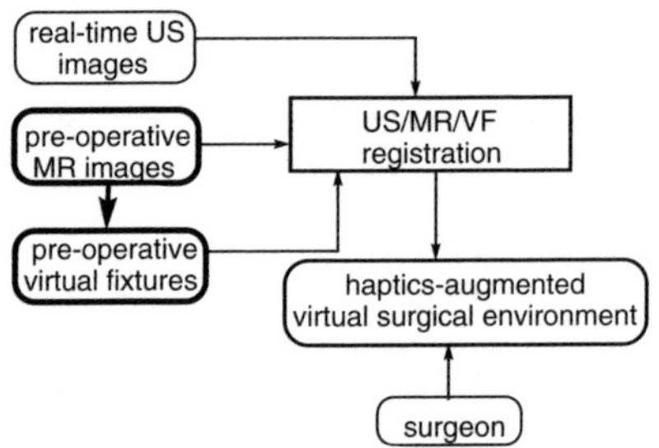

Figure 1. Haptics-augmented intra-cardiac intervention

Our primary objective in this study is to build a force model using MR/CT images and to create a combined virtual visual/haptic model. We apply a potential field-based force model to generate constrained motion on a beating heart phantom. The algorithms uses to generate the surface model and to register MR with US images have been described previously [4,3].

3. Method: Constrained Motion Using Gaussian Functions

In this section, we consider generating virtual fixtures to constrain the surgeon's motion to a predefined region. In this case, the region chosen is the surface of the heart. If we define $q = (x, y, z)$, the potential field based on generalized Gaussian functions can be written as,

$$f(q) = 1 - exp\left(-(\frac{q^2}{2\gamma^2})^m\right) \tag{1}$$

where γ and m are adjustable parameters.

Although continuity in the force model is helpful in order to eliminate undesired oscillations in the surgeon's motion, an ideal virtual fixture should be imperceptible to the operation when the tool is within the desired region. Rather, the user should only feel constraint forces when the tool is about to stray outside the boundary of the desired zone.

In practice, this means that both the slope of the constraint forces through the boundary zone and the location of the boundary zone should be adjustable. By changing the slope, we can change the magnitude of the constraint force that the surgeon feels as the tool approaches the boundary. Altering the location of the boundary zone ensures that the desired region can be made as large as possible, thereby allowing the magnitude of the constraint forces to increase. In our formulation, both of these adjustments are possible through changes to the two parameters m and γ.

Figure 2 illustrates that the feedback force can be easily localized to the boundary of the confined region by adjusting the parameter m. In Figure 2, 0 represents the surface, and $[-11]$ is the planned workspace that is defined by the parameter γ. When we set parameter $m = 1$, the operator will still perceive force even when the surgical tool is close to the surface. This condition can be improved by increasing parameter m. However, an extremely large value of m may result in oscillations near the boundary because the behavior of $f(q)$ is similar to that of an on-off switch control.

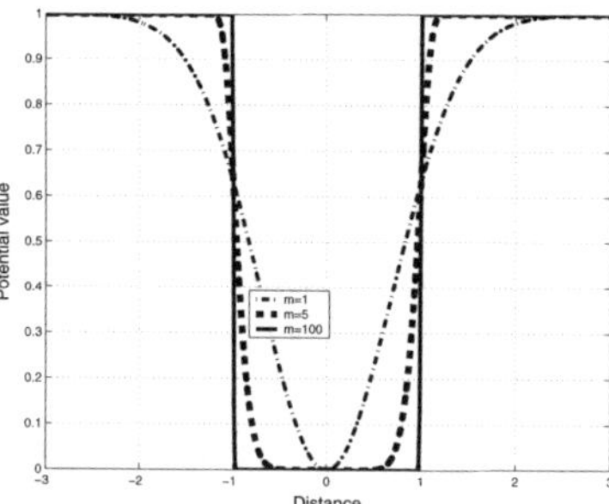

Figure 2. Effect of adjusting m

The parameter γ can be used to adjust the size of the confined area, which ensures that the surgeon does not feel force if the motion of the surgical tool is within the desired area. At the same time, any attempt to move the tool outside the desired area are restricted. Figure 3 illustrates variation in the workspace as a function of γ.

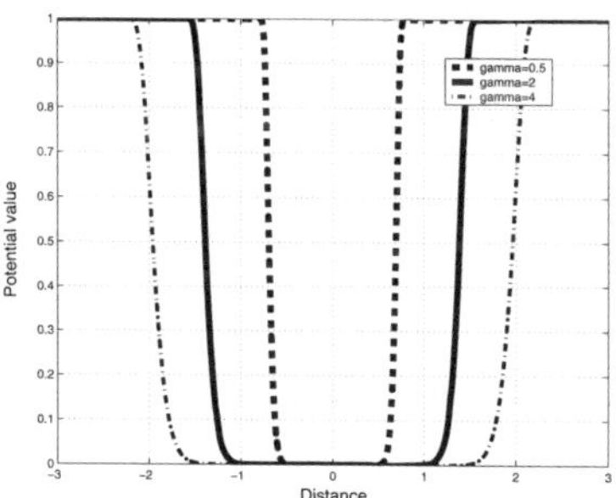

Figure 3. Effect of adjusting γ

The force can be defined as,

$$F_q = f_q(m)\frac{F_q'(m)}{\|F_q'(m)\|} \tag{2}$$

Figure 4 illustrates the potential force model, showing the potential fields for one slice of a heart surface model. The potential fields acquire a value of zero on the heart surface and increase as they move away from the surface.

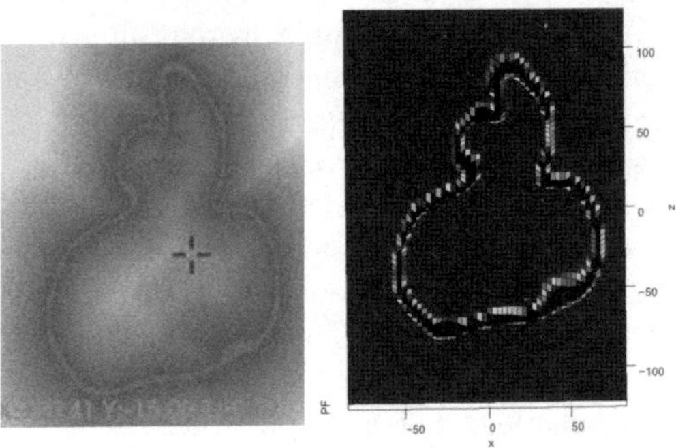

Figure 4. One slice of a heart surface model and its potential fields.

3.1. Evaluation

During robot-assisted cardiac surgery, surgical tools are often inserted to the workspace through small holes and surgeons need to operate with aid of image recorded by endoscope, and displayed in a video monitor. Poor hand-eye coordination, the restricted surgical field, and the low quality of image guidance make it difficult to perform even common procedures such as moving a surgical tool in a straight line or suturing.

However, these challenges can be addressed by our proposed force model. Using our model, we can generate an attractive force around the heart surface. As the user moves away from the pre-defined work area, the vicinity of the heart surface, he/she feels a force pushing the hand back. The force increases as the tool moves further away from the surface, and conversely, it decreases as the tool moves back towards the surface. The force model generates a fixture that is both continuous and soft; it is intended to provide guidance to the surgeon, rather than to restrict the motion of the instrument.

To illustrate the effectiveness of this constrained force, we perform a series of simulated tissue dissection procedures. These procedures use a surgical tool passing through a fixed pivot point in order to simulate the problem of poor hand-eye coordination, which results from the unnatural relationship between the user's hand movements and the motion of the instrument tip during laparoscopic minimally invasive surgery. Figure 5 illustrates a heart with ten pellets close to the surface. Each pellet represents a block of artificial tissue that needs to be removed from a location close to the heart. The goal of this procedure is to remove the tissue rapidly using a rod-like surgical tool.

Two subjects performed this procedure, yielding the results shown in Table 1. We observe that without force guidance, the users finish the task in more than 3 minutes. However, when employing a virtual fixture, the users can remove all ten blocks of tissue in less than half this time. Each observer performed the task ten times over a period of 10.

This decrease in the time to complete the task demonstrate the utility of the haptic-enhanced task. Figure6 illustrates constrained motion on a beating heart surface. Haptic force models are matched and superimposed on US images through the registration of

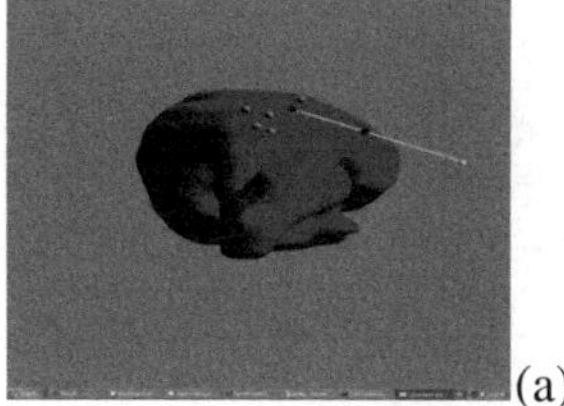
(a)

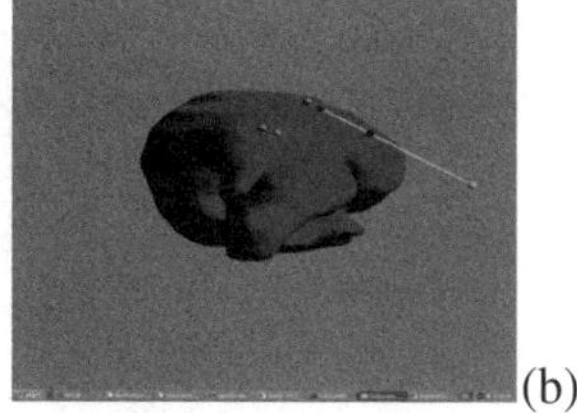
(b)

Figure 5. Evaluation on a simulated tissue dissection task

Table 1. Computation time comparisons

	(no force)	(with force)
1st Person	3'31"	1'30"
2nd Person	3'45"	1'26"

intra operative US and pre-operative MR images. Soft constraints on the heart guide the tip of the tool to the surface and thereby help the user to perform delicate cardiac procedures without restricting their freedom of motion.

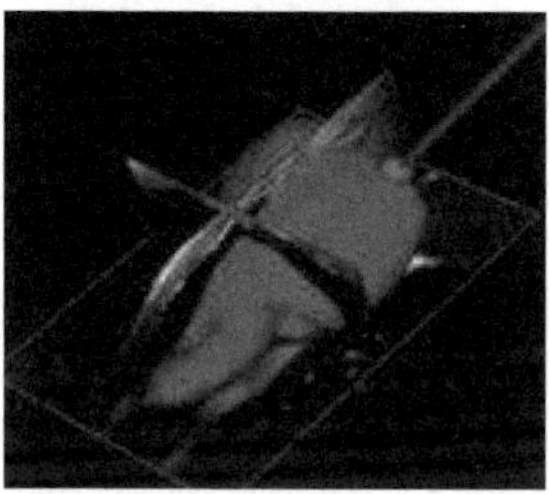

Figure 6. Constrained motion on the beating heart surface

4. Surgical Tools of Non-Point Shapes

In this preliminary work, we simplified the surgical tool to the shape of a point. However, in many applications, it is more reasonable to model the surgical tool as a generic shape rather than as a point: for instance, a cylinder can accurately represent the needle in brachytherapy and a torus is a more realistic model for the valve in mitral valve replacement. In this section, we extend our prior work as it applies to a surgical tool of a generic shape. This approach involves a three-step process; first, we divide the tool into multiple line segments and find the center point of each segment. Secondly, the feedback force is computed for the center point of each segment using the previously described method for points. Finally, we use the tip position to generate feedback force to the operator. The exact method used to divide the surgical tool into multiple line segments depends on the specific application, and it is important to achieve a balance between accuracy and computation time. In order to validate our method, we used a MR data set. The results from this research can be directly used for surgical training and planning. Figure 7 shows a toroidally shaped surgical tool.

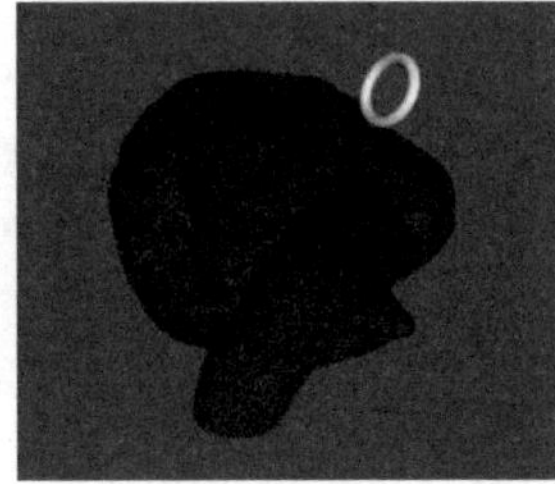

Figure 7. Constrained motion on the beating heart surface with a toroid-shaped tool.

5. Conclusion

In this paper, we have presented a method to augment a surgical guidance system with haptic feedback. Furthermore, we have described a procedure, based on Artificial Potential Fields, for generating constrained motion. Based on the results of our simulations, we believe that this approach has the potential to greatly increase the efficacy of robot assisted image-guided cardiac surgery. In our future work, we will integrate our approach with laboratory research into dynamically registered ultrasound and MR images, which will allow us to evaluate the utility of the virtual fixture model for intervention within the beating heart. We note however that effective utilization of this technique depends critically on robust spatial and temporal image registration of the model to the patient.

References

[1] A. Bettini et al. "Vision-assisted Control for Manipulation using Virtual Fixtures". *IEEE Transaction on Robotics*, vol. 20, pp. 953-966, 2004.

[2] S. Ekvall, D. Aarno and D. Kragic "Online Task Recognition and Real-Time Adaptive Assistance for Computer-Aided Machine Control". *IEEE Transaction on Robotics*, vol. 22, pp. 1029-1033, 2006.

[3] X. Huang, N.A. Hill, J. Ren, G. Guiraudon, D. Boughner and T. M. Peters, "Dynamic 3D Ultrasound and MRI Image Registration of the Beating Heart". *Medical Imaging Computing and Computer-Assisted Intervention (MICCAI)*, 2005

[4] M. Wierzbicki, M. Drangova, G. Guiraudon and T. M. Peters, "Validation of dynamic heart models obtained using non-linear registration for virtual reality training, planning, and guidance of minimally invasive cardiac surgeries", *Medical Image Analysis*, 18(3), pp. 387-401, 2004

Medicine Meets Virtual Reality 15
J.D. Westwood et al. (Eds.)
IOS Press, 2007

Development of a Guiding Endoscopy Simulator

Klaus RIEGER [a] and Reinhard MÄNNER [b]

[a] *Institute for Computational Medicine, University of Mannheim*
[b] *Institute for Computational Medicine, University of Mannheim and Department of Computerscience V, University of Mannheim*

Abstract. Endoscopy simulators get more and more common for the training of physicians. It is important to make simulation as realistic as possible by providing optical, acoustical and haptical feedback. The haptic display of our simulator *EndoSim* allows applying active forces to all degrees of freedom and moving to defined positions. This positioning is used for our automatic guiding system. If the user asks for help, an algorithm calculates how to get over the next barrier, factoring forces and distances. The system is able to decide if it is wise to choose a longer way in order to reduce the force. The user gets either an optical help shown by signs or is guided directly by the automatically moved endoscope. This guiding system is a new possibility for teaching physicians to increase their examination capabilities.

Keywords. EndoSim, Endoscopy simulators, active force feedback, automatic guiding system, training of physicians

Introduction

Endoscopic Examination

Endoscopic devices for gastroscopy and colonoscopy are flexible tubes that are inserted into the digestive system. They are equipped with an optical channel to transmit an image to a video display. For navigation the physician can bend the tip of the endoscope in two orthogonal directions by small wheels attached to the head of the endoscope.

Endoscopy Simulators

There are several reasons why simulators are becoming more and more common in medicine: Hospitals can evaluate the performance of their doctors [1]. Physicians can learn and improve their skills faster. The risk of the treatment can be reduced for patients [2].

For maximum success it is important to make the simulation as realistic as possible. In case of simulating flexible endoscopy it is necessary to give optical, acoustical and haptical feedback. If the trainee gets into trouble, advice should be given to find back to the right way. Help can be provided visually or by leading with active forces.

1. Methods

1.1. The Endoscopy Simulator EndoSim

Learning with our simulator *EndoSim,* the physician moves the flexible endoscope inside a pipe, in which forces are applied to it. In addition the navigation wheels provide force feedback from the bending of the endoscope's tip.

The simulator consists of a haptic interface and a computer. Dependent on the input of the haptic interface, the software calculates the output (force feedback, graphic, sound) using a real-time biomechanical simulation. As a result the physician feels the force by the endoscope, sees the video display and hears if the patient feels unwell.

The haptic display allows to apply active forces to all degrees of freedom. This is important for a realistic force feedback. The second possibility of the haptic display — moving to a defined position — is used for automatic guiding.

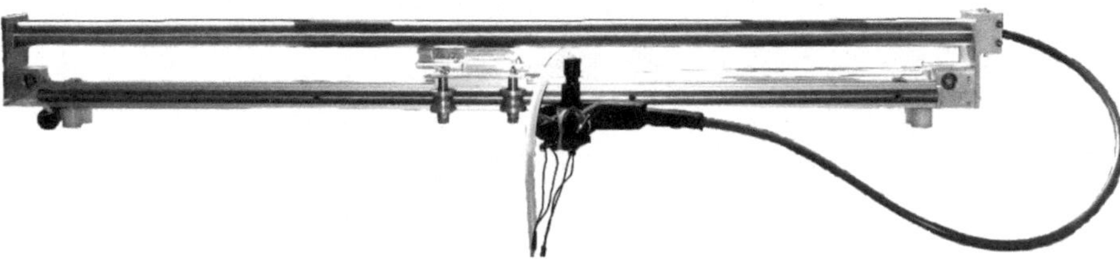

Figure 1. The haptic display of *EndoSim.*

1.2. The Automatic Guiding System

If the user asks for help, an algorithm calculates how to get over the next barrier (mostly an intestinal loop).

The movement of the user has four degrees of freedom and therefore there are eight directions possible. First the algorithm divides the movement into small, discrete steps. Then it calculates the occurring forces for every step. As one big force affects the patient more than many small forces, the different forces between endoscope and colon are summarized quadratically. This is done for all sensible[1] possible ways.

$$Force_{way} = \sum_{s=1}^{Steps} \sum_{f=1}^{Forces} F_{way,s,f}^2 \qquad Distance_{way} = \sum_{s=1}^{Steps} Increment_{way,s} \qquad (1)$$

To find the best way there is a rating: The primary argument is the minimal force, the secondary the minimal distance. The first argument results in forces as low as possible, the second avoids detours.

The best way is provided to the user by the simulator in one of these manners:

1. Successive flashing arrows show how to handle the endoscope.
2. Automatically guiding the user by moving the endoscope of the simulator.

---

[1] By using procedures to eliminate nonsensical ways, it is possible to reduce the order of the algorithm from $O(8^{Steps})$ to a lower order. The result is a faster calculation making more steps possible in a reasonable time.

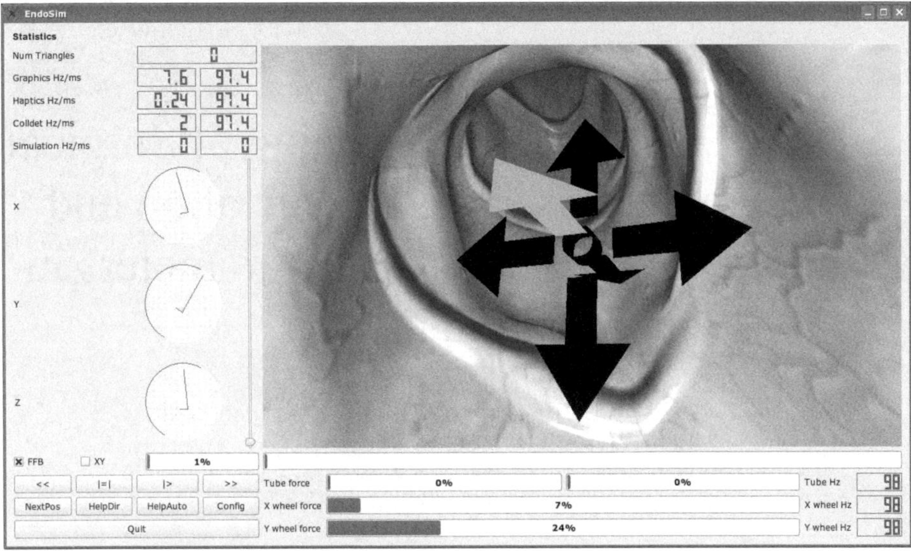

Figure 2. Screenshot of *EndoSim:* Flashing arrows show the best way.

2. Application and Results

Practicing the insertion of an endoscope through the colon up to the caecum is tested
and described as realistic by physicians [3]. Our algorithm for guiding the user is based
upon the well-tried real-time biomechanical simulation. It is able to decide if it is wise to
choose a longer way in order to reduce the force. The output using masking or positioning
works perfectly.

3. Conclusion and Discussion

So far, the algorithm for finding the way depends on our real-time biomechanical simulation [3]. We will generalize our algorithm so that we can use it with other biomechanical
simulations, too. Further optimizations will allow long-distance calculation.

This guiding system is the first step to a new area of supporting learning physicians.
Further trials will show how much this new manner of help will increase their examination capabilities.

References

[1]   A Ferlitsch, P Glauniner, A Gupper, M Schillinger, M Haefner, and A Gangl. Virtual endoscopy simula-
      tion for training of gastrointestinal endoscopy. *Gastrointestinal Endoscopy*, 53, Issue 5, Page 78, 2001.
[2]   D Fregonese, T Casetti, R Cestari, F Chilovi, G D'Ambra, G D Fave, E Di Giulio, G Di Matteo, L Ficano,
      and T Italy. Basic endoscopy training: Usefulness of a computer-based simulator. Cooperative group for
      training in endoscopy. *Gastrointestinal Endoscopy*, 53, Issue 5, Page 78, 2001.
[3]   O Körner and R Männer. Implementation of a haptic interface for a virtual reality simulator for flex-
      ible endoscopy. In B Hannaford and H Tan, editors, *11th Symposium on Haptic Interfaces for Virtual
      Environment and Teleoperator Systems, IEEE–VR2003*, pages 278–284, Los Angeles, March 2003.

Medicine Meets Virtual Reality 15
J.D. Westwood et al. (Eds.)
IOS Press, 2007

A Novel Approach for Training of Surgical Procedures Based on Visualization and Annotation of Behavioural Parameters in Simulators

Mikko J. RISSANEN [a,1], Yoshihiro KURODA [b], Megumi NAKAO [c],
Tomohiro KURODA [d], Keisuke NAGASE [d] and Hiroyuki YOSHIHARA [d]

[a] *Graduate School of Informatics, Kyoto University, Japan*
[b] *Osaka University* [c] *NAIST* [d] *Kyoto University Hospital*

Abstract. Recording performance during training sessions on simulators is becoming a new standard for assessment of surgical skills and thus a significant part of training. Typical simulator-based training can be assessed using criteria that cover the whole procedure to make distinction between skill levels. Studies so far have rarely addressed the challenge of how to provide better feedback about the user's performance on a surgical simulator. Our approach for surgical training is Annotated Simulation Records (ASRs) and visualization of behavioural parameters of interaction in surgery. This paper briefly outlines a framework for building user-defined skill models and presents initial results. We demonstrate the ASR-based approach in force exertion tasks on elastic objects by utilizing a cardiovascular surgeon's recorded interaction on an aorta palpation simulator.

Keywords. Annotation, skill modelling, skill training, haptic

Introduction

Recording performance during training sessions on simulators is becoming the new standard for assessment of surgical skills and thus a significant part of training. Studies have shown how simulator-based training can be assessed using criteria that can make a distinction between skill levels, for example motion analysis of laparoscopic tools [1]. Considering that metrics should be procedure-specific [2], the general metrics in simulators have limited use. Motion analysis does not cover other relevant aspects about the success of the surgical procedure, such as case-specific features of the target organs. Even though the need for novel kinds of feedback in surgical simulation has been presented [3], few studies have introduced methods for enhancing the feedback.

Observation of expert's demonstration is the basis for learning skills in surgery. Some simulators aiming for motion training provide expert's demonstrations within the simulation, for example Just Follow Me [4]. Research on haptic training (e.g. [5]) has been focusing on training of manual skills by using recorded expert's data, but demonstrations of such approaches in medicine are few. Virtual Haptic Back [6]

---

[1] Corresponding Author: Mikko Rissanen, Medical Informatics Division, Kyoto University Hospital, Shogoin Kawahara-cho 54, Sakyo, 606-8507 Kyoto, Japan; E-mail: mikko@kuhp.kyoto-u.ac.jp

introduced training of correct palpation paths along a virtual patient's back, but that approach is not essentially different from the trajectory training applications [5] in terms of real-time feedback.

Training strategies used in surgical training should be supported also in simulator-based training [2]. *Shaping* and *fading* are training strategies that some commercial simulators support [2]. *Shaping* means that the task is built little by little from its subtasks toward the full, complex task. *Fading* is an approach that reduces training aids when the learner's skill level rises.

Our approach for training of surgical skill is based on Annotated Simulation Records (ASRs) and visualization of behavioural parameters of interaction in surgery. In this paper, we summarize the essential concepts behind ASRs. Annotation is viewed as the means for modelling skill into recorded simulation. In order to use the ASRs for training, a novel technique for visualization of skill is presented: only the elements of "skill" are overlaid onto the simulation. An experiment was carried out to evaluate the proposed technique in abstract force exertion task, for which the example interaction was recorded by a cardiovascular surgeon on an aorta palpation simulator.

1. Annotated Simulation Records

The design of ASRs covers two essential aspects of surgical interaction. First, in order to determine what different behavioural parameters of surgical interaction constitute surgical skill, an annotation system has to be introduced. Based on the annotations, a model of surgical skill is constructed. Second, the model has to be presented to the user as a training aid, which is achieved through real-time visualization of the skill's components. The process of creating ASRs includes:

- Recording of example performances
- Authoring of teaching scenarios: mistakes can be corrected and variable approaches created by editing the original recordings.
- Annotation of the examples: elements of skill are defined into the recordings.

Then, the ARS can be used as a training aid. Fig. 1 elaborates this process.

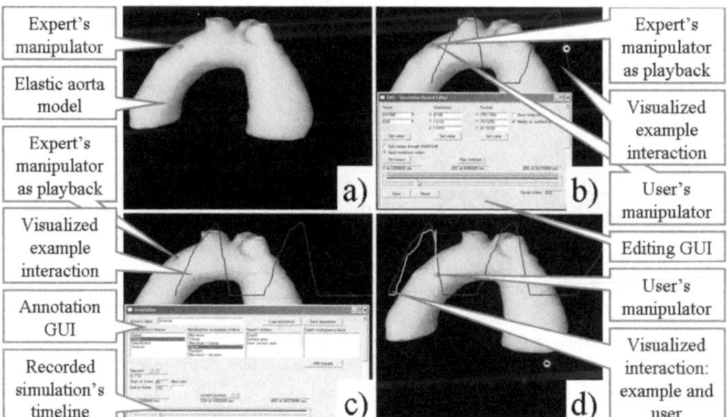

Fig. 1. The process of creating and using ASRs for palpation of the aorta: a) Recording of a simulation. b) Authoring: mistakes are fixed and variations created. c) Annotation: definition of what skill is composed of. d) Self-learning with the aid of SV which can be adjusted to match with the skill definition during training.

1.1. Annotation

Annotation is a common means to input meta-data about a subject. For example annotation of video sequences has made semantic searching of the content possible. Annotation can be thought as giving a meaning to parts or segments of the subject.

Within the ASR concept, annotation covers expert's insight about manipulation-level behavioural parameters of interaction in surgical procedures. The expert is given a means to determine what surgical skill consists of by defining meaningful segments of recorded example performance. Relations between relevant behavioural parameters of the performance are defined. Fig. 2 illustrates the nature of annotation.

1.2. Visualization

The visualization of the behavioural parameters is based on simplicity of 2-dimensional graphs overlaid on a simulator's screen. The example interaction is shown as a template that the user's interaction should match when visualized in real-time. The visualization serves two purposes. First, raw-data is visualized to give an impression of the nature of the interaction. This technique, Visualization of Behavioural Parameters (VBP), presents time-series data as curves. VBP is illustrated in Fig. 3a).

The second technique is a skill training aid: only the elements of skill are visualized. This technique can present the user's desired behaviour by displaying limits for the interaction, and therefore called Skill Visualization (SV). The possibility for this technique exists only in VR. In the real world it is not possible for a novice to perceive the skill as it is, since the skill itself cannot be presented, only the appearance of one of its instances at a time. Fig. 3b-d) elaborates the design of SV. SV serves four purposes:

1. Principle of interaction is directly perceivable.
2. Accurate and exact real-time feedback is achieved during training.
3. Fully proactive training, i.e. the haptic modality is not restricted in any way.
4. Applicable to also indirect effects of interaction, e.g. changes on the target.

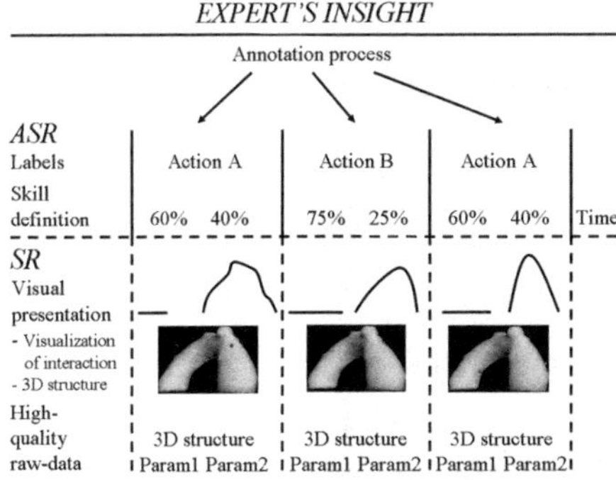

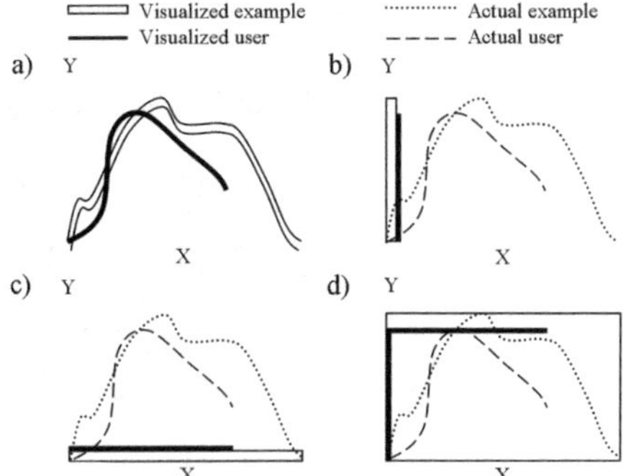

Fig. 2. ASR consists of a Simulation Record (SR) and annotations assigned to the segmented timeline of the recorded simulation: actions' labels and definitions of the elements of skill relevant to the action. Behavioural parameters of interaction (Param1 and Param2) are visualized to ease the annotation process.

Fig. 3. a) VBP: Time-series data is presented as is. b-d) SV: The exact presentation of the example is hidden. Only the 2-dimensional axes indicate what the skill consists of. For example, the axes could be assigned as X=time, Y=maximum power. d) Two axes are combined to display only an approximate of the interaction, yet, showing the limits of the skill.

Fig. 4 explains the role of VBP and SV in the process of creating and using ASRs for simulator-based training. VBP is beneficial for scenario authoring, segmentation of the timeline of the recorded simulation and definition of elements of skill through the annotation process. The intended use of SV covers mainly self-learning of surgical interaction on a simulator, but may be used also in the annotation process, too.

1.3. Training Using Skill Visualization

General skill models can be created by calculating averages or maximum values of ASRs recorded by different experts. The actions that are labelled as the same are grouped and averages are calculated for the annotated components of skill.

The SV technique can draw attention to chosen components of the skill at different phases of the training. When using the *shaping* training strategy, the training of a task can start from just one component, after which another one is introduced.

For the *fading* strategy, SV is capable of presenting all the components of the skill at one time. Then the visual aids are reduced one by one until the user masters the full task. However, human's capability to track several visual cues accurately is limited. Therefore, SV is expected to be beneficial mainly when using the *shaping* strategy.

1.4. Comparison to Earlier Training Systems

The traditional approach to learn motor skills is based on observation and mimicking of expert's performance, which has been incorporated into VR-based training. For example Just Follow Me [4] supports learning from expert's recorded example motions by displaying the examples as a "ghost" that the user follows in the virtual environment. This traditional approach does not draw attention to any components of skill.

Feygin et al. [5] reviewed haptic training systems. Most of them enhance learning by restricting or aiding the novice's motions. Haptic guidance has not yet met a grand theory and sophisticated systems are continuously under development. Haptic training systems have also been introduced to the medical field (e.g. [6]), but a general skill modelling system has not been realized. Since only visual cues are used, the VS technique does not have any restriction to the user's motions on the haptic modality.

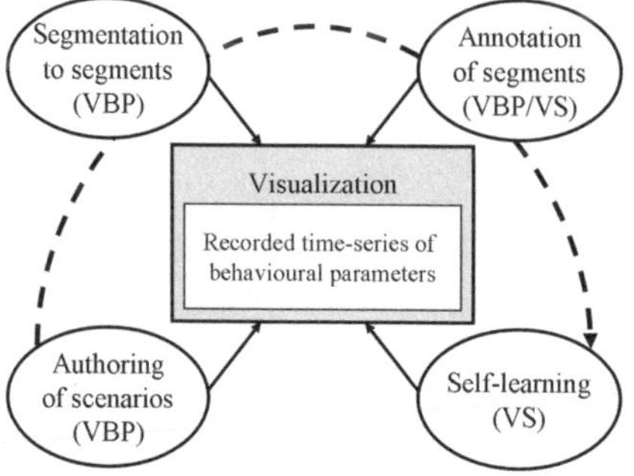

Fig. 4. The role of the visualization techniques in production of ASRs.

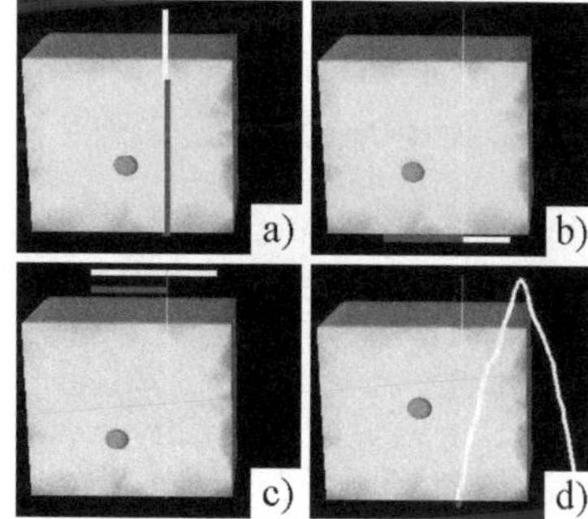

Fig. 5. Visualization conditions in the experiment. White: example. Dark: the user. The example moves from right to left and the user tries to match the lines. a) VS: maximum power b) VS: duration c) VS: maximum power+duration d) VBP: time-series.

2. Experiment

Force exertion was chosen to be a concrete example to demonstrate skill visualization of fundamental interaction in surgery. The experiment was designed to display the difference between VBP and SV, thus to demonstrate the need for the two different visualization techniques. Subjects practised force exertion from expert's pre-recorded example performance. A cardiovascular surgeon from Kyoto University Hospital performed palpation of the aorta on the MVL simulator [7] on a Xeon 3.2 GHz dual CPU with 4 GB RAM desktop platform with a Sensable PHANToM™ device. His example performance was recorded at 100 Hz sampling rate. Two individual pushing excerpts of his interaction were selected from the recorded simulation:

- Example E1: Maximum power 1.25 N, duration 1130 ms.
- Example E2: Maximum power 1.18 N, duration 1930 ms.

In order to see possible differences caused by variable elasticity, two virtual elastic cube mesh models (782 triangles) were prepared with stiffness parameters 1.0 MPa and 0.1 MPa Young's modulus. Poisson's ratio was set to 0.4. The 1.0 MPa model had the same parameters as the aorta model that was used during the expert's recording phase.

Annotation of the recordings was done by the experimenter. In E1, the skill was defined to consist of maximum power as the most important component and duration as the second one. In E2 the order was duration, then maximum power. In this way, the subjects were to *shape* their interaction skill by starting from one component of skill and then adding another one to the task. At first, one of visualizations shown in Fig. 5a) and b) was shown, then another component was "added" as shown in Fig. 5c). For VBP the visualization was always as in Fig. 5d).

6 subjects were divided into Group A and Group B. Their task was to follow the examples E1 and E2 overlaid on the simulator's screen. The examples were evaluated by simply calculating the error between the example's and the user's maximum power as Newtons and duration as milliseconds. Group A practiced the tasks first with VBP and then VS. Group B started with VS. When using VBP the subjects were only told to focus on the specific components, but the curve was always shown. Each evaluated trial consisted of training with the visualized example and repeating from the memory. Each task (E1 and E2) consisted of 7 trial pairs (first: tracking the example, second: repetition from memory) in each training phase, resulting in 42 trials per task, 336 per subject and 2016 in total in the experiment.

3. Results and Discussion

The results are presented briefly in the following. Only the most interesting and statistically significant differences are discussed at this phase of the analysis.

Maximum power was in general easier to be tracked with VS than with VBP. Mean average error was 5.2% when using VS and 11.1% (n=171, p<0.05) with VBP when tracking the example. Every subject's best trial reached less than 1.4% error with both VBP and VS. The ease of following the example affected also the performance from memory: 12.1% with VS and 18.1% with VBP (n=166, p<0.05). The soft cube was the easier target for tracking the example's maximum power: 9.3% on the 0.1MPa model and 14.7% on the 1.0MPa model (n=337, p<0.05). This was suspected to be due to the different distance that the finger had to be pushed in order to exert equal amount of force on both cubes. Use of power was easier to be controlled on the soft cube.

Most subjects reported counting seconds in their minds in order to remember the duration. For this reason, there were no significant findings related to mean average errors of duration. In the second training phase VS was proven better. When tracking the example, mean average errors of maximum power varied from 4.6% (VS) to 7.5% (VBP) (n=340, p<0.05). Performance from memory did not improve with VS, though.

4. Conclusions

A novel approach for simulator-based surgical training was proposed. By annotating experts' recorded performances on a simulator, the skill can be described. Presentation of the skill description to a novice is achieved by overlaying 2D graphs that visualize the chosen behavioural parameters of interaction on the simulator's screen. This paper introduced a technique for visualization of skill, which is only possible in VR. The example "skill" can be displayed component by component, which supports the *shaping* training strategy. The experiment evaluated the skill visualization technique in the case of force exertion and it was found useful for the *shaping* strategy.

Future studies will deal with multiple behavioural parameters of surgical interaction which could also be indirect effects of the surgeon's manipulation, i.e. dynamics in a surgical procedure could be explicitly visualized. Usability of the annotation tool for skill modelling is also a future research subject. Then, more complex skills can be modelled and the models used for assessment of skills.

Acknowledgements

This research is funded by Grant-in-Aid for Scientific Research (S) (16100001), Young Scientists (A) (18680043) and Exploratory Research (18659148) from The Ministry of Education, Culture, Sports, Science and Technology, Japan, and Nakajima Fund.

References

[1] S. Cotin, N. Stylopoulos, M. Ottensmeyer, P. Neumann, D. Rattner and S. Dawson, Metrics for Laparoscopic Skills Trainers: The Weakest Link! In: LNCS Vol 2488: MICCAI, Part I, Tokyo, 2002, Springer, 35-43.

[2] A.G. Gallagher, E.M. Ritter, H. Champion, G. Higgins, M.P. Fried, G. Moses, C.D. Smith and R.M. Satava, Virtual Reality Simulation for the Operating Room: Proficiency-Based Training as a Paradigm Shift in Surgical Skills Training, *Annals of Surgery* **241**:2 (2005), Lippincott Williams & Wilkins, Philadelphia, PA, 364-372.

[3] D. Shaffer, D. Meglan, M. Ferrell and S. Dawson, Virtual Rounds: Simulation-based Education in Procedural Medicine, In: SPIE Vol. 3712: Battlefield Biomedical Technologies, 1999.

[4] U. Yang and G.J. Kim, Implementation and Evaluation of Just Follow Me: An immersive, VR-based, Motion-Training System, *Presence: Teleoperators and Virtual Environments* **11**:3 (2002), MIT Press, Cambridge, MA, 304-323.

[5] D. Feygin, M. Keehner and F. Tendick, Haptic Guidance: Experimental Evaluation of a Haptic Training Method for a Perceptual Motor Skill, In: 10th Symposium on Haptic Interfaces for Virtual Environment and Teleoperator Systems, Orlando, FL, 2002, 40-47.

[6] R.L. Williams II, M. Srivastava, R.R. Conatser Jr. and J.N. Howell, Implementation and Evaluation of a Haptic Playback System, *Haptics-e Journal* **3**:3 (2004). (Online at www.haptics-e.org)

[7] Y. Kuroda, M. Nakao, T. Kuroda, H. Oyama and H. Yoshihara, MVL: Medical VR Simulation Library, In: Medicine Meets Virtual Reality, Long Beach, CA, 2005, IOS Press, 273-276.

Medicine Meets Virtual Reality 15
J.D. Westwood et al. (Eds.)
IOS Press, 2007

NeuroVR: An Open Source Virtual Reality Platform for Clinical Psychology and Behavioral Neurosciences

Giuseppe RIVA [1-2], Andrea GAGGIOLI [1-2], Daniela VILLANI [1], Alessandra PREZIOSA [1], Francesca MORGANTI [1], Riccardo CORSI [3], Gianluca FALETTI [3], Luca VEZZADINI [3]

[1] *Applied Technology for Neuro-Psychology Lab,*
Istituto Auxologico Italiano, Milan, Italy
[2] *ICE-NET, Università Cattolica del Sacro Cuore, Milan, Italy*
[3] *VR Department, Virtual Reality & Multi-Media Park, Turin, Italy*

Abstract. In the past decade, the use of virtual reality for clinical and research applications has become more widespread. However, the diffusion of this approach is still limited by three main issues: poor usability, lack of technical expertise among clinical professionals, and high costs. To address these challenges, we introduce NeuroVR (http://www.neurovr.org – http://www.neurotiv.org), a cost-free virtual reality platform based on open-source software, that allows non-expert users to adapt the content of a pre-designed virtual environment to meet the specific needs of the clinical or experimental setting. Using the NeuroVR Editor, the user can choose the appropriate psychological stimuli/stressors from a database of objects (both 2D and 3D) and videos, and easily place them into the virtual environment. The edited scene can then be visualized in the NeuroVR Player using either immersive or non-immersive displays. Currently, the NeuroVR library includes different virtual scenes (apartment, office, square, supermarket, park, classroom, etc.), covering two of the most studied clinical applications of VR: specific phobias and eating disorders. The NeuroVR Editor is based on Blender (http://www.blender.org), the open source, cross-platform suite of tools for 3D creation, and is available as a completely free resource. An interesting feature of the NeuroVR Editor is the possibility to add new objects to the database. This feature allows the therapist to enhance the patient's feeling of familiarity and intimacy with the virtual scene, i.e., by using photos or movies of objects/people that are part of the patient's daily life, thereby improving the efficacy of the exposure. The NeuroVR platform runs on standard personal computers with Microsoft Windows; the only requirement for the hardware is related to the graphics card, which must support OpenGL.

Keywords: Virtual Reality, Open-Source, Clinical Psychology, Neuroscience

---

[1] Corresponding Author: Prof. Giuseppe Riva, Ph.D., Dipartimento di Psicologia, Università Cattolica del Sacro Cuore, Largo Gemelli 1, 20123 Milan, Italy, e-mail: giuseppe.riva@unicatt.it, web-site: http://www.neurotiv.org

1. Introduction

The use of virtual reality (VR) in medicine and behavioral neurosciences has become more widespread. According to a recent market analysis, in 2003 the medical sector contributed $8.7 billion to worldwide visual simulation/virtual reality systems; in the same year, psychotherapy and medical research were rated among the top ten applications of VR [1]. The growing interest in medical applications of VR is also highlighted by the increasing number of scientific articles published each year on this topic: searching Medline with the keyword "virtual reality", we found that the total number of publications has increased from 45 in 1995 to 246 in 2005, showing an average annual growth rate of nearly 14 per cent (see Figure 1).

One of the leading applications of VR in the medical field is psychotherapy, where it is mainly used to carry out exposure treatment for specific phobias, i.e., fear of heights, fear of flying, and fear of public speaking. In VR exposure therapy, the patient is gradually confronted with the virtual simulation of feared stimuli while allowing the anxiety to attenuate. The main advantage of VR exposure on conventional "in vivo" exposure is that using VR the therapist can control and grade the feared situations with a high degree of safety for the patient [2]. Further applications of VR in psychotherapy include eating disorders [3], posttraumatic stress disorder [4], sexual disorders [5] and nicotine craving [6].

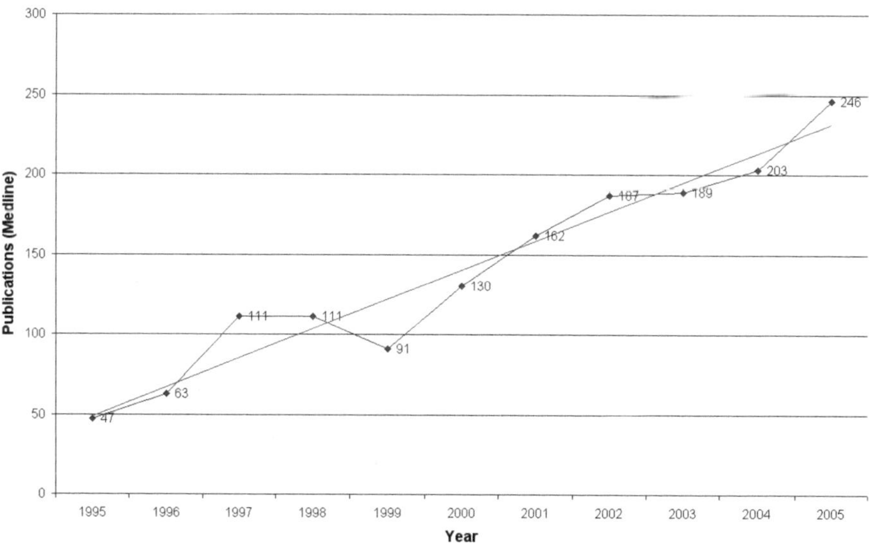

Figure 1. Trend in publications on VR in medicine (Source: Medline; keyword: "virtual reality"; accessed: June 30, 2006)

Another medical field in which VR has been fruitfully applied is neuropsychological testing and rehabilitation. Here, the advantage of VR on traditional assessment and intervention is provided by three key features: the capacity to deliver interactive 3D stimuli within an immersive environment in a variety of forms and sensory modalities; the possibility of designing of safe testing and training environments, and the provision of "cueing" stimuli or visualization strategies designed to help guide successful performance to support an error-free learning approach [7-9].

Beyond clinical applications, VR has revealed to be a powerful tool for behavioral neuroscience research. Using VR, researchers can carry out experiments in an ecologically valid situation, while still maintaining control over all potential intervening variables. Moreover, VR allows to measure and monitor a wide variety of responses made by the subject [10].

Although it is undisputable that VR has come of age for clinical and research applications, the majority of them are still in the laboratory or investigation stage. In a recent review, Riva [11] identified four major issues that limit the use of VR in psychotherapy and behavioral neuroscience:

- the lack of standardization in VR hardware and software, and the limited possibility of tailoring the virtual environments (VEs) to the specific requirements of the clinical or the experimental setting;
- the low availability of standardized protocols that can be shared by the community of researchers;
- the high costs (up to 200,000 US$) required for designing and testing a clinical VR application;
- most VEs in use today are not user-friendly; expensive technical support or continual maintenance are often required.

To address these challenges, we have designed and developed NeuroVR (http://www.neurovr.org), cost-free virtual reality platform based on open-source software, that allows non-expert users to easily modify a virtual environment (VE) and to visualize it using either an immersive or non-immersive system.

The NeuroVR platform is implemented using open-source components that provide advanced features; this includes an interactive rendering system based on OpenGL which allows for high quality images. The NeuroVR Editor is realized by customizing the User Interface of Blender, an integrated suite of 3D creation tools available on all major operating systems, under the GNU General Public License; this implies that the program can be distributed even with the complete source code. Thanks to these features, clinicians and researchers have the freedom to run, copy, distribute, study, change and improve the NeuroVR Editor software, so that the whole VR community benefits.

2. The NeuroVR Editor

The majority of existing VEs for psychotherapy are proprietary and have closed source, meaning they cannot be tailored from the ground up to fit specific needs of different clinical applications [11]. NeuroVR addresses these issues by providing the clinical professional with a cost-free VE editor, which allows non-expert users to easily modify a virtual scene, to best suit the needs of the clinical setting.

Using the NeuroVR Editor (see Figure 2), the psychological stimuli/stressors appropriate for any given scenario can be chosen from a rich database of 2D and 3D objects, and easily placed into the pre-designed virtual scenario by using an icon-based interface (no programming skills are required). In addition to static objects, the NeuroVR Editor allows to overlay on the 3D scene video composited with a transparent alpha channel.

The editing of the scene is performed in real time, and effects of changes can be checked from different views (frontal, lateral and top).

The NeuroVR Editor is built using Python scripts that create a custom graphical user interface (GUI) for Blender. The Python-based GUI allows to hide all the richness and complexity of the Blender suite, so to expose only the controls needed to customize existing scenes and to create the proper files to be viewed in the player.

Currently, the NeuroVR library includes different pre-designed virtual scenes, representing typical real-life situations, i.e., the supermarket, the apartment, the park.

These VEs have been designed, developed and assessed in the past ten years by a multidisciplinary research team in several clinical trials, which have involved over 400 patients [12]. On the basis of this experience, only the most effective VEs have been selected for inclusion in the NeuroVR library.

An interesting feature of the NeuroVR Editor is the possibility to add new objects to the database. This feature allows the therapist to enhance the patient's feeling of familiarity and intimacy with the virtual scene, i.e., by using photos of objects/people that are part of the patient's daily life, thereby improving the efficacy of the exposure [13]. Future releases of the NeuroVR Editor software may also include interactive 3D animations controlled at runtime. A VRML/X3D exporter and a player for PocketPC PDAs are planned Blender features, too.

3. The NeuroVR Player

The second main component of NeuroVR is the Player, which allows to navigate and interact with the VEs created using the NeuroVR Editor.
NeuroVR Player leverages two major open-source projects in the VR field: Delta3D (http://www.delta3d.org) and OpenSceneGraph (http:// www.openscenegraph.org). Both are building components that the NeuroVR player integrates with ad-hoc code to handle the simulations.

The whole player is developed in C++ language, targeted for the Microsoft Windows platform but fully portable to other systems if needed. When running simulation, the system offers a set of standard features that contribute to increase the realism of the simulated scene. These include collision detection to control movements in the environment, realistic walk-style motion, advanced lighting techniques for enhanced image quality, and streaming of video textures using alpha channel for transparency.

The player can be configured for two basic visualization modalities: immersive and non-immersive. The immersive modality allows the scene to be visualized using a head-mounted display, either in stereoscopic or in mono-mode; compatibility with head-tracking sensor is also provided. In the non-immersive modality, the virtual environment can be displayed using a desktop monitor or a wall projector. The user can interact with the virtual environment using either keyboard commands, a mouse or a joypad, depending on the hardware configuration chosen.

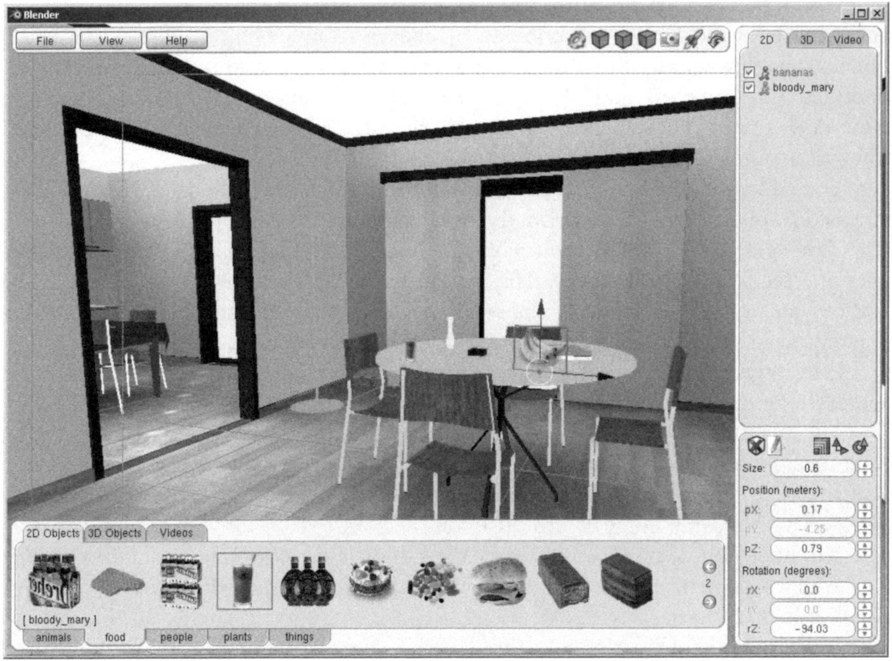

Figure 2. A screenshot taken from the NeuroVR Editor

4. Conclusions

In this paper, we have introduced NeuroVR, an advanced platform designed for the creation and customization of highly flexible VEs for clinical psychology and behavioral neurosciences. Currently, the NeuroVR library includes a limited number of VEs addressing specific phobias (i.e. fear of public speaking, agoraphobia) and eating disorders. However, these pre-designed environments can be easily adapted for targeting other clinical applications. Moreover, it is envisioned that the 250,000 people worldwide Blender user community will contribute to extend the NeuroVR library, developing new VEs which can be tailored by the clinical professionals for a range of clinical and experimental needs.

A future goal is also to provide software compatibility with instruments that allow collection and analysis of behavioral data, such as eye-tracking devices and sensors for psychophysiological monitoring. Beyond clinical applications, NeuroVR provides the VR research community with a cost-free, open source "VR lab", which allows to create highly-controlled experimental simulations for a variety of behavioral, clinical and neuroscience applications.

5. Acknowledgments

The present work was supported by the Italian MIUR FIRB programme (Project "Neurotiv - Managed care basata su telepresenza immersiva virtuale per l'assessment e riabilitazione in neuro-psicologia e psicologia clinica" - RBNE01W8WH - and Project "Realtà virtuale come strumento di valutazione e trattamento in psicologia clinica: aspetti tecnologici, ergonomici e clinici" - RBAU014JE5).

6. References

[1]   CyberEdge, The Market for Visual Simulation/Virtual Reality Systems, Sixth Edition, CyberEdge, Oakland, CA, 2004.

[2]   B.O. Rothbaum, L. Hodges and R. Kooper, Virtual reality exposure therapy, J Psychother Pract Res, **6**, 1997, 219-226.

[3]   G. Riva, M. Bacchetta, G. Cesa, S. Conti and E. Molinari, The use of VR in the treatment of eating disorders, Stud Health Technol Inform, **99**, 2004, 121-163.

[4]   A. Rizzo, J. Pair, P.J. McNerney, E. Eastlund, B. Manson, J. Gratch, R. Hill and B. Swartout, Development of a VR therapy application for Iraq war military personnel with PTSD, Stud Health Technol Inform, **111**, 2005, 407-413.

[5]   G. Optale, A. Munari, A. Nasta, C. Pianon, J. Baldaro Verde and G. Viggiano, Multimedia and virtual reality techniques in the treatment of male erectile disorders, Int J Impot Res, **9**, 1997, 197-203.

[6]   J. Lee, Y. Lim, S.J. Graham, G. Kim, B.K. Wiederhold, M.D. Wiederhold, I.Y. Kim and S.I. Kim, Nicotine craving and cue exposure therapy by using virtual environments, Cyberpsychol Behav, **7**, 2004, 705-713.

[7]   F. Morganti, Virtual interaction in cognitive neuropsychology, Stud Health Technol Inform, **99**, 2004, 55-70.

[8]   A.A. Rizzo and J.G. Buckwalter, Virtual reality and cognitive assessment and rehabilitation: the state of the art, Stud Health Technol Inform, **44**, 1997, 123-145.

[9]   M.T. Schultheis, J. Himelstein and A.A. Rizzo, Virtual reality and neuropsychology: upgrading the current tools, J Head Trauma Rehabil, **17**, 2002, 378-394.

[10] M.J. Tarr and W.H. Warren, Virtual reality in behavioral neuroscience and beyond, Nat Neurosci, **5 Suppl**, 2002, 1089-1092.

[11] G. Riva, Virtual reality in psychotherapy: review, Cyberpsychol Behav, **8**, 2005, 220-230; discussion 231-240.

[12] G. Riva, C. Botella, G. Castelnuovo, A. Gaggioli, F. Mantovani and E. Molinari, Cybertherapy in practice: the VEPSY updated project, Stud Health Technol Inform, **99**, 2004, 3-14.

[13] G. Riva, F. Mantovani and A. Gaggioli, Presence and rehabilitation: toward second-generation virtual reality applications in neuropsychology, J Neuroengineering Rehabil, **1**, 2004, 9.

Medicine Meets Virtual Reality 15
J.D. Westwood et al. (Eds.)
IOS Press, 2007

Cellular phones for reducing battlefield stress: Rationale and a preliminary research

Giuseppe RIVA[1-2], Alessandra GRASSI[2], Daniela VILLANI[1-2], Alessandra PREZIOSA[1]

[1] *Applied Technology for Neuro-Psychology Lab.,*
Istituto Auxologico Italiano, Milan, Italy
[2] *ICE-NET, Università Cattolica, Milan, Italy*

Abstract: Battlefield stress is the consequence of man being exposed to the hostile environment of combat. Combat stress is specifically caused by man's feat of the dangers of combat, and is fueled and tempered by other variables such as morale, cohesion, fatigue, confidence, training and intensity of the combat. Treatment is often as simple as giving soldiers time to rest for a few hours or days, to get a shower and some sleep, to talk about the feelings they have in the presence of a counselor. Only in rare cases soldiers undergo more serious psychological treatment. One of the best strategies for dealing with stress is learning how to relax. However, relaxing is difficult to achieve in a battlefield. In this chapter we suggest the use of mobile multimedia technology – PDA/cellular phones – for the provision of advanced coping techniques suitable to the battlefield context. Specifically, we developed a protocol based on mobile narratives, to be experienced on mobile multimedia technology – 3G cellular phones or PDAs - like the one now under development by the US Army within the "Soldier as a System - SaaS" and "Future Combat Systems - FCS" projects. Mobile narratives are audio-visual experiences, implemented on mobile devices, in which the narrative component is a critical aspect to induce a feeling of presence and engagement. Through the link between the feeling of presence and the emotional state, mobile narratives may be used to improve the mood state in their users. The rationale of the approach and a preliminary test of the proposed method are presented and discussed.

Keywords: Battlefield stress, cellular phones, PDAs, Mobile Narratives

1. Introduction

Battlefield stress is the consequence of man being exposed to the hostile environment of combat [1]. Combat stress is specifically caused by man's feat of the dangers of combat, and is fueled and tempered by other variables such as morale, cohesion, fatigue, confidence, training and intensity of the combat.

The history shows that a stressed soldier may be a significant problem. In the battles of Faid-Kasserine, the first major engagements of US forces in World War II,

---

[1] Corresponding Author: Prof. Giuseppe Riva, Ph.D., Dipartimento di Psicologia, Università Cattolica del Sacro Cuore, Largo Gemelli 1, 20123 Milan, Italy, e-mail: giuseppe.riva@unicatt.it, web-site: http://www.neurotiv.org

20 to 34 percent of the casualties were caused not by direct wounds and disease but by battlefield stress [2]. And the situation is not significantly changed. As demonstrated recently by Morgan and colleagues [3], acute stress may impair working memory and visuo-spatial ability even in elite soldiers. In their study, including 184 Special Operations warfighters, stress exposure impaired visuo-spatial capacity and working memory of the sample, potentialy reducing performance of duty.

For these reasons, stress management is a critical issue for the US Army. As underlined in the Army Regulation 600-63, stress, its effects, and its management is a concern for leaders at every level [4]. Specifically, Field Manual 26-2 provides different techniques and consideration for the management of stress in Army operation [5].

The Field Manual depicts three different and increasing levels of support (Stress Management Module) based on installation resources:

- *Level one*: it is designed as a minimum program that includes placement of pamphlets/brochures/posters around the military community, making sure that welcome packets are provided to all new members and ensuring sponsorship of new arrivals.
- *Level two*: it includes level one plus community education classes (learning new skills and activities) and the use of radio/TV spots.
- *Level three*: it includes level one and level two plus specific intervention programs conducted by qualified health care professionals. These programs include relaxation techniques, problem solving, cognitive restructuring and clarification o of life goals.

Given the limited number of qualified professionals on the battlefield, treatment is often as simple as giving soldiers time to rest for a few hours or days, to get a shower and some sleep, to talk about the feelings they have in the presence of a counselor.
In general, management efforts that emphasize replenishment of physiologic needs, structured occupation, and support of the affected soldier's occupational roles have yielded better results [6]. Nevertheless, only in rare cases soldiers undergo more serious psychological treatment.

Another critical issue is the provision of stress coping techniques. In the civilian sector there is a broad spectrum of techniques available for individual to use. However, the possible techniques are much less when applied in the battlefield. Duration of stress and intensity of battle usually reduce imagination and relaxation abilities. This makes stress coping even more challenging.

In this chapter we suggest the use of mobile multimedia technology – PDA/cellular phones – for the provision of advanced coping techniques suitable to the battlefield context. This technology could be easily integrated in the Future Combat System under development by the US Army.

2. Including Stress Coping Techniques in the Soldier as a System Concept

The "2006 Army Modernization Plan" is an operationally based report that describes the modernization and investment strategies for providing the best capabilities to the Army today, supporting a sustained transformation process [7]. The document serves as a conceptual template for leveraging quality people and technology in order to achieve new levels of effectiveness.

In this report, a critical part is related to the identification of emerging technologies that have the greatest promise for early incorporation into the Soldier as a System (SaaS) concept. Main goal of SaaS is to equip all Soldiers with an integrated modular ensemble based on an open architecture that allows capabilities to be tailored for specific missions. The SaaS related scientific and technological efforts also address technologies for the Mounted Soldier System (MSS), Air Soldier System (ASS), and Core Soldier System (CSS) ensemble. Specifically they pursue a wide range of technologies to enable Soldier systems. These include (p. 39):

- Technologies to provide individual Soldiers with platform-like lethality and survivability.
- Lightweight, long-endurance electric power generation and storage.
- Physiological status reporting and medical response technologies.

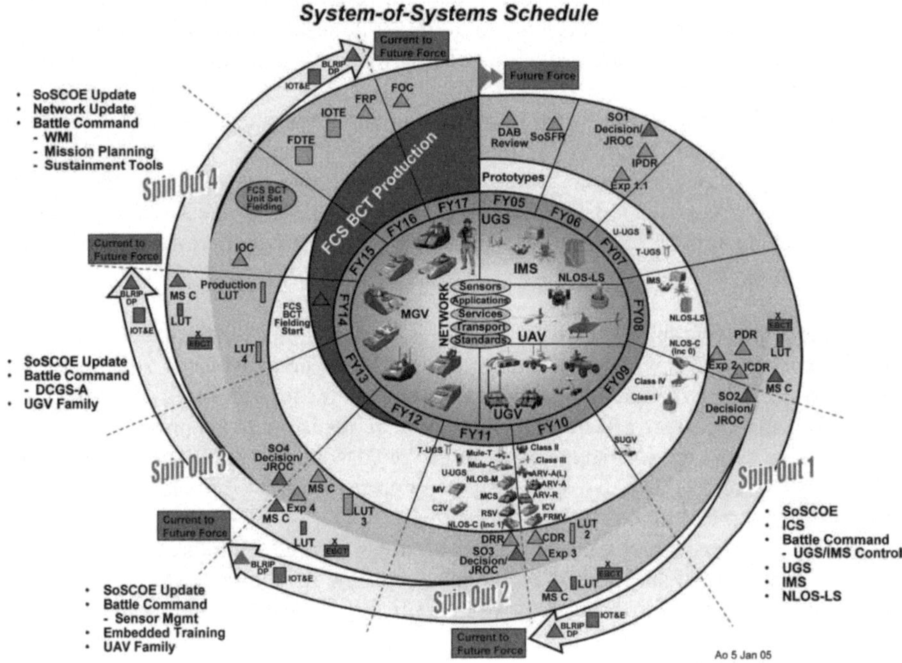

Figure 1. The road towards the Future Combat System

Within the SaaS concept is also included the development of new tools and methodologies for training and leader development (pp. 39-40):

- Training management tools to improve effectiveness of interactive distributed training systems.
- Methodologies utilizing realistic synthetic experience to accelerate the development of critical thinking and interpersonal communication skills.

Our suggestion is to include the development of a new generation of technology supported stress coping techniques within this effort. This should allow the leverage of the different technologies and solutions included in the Future Combat Systems (pp. 41-42, see also Figure 1):

- Networked battle command systems to enable shared situational awareness and improved decision-making.

- Mobile-to-mobile wireless communications networks. The networks will provide large quantities of multimedia information (speech, data, graphics, and video) frompoint to point, and broadcast and multicastover distributed mobile wireless networks.

3. A New Stress Coping Technique: Mobile Narratives

Cellular telephones and hand-held personal digital assistants are multi-purpose computing devices for which 3D content will simply be one more feature, but not necessarily the most important feature (a cell phone, for example, will be used primarily as a phone by most people). Because the combined market size of cell phones and PDAs is massive, however, the financial opportunity for successfully deploying 3D hardware and software to this segment of the market is also potential massive.

A necessary precondition for 3D graphics to make any impact is the availability of open-standard, well-performing APIs that are supported by handset manufacturers, operators and developers alike. Actually, there are two main industry efforts that aim to standardize APIs for animated 3D graphics in mobile phones (see Figure 2): *OpenGL ES* and Mobile 3D Graphics API for J2ME.

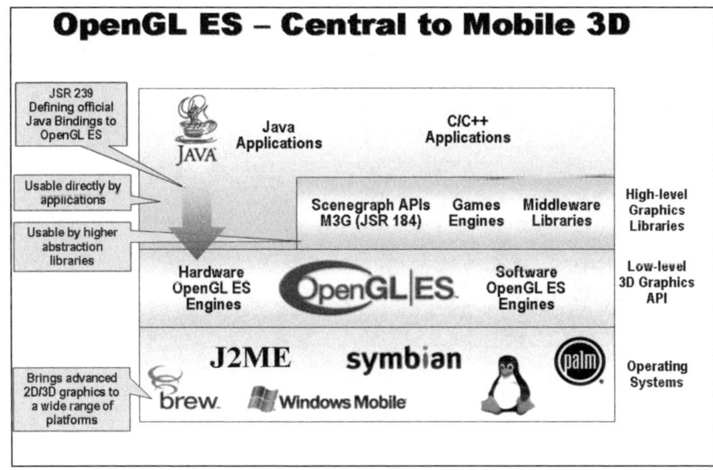

Figure 2: 3D Graphics for mobile devices (courtesy of Khronos, http://www.khronos.org/opengles/)

Although the most significant advances in 3D mobile hardware are yet to come, some cell phones and PDAs are already shipping with enough raw horse power to deliver a good 3D experience today: *Power VR MBX* (Nokia N93, Ericsson P990) and *NVidia GoForce 5500* (Samsung P910/920, HTC Foreseer).

These devices allow the provision of mobile narratives: 3D audio-visual experiences, implemented on mobile devices, in which the narrative component is a critical aspect to induce a feeling of presence and engagement. The developed narratives include different relaxation techniques adapted to the battlefield context: breathing control, progressive relaxation, mindfulness, etc.

Through the link between the feeling of presence and the emotional state, mobile narratives may be used to improve the mood state in their users. Future devices will also allow immersion, through the use of headsets, and tracking.

We developed a specific protocol based on mobile narratives - multimedia narratives experienced on first generation UMTS/3G phones - to reduce stress in non-comfortable situations.

4. Testing the concept: commuting stress

We tested the concept with an experimental sample of 17 male and 16 female commuters (N=33) of the Italian regional train line "Milano-Saronno", aged between 20-25 years (M=23.82+/-0.72). The sample was randomly divided between the following three conditions:

- MN - Mobile narratives: the sample experienced four mobile narratives based on a trip in a desert tropical beach (see Figure 3);
- NA - New age videos: the sample experienced four commercial videos with new age music (see Figure 3). The videos were selected for their similar visual content (a tropical beach) to the mobile narratives;
- CT - Control group: no treatment.

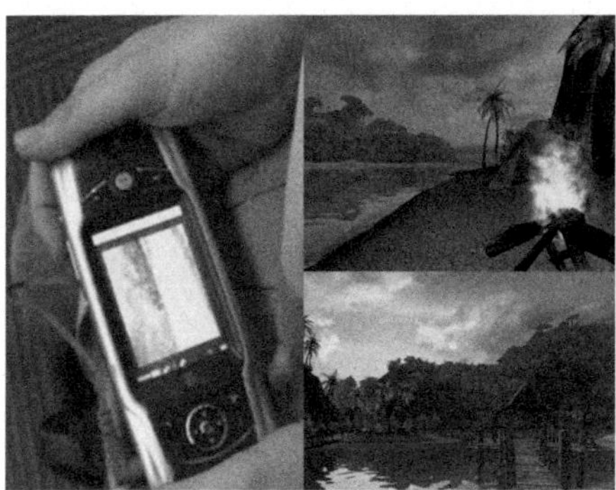 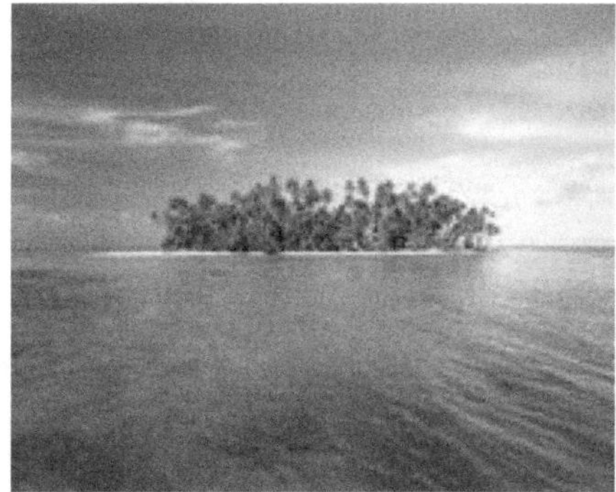

Figure 3. The visual content of the Mobile Narratives (left) and the New Age video (right)

The sample was tracked for two days. During each trip the experimental samples experienced on a Multimedia UMTS cellular phone (screen size: 208x320 pixel) the multimedia content. The total length of each experience was 6 minutes. Before and after each trip the subjects were submitted to the following questionnaires: STAI: State-Trait Anxiety Inventory [8]; VAS: Visual Analog Scale [9]; PANAS: Positive and Negative Affect Schedule [10]; ITC-Sopi: Sense of Presence Inventory [11].

5. Results

The first significant result was the difference in anxiety between the three groups. Only the MN group experienced a significant reduction in the anxiety level (STAI: z=2,943, p<0.01) and an increase in the relax scale (VAS: z=-2,842; p<0.01) at the end of the trial. Also, the anxiety reduction in the MN group was significantly higher than the ones achieved by two groups (STAI: Chi-square: 20.749, p<0.01).

The second relevant result is related to the level of presence experienced by the two experimental groups. The level of "engagement" and "spatial presence" was significantly higher in the MN group. These data suggest that the efficacy of the MN may be related to the higher level of presence induced by mobile narratives.

6. Conclusions

The trials showed the efficacy of mobile narratives in reducing the level of stress experienced during a commute trip. No effects were found in the other groups. These results suggest that 3G mobile handsets, even with their small screens and limited multimedia capabilities, may be used as relaxation tool if backed by a specific therapeutic protocol and an engaging experience. Future research is needed to define and test a specific protocol targeted to battlefield stress. Further, we plan to exploit the forthcoming features of mobile devices – faster 3D graphics, immersion, tracking, etc. – to improve the feeling of presence of the experience and its efficacy.

7. Acknowledgments

The present work was supported by the Italian MIUR FIRB programme (Project *"Neurotiv - Managed care basata su telepresenza immersiva virtuale per l'assessment e riabilitazione in neuro-psicologia e psicologia clinica"* - RBNE01W8WH - and Project *"Realtà virtuale come strumento di valutazione e trattamento in psicologia clinica: aspetti tecnologici, ergonomici e clinici"* – RBAU014JE5).

8. References

[1]   R.J. Hibler, Battlefield stress: management techniques. Mil Med, (1984), 149(1): p. 5-8.

[2]   W.S. Mullins and A.J. Glass, Neuropsychiatry in World War II, Volume 2, Overseas theatres. (1973.

[3]   C.A. Morgan, 3rd, A. Doran, G. Steffian, G. Hazlett, and S.M. Southwick, Stress-induced deficits in working memory and visuo-constructive abilities in special operations soldiers. Biol Psychiatry, (2006), 60(7): p. 722-9.

[4]   T.D.J. West, Army Health Promotion - Army Regulation 600-63. 1996, Washington, D.C.: Headquarters, Department of the Army.

[5]   U.S. Army, Management of Stress in Army Operations - Field Manual 26-2. 1983, Headquarters, Department of the Army: Washington, D.C.

[6]   S.M. Gerardi, The management of battle-fatigued soldiers: an occupational therapy model. Mil Med, (1996), 161(8): p. 483-8.

[7]   U.S. Army, Army Modernization Plan. 2006, Headquarters, Department of the Army: Washington, D.C.

[8]   C.D. Spielberger, R.L. Gorsuch, R. Lushene, P.R. Vagg, and G.A. Jacobs, Manual for the State-.Trait Anxiety Inventor. 1983, Palo Alto, CA: Consulting Psychology Press.

[9]   A. Gift, Visual Analog Scales: Measurement of subjective phenomenon. Nursing Research, (1989), 38(5): p. 286-288.

[10] D. Watson, L.A. Clark, and A. Tellegen, Development and validation of brief measures of positive and negative affect: The PANAS scales. Journal of Personality and Social Psychology, (1988), 54: p. 1063-1070.

[11] J. Lessiter, J. Freeman, E. Keogh, and J. Davidoff, A Cross-Media Presence Questionnaire: The ITC-Sense of Presence Inventory. Presence: Teleoperators, and Virtual Environments, (2001), 10(3): p. 282-297.

Medicine Meets Virtual Reality 15
J.D. Westwood et al. (Eds.)
IOS Press, 2007

Managing Exam Stress Using UMTS Phones: The advantage of Portable Audio/Video Support

Giuseppe RIVA[1-2], Alessandra GRASSI[2], Daniela VILLANI[1-2],
Andrea GAGGIOLI[1-2], Alessandra PREZIOSA[1]
[1] *Applied Technology for Neuro-Psychology Lab.,*
Istituto Auxologico Italiano, Milan, Italy
[2] *ICE-NET, Università Cattolica, Milan, Italy*

Abstract: Test-taking anxiety or stress is very common among university students. It can be very distressing and sometimes debilitating. Exam anxiety involves physical components and emotional components that may be taken into account for managing and reducing anxiety. An approach to control exam anxiety is to learn how to regulate emotions. To help students in managing exam stress we developed a specific protocol based on mobile narratives - multimedia narratives experienced on UMTS/3G phones. 30 female university students (M=23.48; sd=1.24) who were going to perform an exam within a week were included in the trial. They were randomly divided in five groups according to the type and mobility of the medium used: (1) audio only narrative (CD at home); (2) audio only narrative (portable MP3); (3) audio and video narrative (DVD at home); (4) audio and video narrative (UMTS based); (5) control group. Audio/video narratives induced a reduction in exam anxiety in more than 80% of the sample vs 50% of the MP3 sample and 0% of the CD sample. Further, all the users who experienced mobile narratives on UMTS phones were able to relax before the exam, against 50% of DVD users and 33% of audio-only users. The trial showed a better efficacy of mobile narratives experienced on UMTS phones in reducing the level of exam stress and in helping the student to relax. These results suggest that for the specific sample considered – Italian university students – the media used for providing an anti-stress protocol has a clear impact on its efficacy.

Keywords: Exam stress, cellular phones, UMTS, Mobile Narratives

1. Introduction

Test-taking anxiety or stress is very common among university students. It can be very distressing and sometimes debilitating. Exam anxiety involves physical components and emotional components that may be taken into account for managing and reducing anxiety.

A common approach to control exam anxiety is Stress Inoculation Training (SIT). SIT [1, 2] has been employed on a treatment basis to help individuals cope with the aftermath of exposure to stressful events and on a preventive basis to "inoculate" individuals to future and ongoing stressors.

Typically a SIT protocol is based on a three-phase intervention [3, 4]:

---

[1] Corresponding Author: Prof. Giuseppe Riva, Ph.D., Dipartimento di Psicologia, Università Cattolica del Sacro Cuore, Largo Gemelli 1, 20123 Milan, Italy, e-mail: giuseppe.riva@unicatt.it, web-site: http://www.neurotiv.org

- *conceptualization phase*: A Socratic-type exchange is used to educate clients about the nature and impact of stress;
- *skills acquisition and rehearsal:* The specific coping skills are taught to the clients;
- *application and follow through*: provides opportunities for the clients to apply the variety of coping skills across increasing levels of stressors.

2. A SIT Protocol for Cellular Phones

To help students in managing exam stress we developed a specific protocol based on mobile narratives - multimedia narratives experienced on UMTS/3G phones (Nokia 6680). Following the SIT protocol, our one is composed by six sessions:
- *session 1 and 2* target the psycho-physiological reactions to the exam;
- *session 3 and 4* target the psycho-physiological reactions and coping strategies;
- *session 5 and 6* present the stressful situation (an exam) to test and eventually tune the learned strategies.

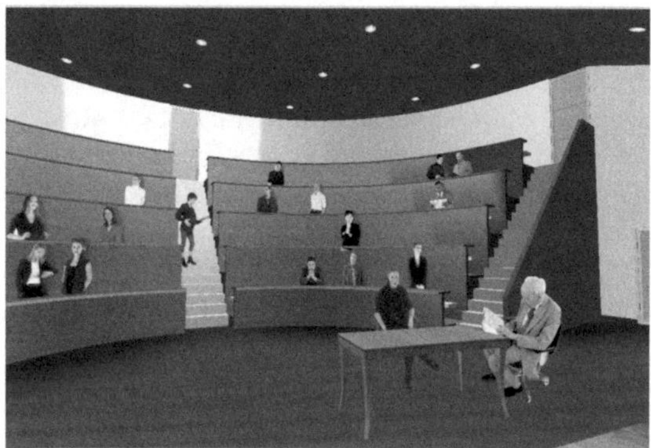

Figure 1. A screen shot of the simulated exam

30 female university students (M=23.48; sd=1.24) who were going to perform an exam within a week were included in the trial. They were randomly divided in five groups according to the type and mobility of the medium used: (1) audio only narrative (CD at home); (2) audio only narrative (portable MP3); (3) audio and video narrative (DVD at home); (4) audio and video narrative (UMTS based); (5) control group.

At the start of the treatment, before and after the exam, subjects were submitted to the following questionnaires: STAI: State-Trait Anxiety Inventory [5]; VAS: Visual Analog Scale [6] and PANAS: Positive and Negative Affect Schedule [7].

3. Results

Audio/video narratives induced a reduction in exam anxiety in more than 80% of the sample vs 50% of the MP3 sample and 0% of the CD sample (STAI Questionnaire – $X^2=11.25; p<.05$ - Figure 2). Further, all the users who experienced mobile narratives on UMTS phones were able to relax before the exam, against 50% of DVD users and 33% of audio-only users (VAS Questionnaire – $X^2=13.33$, p<.05 - Figure 3).

Finally, a negative correlation was found between the level of anxiety – as assessed by VAS Questionnaire - and exam marks (r: -.340, p< .05).

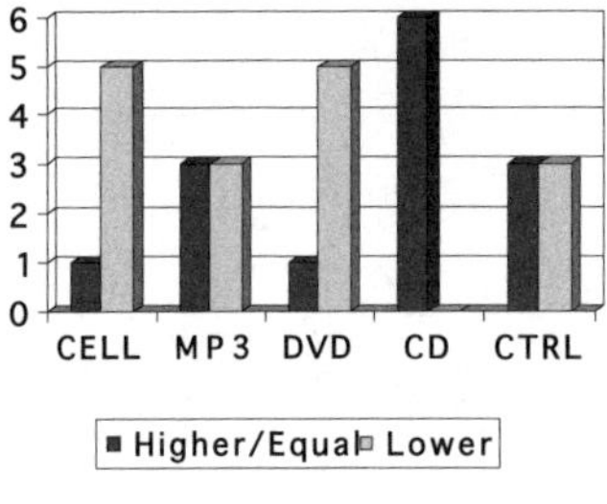

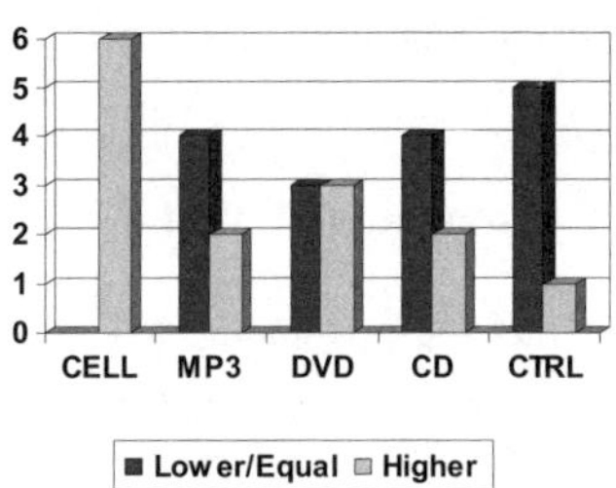

Figure 2. Anxiety level during exam

Figure 3. Relaxation level before exam

4. Conclusions

The trial showed a better efficacy of mobile narratives experienced on UMTS phones in reducing the level of exam stress and in helping the student to relax. These results suggest that for the specific sample considered – Italian university students – the media used for providing an anti-stress protocol has a clear impact on its efficacy.

Further, the data confirm that 3G mobile handsets may be used as relaxation tools when backed by a specific therapeutic protocol and meaningful narratives.

5. Acknowledgments

The present work was supported by the Italian MIUR FIRB programme (Project *"Neurotiv - Managed care basata su telepresenza immersiva virtuale per l'assessment e riabilitazione in neuro-psicologia e psicologia clinica"* - RBNE01W8WH - and Project *"Realtà virtuale come strumento di valutazione e trattamento in psicologia clinica: aspetti tecnologici, ergonomici e clinici"* – RBAU014JE5).

6. References

[1] T. Saunders, J.E. Driskell, J.H. Johnston, and E. Salas, The effect of stress inoculation training on anxiety and performance. J Occup Health Psychol, (1996), 1(2): p. 170-86.

[2] A.A. Hains, A stress inoculation training program for adolescents in a high school setting: a multiple baseline approach. J Adolesc, (1992), 15(2): p. 163-75.

[3] J. Coburn and M.A. Manderino, Stress inoculation: an illustration of coping skills training. Rehabil Nurs, (1986), 11(1): p. 14-7.

[4] D. Meichenbaum, Stress inoculation training for coping with stressors. The Clinical Psychologist, (1996), 49: p. 4-7.

[5] C.D. Spielberger, R.L. Gorsuch, R. Lushene, P.R. Vagg, and G.A. Jacobs, Manual for the State-.Trait Anxiety Inventor. 1983, Palo Alto, CA: Consulting Psychology Press.

[6] A. Gift, Visual Analog Scales: Measurement of subjective phenomenon. Nursing Research, (1989), 38(5): p. 286-288.

[7] D. Watson, L.A. Clark, and A. Tellegen, Development and validation of brief measures of positive and negative affect: The PANAS scales. Journal of Personality and Social Psychology, (1988), 54: p. 1063-1070.

Medicine Meets Virtual Reality 15
J.D. Westwood et al. (Eds.)
IOS Press, 2007

Employing Graphics Hardware for an Interactive Exploration of the Airflow in the Human Nasal Cavity

Marc SCHIRSKI [a,1], Christian BISCHOF [b] and Torsten KUHLEN [a]

[a] *Virtual Reality Group, RWTH Aachen University, Germany*
[b] *Institute for Scientific Computing, RWTH Aachen University, Germany*

Abstract. This paper presents an interactive method for the intuitive exploration of airflow within the human nose. Employing the computational power of modern graphics hardware allows for computing the movement of large numbers of particles through the flow domain. By using tetrahedral grids, we preserve the precision of the numerical flow simulation even for irregular flow domains. For rendering, we employ billboard-based visualization methods, which result in a high visual quality at little computational cost and highly interactive frame rates.

Keywords. Virtual Reality, Flow Visualization, Particle Tracing, GPGPU

1. Introduction

As the analysis of flow processes within the human body gains more and more attention, a simulation thereof through computational fluid dynamics (CFD) becomes increasingly important. For example, the airflow within the human nose exhibits quite complex structures [1], an understanding of which is hampered by its complexity. However, due to the diversity of the nose's functions, including respiration, smelling, and moistening, tempering and cleaning the air, a thorough understanding and evaluation of the corresponding flow field is a difficult process, which can be facilitated by employing virtual reality (VR) techniques [2]. An immersive stereoscopic projection and an intuitive user interface are the main advantages over conventional, desktop-based visualization systems.

In order to gain insight into such simulation results, a variety of visualization approaches are being employed. A very intuitive method is the depiction of particle movement inside the flow field as in [3], where a particle-based visualization is used for the analysis of arterial blood flow, but the computational cost complicates its use within a virtual environment with its non-trivial real-time constraints. With the advent of powerful and flexible graphics hardware, an additional resource is available, which helps alleviating this problem [4].

---

[1]Corresponding Author: Marc Schirski, Virtual Reality Group, Center for Computing and Communication, RWTH Aachen University, Seffenter Weg 23, 52074 Aachen, Germany; E-mail: schirski@rz.rwth-aachen.de

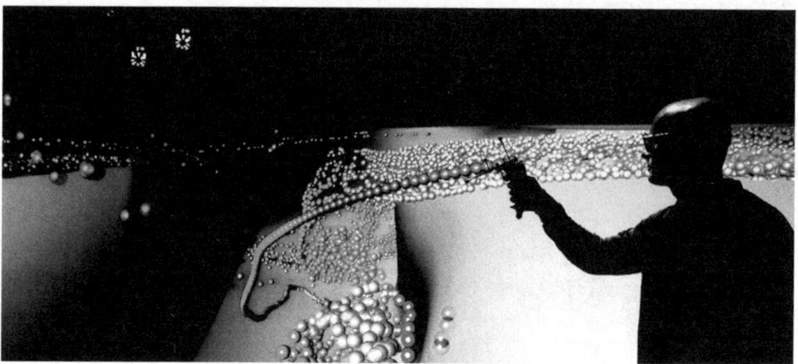

Figure 1. Flow field exploration via interactively seeded particles.

2. Using the GPU for Particle Trajectory Computation and Depiction

We employ a similar approach by storing the flow field and the particles to be traced in graphics memory and computing the particles' movement directly on the graphics processing unit (GPU). Unlike previous work, we do not resample the simulation grid into a regular structure. Instead, we work directly with a tetrahedral grid, thus effectively preserving the optimized discretization of the flow domain as used for the fluid solver. Then, we encode it into a variety of textures, including vector and scalar data, vertex positions, cell topology and cell neighborhoods. Particle data is stored in additional textures. The particles' movement is computed by numerical integration through the flow field. After each iteration, billboarded spheres or Virtual Tubelets [5] are generated from the particle data and rendered with per-pixel shading, resulting in a convincing illusion of rounded geometry and, therefore, a high-quality depiction of particle data.

For now, the user interface consists mainly of an input device with 6 degrees-of-freedom, which allows the user to directly release particles into the flow field (see Figure 1). This results in a very intuitive method for flow field exploration, which helps in understanding even complex flow structures and dynamics by allowing users to interact with the flow as they see fit.

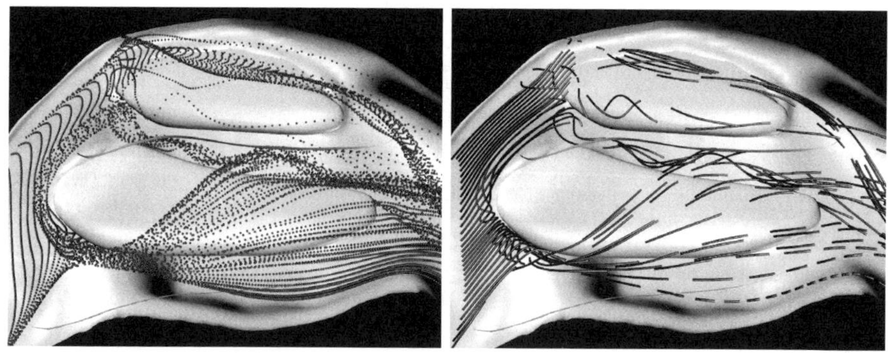

Figure 2. Depicting the movement of particles as instantaneous particles (left) or tracers (right) allows for an intuitive understanding of the underlying airflow.

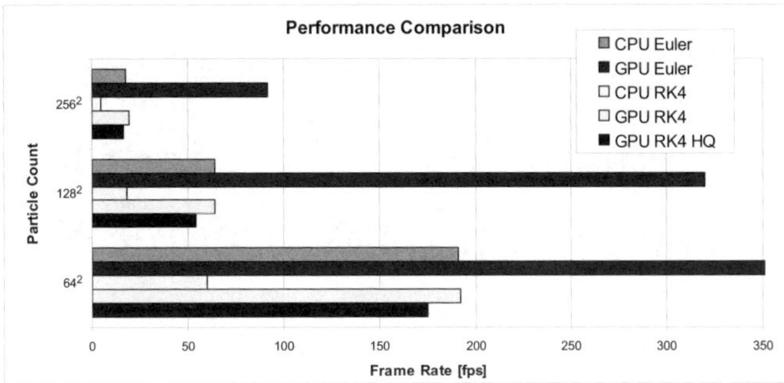

Figure 3. Framerate comparison for interactive particle tracing on the CPU and on the GPU.

3. Results and Future Work

The depiction of particle trajectories either as billboarded particles or Virtual Tubelets provides an easily understandable depiction of underlying flow structures (see Figure 2). Compared to conventional techniques like streamlines, this approach conveys a much better sense of flow dynamics and direction. Employing the GPU for the computation of particle movement is significantly faster despite a better visual quality than a CPU-based reference implementation, which is not suited for an interactive tracing of large numbers of particles (see Figure 3).

While the direct interaction with the flow field via the 3D input device is one of the main advantages, it might result in a relatively volatile visualization. Depending on the flow field, particles tend to leave the flow domain quite quickly, thus reducing the expressiveness of the visualization. This is alleviated by automated seeders, which can be placed near interesting flow features, and which continuously release new particles, effectively maintaining a meaningful depiction of the flow field.

This work concentrates on the visualization of stationary flows. In a next step, the visualization of unsteady data is planned. However, it is still to be determined, whether internal bandwidth restrictions prohibit an interactive processing of time-dependent data.

References

[1] I. Hörschler, C. Brücker, W. Schröder, M. Meinke. Investigation of the Impact of the Geometry on the Nose Flow. *European Journal of Mechanics-B/Fluids*, 25(4):471–490, 2006.

[2] B. Hentschel, T. Kuhlen, C. Bischof. Flow Field Visualization inside the Human Nasal Cavity. In *Proceedings of IEEE VR 2005*, pp. 233–236, 2005.

[3] J. Sobel, A. Forsberg, D.H. Laidlaw, R. Zeleznik, D. Keefe, I. Pivkin, G. Karniadakis, P. Richardson, S. Swartz. Particle Flurries: Synoptic 3D Pulsatile Flow Visualization. *IEEE Computer Graphics and Applications*, 24(2):76–85, 2004.

[4] J. Krüger, P. Kipfer, P. Kondratieva, R. Westermann. A Particle System for Interactive Visualization of 3D Flows. *IEEE Transactions on Visualization and Computer Graphics*, 11(6):744–756, 2005.

[5] M. Schirski, T. Kuhlen, M. Hopp, P. Adomeit, S. Pischinger, C. Bischof. Virtual Tubelets – efficiently visualizing large amounts of particle trajectories. *Computers & Graphics*, 29(1):17–27, 2005.

Medicine Meets Virtual Reality 15
J.D. Westwood et al. (Eds.)
IOS Press, 2007

Task Sequencing Effects for Open and Closed Loop Laparoscopic Skills

Elizabeth A. SCHMIDT[a]   Mark W. SCERBO[a]
Gayatri KAPUR[b]   Adair R. HEYL[b]

[a] *Old Dominion University*
[b] *Eastern Virginia Medical School*

Abstract. The present study examined laparoscopic skill acquisition on a simulator for different sequences of open and closed loop tasks. Sixteen medical students were divided into four groups distinguished by their initial training task and subsequent transfer task. Group 1 practiced instrument navigation, an open loop task, and then transferred to grasping, a closed loop task. Group 2 practiced grasping, and then transferred to the instrument navigation task. Group 3 practiced instrument navigation and then transferred to a complex cutting task that involved both open and closed loop components. Group 4 practiced grasping and then transferred to the cutting task. The results showed distinct task sequencing effects in favor of initial practice on a closed loop task. Specifically, task completion times declined significantly when participants practiced the closed loop task followed by the open loop task. The benefits of initial practice on a closed loop task, however, were limited primarily to accuracy measures when participants transferred to the complex cutting task. The findings indicate that task order is important and that training on one task can either facilitate or impede skill acquisition on a subsequent task and that these differences reflect fundamental psychomotor characteristics of the tasks.

1. Introduction

Patient safety during hospital care has become a national problem. In 1999 the Institute of Medicine estimated that between 44,000 and 98,000 deaths in U.S. hospitals could be attributed to medical errors [1]. In an effort to reduce hospital-related health care errors, the American Medical Association limited resident work hours to 80 per week. The reduction in work hours likely alleviated some fatigue among residents. However, the work week restrictions created another problem. Residents now have less time available to devote to their educational training [2,3]. The decreased time available for formal training can result in fewer opportunities for patient contact and sub-standard technical abilities [4,5]. Thus, there exists a greater need for resident training to be more effective and efficient. The recent availability of simulator training systems for medical procedures may help residents overcome some of the lost opportunities for training due to the reduced patient-contact hours.

Medical simulator-based training currently offers an alternative way for residents to acquire necessary procedural skills. Medical virtual reality simulators are computer-based simulators that offer real-time interaction with computer generated anatomy and objective performance feedback. The majority of medical virtual reality simulators currently available address laparoscopic procedures. Laparoscopic surgical skills are difficult to master and require hours of practice. Commercial laparoscopic simulators often provide different training exercises aimed at developing a variety of laparoscopic skills (e.g., camera navigation, cutting, diathermy, etc.). However, most training programs incorporating virtual reality simulators are not based on principles of psychomotor skill acquisition [6].

Skills have been described as an individual's learned capability to perform specific acts [7]. Skills reflect a relatively permanent change in performance attributable to the learning process. High performance skills, including laparoscopic skills, have three defining characteristics [8]. First, they require the trainee to invest considerable time and effort to acquire the skills. Second, despite the time and effort devoted to acquiring the skills, some individuals may never attain competent levels of performance. Third, a discernable difference exists between novice and expert performance.

Schneider argues that there are common misconceptions when it comes to training high performance skills [8]. One such misconception is to train the total skill. Often training on the whole task is not required. Instead, part-task training may be sufficient and in many instances, even optimal. Once fundamental skills are acquired during part-task training, the parts can be recombined to practice the entire procedure.

An understanding of the basic types of movements underlying psychomotor skills is necessary for structuring training programs. Schmidt and Lee [9] describe fundamental types of movements that represent different points along a continuum of psychomotor skills and can be characterized by attentional control mechanisms. *Closed loop* movements are generally considered to be slow and require continuous attentional monitoring to minimize the error between desired positioning and movements. By contrast, *open loop* movements utilize mental motor programs and require attention before they are executed. They are performed quickly and once initiated, are difficult to interrupt.

Laparoscopic tasks draw upon both closed and open loop motor skills. However, little information in the literature describes optimal ways to sequence the training for both types of skills. Thus, the present study represents an initial effort to address laparoscopic skill acquisition from a psychomotor skills perspective by examining the impact of sequencing different fundamental tasks. Specifically, two laparoscopic tasks representing each end of the continuum were examined: instrument navigation (open loop) and grasping (closed loop). In addition, a third cutting task that includes both types of movements and was used to determine how training on the individual skills transfers to more complex movements. Thus, the goal of the present study was to examine the effects of task order on the acquisition of two fundamental laparoscopic skills.

2. Method

2.1 Participants

Participants were 16 medical students from the Eastern Virginia Medical School. Their ages ranged from 22-29 years old ($M = 25.4$, $SD = 1.6$). Four participants had experience with another medical simulator. Three reported using a box trainer for a maximum of 20 minutes, and one reported using a laparoscopic virtual reality simulator for one hour. The same participant who used the laparoscopic virtual reality simulator also reported using a driving simulator for approximately 5 hours. All participants reported using a computer for education or recreational use ($M = 11.7$, $SD = 8.8$). All students participated voluntarily.

2.2 LapSim Simulator

The LapSim virtual reality laparoscopic skills trainer produced by Surgical Science was used in this study (see Figure 1). It is a PC-based training system and contains multiple software modules designed to foster the development of laparoscopic skills. The LapSim also records a variety of performance-based metrics. The surgical workstation is made by Immersion Medical Inc., and it tracks and records movement of the simulated laparoscopic instruments. The instrument interface contains two handles for instruments that use a five degree-of-freedom tracking system. The tasks were displayed on a 20-in monitor. A single processor PC with 512 MB of RAM and 40 BG of hard disk is required. The software requires a windows operating system of 2000 or XP professional.

Figure 1. Participant practicing the closed loop (grasping) task on the LapSim system.

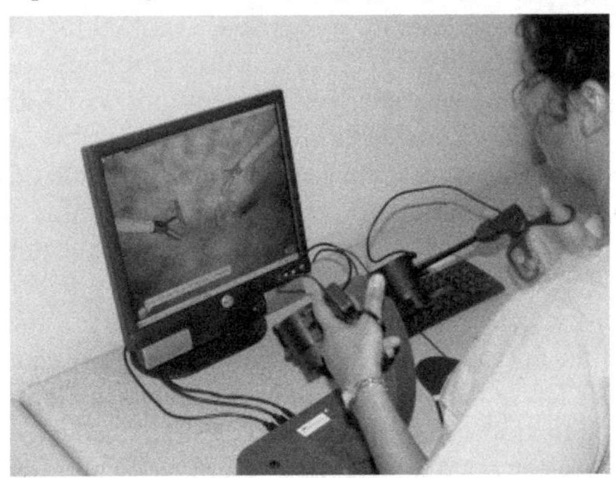

Three of the tasks from the LapSim Basic Skills module were chosen for this study. Instrument navigation was chosen as a representative task for open loop movements. The task consists of maneuvering each instrument (right and left), one at a time, into a position where a simulated probe touches a simulated ball. Each probe must touch five balls, for a total of ten targets. The grasping task represents closed loop movements and requires the trainees to maneuver each instrument (i.e., a grasper is in each hand), one at a time, toward a cylindrical target. The target must then be grasped and placed into another smaller target area that is highlighted in red. A total of 10 cylindrical targets had to be grasped and were evenly balanced for the right and left instruments. The third task was a cutting task selected because it includes both open and closed loop movements. The cutting task requires the trainee to hold a grasper in the left hand and make three successive cuts to a cylindrical target with the right hand diathermy cutter. Cuts were performed by grasping the correct segment of the target with the diathermy instrument and depressing the foot pedal until the segment was removed. After each cut, the excised target area had to be placed into a smaller circular target.

The order of stimulus presentation within the LapSim tasks had to be altered for this study. The default mode in the LapSim fixes targets in the same locations over successive trials. In the present study, the placement of targets was adjusted to vary at random across the 48 trials for each participant to guard against trial-specific order effects. Thus, participants never encountered the same sequence of target locations over trials. Also, the LapSim allows tasks to be practiced at three different levels of difficulty: easy, medium, and hard. In the present study, all tasks were set to the highest level of difficulty. Unfortunately, the specific difficulty criteria for each task are not objectively defined in the LapSim. For example, target sizes decrease as difficulty increases; however, absolute target sizes (or proportional changes among sizes) are not available nor are they consistent across all tasks. Thus, no specific details regarding task difficulty can be provided.

2.3 Procedure

Participants were recruited with flyers posted in the medical school. Participation was strictly voluntary and involved two experimental sessions spread over the course of one week. Both sessions lasted approximately 60 minutes. When participants reported for the experiment, they were randomly assigned to one of four groups. Group 1 practiced the instrument navigation (open loop) task and then transferred to the grasping (closed loop) task. Group 2 practiced the grasping (closed loop) task and then transferred to the instrument navigation (open-loop) task. Group 3 practiced instrument navigation (open loop) and then transferred to the cutting (complex) task. Group 4 practiced the grasping (closed loop) task and then transferred to the cutting (complex) task. Participants were given a total of 48 trials across the two sessions to acquire skills for either the instrument navigation or grasping task. Immediately upon completion of the practice trials, participants were assessed on the transfer task. An experimenter was present at all times to ensure that the trials were completed.

3. Results

Performance was assessed by both completion time and accuracy measures. The results were analyzed by comparing data from the last five practice trials of the acquisition task with the first five trials of the transfer task. The completion time results show distinct task sequencing effects (see Table 1). Specifically, when an open loop task (instrument navigation) was practiced first, there were significant increases in the task completion times when participants performed a subsequent closed loop task (grasping), $t(19) = 8.64$, $p < .0001$, or a complex task (cutting) that had both open and closed loop components, $t(18) = 5.44$, $p < .0001$. By contrast, practice on a closed loop task (grasping) reduced performance times when students transferred to the open loop task (instrument navigation), $t(19) = 10.28$, $p < .0001$. The benefits of initial practice on a closed loop task, however, were not observed when participants transferred to the complex cutting task. Instead, completion times for the cutting task increased over the initial completion times for the grasping task, $t(19) = 4.53$, $p < .0001$.

The accuracy measure was based on the tissue damage scores (in mm) provided by the LapSim. The results showed an overall tendency for increased tissue damage when participants transferred to the second task in all conditions; however, only one significant result was observed. Specifically, participants who initially practiced the grasping (open loop) task and then transferred to the complex cutting task caused significantly more tissue damage during the cutting task.

Table 1. Mean Completion Times and Tissue Damage Scores for Each Group on the Acquisition and Transfer Tasks. (Standard Deviations in Parentheses.)

Group	Mean Task Time (in Sec.) and Tissue Damage Scores on the Acquisition Task	Mean Task Time (in Sec.) and Tissue Damage Scores on the Transfer Task
Navigation → Grasping	32.4 s (4.8 s) 1.6 (1.6)	101.9 s (34.4 s) * 2.6 (3.3)
Grasping → Navigation	63.5 s (10.2 s) 0.85 (1.3)	38.1 s (8.4 s) * 1.4 (1.4)
Navigation → Cutting	40.8 s (7.7 s) 0.7 (0.9)	183.7 s (116.4 s) * 3.3 (4.4) *
Grasping → Cutting	57.3 s (11.3 s) 1.3 (1.6)	174.6 s (70.0 s) * 2.1 (2.8)

* $p < .05$, difference between initial task and transfer task

4. Discussion

The primary goal of the present study was to examine laparoscopic skill acquisition for open and closed loop tasks under different task sequencing paradigms. The results show that task order is important and that training on one task can either facilitate or impede skill acquisition on a subsequent task. The findings showed a significant decrease in completion times for an open loop task (instrument navigation) when participants initially practiced a closed loop task (grasping). However, the opposite pattern was observed when the open loop task was *followed* by the closed loop task. These findings suggest that the continuous motor control movements needed for the grasping task may have helped establish the motor schema needed for the simple "ballistic" movements involved in the subsequent camera navigation task. By contrast, the motor schema developed through initial practice on the instrument navigation (open loop) was of no benefit on a subsequent task requiring continuous attentional control (grasping).

The results also showed that the benefits of initial practice on a closed loop task were primarily limited to simple tasks. Participants who initially practiced the closed loop (grasping) task produced longer completion times when transferred to the complex (cutting) task involving both closed and open loop components. However, it should be noted that there was still an advantage for practicing the closed loop (grasping) task first in the sequence even when transferring to the more complex cutting task. As can be seen in Table 1, there was a substantial increase in completion times on the complex cutting task irrespective of which task (closed or open loop) was practiced initially. However, the group that initially practiced the open loop navigation task was also less accurate (i.e., they had significantly higher tissue damage scores) and had slightly higher completion times when transferred to the complex cutting task than those who initially practiced the closed loop grasping task. It is possible that the much higher completion times observed for those who transferred to the complex task as opposed to simple tasks is due to the need to learn a new task while simultaneously coordinating components of *both* the previously learned task and the task undergoing training. Again, the slight advantage observed for initial practice on the closed loop grasping task when transferring to the complex task may be due to learning continuous motor control movements that help establish a motor schema for simple ballistic movements involved in the complex task.

Although the results from the present study shed some light on the importance of task sequencing, additional research is still needed. There are several characteristics of practice schedules (e.g., task duration, inter-trial spacing, frequency and type of feedback, etc.) that need to be examined in concert with sequencing open and closed loop tasks. Also, from a simulator-specific perspective only 3 of 8 practice tasks available on the LapSim were studied. Guidelines for structuring a training regimen would require a more comprehensive examination of practice tasks.

Incorporating simulators into medical training has been heralded as one of the primary ways to close the gap between classroom instruction and skill acquisition for medical personnel [4,10]. Medical schools are adopting simulation-based training into their curriculum to supplement resident training. Simulation-based training can provide a valuable way to acquire the high performance skills needed for laparoscopic procedures. When simulator designers and instructors capitalize on the fundamental principles of psychomotor skill acquisition, the full benefits simulation-based training will be realized.

Acknowledgements

This study was a collaborative project between Old Dominion University and the Obstetrics and Gynecology department at the Eastern Virginia Medical School in Norfolk Virginia.

References

[1]   Kohn, L., Corrigan, J., Donaldson, M. (Eds.) (1999). *To Err is Human: Building a Safer Health System.* Institute of Medicine. Washington DC: National Academy Press.

[2]   Scerbo, M.W. (2006). Medical virtual reality simulators. In W. Karwowski (Ed.), *International Encyclopedia of Ergonomics and Human Factors, 2nd Ed.* (pp. 1181-1185). Boca Raton, FL: CRC Press

[3]   Gelfand, D. V., Podnos, Y.D., Carmichael, J.C., Saltzman, D.J., Wilson, S.E., & Williams, R.A. (2004). Effect of the 80-hour workweek on resident burnout. *Archives of Surgery, 139,* 933-940.

[4]   Kauffman, C. R. (2001). Computers in surgical education and the operating room. *Annales Chirurgiae et Gynaecologiae, 90,* 141-143.

[5]   Feldman, L.S., Sherman, V., & Fried, G.M. (2004). Using simulators to assess laparoscopic competence: Ready for widespread use? *Surgery, 135,* 28-42.

[6]   Schmidt, E., & Scerbo, M.W. (in press). Simulation advances in medical education and training: Laparoscopic skill acquisition. In D.A. Vincenzi, M. Mouloua, & J.A. Wise (Eds.), *Human factors in simulation and training.* Mahwah, NJ: Erlbaum.

[7]   Farmer, E., van Rooij, J., Riemersma, J., Jorna, P., & Moraal, J. (1999). *Handbook of simulator-based training.* England: Ashgate.

[8]   Schneider, W. (1985). Training high-performance skills: Fallacies and guidelines. *Human Factors, 27,* 285-300.

[9]   Schmidt, R. A., & Lee, T. D. (2005). *Motor control and learning: A behavioral emphasis, 4th Ed.* Champaign, IL: Human Kinetics.

[10] Kauffman, C. R. (1999). Role of surgical simulators in surgical education. *Asian Journal of Surgery, 22,* 398-401.

Medicine Meets Virtual Reality 15
J.D. Westwood et al. (Eds.)
IOS Press, 2007

Evaluating Tool-Artery Interaction Force during Endovascular Neurosurgery for Developing Haptic Engine

Anindita Sengupta[1] (as225@buffalo.edu), T Kesavadas[1], Kenneth R Hoffmann[2, 1], Robert E. Baier[1], S. Schafer[2, 1]

[1] *Virtual Reality Laboratory, Department of Mechanical and Aerospace Engineering*
[2] *Toshiba Stroke Research Center, University at Buffalo, Buffalo, NY 14260*

Abstract: Endovascular neurosurgery has gained acceptance as the best method of treatment of vascular abnormalities like cerebral aneurysms. However, the procedure is associated with difficulties in tool/tissue manipulation. Navigation of stent, catheter and, guide wire through complex arteries without any force information often causes stent snagging, plaque dislocations and formation of thrombosis caused by the damage of the arterial wall. Currently, there is no haptic device available which can provide the surgeons with the force information, related to stent placement procedure. The goal of this work is to create a data base for a fast synthetic endovascular force simulator, which will provide the surgeon with force information during tool-artery interaction, based on the various combinations of tool sizes and vessel complexity, [1, 2] to facilitate better pre-operative planning, safer interventions, and advanced training of new surgeons.

1. Introduction

The challenge of endovascular procedures lies in the fact that it is dependent on intuition due to the lack of sufficient visual information and absence of almost any force feedback. Recent development in the reconstruction of CT images of arteries into 3D vasculature, instead of using 2D angiograms under fluoroscopic guidance, has improved the visual aspect to a great extent; however, this alone is insufficient to improve the quality of surgery. Surgeons performing the operation report they feel some force feedback from the endovascular tools. This is the resultant of the different forces occurring in the system during the process of tool movement and tool placement [3]. Based on this, we intend to develop a force simulator, which will produce a parametric force equation to predict the forces experienced by surgeons at a particular location during endovascular navigation based on the vessel tortuosity and size of tools.

2. Force Measurements and determination of tortuosity

Experiments were conducted to find forces occurring at different tortuous regions of the arterial complex, in vitro, using silicone phantom vessels. The phantoms were made from the 3D reconstructed images of actual vasculature, having different shape and tortuosity, obtained from the CT scans or angiograms. A guide wire was inserted into the phantom, and a stent catheter was moved in it. Based on a previous study done within the group [4], which reported that after insertion the guide wire always attains the same position, it was assumed that the stent catheter always follows the same path over the guide wire inside the phantom. Rotational angiograms of the phantom with the guide wire were taken and the path of the guide wire extracted to define the path of tool movement. Tool/vessel interaction forces were evaluated using a combination of force and torque sensors as a stent catheter was moved in increments of 1.2cm from one end of the phantom to the other. The complexity of the vasculature as a measure of tortuosity was calculated using the in-plane angles and the torsional angles along the path of navigation, obtained from the rotational angiograms. The areas of concern for navigating tools in each of the phantoms were determined using Configuration Space (C-Space) techniques [3]. Experiments were repeated using umbilical cord vein grafts as surrogate tissues to compare the force values in actual tissues, to that in the silicone phantoms. The forces experienced while navigating the stent into the phantom were plotted against the lengths of insertion. (sample data shown Figure 1a). Using 3D reconstructions, from the rotational angiograms of the phantom, the guide wire path, and its distance from the wall were determined. It was seen that the contact points between the guide wire and the phantom depended on the shape of the phantom vessels. It was concluded that high forces were encountered at the points where the tool tip had to dislodge the guide wire from the wall and also where the tortuosity of the path was high. The forces when plotted along the path of the guide wire using a color code is shown below in figure 1b.

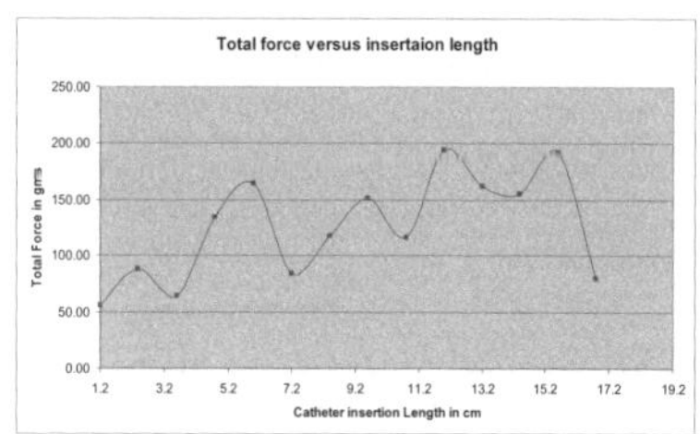

Figure 1(a) 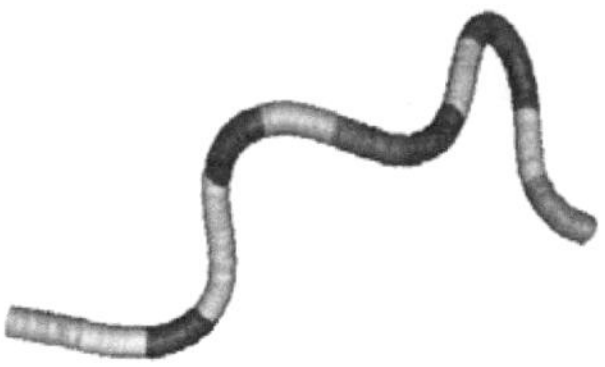   Figure 1 (b)

Figure 1a: Typical force over insertion length graph 1b: Force mapping along the path of stenting (dark patches show regions of higher forces and light ones, the areas of minimum).

3. Data Base

Tortuosity of the vessel was calculated using the techniques of Distance Matrix [1, 5] and Sum of Angle Matrix [5]. The contact points of guide wire along the vessel were determined and correlated with vessel geometry. The forces measured vary from 10 grams force to about 190 grams force depending on the phantom vessel configuration and from 10 grams to about 150 grams in the surrogate tissues. These forces at a given position were related to the geometry of the vessel and compared to the areas of concern evaluated from the configuration space (C-Space) technique [2]. A data base of forces for different shapes and sizes of vasculature and tools was developed.

4. Predictive Force Equation

Currently, we are developing a mathematical correlation and a predictive equation of the force for known geometry and shape of the vasculature and tool dimensions. Using the data base of the predictive interpolation equation, we can expect to obtain the force ranges that the surgeon experiences at a particular location in the artery during intervention using 3D reconstruction techniques from CTs and MRI images. This force database will be used to enhance a real-time endovascular simulator that was developed before [1]. The predictive force experiments will help us to identify the critical areas in the tool-vasculature interaction using the combination of tool-artery size, even without performing the C space techniques for every vasculature model.

Future work

The haptic device will be developed based on the data base and the predictive equation. Experiments will be conducted to estimate the amount of force required for plaque dislocation, intimal layer damage and puncture. From these values and depending on the size and shape of the tool and vasculature the haptic device will be eventually modified to provide a go/ no-go decision to the surgeons in the surgical room.

Acknowledgements

This work was supported by NIH grant number R01-EB02916.

We would also like to thank Dr. Anne E. Meyer and Dr. Robert E. Baier to allow us to use the facility of University/Industrial Center for Biosurfaces.

References

[1] Subramanian N, Kesavadas T, Hoffmann KR, "A Prototype Virtual Reality System for Preoperative Planning of Neuron-Endovascular Interventions": Proceedings of Medicine meets Virtual Reality 12, 2004, pg 376-381
[2] Kesavadas K, Agrawal R, Hoffmann KR. Configuration-space technique for calculating stent-fitness measures for the planning of neuro-endovascular interventions, SPIE Medical Imaging 5744: 191-199, 2005.
[3] Mitsutaka Tanimoto, Fumihito Ami, Toshio Fukuda, Hitoshi Iwata, Kouichi Itoigawa, Yasuhiro Gotoh, Masashi Hashimoto, and Makoto Negoro, "Micro Force Sensor for Intravascular Neurosurgery": Proceedings of the 1997 IEEE, International Conference on Robotics and Automation, 1997, Pg1561-1566
[4] Schaefer S, Hoffmann KR, Noel P, Walczak AM: Reproducibility of guidewire positioning and stent path for endovascular interventions. Medical Physics, 32: 1918, 2005. Presented at AAPM 2005, July 24-28, 2005, Seattle, Washington.
[5] Elizabeth Bullitt, Guido Gerig, Stephen M. Pizer, Weili Lin, and Stephen R Aylward et al., "Measuring Tortuosity of the Intracerebral Vasculature From MRA Images" IEEE Transactions on Medical Imaging, Vol. 22, No. 9, September 2003 , pg 1163-71

Medicine Meets Virtual Reality 15
J.D. Westwood et al. (Eds.)
IOS Press, 2007

Validating Metrics for a Mastoidectomy Simulator

Christopher SEWELL [a], Dan MORRIS [a], Nikolas H. BLEVINS [b], Sumit AGRAWAL [b],
Sanjeev DUTTA [c], Federico BARBAGLI [a], Kenneth SALISBURY [a]
[a] *Department of Computer Science, Stanford University*
[b] *Department of Otolaryngology, Stanford University*
[c] *Department of Surgery, Stanford University*

Abstract. One of the primary barriers to the acceptance of surgical simulators is that most simulators still require a significant amount of an instructing surgeon's time to evaluate and provide feedback to the students using them. Thus, an important area of research in this field is the development of metrics that can enable a simulator to be an essentially self-contained teaching tool, capable of identifying and explaining the user's weaknesses. However, it is essential that these metrics be validated in able to ensure that the evaluations provided by the "virtual instructor" match those that the real instructor would provide were he/she present. We have previously proposed a number of algorithms for providing automated feedback in the context of a mastoidectomy simulator. In this paper, we present the results of a user study in which we attempted to establish construct validity (with inter-rater reliability) for our simulator itself and to validate our metrics. Fifteen subjects (8 experts, 7 novices) were asked to perform two virtual mastoidectomies. Each virtual procedure was recorded, and two experienced instructing surgeons assigned global scores that were correlated with subjects' experience levels. We then validated our metrics by correlating the scores generated by our algorithms with the instructors' global ratings, as well as with metric-specific sub-scores assigned by one of the instructors.

Keywords. Surgical simulation, automatic performance evaluation, metrics, temporal bone, tutoring, mastoidectomy

Introduction

The existing "apprenticeship" model of surgical training relies on real-life patient encounters as the substrate for learning. Inherent to this opportunistic approach is the assumption that enough patient encounters will take place within the set period of time (the "residency") to effect proficiency. Assessment of this cognitive and technical proficiency is based on the subjective impressions of the surgical educators, and is often erroneous [1].

The economics [2], efficiency [3], effectiveness, degree of responsibility and ethics [4] of this traditional approach have come into question in recent years, particularly for physicians in the early stages of training. With recent data on unacceptable rates of medical error nationwide to fuel this criticism, medical interest groups and governing bodies have called for accountability. Finally, educators are concerned over the validity of a training system that relies on chance patient encounters to fulfill learning objectives.

To address these challenges some surgical educators have moved toward enhancing, or perhaps replacing, the apprenticeship model with a competency-based curriculum [5]. Within such a system, proficiency is determined by successive mastery of skills as opposed to a prescribed length of training. Mastery is assessed not only by the subjective assessment of the surgeons that are responsible for training, but also by objective and standardized assessment tools. Furthermore, opportunities are put in place for repetitive practice of the necessary cognitive and technical skills in a non-threatening environment where errors are opportunities for learning rather than precursors to adverse outcomes. Finally, trainees are required to meet a rigorous standard of proficiency before being allowed to enter the workforce.

Recognizing that the current system of training cannot accommodate the above criteria, surgical educators have turned to simulation as a novel approach to instruction. Simulators are devices, often technologically intensive as in the case of virtual reality, that provide an ideal platform for repetitive practice, a key component to building expertise [6]. Tutorials that are developed through established methods of expert knowledge extraction (e.g. cognitive task analysis) can be programmed into simulators to teach the learner the preferred way of performing a procedure that they are then required to replicate. The simulators can be programmed to gradate difficulty of tasks to suit the level of the learner. The learner can "test" a variety of approaches to solving the same problem, promoting reflection and analysis of alternative strategies.

A key aspect of training by repetitive practice is constructive feedback. Without it, trainees are not able to improve upon their performance, and may reinforce substandard techniques. However, real-time or offline expert assessment of trainee performance on simulated tasks can be time consuming and costly. As such, it is crucial that virtual reality simulators automatically generate valid and reliable performance metrics that can be used by the trainee to gauge their progress. This study attempts to establish construct validity and inter-rater reliability for performance metrics generated by a novel mastoidectomy virtual reality simulator.

1. Simulator and Metrics

In close collaboration with an otolaryngologist, we have developed a visuohaptic mastoidectomy simulator [7]. In the simulator, a hybrid data structure is maintained that allows computation of appropriate drill forces using rapid collision-detection in a spatially-discretized volumetric voxel representation while graphically rendering a smooth triangular mesh that is modified in real-time as the voxels are drilled away. Other features include realistic drill sounds, bone dust (which can be removed using a suction controlled by a second haptic device), shadows, detailed anatomical models of surrounding structures and the inner ear, stereo graphics, a tool selection menu, networking for haptic mentoring, and a simulated neurophysiology monitor.

In order to take advantage of the opportunities for automated evaluation and intelligent tutoring made possible by a computer simulator's ability to record and analyze all of a user's actions, we have been particularly interested in developing performance metrics for our simulator. During a run of the simulator, all of the data is logged. A video can then be rendered, and the data can be loaded into a console that provides extensive calculation and visualization of all metrics (see Figure 1). The details of the implementations for each of these metrics are discussed in other papers [8][9][10], and are numbered here as listed in Table 1. The numerical "threshold" values given in the subsequent descriptions and used in this study are based on our informal adjustments using training data and feedback from surgeons, but are all easily modifiable in the console.

Metric 1 reports the percent of voxels that were removed while maintaining proper visibility, since it is important to keep the drilled bone within the line of sight so as to be able to notice visual cues and avoid underlying vulnerable structures. Metric 2 reports the percent of voxels removed using a 6mm drill burr when more than 75% of experts used a 3mm burr for that voxel, since using a large burr is dangerous near certain structures (while using a small burr in safe areas can prolong the procedure). Metric 3 reports the frequency of drill "jumps": the number of removed voxels per thousand that were more than 1 cm away from the previously removed voxel, since smooth, continuous drill strokes reflect expertise and confidence. Metric 4 reports the percent of voxels removed with the drill and suction more than 2 cm apart, since the suction should be kept near the drill to remove obscuring dust and provide irrigation. Metric 5 reports the percent of voxels removed while the surgical field was obscured by more than 300 bone dust particles, since this can reduce visibility. Each voxel of the bone is associated with a probability that an expert removes it, learned from expert training data, since removing all and only the correct bone is essential for a complete yet safe procedure. Metric 6 reports the mean of this probability for all voxels removed by the user. Metric 7 reports the sum of the number of voxels with expert probability over 0.8 not removed by the user and the number of voxels with expert probability under 0.2 that were removed by the user. Metric 8 reports the percentage of voxels removed while applying a drill force magnitude above 0.2 N (using a sliding-window average over 20 milliseconds), as pushing too hard could result in popping through bone and harming underlying structures. Metrics 9 through 12 report the percentage of voxels within 1 cm of, respectively, the dura, sigmoid, facial nerve, and inner ear, that were removed while applying a drill force above 0.2 N, since it is especially critical to be careful around these. Metric 13 reports the percentage of voxels removed while moving the drill faster than 2 cm/s (using a sliding-window average over 20 milliseconds), since moving too quickly can result in a loss of control. Metrics 14 through 17 report the percentage of voxels within 1 cm of, respectively, the dura, sigmoid, facial nerve, and inner ear, that were removed while moving the drill faster than 2 cm/s. Metric 18 reports the percentage of the facial nerve that has been properly exposed: the bone sufficiently thinned over it so that it can be seen, located, and safely avoided. Metric 19 reports the percentage of the facial nerve that has either been directly exposed or can be inferred from the directly exposed area. Metric 20 reports the percentage of the facial that has been overexposed: too much bone has been removed, allowing it to be contacted and harmed.

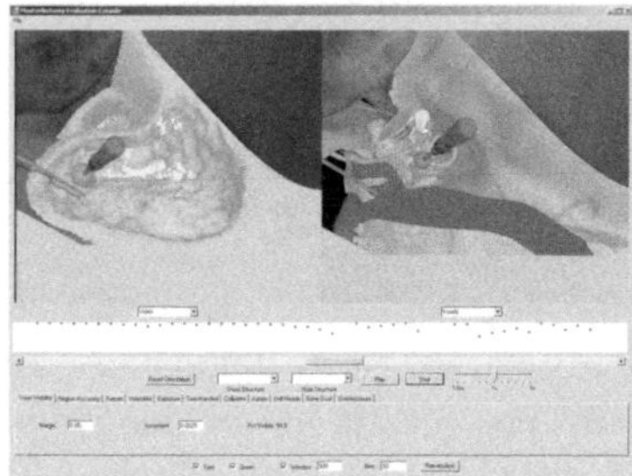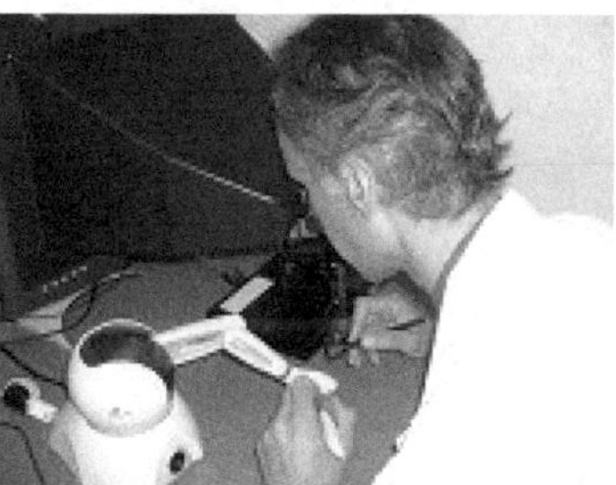

Figure 1. At left, a run of our simulator being replayed in the metrics console. At right, our simulator set-up.

2. Experimental Design

Fifteen right-handed participants were asked to perform a mastoidectomy (removal of a portion of the temporal bone and exposure of relevant anatomy) in our simulator. Participants included four experienced surgeons, four residents in head and neck surgery with surgical experience, and seven novices with no surgical experience.

Participants were presented with a tutorial of the simulator and were given fifteen minutes to practice using the haptic devices and the simulator's user interface. Participants were then presented with an instructional video describing the target procedure, and were given access – before and during the procedure – to still images indicating the desired appearance of the bone model at various stages in the procedure (Figure 2, left). Participants were asked to perform the same procedure twice.

Each participant's hand movements, haptic forces, and surgical interactions were logged to disk, then later rendered to video. Videos were assigned a global score on a scale of 1 to 5 by two experienced head and neck surgery instructors; the instructors were not aware of which videos came from which subjects and viewed them in randomized order. In addition, one of the instructors also assigned sub-scores (also on a scale of 1 to 5) to each of the videos according to several specific criteria directly related to individual metrics included in the simulator.

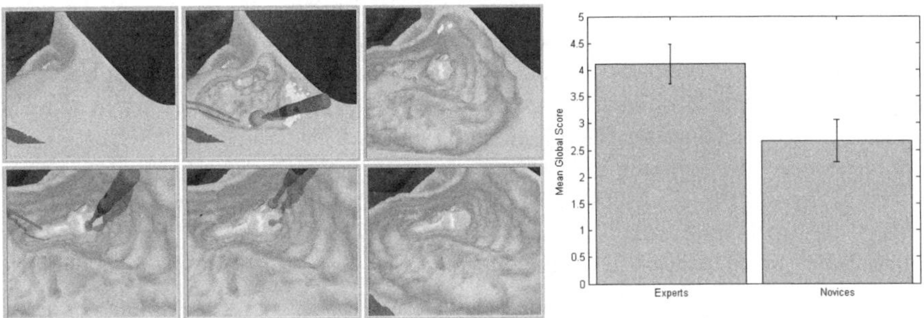

Figure 2. At left, still images presented to experimental participants, indicating the stages of the procedure. At right, expert and novice mean global scores, with 95% confidence interval error bars.

3. Results

The mean of the global scores received by the participants with prior surgical experience was found to be significantly different (p<0.0001 using one-tailed t-test) from the mean of the global scores received by the novices, whether considering the scores assigned by either of the instructors separately or considering the average of the two scores for each participant, thus establishing construct validity of our simulator (Figure 2, right). The scores assigned by the two instructors were well correlated (r=0.718, p<0.0001), demonstrating inter-rater reliability (Figure 3, left). The correlations of each of the metrics with the average of the two global scores assigned by the instructors are shown in Table 1. Table 2 presents the correlations of metrics for which one of the instructors assigned metric-specific sub-scores. A plot of instructor rating versus simulator score is shown for Metric 1 (visibility) in Figure 3, right side.

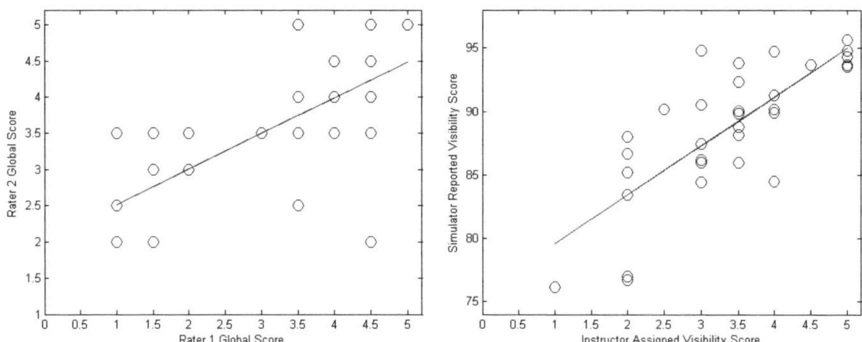

Figure 3. At left, correlation of the two instructors' scores. At right, correlation between instructor and computer assigned visibility scores (Metric 1).

Table 1. Correlations of metrics with the average of the global scores assigned by two instructors.

Metric	r	p	Metric	r	p
Drilling Technique			**Drill Forces**		
Pct Bone Visible at Removal (1)	0.728	<0.001	Pct Excessive Forces (8)	-0.355	0.046
Pct Removed with Burr Too Large (2)	-0.405	0.022	Near Dura (9)	-0.471	0.007
Jump Frequency (3)	-0.226	0.213	Near Sigmoid (10)	-0.420	0.017
Suctioning Technique			Near Facial Nerve (11)	-0.563	<0.001
Pct Excessive Inter-Tool Distance (4)	-0.469	0.007	Near Inner Ear (12)	-0.468	0.007
Pct Excessive Dust (5)	-0.365	0.040	**Drill Velocities**		
Bone Removal			Pct Excessive Vel. (13)	-0.131	0.474
Mean Removal Probability (6)	0.337	0.059	Near Dura (14)	-0.152	0.407
Pct Improbable (Non)Removals (7)	-0.794	<0.001	Near Sigmoid (15)	-0.143	0.434
Facial Nerve Exposure			Near Facial Nerve (16)	-0.387	0.029
Pct Directly Exposed (18)	0.469	0.007	Near Inner Ear (17)	-0.339	0.058
Pct Direct or Indirect Exposed (19)	0.519	0.002			
Pct Overexposed (20)	-0.536	0.002			

4. Discussion

Most of the metrics (1,2,4,5,7,8-12,16,18-20) correlated strongly ($p < 0.05$) with assigned global scores. While the avoidance of applying excessively large drill forces (8-12) did strongly correlate with performance, there was little such correlation for overall drill velocities (13), or for velocities when near the dura or sigmoid (14, 15), but there was a moderate correlation for velocities when near the facial nerve and inner ear (16, 17). This may reflect a tendency for skilled participants to always avoid applying large forces while still working quickly and confidently in relatively safe areas and exercising extreme caution in the particularly dangerous regions near the facial nerve and inner ear.

Table 2. Correlations of metrics with global scores and with metric-specific sub-scores.

	Specific Score		Global Score	
Metric	**r**	**p**	**r**	**p**
Pct Bone Visible at Removal (1)	0.777	<0.001	0.728	<0.001
Jump Frequency (3)	-0.355	0.046	-0.226	0.213
Pct Excessive Distance Between Tools (4)	-0.737	<0.001	-0.469	0.007
Pct Excessive Dust (5)	-0.681	<0.001	-0.365	0.040
Mean Removal Probability (6)	0.323	0.072	0.337	0.059
Pct Improbable Choices of Removal Regions (7)	-0.736	<0.001	-0.794	<0.001
Pct of Facial Nerve Directly Exposed (18)	0.400	0.023	0.469	0.007
Pct of F.N. Directly or Indirectly Exposed (19)	0.411	0.019	0.519	0.002
Pct of Facial Nerve Overexposed (20)	-0.500	0.004	-0.536	0.002

Several metrics correlated much more strongly with specific sub-scores than with the global scores. The frequency of drill jumps (3) was found to be closely related to the instructor's assessment of making "purposeful, confident motions", while the distance between instruments while drilling (4) and the percent of time drilling with excessive bone dust in the surgical field (5) closely correlated with the assessment of "two-handed and suctioning technique". However, for most metrics, the correlations with sub-scores were fairly similar to their correlations with the global scores, probably due to the tendency of most participants to score either relatively high on nearly all scores or relatively low on nearly all scores.

References and Acknowledgements

Support was provided by NIH LM07295.

[1] Paisley AM, Baldwin PJ and Paterson-Brown S: Accuracy of medical staff assessment of trainees' operative performance. Med Teach 27:634-8, 2005.
[2] Bridges M and Diamond DL: The financial impact of teaching surgical residents in the operating room. Am J Surg 177:28-32, 1999.
[3] Anastakis DJ, Wanzel KR, Brown MH, et al: Evaluating the effectiveness of a 2-year curriculum in a surgical skills center. Am J Surg 185:378-85, 2003.
[4] Gates EA: New surgical procedures: can our patients benefit while we learn? Am J Obstet Gynecol 176:1293-8; discussion 98-9, 1997.
[5] Sidhu RS, Grober ED, et al: Assessing competency in surgery: where to begin? Surgery 135:6-20, 2004
[6] Ericsson K: The acquisition of expert performance: An introduction to some of the issues, in Ericsson KA (eds): The road to excellence: The acquisition of expert performance in the arts and sciences, sports, and games. Mahwah, N.J., Erlbaum, 1996, pp 1 – 50.
[7] Morris D, Sewell C, Barbagli F, Blevins NH, Girod S, Salisbury K: Visuohaptic simulation of bone surgery for training and evaluation. To appear in IEEE Tran. on Comp. Graph. & App, Nov 2006.
[8] Sewell C, Morris D, Blevins N, Barbagli F, Salisbury K: Quantifying risky behavior in surgical simulation. Medicine Meets Virtual Reality, Long Beach, CA, January 2005, IOS Press, pp. 451-457.
[9] Sewell C, Morris D, Blevins N, Barbagli F, Salisbury K: Achieving proper exposure in surgical simulation. Medicine Meets Virtual Reality, Long Beach, CA, January 2006, IOS Press, 497-502.
[10] Sewell C, Morris D, Blevins N, Barbagli F, Salisbury K: Evaluating drilling and suctioning technique in a mastoidectomy simulator. To appear in Medicine Meets Virtual Reality, February 2007.

Medicine Meets Virtual Reality 15
J.D. Westwood et al. (Eds.)
IOS Press, 2007

Evaluating Drilling and Suctioning Technique in a Mastoidectomy Simulator

Christopher SEWELL [a], Dan MORRIS [a], Nikolas H. BLEVINS [b], Federico BARBAGLI [a], Kenneth SALISBURY [a]

[a] *Department of Computer Science, Stanford University*
[b] *Department of Otolaryngology, Stanford University*

Abstract. This paper presents several new metrics related to bone removal and suctioning technique in the context of a mastoidectomy simulator. The expertise with which decisions as to which regions of bone to remove and which to leave intact is evaluated by building a Naïve Bayes classifier using training data from known experts and novices. Since the bone voxel mesh is very large, and many voxels are always either removed or not removed regardless of expertise, the mutual information was calculated for each voxel and only the most informative voxels used for the classifier. Leave-out-one cross validation showed a high correlation of calculated expert probabilities with scores assigned by instructors. Additional metrics described in this paper include those for assessing smoothness of drill strokes, proper drill burr selection, sufficiency of suctioning, two-handed tool coordination, and application of appropriate force and velocity magnitudes as functions of distance from critical structures.

Keywords. Surgical simulation, automatic performance evaluation, metrics, temporal bone, tutoring, mastoidectomy

Introduction

In order to move towards the goal of enabling simulators to serve as intelligent, mostly-autonomous virtual instructors of surgical skill, we have previously proposed [1, 2] a number of metrics intended to capture some of the most important aspects of good technique that a real instructor tries to teach his/her residents in the field of temporal bone surgery, using our simulator [3]. In this paper we present several new metrics related to bone removal and suctioning technique.

Most existing surgical simulators, especially laparoscopic skill trainers, have attempted to incorporate a small number of simple metrics [4]. Most assume a simple global optimum value, such as minimize wall collisions, maximize path efficiency, or minimize completion time, and do not attempt to learn from runs of the simulators by experts or novices. Several have used learning algorithms such as Markov Models [5] or neural nets [6] to evaluate surgical performance.

1. Naïve Bayes Classifier for Removed Bone Voxels

One of the most obvious criteria for the evaluation of a mastoidectomy, a procedure in which part of the temporal bone is drilled away in order to access the inner ear, is whether correct decisions were made as to which regions of bone to remove and which to leave intact. A simple method is to have an instructing surgeon label which regions should and should not be removed, or to automatically label the voxels (used as the underlying representation of the bone volume in our simulator) drilled away by the instructor, and then compare the set of voxels removed by the trainee to this model. However, there is not necessarily a single correct technique; different experts may make somewhat different choices as to which bone to remove, and a given expert may vary somewhat between runs. In addition, not all regions are of equal importance; in some regions, it does not matter much exactly what is removed, while the choices may be much more critical in other areas, especially near nerves and other critical structures.

Thus, similar to how many e-mail spam classification algorithms assume that words from a dictionary are chosen for an e-mail message according to separate distributions by spammers and non-spammers [7], we have made an assumption that voxels from the full voxel mesh are chosen for removal according to separate distributions for experts and novices. We have implemented a Naïve Bayes classifier that calculates the maximum likelihood estimates for the probabilities that each voxel is removed by an expert and by a novice, and uses these to determine the probabilities that a given mastoidectomy was performed by an expert or by a novice.

If $y \in \{0,1\}$ are the class labels (0 = novice, 1 = expert), there are n voxels in the temporal bone model, and $\mathbf{x} \in \{0,1\}^n$ is an n-dimensional vector encoding whether each of the n voxels was (1) or was not (0) removed in a particular simulator run, then, making the Naïve Bayes assumption that the x_i's are conditionally independent given y, the probability of a particular set of choices for removal or non-removal for each voxel, given the class which generated it, can be written

$$p(\mathbf{x} \mid y) = \prod_{i=1}^{n} p(x_i \mid y)$$

The model is parameterized by $\phi_{i|y=k} = p(x_i=1 \mid y=k)$, the probabilities for each voxel i that it is removed in a run performed by a member of class y=k, and $\phi_y = p(y=1)$, the prior probability that a run was performed by an expert (y=1). We assume no prior probabilities, so we set $\phi_y = 1/2$. Given a set of m training examples, the maximum likelihood estimates for the other parameters, using Laplace smoothing (adding one phantom example that removes every voxel and one that removes none in each class, so as to avoid zero probabilities for any voxel), and denoting 1{s} as the function that returns 1 if s is true and 0 if s is false, are simply the fractions of examples in each class in which the voxels were removed:

$$\phi_{i|y=k} = \frac{\sum_{j=1}^{m} 1\left\{\left(x_i^{(j)} = 1\right) \wedge \left(y^{(j)} = k\right)\right\} + 1}{\sum_{j=1}^{m} 1\left\{y^{(j)} = k\right\} + 2}$$

Then, given a new set $\mathbf{x}$ of voxel removal choices, the probability that this was generated by an expert can be estimated using Bayes' Rule as:

$$p(y=1\mid\mathbf{x})=\frac{p(\mathbf{x}\mid y=1)p(y=1)}{p(\mathbf{x})}=$$

$$\frac{\left(\prod_{i=1}^{n}p(x_i\mid y=1)\right)\left(\frac{1}{2}\right)}{\left(\prod_{i=1}^{n}p(x_i\mid y=1)\right)\left(\frac{1}{2}\right)+\left(\prod_{i=1}^{n}p(x_i\mid y=0)\right)\left(\frac{1}{2}\right)}=$$

$$\frac{\prod_{i=1}^{n}\left(1\{x_i=1\}\phi_{i\mid y=1}+1\{x_i=0\}(1-\phi_{i\mid y=1})\right)}{\prod_{i=1}^{n}\left(1\{x_i=1\}\phi_{i\mid y=1}+1\{x_i=0\}(1-\phi_{i\mid y=1})\right)+\prod_{i=1}^{n}\left(1\{x_i=1\}\phi_{i\mid y=0}+1\{x_i=0\}(1-\phi_{i\mid y=0})\right)}$$

However, since the bone mesh is so large, and so many voxels are likely to not be very informative (i.e., will almost always be removed or not be removed, regardless of the subject's expertise), we calculated the mutual information (equivalent to a Kullback-Leibler divergence) for each voxel and built the classifier using only the $n=1000$ most informative voxels. The mutual information between each voxel x_i and the class labels y was calculated as

$$\mathrm{MI}(x_i,y)=\sum_{x_i\in\{0,1\}}\sum_{y\in\{0,1\}}p(x_i,y)\log\frac{p(x_i,y)}{p(x_i)p(y)}$$

with each of the probabilities estimated using their empirical distributions in the training set.

We then evaluated this metric by performing leave-one-out cross validation with our classifier. There was a statistically significant correlation ($r = 0.740$, $p<0.00001$) between the calculated probability estimates and a one-to-five subjective global score assigned by an instructing surgeon who watched video replays of the procedures (Figure 1).

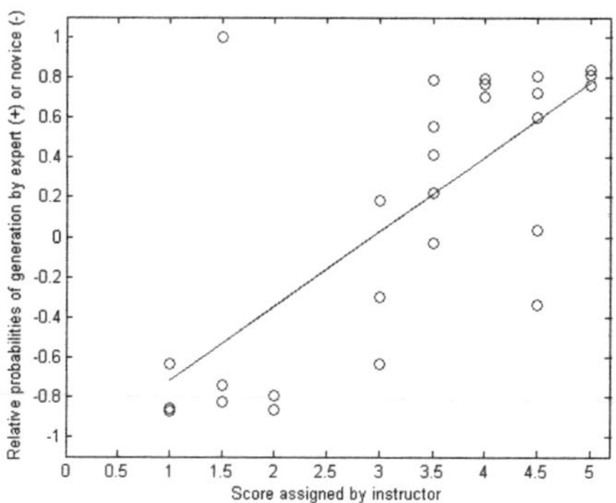

Figure 1. Correlation between instructor-assigned score and calculated probability of being in expert class.

This metric, along with all of our others, has been incorporated into our metrics console. When the simulator is run, all of the data is logged and can then be rendered to video or loaded into the console, which computes metric scores and provides a number of visualizations intended to help the user highlight potential problem areas. The user can be shown dots at the locations of each voxel he/she removed for which the expert removal probability was below a specified threshold value (Figure 2, left), or dots for each voxel not removed for which the expert removal probability was above a specified threshold value (Figure 2, right). The percentage of low-expert-probability voxels removed can be plotted at specified intervals on a timeline, allowing the user to quickly fast-forward to mistakes.

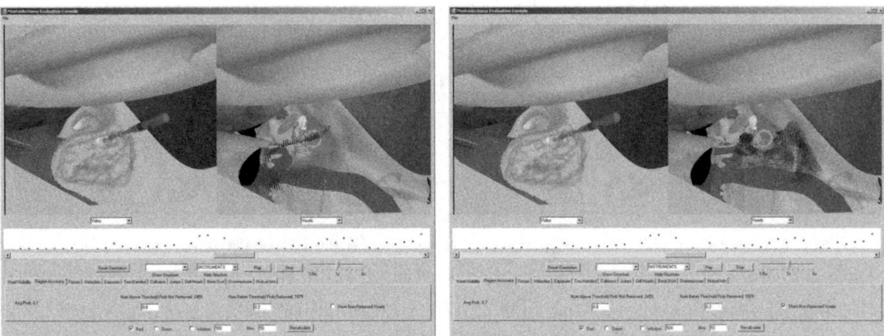

Figure 2. At left, improperly removed voxels shown with dots. At right, improperly remaining voxels.

This analysis can also yield an interesting visualization of the most informative voxels, which provides useful insight into the regions of bone most likely to be removed by experienced surgeons but left by novices and vice versa. In Figure 3, the 1000 most informative voxels (based on the training data) are shown. Those more likely to be removed by experts are in gray (brighter corresponds to greater expert-novice discrepancy), while those more likely to be removed by novices are in dark color. There are more voxels of the former case presumably due to greater uniformity among experts than among novices.

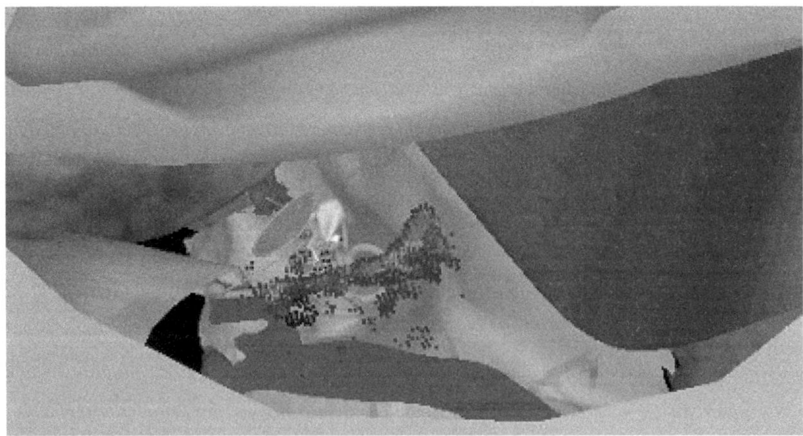

Figure 3. The 1000 most informative voxels (likely expert removals in gray, likely novice removals in black).

2. Other Metrics for Drilling Technique

Another key indicator of surgical skill is the exhibition of "purposeful" movements in drilling. An expert will almost invariably work locally, accomplishing a specific sub-goal (such as exposing a certain structure), and then move on to another task, and make smooth, continuous motions with the drill. A novice, on the other hand, is more likely to move around haphazardly without recognition for the localized subtasks that should be completed. Therefore, we have included a metric that reports the frequency of drill "jumps": the number of removed voxels per thousand that were more than a specified distance away from the previously removed voxel.

It is also important for a surgeon to know when to use each of his/her tools. In our simulator, the user can switch between 6mm and 3mm drill burrs. The smaller burr is intended for use near delicate structures, while the larger burr allows for quicker drilling in safer areas. The fraction of the time each burr is used to remove each voxel is learned from expert training data, and the user can be shown voxels he/she removed with the burr opposite the one used by the experts more than a specified fraction of the time for that voxel.

3. Metrics for Suctioning Technique

Good technique in the use of the suction involves removing bone dust as it is created in order to maintain visibility of the bone surface. In our simulator, particles of bone dust are generated as bone is removed, and a suctioning device (a second haptic device held in the opposite hand as the drill) is used to remove these particles. We have included a metric that highlights times in which the user was drilling while more than a specified number of dust particles obscured the surgical field. An example of excessive bone dust accumulation in the simulator is shown in Figure 4 (left side).

The coordination of the drill and the suction is an important element of good "two-handed technique." The suction should be kept near the drill when removing bone in order to prevent accumulation of bone dust and to properly cool the drilling surface (since the suction tool also provides irrigation). Therefore, another metric identifies voxels removed with the drill and suction more than a specified distance apart.

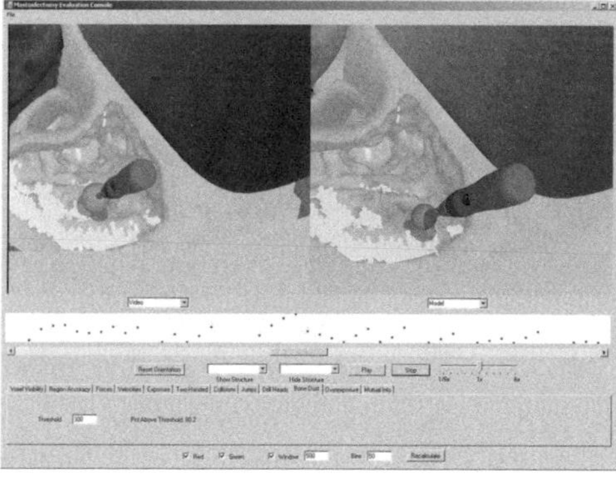
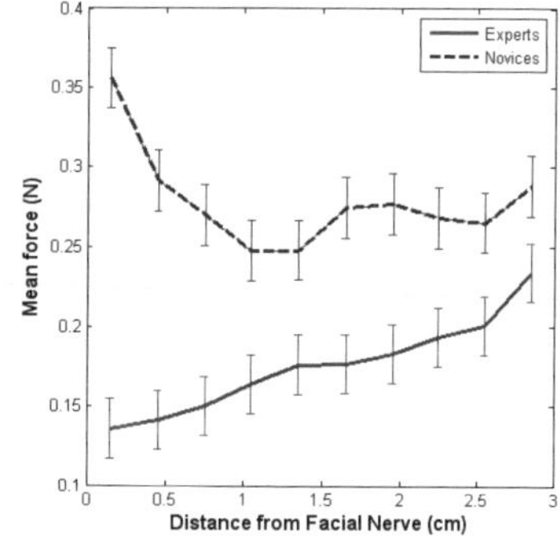

Figure 4. At left, excessive accumulated bone dust. At right, mean drill forces as facial nerve approached.

4. Metrics for Forces and Velocities

Applying appropriate forces and operating the drill at appropriate velocities are critical to safe drilling practice. In general, the magnitudes of these forces and velocities should decrease as vulnerable structures, such as the facial nerve, are approached, as shown in Figure 4 (right side), which shows force magnitudes as a function of distance from the facial nerve for experts and novices in our training data. The metrics console can highlight all voxels removed while applying force or velocity magnitudes above specified thresholds, or just such voxels within specified distances of critical structures. The values of these "safety thresholds" for forces and velocities can be assigned by an instructor or estimated from the expert training data.

5. Discussion

By considering all of these metrics together, as well as those we have previously proposed and ones yet to be developed, it is hoped that eventually the virtual instructor may be an adequate stand-in for the real instructor throughout much of the learning process, greatly reducing the time demands on instructors. It is therefore essential that we be able to establish that the feedback provided by these metrics mirrors that given by live instructors. We have conducted a study in which we have correlated the scores returned by these metrics with instructors' evaluations, the results of which are reported in [8]. We are also exploring additional metrics, including analyses of force, positional, and velocity profiles using time series classification.

References and Acknowledgements

Support was provided by NIH LM07295.

[1]   Sewell C, Morris D, Blevins N, Barbagli F, Salisbury K: Quantifying risky behavior in surgical simulation. Medicine Meets Virtual Reality, Long Beach, CA, January 2005, IOS Press, pp. 451-457.
[2]   Sewell C, Morris D, Blevins N, Barbagli F, Salisbury K: Achieving proper exposure in surgical simulation. Medicine Meets Virtual Reality, Long Beach, CA, January 2006, IOS Press, 497-502.
[3]   Morris D, Sewell C, Barbagli F, Blevins NH, Girod S, Salisbury K: Visuohaptic simulation of bone surgery for training and evaluation. To appear in IEEE Transactions on Computer Graphics and Applications, November 2006.
[4]   Cotin S, Stylopoulos N, Ottensmeyer M, Neumann P, Rattner D, Dawson S: Metrics for laparoscopic skills trainers: the weakest link! Proc of MICCAI, Lecture Notes in Computer Science 2002, 288: 35-43.
[5]   Rosen J, Solazzo M, Hannaford B, Sinanan M: Objective laparoscopic skills assessments of surgical residents using Hidden Markov Models based on haptic information and tool/tissue interactions. Proc of MMVR 2001.
[6]   Huang J, Payandeh S, Doris P, Hajshirmohammadi I: Fuzzy classification: towards evaluating performance on a surgical simulator. Proc of MMVR 2005, pp. 194-200.
[7]   Sahami M, Dumais S, Heckerman D, Horvitz E: A bayesian approach to filtering junk e-mail. AAAI Workshop on Learning for Text Categorization, 1998.
[8]   Sewell C, Morris D, Blevins N, Agrawal S, Dutta S, Barbagli F, Salisbury K: Validating metrics for a mastoidectomy simulator. To appear in proceedings of Medicine Meets Virtual Reality, February 2007.

Medicine Meets Virtual Reality 15
J.D. Westwood et al. (Eds.)
IOS Press, 2007

433

Patient Specific Simulation and Navigation of Ventriculoscopic Interventions [1]

R. SIERRA [a,2], S.P. DIMAIO [a], J. WADA [b], N. HATA [a], G. SZÉKELY [c],
R. KIKINIS [a], F. JOLESZ [a]

[a] *Brigham and Women's Hospital, Harvard Medical School, USA*
[b] *Department of Neurosurgery, Tokyo Medical University*
[c] *Computer Vision Laboratory, ETH Zurich, Switzerland*

Abstract. In this paper a comprehensive framework for pre-operative planning, procedural skill training, and intraoperative navigation is presented. The goal of this system is to integrate surgical simulation with surgical planning in order to improve the individual treatment of patients. Various surgical approaches and new, more complex procedures can be assessed using a safe and objective platform that will allow the physicians to explore and discuss possible risks and benefits prior to the intervention. A simulation environment extends the pre-operative planning in a natural way, as it allows for direct evaluation of the surgical approach envisioned for each case. In addition, by providing intraoperative navigation based on this simulation, surgeons can carry out the previously optimized plan with higher precision and greater confidence.

Keywords. patient-specific simulation, ventricles, fluid simulation, neurofiberscopic surgery, endoscope navigation

1. Introduction

To date, research has focused on either surgical training simulation or surgical planning, which have in some cases been combined with intraoperative guidance [1]. Surgical interventions are becoming increasingly complex in order to treat a broader range of diseases with minimal invasiveness while trying to reduce iatrogenic injuries. In particular, technological advances, e.g., in the miniaturization of devices, have provided the necessary means to reach remote areas in the human body through small incisions and to perform complex operations with appropriately adapted manipulators. For the success of these interventions, it is crucial that the surgery is not only thoroughly planned, but also that an appropriate environment is provided for the surgeons to practice and test the necessary skills.

Ventriculoscopy – the minimally invasive endoscopic inspection and treatment of the ventricles of the brain – serves as a driving application for this research. From the large range of ventriculoscopic procedures performed nowadays, ventriculostomy (the surgical

---

[1]This work was partially funded by NIH (U41-RR019703) and the Swiss National Science Foundation Fellowship (PBEZ2-110771)
[2]Correspondence to: Raimundo Sierra, rsierra@bwh.harvard.edu

establishment of an opening in a ventricle, e.g., for the treatment of hydrocephalus) and tumor biopsy are particularly challenging tasks, as evidenced by the high rates of failure and complication [2].

The long term goal of this research is to enable endoscopic, trans-ventricular in-traparenchymal brain tumor resection. Our vision is to provide a system for the safe treatment of pathologies that are unreachable using current techniques; where their re-moval would cause unacceptable morbidity when targeted directly from the skull. For such an intervention, accurate planning – including patient-specifi c training of skills and complication management – as well as intraoperative navigation, will be indispensable. Bleeding, for example, can impede the direct visualization of the surgical site through the endoscopic camera, thus requiring enhanced navigation in a simulated environment.

2. Materials and Methods

The position of the camera and the instruments, located at the tip of the flexible en-doscope, is tracked using a miniaturized tracking coil introduced through the working channel of the endoscope. The position and heading direction of the coil, i.e., 5 degrees of freedom (DOF), are measured by the NDI Aurora tracking system [3]. In our experi-ments, the complete ventricular system consisting of both lateral, the third and the fourth ventricle were segmented based on the patient's pre-operative MR data using an active contour segmentation tool using a level set approach as implemented in the 3D Slicer [4]. The resulting surface meshes were in excellent agreement with a manual segmentation performed by a clinical expert. A corresponding hollow plastic model was built by stere-olithography and fi xed inside a Styrofoam head model. The resulting anthropomorphic phantom was imaged in a CT scanner. The resulting images were registered with the head phantom – within the tracker's coordinate frame – and the endoscope position was tracked in order to be able to generate virtual endoscopic views from the image data. The underlying software framework is based on a high fi delity surgical simulator developed for procedural training of hysteroscopic interventions [5]. In the current implementation, the cerebrospinal fluid flow, bleeding, and soft tissue deformations can be simulated in real-time; however, given the complexity of the anatomical structures and the size of the meshes (approx. 175,000 triangles), tissue deformation had to be limited to a region of interest in order to maintain real-time performance.

3. Results

The current system is illustrated in Figure 1, where the fi eld generator of the Aurora tracker can be seen on the left side. The true endoscopic camera view is presented on the left screen, while the virtual environment is illustrated on the right screen with the navigation view on the left side and the simulated endoscopic perspective on the right side.

A subjective assessment of the real and virtual view shows excellent agreement. The missing information of the 6th degree of freedom is clearly visible as a rotation of the virtual view around the camera axis with respect to the actual camera view. This problem will be solved by using a new generation of coils which will allow for tracking of 6 DOF. The accuracy of endoscope localization was measured at a number of known landmarks visible in the CT images, yielding a mean overall error of 1.25mm (1.36mm RMS), which includes image registration errors [6]. Distortion due to camera optics has been

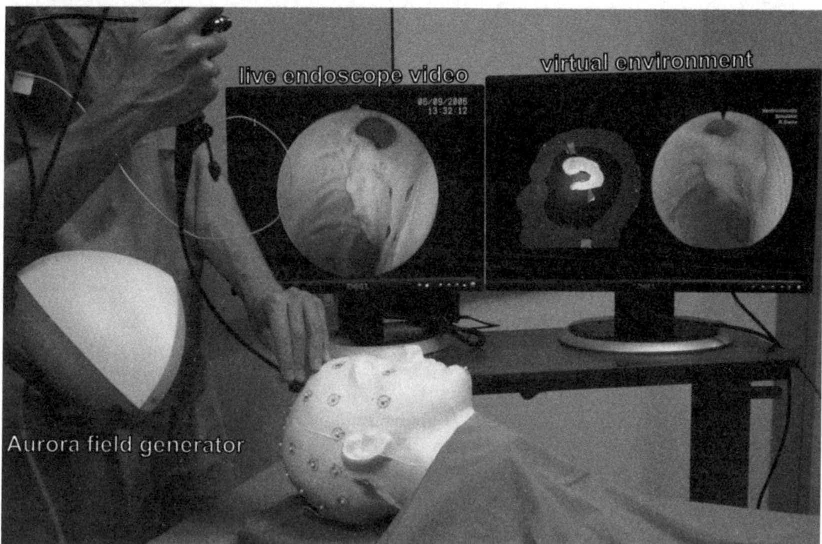

Figure 1. Ventriculoscopy navigation and simulation system.

measured separately. Lighting parameters and depth of view have been set empirically but will be measured in the future.

4. Discussion

Several aspects of navigated endoscopy can be explored using the framework developed here. By leaving out the real camera and navigation view, surgical skills can be trained in a realistic virtual, simulated environment. In addition, different entry points and instrument workspace traversals can be evaluated for planning and procedure prototyping. Intra-procedural brain shift is less pronounced in endoscopic procedures as compared to open surgeries; nevertheless, the system will have to account for this. Several options will be investigated, including image-based registration of the intraoperative view with the simulation or the control of the cerebrospinal fluid volume to maintain a constant fluid pressure and thus a constant ventricle shape. The ability to track the position of the instruments during surgery will be crucial in order to relate the video sequence to the virtual model which is necessary to quantify the predictive capabilities of the simulator.

References

[1] D. T. Gering et al. An Integrated Visualization System for Surgical Planning and Guidance Using Image Fusion and an Open MR. J. Mag. Res. Imag., 13:967–975, 2001.

[2] D. Hellwig et al. Endoscopic third ventriculostomy for obstructive hydrocephalus. Neurosurg Rev, 28:1–34, 2005.

[3] http://www.ndigital.com/aurora.php

[4] K. Krissian et al. Fast Sub-Voxel Re-initialization of the Distance Map for Level Set Methods. Pattern Recognition Letters, 26:10,1532–1542, 2005.

[5] http://www.hystsim.ethz.ch

[6] J. Wada et al. Development of a Slicer-based Navigation System for Neurofiberscopic Surgery. Symp. of the Int. Brain Mapping and Intraoerative. Surgical Planning Society, 2005.

Medicine Meets Virtual Reality 15
J.D. Westwood et al. (Eds.)
IOS Press, 2007

Developing Performance Criteria for the e-Pelvis Simulator Using Visual Analysis

Jonathan SILVERSTEIN[1], MD, MS, Gene SELKOV[1], Jr., Lawrence SALUD[2], MS,
Carla PUGH[2], MD, PhD
[1]*Department of Surgery, University of Chicago, Chicago IL, USA*
[2] *Department of Surgery, Northwestern University*
E-mail: jcs@uchicago.edu and drpugh@northwestern.edu

Abstract. The e-Pelvis is an inanimate simulator for clinical uterine examination. Data from the e-Pelvis has been studied extensively yet the clinical characteristics of palpation remain elusive. We describe our use of visual representation of the data that enabled expert physician/investigators to discover patterns of palpation.

Keywords. Visual Analysis, Clinical Examination, Simulation, Education.

1. Introduction

This paper describes our initial use of visualization and analysis to assist physician/investigators in the discovery of patterns in e-Pelvis sensor data. By looking for and finding patterns in the sensor data, we have identified latent measures that may be used as clinical performance criteria during simulated female pelvic examinations.

2. Background

The e-Pelvis is an inanimate teaching and assessment simulator for clinical uterine examination developed in an academic environment and then commercialized [1-3]. The system consists of a physical model instrumented with five force-sensing resistors on the simulated uterus. There are four sensors on the cervix (left posterior, right posterior, os, and anterior) and one sensor on the apex of the fundus. Each of these sensors independently records, at high fidelity, subjects' compression at various anatomic locations. Prior studies have generated much sensor and quiz data for specific clinical examples. Data was reduced to exam completion times, number of anatomical areas palpated, palpation frequencies and average palpation pressures. Statistical analyses using these variables have shown that students palpate the same number of areas as clinicians but with greater pressure and frequency and have longer examination times [4]. Markov Models have been successfully used to classify over 90% of subjects as students or clinicians. Palpation pressures in specific anatomical areas and certain palpation sequences appear to be skill dependent [5]. Despite these successes, prior analyses have not completely clarified the clinical characteristics of palpation techniques used during an exam. Hence, other methods are needed to more fully understand the data generated during simulated examinations.

3. Methods

Anonymous historical data was used with human subjects review exemption. All data from one day for one clinical example was used including two groups: 362 clinicians and 79 students. The data consisted of pressure values calculated from the force on each sensor for each subject sampled at 30 Hz for 2.2 min. Baseline was determined for each sample by using the most common value for each sensor. Start and end time for each subject was determined by detecting the first and last 5% deviation from baseline among all sensors (100% is the highest pressure recorded of all sensors). The mean value at each time point for each sensor for each group was calculated. The denominator was the number of subjects who had not yet reached their end time. We used custom software to generate "arc graphs" that summarize the data.

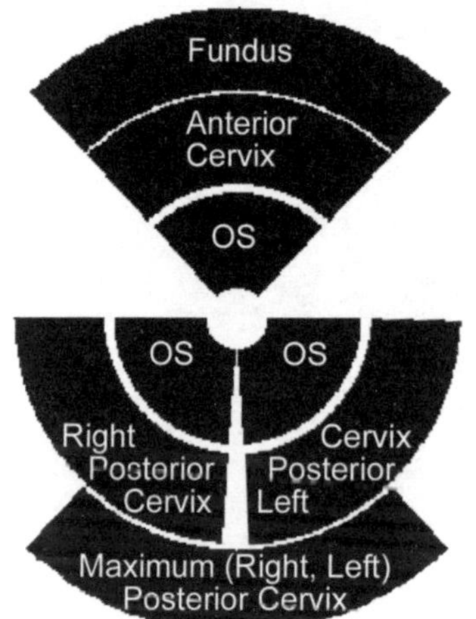

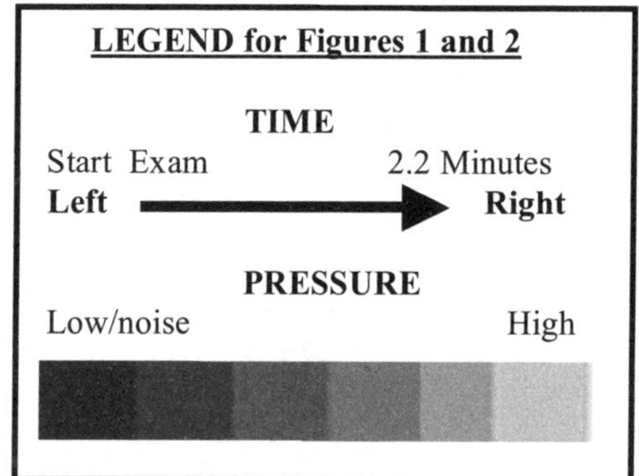

Figure 1. Arc graph representation of 2.2 minutes at baseline indicating the corresponding anatomical areas with overlaid text. The legend reveals time series direction and duration and gray scale correlation with amount of pressure applied to each sensor.

Each arc on each of Figures 1 and 2 is a clinically derived visual representation of a mean time series. They are intended to allow clinician/investigators to meaningfully view summarized data across many subjects simultaneously and correlate the sensor data with its spatial and temporal origin. Noise-level values (5% from baseline) are shown in black. Higher averages are shown in correspondingly brighter gray bands. Time progresses from left to right (clockwise above center white dot and counterclockwise below). Layout of the arcs conceptually represents locations of the sensors on the simulated uterus. The top arc shows the fundus data; the next lower arc (in the upper middle ring) shows the anterior fornix data; the lower middle arcs show left and right posterior fornix data (viewpoint of a clinical examiner); the bottom arc shows the maximum of the two posterior sensors (to correspond in time in the visualization with the fundus data). Three innermost arcs show three copies of the os data repeated for convenient juxtaposition in viewing with the other arcs.

4. Results

If one carefully reviews the arc graphs in Figure 2, a summary of the sensor data as two icons, a number of observations appear. First, one can see that the students spent much time pressing on the os throughout the exam (right center arcs are bright) whereas the clinicians applied less pressure for less time (left center arcs are first gray and then dark). Further, for each sensor, the clinicians, on average, discretely apply increasing pressure and then stop whereas the student average data is more random in nature for each sensor. One can also appreciate that on average clinicians moved counterclockwise and superiorly throughout the exam (to peak pressure at each location): left posterior, then right posterior, then os, then anterior, then fundus and then concluding with simultaneous fundus and right posterior pressure again.

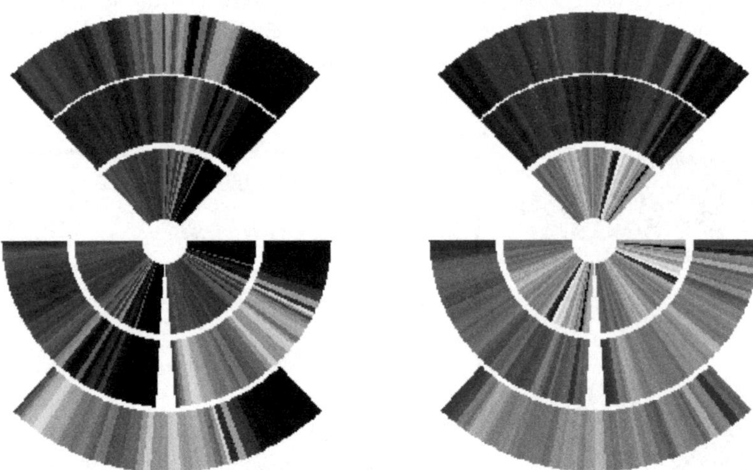

Figure 2. Arc graphs of mean pressure among all participants for the first 2.2 minutes of their exam. Clinicians data is averaged in the left arc graph and students in the right arc graph. Note that 2.2 minutes was selected as the cutoff time because all clinicians were finished (some student exams exceeded that time).

5. Conclusions

We have demonstrated that unique visual representations of time series from palpation data can enable discovery of clinical exam characteristics from expert examiners. These discoveries should now enable development and confirmation of statistical classifiers and performance criteria for each. This may enable a new class of physical exam simulators with criterion performance measures because the pressure sensors are also being used for breast exam, endotracheal intubation and other simulators.

References

[1]   Pugh C., Srivastava S., Shavelson R., Walker D., Cotner T., Scarloss B., et al. The effect of simulator use on learning and self-assessment: the case of Stanford University's E-Pelvis simulator. Stud Health Technol Inform. 2001;81:396-400.

[2]   Pugh C., Rosen J. Qualitative and quantitative analysis of pressure sensor data acquired by the E-Pelvis simulator during simulated pelvic examinations. Stud Health Technol Inform. 2002;85:376-9.

[3]   Pugh C., Youngblood P. Development and validation of assessment measures for a newly developed physical examination simulator. J Am Med Inform Assoc. 2002 Sep-Oct; 9(5):448-60.

[4]   Pugh CM, Heinrichs WL, Dev P, Srivastava S, Krummel TM. Use of a mechanical simulator to assess pelvic examination skills. JAMA. 2001 Sep 5;286 (9):1021-3.).

[5]   Mackel T., Rosen J., Pugh C. Data Mining of the E-Pelvis Simulator Database: A Quest for a Generalized Algorithm Capable of Assessing Medical Skill.   Stud Health Technol Inform 2003;119:355-360.

Medicine Meets Virtual Reality 15
J.D. Westwood et al. (Eds.)
IOS Press, 2007

439

Immersive Virtual Anatomy Course using a Cluster of Volume Visualization Machines and Passive Stereo

Jonathan C. SILVERSTEIN[1,2], Colin WALSH[1], Fred DECH[1], Eric OLSON[2],
Michael E. PAPKA[2], Nigel PARSAD[1], Rick STEVENS[2]
[1]Department of Surgery, University of Chicago, Chicago IL, USA
[2] Computation Institute, University of Chicago and Argonne National Laboratory
E-mail: jcs@uchicago.edu

Abstract. For more than a decade, various approaches have been taken to teach anatomy using immersive virtual reality. This is the first complete anatomy course we are aware of which directly substitutes immersive virtual reality via stereo volume visualization of clinical radiological datasets for cadaver dissection. The students valued highly the new approach and the overall course was very well received. Students performed well on examinations. The course efficiently added human anatomy to the University of Chicago undergraduate biology electives.

Keywords. Immersive Virtual Reality, Volume Rendering, Stereo Visualization, Education, Anatomy.

1. Background/Problem

Much has been presented at Medicine Meets Virtual Reality and elsewhere over the last decade regarding the theory and technical approaches toward using *immersive virtual reality as a cognitive teaching tool for clinical anatomy*. There are also numerous non-immersive virtual approaches for enhancing anatomy education via the Internet, commercial applications, books, dissection videos, virtual models, etc. A recent review of the theory behind using virtual materials for anatomic teaching and its potential future is instructive [1]. However, in the context of a formal anatomy course with discrete educational objectives, publications of *assessments of the value* of immersive virtual technologies are rare excluding our own work [2, 3].

Our prior assessment studies used geometric models to teach surgical anatomy in medical school and residency curricula [4, 5]. In this paper we highlight another novel technical approach to teaching human anatomy in a class taught Spring Quarter 2006 in the undergraduate biology curriculum at the University of Chicago. More importantly, we present our assessment of its first use. This comprehensive anatomy course was instructed using a "cover-to-cover" methodology with the same human anatomy textbooks used in our medical school (including web-based media) [6, 7]. However, in a small group setting, large format stereo volume visualization of high-resolution clinical radiological data was completely substituted for human cadaver dissection laboratory experience. To clarify, we did not have an extant undergraduate human anatomy course or access to cadavers nor was there sense of equipoise among the investigators to warrant a "trial".

2. Tools and Methods

Use of anonymous clinical radiological (CT and MR) and Visible Human Female [8] imaging data and reporting of educational practice in a formal course was exempt from human subjects review.

The datasets, normal clinical studies, were obtained directly from the clinical imaging scanners in the DICOM standard. Studies were chosen to contrast anatomic structures in all body regions. For the hand and some features of the head and neck, not normally well contrasted in clinical radiological studies, specialized reformatting of Visible Human data to DICOM was used (which has similar pixel resolution to our Philips 64-slice CT scanner from which the CT data originated). Clinical studies were not pre-processed. In general, studies had highest available clinical resolution.

The volume visualization system is a customized cluster of nine commodity computer graphics Linux servers running our home-grown scalable libraries (parallelized ray casting of volumetric data using MPI) written in OGL Shader Language, coupled with the VTK DICOM loader class, and a GUI written in the wxWidgets C++ cross-platform GUI library. The library includes a custom designed automatic coloring algorithm that gives the anatomy a life-like appearance in many regions and provides full-volume dataset rendering control at interactive rates (window, level, cut, pan, zoom, rotate, color, etc.). The system can display directly to left and right VGA outputs or via Access Grid to remote participants (in stereo). The display used in the course was a passive stereo wall, approximately 6' by 5', with back projection of left and right images separated via linear polarization filters. Figure 1 shows three different renderings of the same data by simply adjusting the window level and moving in a cutting plane.

The class size was small, seven undergraduate students, and was held in a conference room seminar environment with immersive system display on one wall and standard projection on the perpendicular wall for live web-based textbook materials (see Figure 2). The stereo volume renderings and web-based textbook materials were interspersed, as the instructor deemed most productive during each session. Student questions and comments in this open forum drove the type of media used at any given time. The class was intense, covering the whole body in one 10-week quarter with two 110-minute sessions per week including quizzes for each body region (30 "contact hours"). Weekly student exams by body region were quite similar to medical school course exams using cadavers. These included fill-in, essay, matching, and much structure identification (via blinded use of the extensive photographic atlas).

Assessments included student exams, specific assessments of the various elements of the course (textbook, atlas, and immersive virtual reality), and the standard University of Chicago ratings of undergraduate courses by students.

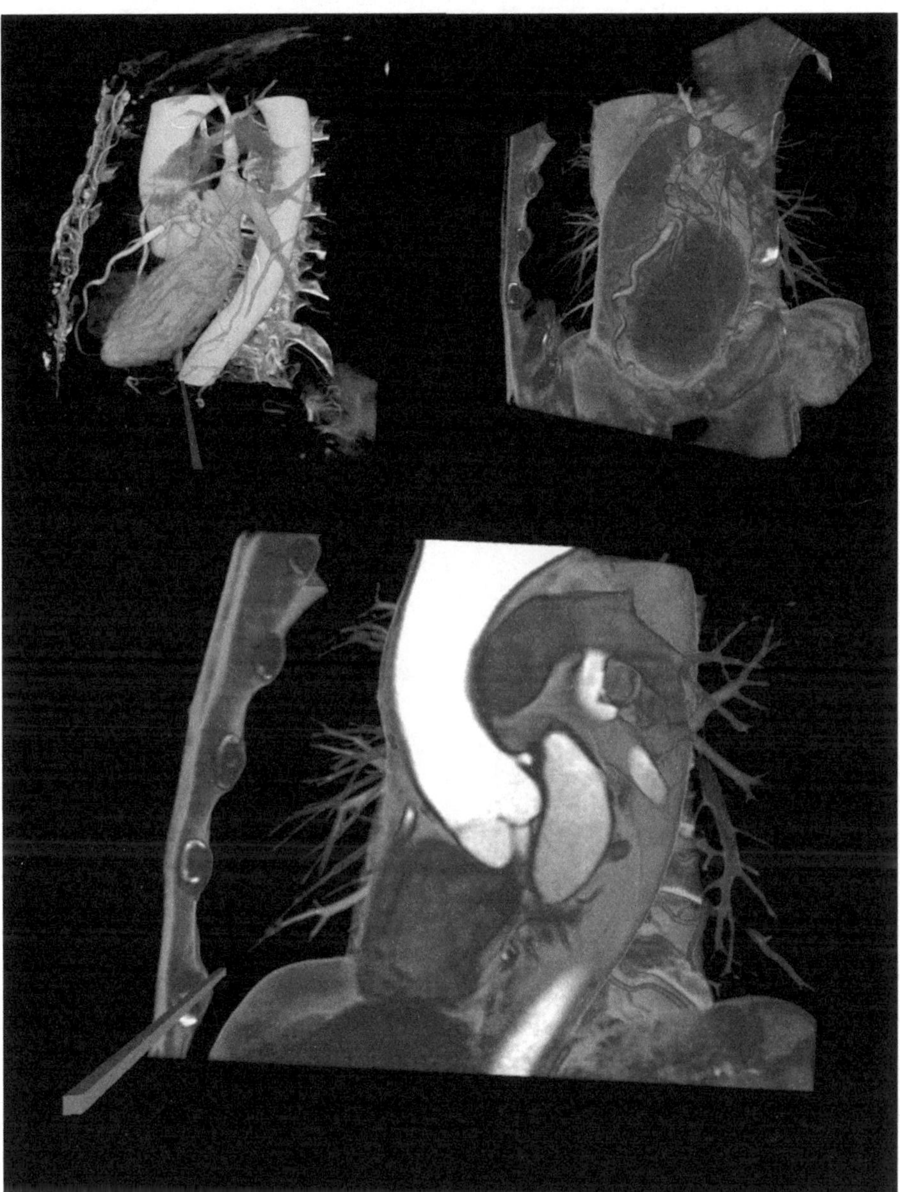

Figure 1: Renderings of high resolution CT data of the Heart. The first (upper left) pane is at high window level showing vascular contrast. The second (middle) pane shows a mid-range window level. The lower pane shows a cut plane view and a virtual pointer.

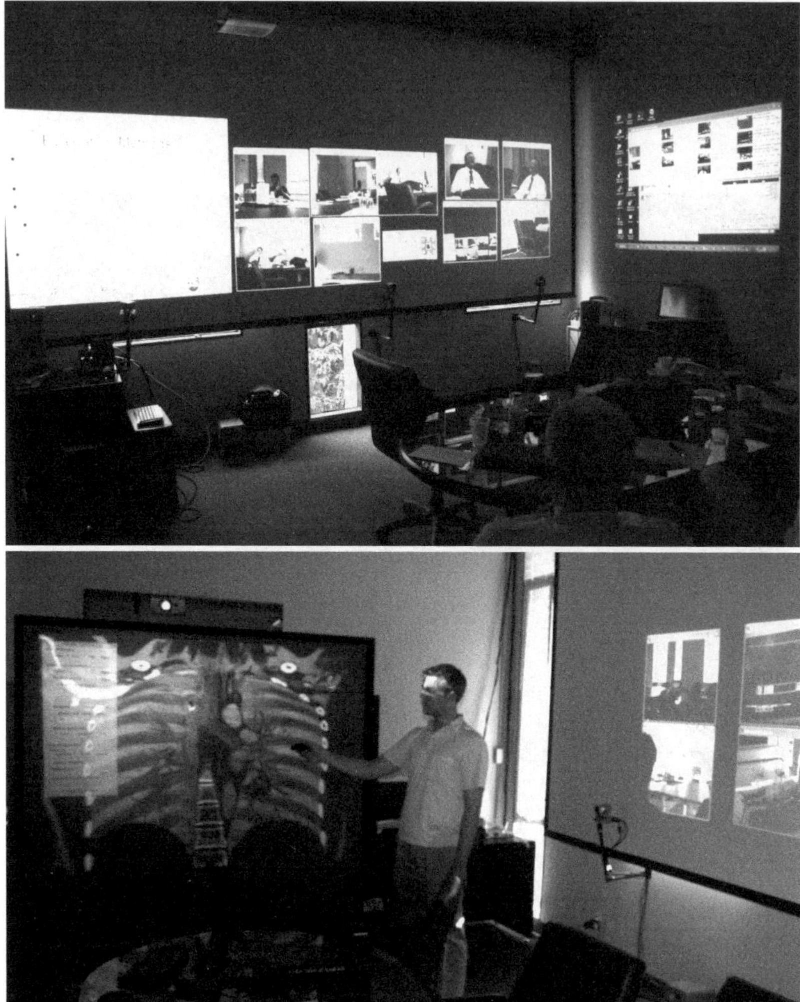

Figure 2: Layout of the classroom. The first (upper) pane is a room view from the entrance doorway showing a small conference table and two standard (2-D) multi-projection walls. Here they show an Access Grid session. The second (lower) pane looks left at the third projection wall, the stereo rendering wall.

3. Results

Each weekly exam was completed in approximately 20 to 30 minutes of class time. Excellent learning was achieved as demonstrated by the exam scores among the students, typically ranging from 60% to 95% correct answers. No student had significant prior experience with human anatomy. Students reported an average of 6.6 (s.d. 1.82) hours of preparation per week.

Because materials (textbook, atlas, immersive virtual reality) were used in interspersed, sometimes seemingly random, fashion in each educational session, direct observation and analysis of how each type of material contributed to the knowledge gained was not possible. However, the course-specific assessment of each element of the course did enable some stratification of the students' value judgments according to course elements. Table 1 demonstrates that overall the virtual reality system was deemed equally or more valuable than the standard materials. The system contributed equally or more than other materials in enjoyment and in the framework of learning, but not in ultimate understanding or learning value (which we have seen before [4]).

Value Element Assessed	Enjoyment	Value in learning	Efficiency in learning	Contribution to mental model or framework of learning	Contribution to ultimate understanding	Total Value (calc)
Paper Textbook	3.9 (0.3)	4.4 (0.5)	3.7 (0.7)	4.1 (0.3)	4.6 (0.5)	4.1 (0.3)
Paper Atlas	3.9 (0.6)	4.6 (0.7)	3.7 (1.2)	4.4 (0.5)	4.8 (0.4)	4.3 (0.4)
Virtual Reality	4.9 (0.3)	4.3 (0.5)	3.6 (0.9)	4.4 (0.7)	4.4 (0.5)	4.3 (0.4)

1 = poor, 2=fair, 3=good, 4=very good, 5=excellent
Table 1: Mean (s.d.) value element assessments (N=7)

The standard course assessments (Table 2) demonstrated that the course was valued well above the average rating for all University of Chicago Biological Sciences Collegiate Division courses in all factor areas and in all sub-areas (not shown).

Factor Assessed	Immersive Virtual Anatomy Course	Average Rating for all Courses Spring 2005-06
Organization of Course	4.5	4.2
Value of Material	4.9	4.2
Demands and Expectations	4.5	4.2
Overall Rating	4.4	4.1

5=Strongly Agree. Note that students also reported Mean (s.d.) of 6.6 (1.82) hours preparation per week.
Table 2: Ratings of Undergraduate Course by Students. Includes all University of Chicago Biological Sciences Collegiate Division courses (N=5)

4. Conclusions/Discussion

The combination of the technology and data was so compelling that students invited colleagues, friends and other professors to class and requested that they incorporate the method into other courses. This course has now added human anatomy to the undergraduate biology electives, and has done so efficiently in that there is very low cost of materials (essentially zero because the room and computers are infrastructure).

There were some difficulties encountered in the course worth noting. Some key structures, particularly peripheral nerves, cannot be contrasted yet in today's best radiological studies. The approach of simply exploring the data ad hoc during class coupled with the complexity of selecting optimal windows, levels, and cut planes did certainly sometimes make inefficient use of class time. More pre-planning of the use of each dataset was needed (and is generally good educational practice). Unfortunately, pre-planning of each use was often not done because the system and data was frequently available just in time throughout this first instance of the course.

Student exams and course assessments demonstrated that the new approach was very valuable. The value element assessment results and course ratings suggests a clear role for systems of this type in enhancing the learning experience and as an adjunct to gaining a framework or mental model of the material, but not at this stage as a replacement of traditional materials. It would be interesting to see how cadaver dissection performed on similar measures, but this is not available to us. We suspect the lower results for value and efficiency of learning relates to the system being used as a demonstration tool throughout the course rather than as a self-study element and to the complexity of the early version visualization interface (not shown). We suspect more mature deployments would further improve value.

We are working toward a manuscript fully characterizing the underpinning technology and open source release of the code.

Acknowledgement

This work was supported in part by the National Institutes of Health/National Library of Medicine, under Contract N01-LM-3-3508 and by the U.S. Department of Energy under Contract W-31-109-Eng-38. The authors also wish to acknowledge the support of Drs. Dianna Bardo and Michael Vannier in identifying and providing suitable radiological studies for the course as well as Matt McCrory and Justin Binns for early work on our volume rendering library and cluster systems.

References

[1]   V.M. Spitzer, A.L. Scherzinger. Virtual Anatomy: an anatomist's playground. *Clinical Anatomy*. 2006 Apr;19(3):192-203.
[2]   H. Hoffman, M. Murray. Anatomic VisualizeR: realizing the vision of a VR-based learning environment. *Stud Health Technol Inform*. 1999;62:134-40.
[3]   Issenberg SB, McGaghie WC, Petrusa ER, Lee Gordon D, Scalese RJ. Features and uses of high-fidelity medical simulations that lead to effective learning: a BEME systematic review. *Med Teach*. 2005 Jan;27(1):10-28.
[4]   Silverstein JC, Dech F, Edison M, Jurek P, Helton WS, Espat NJ. Virtual Reality: Immersive Hepatic Surgery Educational Environment (IHSEE). *Surgery*. 2002;132(2):274-7.
[5]   Silverstein JC, Ehrenfeld JM, Croft D, Dech F, Small S, Cook S. Tele-Immersion: Preferred Infrastructure for Anatomy Instruction. *Journal of Computing in Higher Education*. 2005;18(1):80-93.
[6]   R.L. Drake, W. Vogl, A.W.M. Mitchell. *Gray's Anatomy for Students*. Elsevier. Philadelphia. 2005.
[7]   J.W. Rohen, C. Yokochi, E. Lutjen-Drecoll. *Color Atlas of Anatomy*. Lippincot Williams &Wilkins. Philadelphia. 2002
[8]   M.J. Ackerman. The Visible Human Project: a resource for education. *Acad Med*. 1999;74:667-70.

Medicine Meets Virtual Reality 15
J.D. Westwood et al. (Eds.)
IOS Press, 2007

445

Virtual Open Heart Surgery: Obtaining Models Suitable for Surgical Simulation

Thomas Sangild SØRENSEN [a], Jean STAWIASKI [b] and Jesper MOSEGAARD [c]
[a] CAVI and [c] Dept. of Computer Science, University of Aarhus, Denmark
[b] Centre for Mathematical Morphology, Ecole des Mines de Paris, France
sangild@cavi.dk

Abstract. We present a pre-processing strategy including imaging, segmentation, and model reconstruction that is well suited for previously published GPU-accelerated techniques for surgical simulation. In particular we describe these modeling steps as a prerequisite for our virtual open heart surgery simulator. A short description including relevant references is presented for each of the steps.

Keywords. Segmentation, surgical simulation, congenital heart disease

Introduction

The modern graphics processing unit (GPU) has provided a new computational platform suitable for surgical simulation [1]. Using the GPU for both simulation and visualization, the deformation of complex morphology can now be simulated interactively [2-4]. While [1-4] introduce the technical aspects behind a GPU-based surgical simulator, this paper presents a method to obtain simulation suitable, high resolution morphological volumes and surfaces – a prerequisite for realistic simulation of e.g. open heart surgery [5].

1. Materials, Methods and Results

Our aim is to obtain a volumetric segmentation of the heart muscle (the myocardium) and vessel walls. A spring-mass based physical simulation is then used to interactively deform this volume [2]. Visualization of the deformed heart is fully decoupled from the underlying simulation [3], and surfaces are thus reconstructed independently of the resolution of the spring-mass system.

1.1. Imaging and segmentation

All models are reconstructed from isotropic 3D MRI covering the whole heart (Figure 1, left). An operator-independent acquisition lasting from six to twelve minutes results in 50 to 120 slices. The voxel resolution ranges from 1.5^3 mm^3 to 2.0^3 mm^3 depending on the heart rate, size, and general cooperation of the patient [6-7]. A watershed-based segmentation algorithm was used to segment the blood pool and myocardial volume semi-automatically (Figure 1, middle left) using the Cardiac3D software (Systematic Software Engineering, Denmark). The user interactively inserts colored markers in the MRI and the resulting segmentation is presented instantly (transparent red/green colors) [8-10]. Some manual adjustments are always necessary, and a "drawing stencil" is provided to support this operation. The tissue bordering major blood vessels (i.e. the

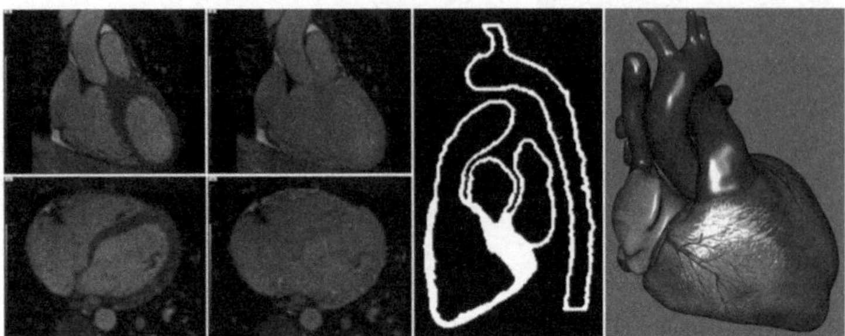

Figure 1. MR image acquisition (left), segmentation (middle left), smoothing and
vessel wall growing (middle right), and surface reconstruction (right).

aorta, the pulmonary arteries and veins, and the caval veins), the atria, and parts of the
right ventricle is too thin to be clearly visible on the MRI. To overcome this problem,
(vessel) walls are automatically grown to constitute the blood pool borders in areas
where the segmented blood pool is not bordered by segmented tissue (Figure 1, middle
right). We tend to smooth the epicardium (the outmost myocardial border) more than
the endocardium (the innermost myocardial border) as we extract the segmentation.
This is achieved by restoring the segmented blood pool and hereby the endocardium
some user-defined fraction through the smoothing process. The endocardium is
consequently only affected in the remaining smoothing iterations.

1.2. Obtaining the volumetric simulation grid

A typical 3D MRI dataset contains 256 x 256 x 100 voxels [6-7]. The number of voxels
classified as tissue by the segmentation process is in the order of 250.000. Ideally, each
of these tissue voxels should be treated as one particle in the spring-mass simulation.
The simulation and convergence rates for such large systems are too slow however,
even with for GPU-accelerated implementations. We consequently downsample by a
factor of 2^3 to obtain approximately 30.000 simulation nodes in a regular three-
dimensional grid [2]. The binary image in Figure 1 (middle right) shows one slice from
such a simulation grid.

1.3. Surface visualization processing

A highly detailed surface is extracted from the segmented endocardium-, epicardium-,
and vessel borders at full resolution by the marching cubes algorithm [11]. The
resulting model easily contains 1.000.000 triangles. We represent each vertex by an
offset from the nearest simulation grid node [3]. It is necessary to express each offset in
a vector basis local to the simulation node to have the offset vector deform according to
the spring-mass system's deformation. This requires some per vertex processing in
each frame. As this is a relatively costly operation we reduce the triangle count in the
high-resolution surface model to avoid a visualization bottleneck. Normal maps are
used to conserve the details of the high-resolution mesh in the simplified model of
50.000-100.000 faces (Figure 1, right).

Our implementation of force feedback is realized by a GPU based picking and
force calculation technique [4]. It requires off-screen rendering of a low-resolution
model with a vertex for each "surface mass point" in the simulation grid. This model is
again obtained from the marching cubes algorithm [11].

2. Discussion

We see two potential scenarios for the current simulator prototype; patient-specific preoperative planning, and surgical education [5]. In the first scenario we can segment the blood pool, the left sided myocardium and grow vessel walls in one to two hours in good quality datasets. The right sided epicardium remains a challenge to segment rapidly, but could be "grown" to a certain thickness surrounding the blood pool by a dedicated volume paint application instead. Generally, any thin borders are invisible on the MRI due to partial volume effects, which makes the "tissue growing mechanism" a necessity. While some manual corrections are needed at the segmentation stage, the remaining pre-processing steps can be fully automated. We are currently evaluating the required segmentation time on a larger number of patients.

When working in the educational scenario, we have no time constraints creating each model. In Figure 1, right 2 we consequently normal mapped the myocardial surface with the coronary arteries – drawn manually by a graphics artist. We could also have encoded information on e.g. the electrical induction system in such texture maps. These need not be visible to the user but can be used instead to detect and report the likelihood of each incision damaging in this case the induction system.

3. Acknowledgments

Funding received from the Danish Research Council (grant #2059-03-0004), The Danish Heart Foundation (grant #05-10-B359-A657-22265), and an EU Marie Curie Host Fellowship.

4. References

[1]　T.S. Sørensen, J. Mosegaard. An Introduction to GPU Accelerated Surgical Simulation. 3rd Symposium on Biomedical Simulation. Zurich, Switzerland. Lecture Notes in Computer Science (4072) 2006; 93-104.

[2]　J. Mosegaard, P. Herborg, T.S. Sørensen. A GPU accelerated spring-mass system for surgical simulation. 13th Medicine Meets Virtual Reality 2005. Stud Health Technol Inform; 111:342-8.

[3]　J. Mosegaard, T.S. Sørensen. Real-time Deformation of Detailed Geometry Based on Mappings to a Less Detailed Physical Simulation on the GPU. Eurographics Virtual Environments Workshop 2005; 105-10.

[4]　T.S. Sørensen, J. Mosegaard. Haptic Feedback for the GPU-based Surgical Simulator. 14th Medicine Meets Virtual Reality 2006. Stud Health Technol Inform; 119:523-8.

[5]　T.S. Sørensen, G.F. Greil, O.K. Hansen, J. Mosegaard. Surgical simulation - a new tool to evaluate surgical incisions in congenital heart disease? Interactive Cardiovascular and Thoracic Surgery 2006; 5:536-539.

[6]　T.S. Sørensen, H. Körperich , G.F. Greil, J. Eichhorn, P. Barth, H. Meyer, E.M. Pedersen, P. Beerbaum. Operator-independent isotropic three-dimensional magnetic resonance imaging for morphology in congenital heart disease: a validation study. Circulation. 2004; 110(2):163-9.

[7]　M. Fenchel, G.F. Greil, P. Martirosian, U. Kramer, F. Schick, C.D. Claussen, L. Sieverding, S. Miller. Three-dimensional morphological magnetic resonance imaging in infants and children with congenital heart disease. Pediatr Radiol. 2006; In press.

[8]　L. Vincent, P. Soille. Watersheds in Digital Spaces: An efficient Algorithm based on Immersion Simulations. IEEE Transactions on Pattern Analysis and Machine Intelligence 1991; 13(6): 583-98.

[9]　T.S. Sørensen, E.M. Pedersen, O.K. Hansen, K. Sørensen. Visualization of morphological details in congenitally malformed hearts: Virtual, three-dimensional reconstruction from magnetic resonance imaging. Cardiol Young. 2003; 13(5):451-60.

[10]　J. Stawiaski, J. Mosegaard, T.S Sørensen. Virtual Open Heart Surgery: Segmentation. 15th Medicine Meets Virtual Reality 2007. In press.

[11]　W.E. Lorensen, H.E. Cline. Marching cubes: A high resolution 3D surface construction algorithm. Proceedings of the 14th annual conference on Computer graphics and interactive techniques, Siggraph 1987; 163-69.

Medicine Meets Virtual Reality 15
J.D. Westwood et al. (Eds.)
IOS Press, 2007

Virtual Open Heart Surgery Segmentation

Stawiaski Jean [a], Mosegaard Jesper [b], Sørensen Thomas [b]
[a] *Ecole des Mines de Paris, Centre de Morphologie Mathématique*
[b] *Aarhus University, Centre for Advanced Visualization and Interaction*

Abstract. We have developed a semi-automated segmentation method based on the Watershed transform [1]. The watershed transform is a fast and intuitive segmentation method. It is applied to 3D cardiac MRI to interactively produce patient-specific models for pre-operative planning and virtual heart surgery [2]. Our software offers a detailed exploration of the data-set via combination of many visualization techniques such as volume rendering, multiple overlays, and surface rendering.

Keywords. Virtual heart surgery, watershed segmentation.

Introduction

Segmentation of the heart remains a challenging task as the heart morphology is known to be very complex. Particularly in congenitally malformed hearts, where the morphology varies significantly from individual to individual, any approach relying on prior knowledge from normal morphology will fail. We propose an interactive solution to the problem of the heart segmentation: the marker constraint watershed transform. Our process needs some markers on different parts of the organ to be segmented. The markers are then growing according to the watershed algorithm [3]. These markers can be seen as patient-specific prior information that constraint the watershed transform to include some specific parts of the image.

1. Algorithm

The watershed transform uses an intuitive description of boundary in an image: It considers an image as a topographic surface where the height of each point is directly related to its gray level. The algorithm then simulates a flooding of this surface from a finite set of points. To avoid mixing of water of different sources, a watershed line is constructed where they meet. The watershed line computed on the gradient of an image finds the high gradient points which are related to boundaries in the image. In cardiac MRI this corresponds to e.g. the border between the blood pool and the myocardium. To avoid over-segmentation due to noise in the images, the set of points from which the flooding process starts is defined interactively by the user [3]. Details of the implementation can be found in [1].

2. Segmentation

All models are reconstructed from 3D MRI acquired with isotropic voxels at a resolution of approximately $1.7^3 mm^3$, which forms a data-set of 256x256x100 voxels. The images are first filtered using anisotropic diffusion [4]. The user then specifies the different objects of interest in the image by inserting a few markers from which the watershed transform is invoked. The user can place markers interactively by drawing on 2D slices. This method was used to segment the blood pool and myocardium volume semi-automatically (see Figure 1). After the segmentation step, the user can add or delete markers if it is necessary.

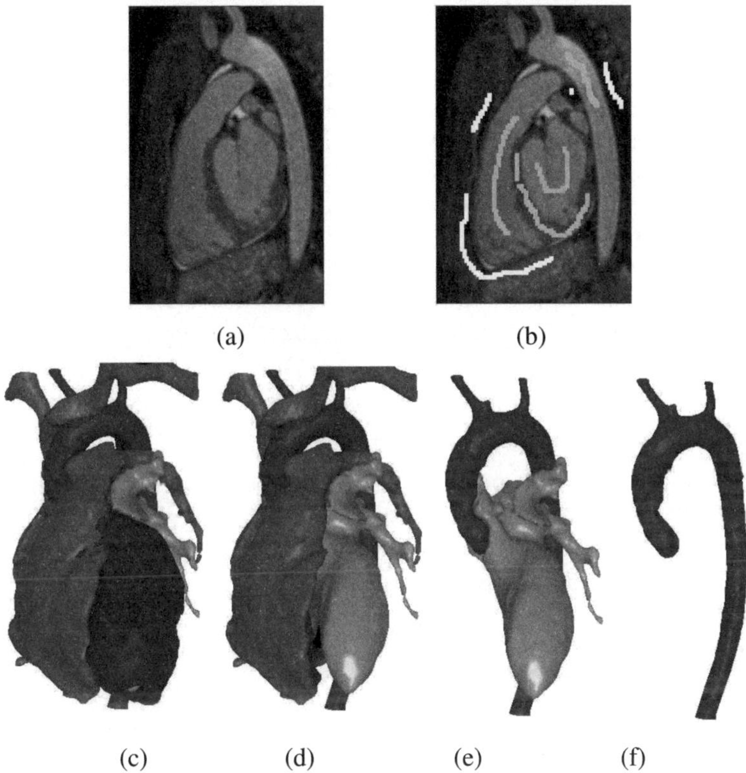

Figure 1. (a) Original MRI Data.(b) User specifies interactively some markers by drawing on a slice. (c-f) Different parts of the segmented data. The segmented images are drawn as surfaces. The software enables the user to select surfaces to hide it or to overlay it with the original data.

3. Image Visualization

We have developed a software dedicated to heart MRI segmentation and visualization. Our software allows the user to explore a highly detailed view of the data-set for easy interpretation. This is important for validation purposes. The user can visualize the segmented image as a set of surfaces, one surface for each region. The marching cubes algorithm was used to extract detailed surfaces of the segmented image. Users can also overlay the surfaces on the original image. It is possible to view 2D slices of both segmented and original image as well as 3D volume rendering. Combination of all this visualization methods allows an easy and fast interpretation of the segmentation. Complex morphologies can therefore be explored easily and interactively.

4. Conclusion

We encounter problematic issues with the segmentation of the right ventricular epicardium due to bad contrast of the bordering tissue. The resolution of the images is often too small to distinguish clearly this part of the heart. However we have partially solved this problem via new segmentation methods based on graph-cuts and minimal surfaces [5]. Graph-cuts is a combinatorial optimization method which is today considered as a leading method for image segmentation. Its combination with the watershed transform offers a stable segmentation that can be used interactively [6].

Acknowledgements

We would like to thank Marie Curie Fellowship Association and the European community for funding our research on medical image segmentation.

References

[1] L. Vincent and P. Soille, Watersheds in digital spaces: an efficient algorithm based on immersion simulations, IEEE Transactions on Pattern Analysis and Machine Intelligence, 13(1991) 583-598.

[2] T.S. Sørensen, G.F. Greil, O.K. Hansen, J. Mosegaard. Surgical simulation - a new tool to evaluate surgical incisions in congenital heart disease. Interactive Cardiovascular and Thoracic Surgery 5(2006) 536-539.

[3] S. Beucher and F. Meyer, the Morphological approach of segmentation: the watershed transformation. In Dougherty E. (Editor), Mathematical Morphology in Image Processing, Marcel Dekker, New York, 1992.

[4] J. Weickert, Nonlinear diffusion filtering, B. Jähne, H. HauSSecker, P. GeiSSler (Eds.), Handbook on Computer Vision and Applications, Vol. 2: Signal Processing and Pattern Recognition, Academic Press, San Diego, (1999) 423-450.

[5] Yuri Y. Boykov and Vladimir Kolmogorov, Computing geodesics and minimal surfaces via graph cuts, International conference on computer vision, Nice, France 1(2003) 26-33.

[6] Y. Li, J. Sun, C. Tang, H. Shum. Lazy snapping. SIGGRAPH 2004. ACM Transaction on Graphics 23(2004) 303-308.

Medicine Meets Virtual Reality 15
J.D. Westwood et al. (Eds.)
IOS Press, 2007

A Virtual-Reality Approach for the Treatment of Benign Paroxysmal Positional Vertigo

Karl V. STEINER, PhD[1,2,*], Michael TEIXIDO, MD[3,4], Brian KUNG, MD[3],
Mads SORENSEN[5], MD, Robert FORSTROM[1,2], and Patrick COLLER[1,6]

[1] *Delaware Biotechnology Institute, University of Delaware, Newark, DE*
[2] *Department of Electrical and Computer Engineering, University of Delaware*
[3] *Christiana Care Health System, Newark, DE*
[4] *Jefferson Medical College, Department of Otolaryngology, Philadelphia, PA*
[5] *Department of Otolaryngology, Rigshospitalet, Copenhagen Denmark*
[6] *Department of Computer Information Sciences University of Delaware*

Abstract. Benign Paroxysmal Positional Vertigo (BPPV) is a common cause of dizziness caused by debris, which has collected within the semicircular canals of the inner ear. Stereoscopic representations of the human labyrinth are constructed and incorporated into a downloadable viewing platform to allow visualization of straightforward and complex variations of BPPV.

Keywords. Benign Paroxysmal Positional Vertigo, Inner Ear, Visualization, Treatment

1. Background

We present a new virtual-reality based approach to aid clinicians in the treatment of BPPV. This approach utilizes a downloadable 3-D model of the inner ear utilizing true anatomical representations of the human semicircular canals shown in correct spatial relation to the human head.

Benign Paroxysmal Positional Vertigo (BPPV) is a clinical syndrome characterized by short bursts of severe vertigo associated with changes in head orientation. This most commonly diagnosed clinical syndrome [1] may account for up to 20% of all dizziness [2]. 9% of all older persons have BPPV [2]. Despite the prevalence of this problem and the frequency with which primary care physicians are confronted with it, considerable confusion persists regarding the prescription of effective physical maneuvers for its treatment and the actual effects of the maneuvers on the inner ear.

In BPPV, calcium carbonate crystals (otoliths) interfere with the normal function of the semicircular canals. Characteristic eye movements can be seen with the abnormal presence of otoliths in the horizontal, posterior, and superior canals (canalithiasis). Particles may also cause symptoms if attached abnormally to the cupula of any canal (cupulolithiasis). Perhaps even more confusing is the common occurrence of multiple canal BPPV in an individual patient. This complex range of possibilities may make diagnosis and treatment quite difficult. Because the actual canals, the cupulae, and the otoliths cannot be seen directly by any examiner, the presence of pathologically

---

* Corresponding Author: Karl V. Steiner; Delaware Biotechnology Institute; University of Delaware;
15 Innovation Way; Newark, DE 19711; E-mail: steiner@dbi.udel.edu; www.dbi.udel.edu

displaced otoliths is inferred by eye movements provoked in response to changes in head position.

The treatment of this common vestibular disorder involves head movements designed to 1) displace the otoliths from the affected semicircular canal(s) back into the vestibule, where there is an active mechanism for their resorption, and/or 2) to move the otoliths back and forth within the canal to promote their dissolution. Confidence in these maneuvers can only arise after the clinician achieves the ability to visualize the position of the affected vestibule and its semicircular canals within the patient.

2. Tools and Methods

The stereoscopic representation of the inner ear, in particular the human membranous labyrinth, was segmented from human temporal bone histopathology sliced at 20 μm thickness. Every fifth slice was digitally scanned and selected anatomy segmented using AMIRA® 4.1 [3]. A 3-D representation of the right membranous labyrinth was created and positioned according to anatomic norms within the CT data representing the skull and skin surface of a human head. By reversing the X-axis values for the surface files of the right membranous labyrinth, a mirror image of the left membranous labyrinth was created and positioned according to anatomic norms (Fig. 1a).

The surface files were loaded into a stand-alone downloadable cross-platform software, the 3-D Surface Viewer [4]. The viewer allows rotation of the surface models in any angle using simple mouse controls. The degree of transparency of each structure can be changed to view structures normally obscured by one another. Artificial spherical surfaces representing otoliths can be loaded on the cupulae, the semicircular canals, and vestibules in any combination (Fig. 1b). The otoliths move toward the most dependent position of the labyrinth according to a gravity field created for this model. The model is useable across platforms, including Mac, Windows XP, and Linux, and can be downloaded from our website: www.dbi.udel.edu/People/teixido.html

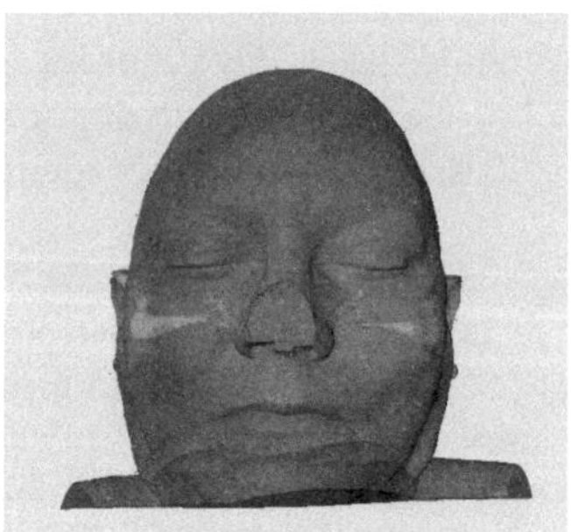
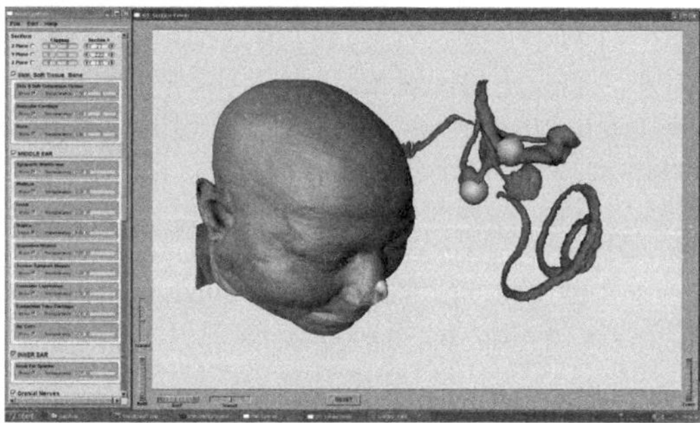

Figure 1. A: Left: Anatomical location of membranous labyrinths inside head; B: Right: During exercise to reposition otoliths, labyrinths and spherical otolith markers are located outside head and amplified for clarity.

The implementation of the otoliths moving throughout the canal was achieved through altering portions of Molofee's particle system source [5]. The system models a ball-on-string method coupled with a gravitation force. The spheres representing the otoliths obey the law of gravity but are limited to travel along specified positions, creating a string path for the particles to follow. This gives the appearance of particle independence and allows for faster simulation. Therefore, the selected string-path method is preferred over a per-frame triangle collision detection method.

The user can load otoliths into one or more canals and observe the appropriate combination of head movements required to treat the patient. Future enhancements will include a display of predicted eye movements and downloadable stereo viewing.

3. Conclusions/Discussion

Over the past 15 years several investigators have approached 3-D reconstruction of the complex anatomy of the inner ear. Some models have relied on photographic information [6,7] and others have used digital reconstruction to study specific structures of interest [8,9]. The first widely available 3-D temporal bone model in downloadable form was just recently developed [4]. It owes its wide circulation to the development of the 3-D Surface Viewer, a cross-platform compatible tool that is inexpensive and easy to use. Adapted to this viewer, our 3-D model of the human labyrinths provides an effective teaching tool for students and clinicians treating patients with balance disorders.

The model will allows basic orientation for the novice clinician as well as complex clinical hypothesis testing for experts (i.e., multiple canal BPPV and bilateral BPPV). We have used this model to demonstrate the efficacy of established maneuvers for the treatment of BPPV, such as the canalith repositioning maneuver (Epley), the Brandt-Daroff exercise, and the liberatory maneuver of Semont. The model lends itself well to both clinical hypothesis generation and testing. The enhanced visualization afforded by the model has presented potential enhancements of these standard treatments, which are currently undergoing clinical trial. If the physician can successfully diagnose the location of abnormally positioned otoliths by careful observation of the eye movements of the patient as they perform specific head motions, this virtual-reality simulator will allow them to demonstrate and practice the appropriate combination of head movements required to treat the affected semicircular canal or canals.

4. Acknowledgements

This project is partially supported by NIH Grant 2 P20 RR016472–06 under the Delaware INBRE Program of the National Center for Research Resources (NCRR).

References

[1]　Brandt, *Vertigo: its multisensory syndromes*. 1991, London: Springer-Verlag.

[2]　Oghalai, J.S., et al., *Unrecognized benign paroxysmal positional vertigo in elderly patients*. Otolaryngol Head Neck Surg, 2000. **122**(5): p. 630-4.

[3]　Amira - Mercury Computer Systems, San Diego, CA, www.amiravis.com, 2006.

[4]　Wang, H., et al., *Three-dimensional virtual model of the human temporal bone: a stand-alone, downloadable teaching tool*. Otol Neurotol, 2006. **27**(4): p. 452-7.

[5]　Molofee, J., Particle System, Gravity Field Source Code, optimized by Fredric Echols, nehe.gamedev.net, 2000.

[6]　Takahashi, H. and I. Sando, *Stereophotography of computer-aided three-dimensional reconstructions of the temporal bone structures*. Otolaryngol Head Neck Surg, 1992. **106**(1): p. 110-3.

[7]　Harada, T., S. Ishii, and N. Tayama, *Three-dimensional reconstruction of the temporal bone from histologic sections*. Arch Otolaryngol Head Neck Surg, 1988. **114**(10): p. 1139-42.

[8]　Mason, T.P., et al., *Virtual temporal bone: creation and application of a new computer-based teaching tool*. Otolaryngol Head Neck Surg, 2000. **122**(2): p. 168-73.

[9]　Qiu, M.G., et al., *Plastination and computerized 3D reconstruction of the temporal bone*. Clin Anat, 2003. **16**(4): p. 300-3.

Medicine Meets Virtual Reality 15
J.D. Westwood et al. (Eds.)
IOS Press, 2007

Medical Student Evaluation using Augmented Standardized Patients: New Development and Results

Bo Sun[1] Frederic D. McKenzie[1*] Hector M. Garcia[1]
Thomas W. Hubbard[2] John A. Ullian[2] Gayle A. Gliva[2]

[1]*Old Dominion University* [2]*Eastern Virginia Medical School (EVMS)*
**fmckenzi@ece.odu.edu*

Abstract. Standardized patients (SPs), individuals who realistically portray patients, are widely used in medical education to teach and assess communication skills, eliciting a history, performing a physical exam, and other important clinical skills. They are typically healthy individuals with few or no abnormal physical findings. One limitation is that each SP can only portray a limited set of physical symptoms. We have developed a functioning prototype that uses sound-based augmented reality (AR) to expand the capabilities of an SP to exhibit physically-manifested abnormalities. The previous research and evaluation of this prototype have been published in medicine meets virtual reality conference in January 2006. Current research has combined a virtual crackle sound with a healthy SP's real breath sound at end of inspiration in real time. The technology used is intended to correlate the inspiration timing of SP's. A learner will hear this simulated sound through an electronic-stethoscope wirelessly.

Keywords. Virtual reality, augmented reality, standardized patients, medical assessment, OSCE

1. Introduction

To become clinically competent physicians, medical students must develop knowledge and skills in many areas of both the art and science of medicine. Three areas are emphasized in medical students' early clinical training: doctor-patient communication, eliciting the history, and performing the physical exam. Standardized patients (SPs), individuals trained to realistically portray patients, are commonly used to teach and assess medical students in those three areas.

Working with them provides students the opportunity to learn doctor-patient communication, the history, the physical exam, and other clinical skills in a safe setting. SPs also provide a way to reliably test students' clinical skills in a realistic setting, interacting with a person. The range of clinical problems an SP can portray, however, is limited. They are typically healthy individuals with few or no abnormal physical findings. While some can be trained to simulate physical abnormalities (e.g., breathing through one lung, voluntarily increasing blood pressure, etc.), there are many abnormalities they cannot simulate.

The previous phase of this research involves simulating abnormal heart or lung sounds in an SP, thus expanding the breadth of sounds that can be heard in an SP. A learner will listen to an SP's heart and lungs through a modified stethoscope and hear pre-recorded sounds rather than the SP's. This work has been documented in paper [1] and [2]. The current research overlays fine crackles along with the real breath of the SP's. A learner will hear this sound at the anterior lung bases after a maximal expiration or after prolonged recumbency [3]. The pre-recorded crackle and real breath sound is combined in real time and played out through a modified electric-stethoscope.

2. Methods

We have created a functional prototype that augments the reality of the SP by adding virtual sounds to his/her breath. The intent is to impart abnormal pathology that could not be faked or reproduced by the SP alone. This technique could greatly enhance the repertoire of lessons that can be hands-on trained by the SP and not experienced for first time on actual patients.

Since fine crackles should be heard most prominently at the end of inspiration, synchronizing the virtual crackle sound with the SP's real breath sound is the main research of this simulation. Moreover, crackle sound is usually heard at specified locations upon chest auscultation. Instead of employing a tracking system as in the previous work, we chose to utilize a simple but effective method of identifying correct point of inspiration to combine the virtual crackles along with the correct location on the body at which the sounds should be combined.

For this new method, we use a SP controlled actuator, which is a wireless remote controller (see figure1), to allow the SP to signal the correct timing of respiration. SP clicks the controller towards the end of his/her inspiration. When the computer program detects this signal event, it will play the virtual crackle sound to computer audio. A learner will hear the combined virtual sound with real breath sound through a modified electric-stethoscope (see figure1). The original electronic-stethoscope has auscultation function as well as hearing computer audio by connected via a cable. After our modification, the electronic-stethoscope connects to the computer using wireless transducer and receiver. In this way, the real breath sound directly coming from SP is actually combined with pre-recorded crackle sound at SP's end of inspiration upon chest auscultation in real time.

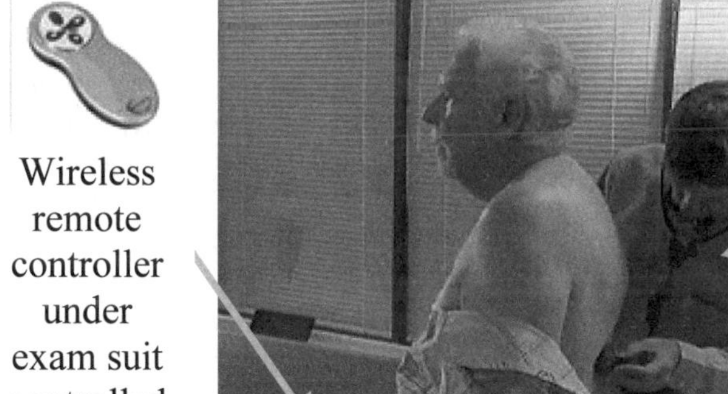

Figure 1: OSCE ASP Assessment Configuration

3. Conclusions

This new development of ASP system has been evaluated in an annual Objective Structured Clinical Examination (OSCE). The crackle simulation is used in a case called heart failure. Fourth year medical students were the study subjects. The main objective of the study was to determine the validity of using augmented SPs as a reliable assessment tool by presenting abnormal pathology – crackles.

Two SPs were provided with the augmentation in two separate rooms; however, only one SP at a time had an audible crackle to keep students unaware of the purpose of the augmentation. Figure 1 shows the configuration of one of the ASP rooms. In the picture, the medical student listens to the back of the sitting patient with the electronic stethoscope.

Our project was successful in its attempt to combine simulated crackles into a real SP' breath sound. A real human (SP) is augmented with our system just as easily as clicking a mouse in order to synchronize her/his breath. The initial proof-of-concept evaluation of the system was performed by an EVMS doctor experienced in SPs and the training of auscultation. It was evident that the concept works, and the system could become a useful and integral part of auscultation education with expanded fields of interest with abnormalities.

4. Acknowledgements

This project was a collaborative effort between the Virginia Modeling, Analysis and Simulation Center (VMASC) at Old Dominion University and the Eastern Virginia Medical School. Partial funding was provided by the Stemmler Medical Education Research Fund. Partial funding was also provided by the Naval Health Research Center through NAVAIR Orlando TSD under contract N61339-03-C-0157, and the Office of Naval Research under contract N00014-04-1-0697, entitled "The National Center for Collaboration in Medical Modeling and Simulation." The ideas and opinions presented in this paper represent the views of the authors and do not necessarily represent the views of the Department of Defense.

References

[1] Frederic D. McKenzie, Thomas W. Hubbard, John A. Ullian, Hector M. Garcia, Reynel J. Castelino, Gayle A. Gliva. "Medical Student Evaluation using Augmented Standardized Patients: Preliminary Results", Medicine Meets Virtual Reality 14: Accelerating Change in Healthcare: Next Medical Toolkit, San Diego, CA, Jan, 2006

[2] McKenzie, Frederic D., Hector M. Garcia, Reynel Castelino, Thomas Hubbard, John Ullian, Gayle Gliva. "Augmented Standardized Patients Now Virtually a Reality." In *Proceedings of the Third IEEE and ACM International Symposium on Mixed and Augmented Reality (ISMAR 2004)*. Arlington VA, Nov. 2 – Nov. 5 2004.

[3] Breath Sound. Last accessed at http://rnbob.tripod.com/breath.htm in June, 2006.

Medicine Meets Virtual Reality 15
J.D. Westwood et al. (Eds.)
IOS Press, 2007

457

Design of the Next-Generation Medical Implants with Communication and Energy Ports

Mingui SUN [a,b,1]   Steven A. HACKWORTH [a,b]   Zhide TANG [a]   Jun ZHAO [a]
Daliang LI [a,b]   Sharon E. ENOS [b]   Brian ERRIGO [b]   Gary GILBERT [c]
Ronald MARCHESSAULT [c]   Sylvain CARDIN [c]   Troy TURNER [c] and
Robert J. SCLABASSI [a,b]

[a] *Laboratory for Computational Neuroscience, Department of Neurosurgery,
University of Pittsburgh, Pittsburgh, PA, 15260*
[b] *Computational Diagnostics, Inc., Pittsburgh, PA 15213*
[c] *Telemedicine and Advanced Technology Research Center (TATRC), US Army
Medical Research & Material Command (USAMRMC) Fort Detric, Frederick MD
21702*

Abstract. In this work, we provide an effective solution to the communication and power supply problems in miniature medical devices implanted
within the human body. The volume conduction property of the human tissue is utilized as a natural cable for the delivery of both information and
energy. A practical design is presented consisting of a small, simple, and
convenient external device called an energy pad.

Keywords. Communication, Energy Delivery, Implantable Device, Recharging

Introduction

Two critical problems exist in the engineering design of minimally invasive
implantable devices: power supply and communication[1,2]. These problems are
currently approached by using percutaneous wire connection[1] and transcuta-
neous radio-frequency (RF) magnetic induction through the skin. Percutaneous
wire connection has oblivious drawbacks of high infection risk and severe mobility limitation. RF magnetic induction can deliver both signal and energy without wires. However, when the size of the implant decreases, this method has a
low magnetic coupling efficiency between the primary and secondary coils, the
implanted device is subject to interference, and can cause interference itself. Existing commercial implants utilize large, non-rechargeable batteries as the power
source (e.g., cardiac pacemaker). This battery power leads to device-related complications due to the use of subcutaneous cabling and involves high costs and
increased risk from surgical replacements of batteries.

---

[1]Corresponding Author: Mingui Sun, Department of Neurosurgery, University of Pittsburgh,
Pittsburgh, PA 15261; E-mail: mrsun@neuronet.pitt.edu.

1. Methods

We have developed a different method to provide future implants with both energy supply and communication capacities using the volume conduction property of the biological tissue[2,3]. Our method uses the human body as a natural cable to deliver both signal and power. We have designed a convenient de-

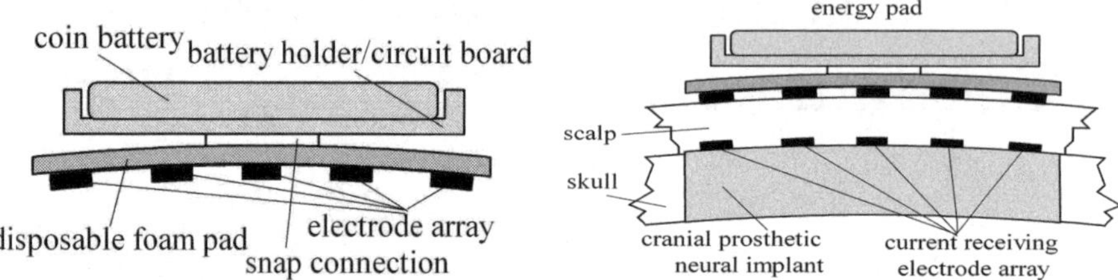

Figure 1.: LEFT: Fundamental design of energy pad; RIGHT: Coupling between energy pad and implanted device

vice for practical application of the volume conduction technology[2]. This device is called an energy pad about the size of an American quarter (see Fig. 1). It consists of a disposable foam pad embedded with electrodes and coated with adhesive to be easily pasted on the skin. The energy pad also contains a thin-profile button battery, and a dual-use battery holder/circuit board. The main function of the energy pad is to recharge a novel power system within the implant containing a miniature Lithium-ion polymer battery and a supercapacitor[2]. During operation, an AC current is transmitted from the electrodes on the foam pad to the reception electrodes on the surface of the implant below the skin, through the electrically conductive tissue (right panel in Fig. 1). For low power applications of medical implants, the recharging process is required infrequently (e.g. once a week at nighttime), causing little inconvenience to patients. The energy pad can also communicate with the implant, allowing tasks such as acquiring data and transmitting control signals. A modified version of the energy pad can perform more complex communication functions.

2. Results

In order to facilitate analysis, we constructed an equivalent 2-port linear circuit model shown in Fig. 2, where the battery polarities (V_1 and V_2) are instantaneous since, in practice, both the recharging and communication signals are AC signals. Using this model, it can be shown that, for recharging to take place, the following condition must be satisfied:

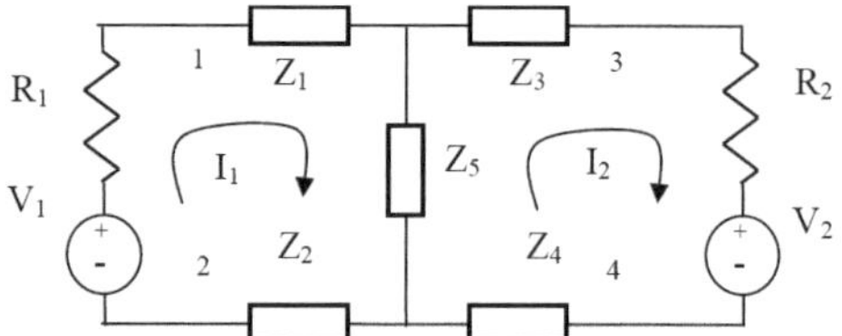

Figure 2.: Equivalent circuit model of the volume conduction system

$$\frac{V_{1m}}{V_2} > \left| \frac{R_1 + Z_1 + Z_2 + Z_5}{Z_5} \right| > 1. \tag{1}$$

where V_{1m} is the maximum voltage amplitude of exterior voltage V_1, and V_2 is the battery voltage inside the implant. From Eq. (1), The following features can be observed: 1) for recharging to take place, the maximum amplitude of the external voltage source must be higher than the voltage of the internal battery; and 2) the equivalent series resistor (ESR) of the internal battery does not affect the condition for recharging, but the ESR of the external voltage source does.

In order to evaluate our system further, we have constructed a physical head model (Fig. 3) which has both an accurate head geometry and correct conductivity values for the brain, skull and scalp in the top portion of the head model. Both the brain and scalp were made of agar and NaCl, and the skull was made from a mixture of carbon black epoxy and barium titanate ($BaTiO_3$). We implanted our prototype device within the conductive epoxy skull and covered the skull with the simulated agar scalp. We utilized an energy pad, implemented on a breadboard, to communicate with and deliver power to the implanted device.

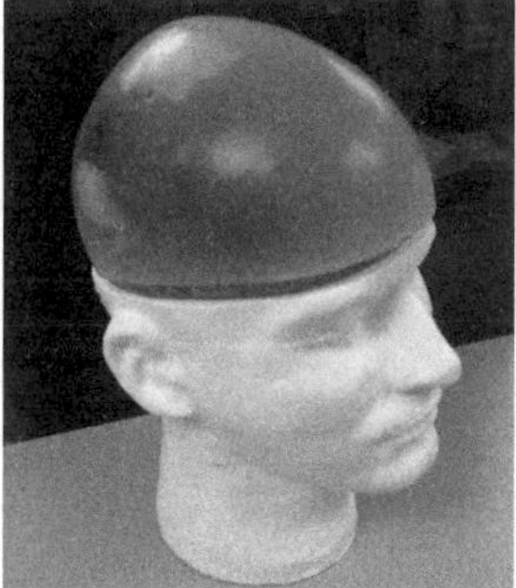

Figure 3.: Physically constructed head model

For the communication tasks, we were able to reliably control 16 different functions by sending commands and receiving responses, and to deliver sufficient current for battery recharging. Our system also verified the linear system model presented previously.

3. Conclusion

We have investigated the communication and power supply problems in implantable devices. A novel design of an energy pad has been presented using the volume conduction property of the human tissue. This device is lightweight and self-adhesive, the skin-contact portion is disposable, and the use of the device is very convenient.

Acknowledgments

This work was supported in part by US Army Medical Research and Materiel Command contract No. W81XWH-050C-0047, National Institutes of Health grant No. EB002099, and Computational Diagnostics, Inc.

References

[1]   L.R. Hochberg, M.D. Serruya, G.M. Friehs, J.A. Mukand, M. Saleh, A.H. Caplan, A. Branner, D. Chen, R.D. Penn and J.P. Donoghue, Neuronal ensemble control of prosthetic devices by a human with tetraplegia, *Nature*, **442** (1996), 164-171.

[2]   M. Sun, S. A. Hackworth, Z. Tang, J. Zhao, D. L. Li, S. E. Enos, B. Errigo, G. Gilbert, R. Marchessault, S. Cardin, T. Turner, and R. J. Sclabassi, Platform Technologies for Minimally Invasive Physiological Monitoring, Proc. *25th Army Science Conference*, Orlando, FL, Nov. 2006.

[3]   M. Sun, G. A. Justin, P. A. Roche, J. Zhao, B. L. Wessel, Y. Zhang and R. J. Sclabassi, Passing data and supplying power to neural implants, *IEEE EMBS Magazine*, Sept/Oct issue, (2006), 39-46.

Medicine Meets Virtual Reality 15
J.D. Westwood et al. (Eds.)
IOS Press, 2007

Development of a surgical robot system for endovascular surgery with augmented reality function

Naoki Suzuki, Asaki Hattori, Shigeyuki Suzuki, Yoshito Otake
*Institute for High Dimensional Medical Imaging, The Jikei University School of
Medicine, 4-11-1 Izumihoncho, Komae-shi, Tokyo, Japan*

Abstract. We started the project of the surgical robotic system in 2001 as an application for abdominal surgery. The robot enables a surgeon to perform various surgical procedures in abdominal region as in open surgery. We have extended the concept of the robotic surgery system and developed a new robotic system for cardiac and endovascular surgery. The new robot has a stereo video camera system, two manipulators and a flexible tube, 3 mm in diameter, used as an instrument channel. The maximum diameter of the robot is 6 mm. We also applied 4D ultrasound imaging system to the robot system, that enabled to observe a situation of the robot and surgical field in a blood flow. In this paper, we describe a detail of the robot system and results of phantom experiment.

Keywords. Surgery robot, Cardiac surgery, Endovascular surgery, 4D ultrasound imaging system

1. Purpose

The aim of the project is to develop a new surgical robot system that enables a surgeon to perform surgical procedures on the heart and aorta as in open cardiovascular surgery. We have been developing an endoscopic robot system for abdominal surgery since 2001[1-5]. The abdominal robot has endoscopic eye and two manipulators to grasp the soft tissue or hold surgical tools in a limited space of the body. Clinical feasibility of the robot has been evaluated in animal experiments: endoscopic mucosal resection (EMR) and other various surgical procedures were carried out by cooperative works of the robot manipulators. We have extended the concept of the robotic surgery system and developed a new robotic system for cardiac and endovascular surgery.

2. Method

Basic man/machine interface of the robotic system is the same as in our endoscopic robotic system with two manipulators that enable arbitrary surgical procedures to be performed in a limited space as proficiently as done by a surgeon. However, two problems had to be overcome in order to complete the system for cardiovascular surgery. The first was smooth mobility of the robot in an arterial lumen of ascending aorta, descending aorta or iliac artery without perforating or tearing the arterial wall. To

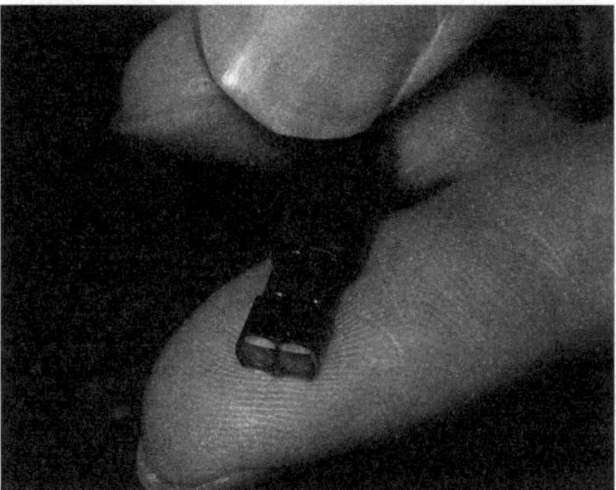

Figure 1. An appearance of the stereo CCD video camera system

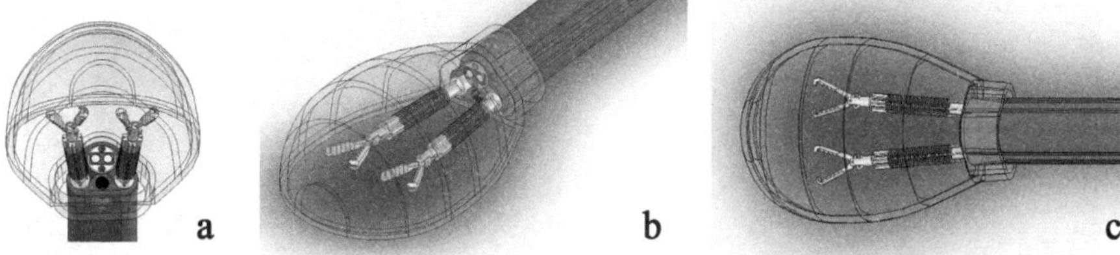

Figure 2. 3D CAD model of the robot

solve this problem, we developed a new video camera system instead of the endoscope applied in the previously constructed robotic system. The video camera system was 3mm in diameter and has two small CCD cameras embedded in its body to enable stereoscopic view (Figure 1). The manipulator diameter was also reduced from 6 mm to 3 mm. We completed the robot by assembling the stereo video camera system, two manipulators and a flexible tube, 3 mm in diameter, used as an instrument channel. Consequently, the maximum diameter of the robot could be reduced in size from 20 mm to 6 mm, compared to the endoscopic robot. Figure 2 shows a 3D CAD model of the robot.

The second problem was the surgical field view acquisition from within the artery. Because the robot system was equipped with the navigation system same as in the endoscopic robot system, surgeon was able to recognize the location and direction of the robot tip. In order to perform detailed surgical procedures, however, a new real-time imaging system was required to obtain clear field of view within opaque blood flow. Injecting saline into the artery through the instrument channel was the most effective for acquiring clear surgical field image. We designed an acrylic cover and attached it to the tip of the robot to keep saline enough time in the surgical field. However, the injection frequency was limited. Therefore, a four-dimensional (4D) ultrasound imaging system using two dimensional array probes was applied. The probe was attached to the body surface and the target area within the arterial lumen could be visualized with time sequential (4D) images in real time. The viewpoint of 4D images could be interactively changed or fixed to the viewpoint of the video camera. Furthermore, because the ultrasound imaging system was linked to the navigation system, the surgeon could simultaneously obtain information on navigation and real-

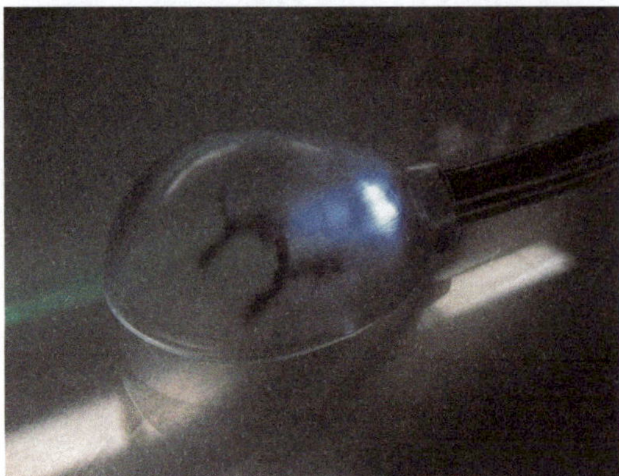

Figure 3. An appearance of the robot

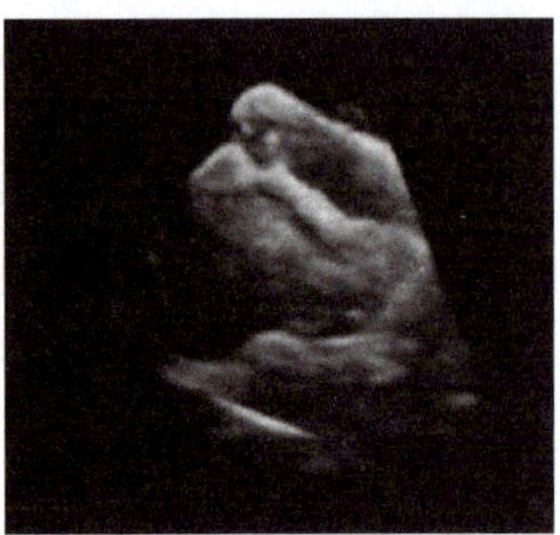

Figure 4. Measured image of the manipulator by 4D ultrasound imaging system

time operative procedures in the surgical field. We examined the robot movement and function in a phantom experiment.

3. Results and conclusions

Figure 3 shows the assembled robot. Using the robotic system, we performed the phantom experiment with an acrylic tube. A model of detached inner membrane of arterial wall was attached to the interior wall of the tube. The experiment was carried out in a water tub. First, the robot movement in the water tub was assessed and we were able to control the manipulators accordingly with the direction of the master device.

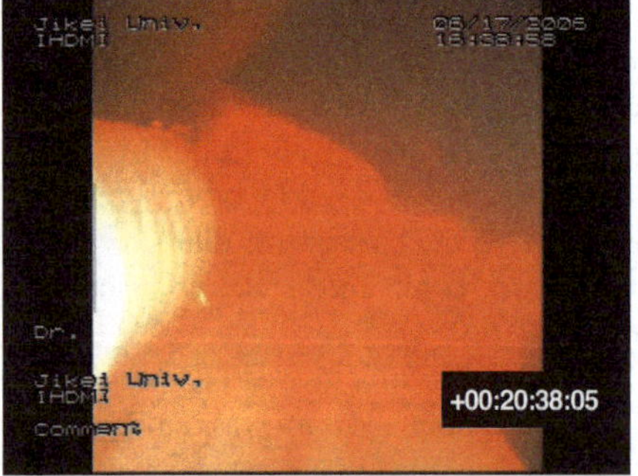

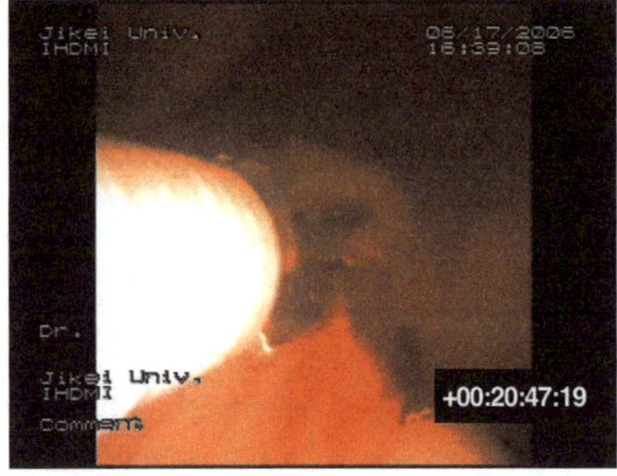

Figure 5. CCD video camera images during injecting saline in the phantom experiment

Second, we evaluated the 4D ultrasound imaging system. After inserting the robot into the tube, we monitored the movement of the manipulators and condition within the surgical field. The shape of the manipulators and the arterial lesion model were reconstructed as 4D images in real time and the view point of the images could be interactively changed (Figure 4). We tried to perform the elimination of the arterial lesion with two manipulators and electric knife with viewing 4D ultrasound images. The frame rate of the reconstructed images was about 15 frames / sec. Figure 5 shows a scene of injecting saline. According to the injection, the view of the surgical field became clear gradually and we could continue surgical procedures by manipulators.

By expanding our concept of robotic surgery, we have developed a new robotic system with navigation and monitoring features. The phantom experiment results indicate that the system can be applied in cardiac and endovascular surgery. Currently we are adding data fusion functionality for the robotic system: a three-dimensional model providing color information of the surgical filed from the stereoscopic CCD camera images during saline injection. The reconstructed model will be superimposed onto navigation images.

Following safety evaluations by animal experiments, we plan to apply the system in clinical settings and examine its efficiency.

References

[1]   N. Suzuki, K. Sumiyama, A. Hattori et al., Development of an endoscopic robotic system with two hands for various gastric tube surgeries, MMVR 11 2003, 349-53.

[2]   N. Suzuki, M. Hayashibe, S. Suzuki et al., Dual manipulator endoscopic robotic system for intraluminar gastrointestinal surgery, World Congress on Medical Physics and Biomedical Engineering 2003, 3916.pdf (CD-ROM)

[3]   F.A.Y Murakami, N. Suzuki, A. Hattori et al., Design and evaluation of a man-machine interface for endoscopic surgery robot, World Congress on Medical Physics and Biomedical Engineering 2003, 3973.pdf (CD-ROM)

[4]   A. Hattori, N. Suzuki, M. Hayashibe et al., Navigation system for a developed endoscopic surgical robot system, International Congress Series 1268 2004, 539-44.

[5]   A. Hattori, N. Suzuki, M. Hayashibe et al., Development of a navigation function for an endoscopic robot surgery system, MMVR 13 2005, 167-171.

Medicine Meets Virtual Reality 15
J.D. Westwood et al. (Eds.)
IOS Press, 2007

Surgery simulation using patient-specific models for laparoscopic colectomy

Shigeyuki SUZUKI [a,1], Ken ETO [b], Asaki HATTORI [a],
Katsuhiko YANAGA [b] and Naoki SUZUKI [a]

[a] *Institute for High Dimensional Medical Imaging, The Jikei University School of Medicine, Tokyo, JAPAN*
[b] *Department of Surgery, The Jikei University School of Medicine, Tokyo, JAPAN*

Abstract. Laparoscopic surgery has become an option for patients. However there have been some difficulties common to all laparoscopic procedures. Surgery simulation system for surgical planning and training is necessary and important in order to increase the safety of this surgery. We have been developing a surgery simulation system for laparoscopic assisted colorectal surgery utilizing patient-specific anatomy. In this system, we focused on the tissue deformation caused by laparoscopic right hemicolectomy manipulations, and applied a soft tissue model with anisotropic properties and a sphere-filled method. The sphere-filled model enables visualization of real-time deformations and is based on patient-specific data obtained from CT angiograms. The virtual laparoscopic instruments were emulated by manipulation of two PHANToM devices. As a result, the surgical maneuvers involved in laparoscopic colectomy, such as pushing and grasping of the mesentery and its vessels, were effectively simulated in real-time. In addition, surgeons are able to practice dissecting, isolating and dividing vessels with the virtual laparoscopic instruments.

Keywords. Surgery simulation, Patient-specific model, Laparoscopic colectomy

1. Introduction

Laparoscopic surgery allows surgeons to conduct minimally invasive surgery. However, the surgery is operator-driven and unlike laparotomy, the help of a surgical assistant is rather difficult. Furthermore, surgeons cannot manipulate organs and lesions directly. Laparoscopic colorectal surgery is an option for patients with colorectal lesions, but some difficulties common to all laparoscopic procedures remain. Therefore, a simulation system that would enable surgical procedures to be practiced repeatedly would be both important and indeed necessary for many surgeons. This study aimed to develop a simulation system for laparoscopic assisted colorectal surgery that would allow for a safer operation by enabling surgeons to visualize the patient anatomy pre-operatively and practice the surgical maneuvers for the specific patient. In this paper, we demonstrate tissue deformation effects of the mesentery and the ileocolic vessels caused by laparoscopic right hemicolectomy manipulations.

---

[1] Correspondence to: Shigeyuki Suzuki, Institute for High Dimensional Medical Imaging, The Jikei University School of Medicine, Tokyo, Japan. Tel.:+81-3-3480-1151(ext.2335); Fax.:+81-3-5438-8380; E-mail: sshige@jikei.ac.jp

2. Method

We have developed a surgery simulation system for open surgery [1],[2] as well as a tele-surgery simulation system for liver surgery and cholecystectomy [3]. With these systems, surgical maneuvers such as cutting, resection and dissection could be performed in real-time. Based on these simulation systems, we have proposed a sphere-filled organ model that is able to demonstrate organ deformations interactively and quantitatively. In this study, we propose a real time deformable model based on anisotropic elasticity and sphere-filled method. Models for the mesentery, the pancreas, the duodenum and mesenteric artery/vein were created using the sphere-filled method based on patient-specific data. To include in the model features of tissue properties, especially anisotropic elasticity, the algorithm used for model deformation was improved. At first, the collision between the spheres of the mesentery model and virtual instrument were detected, by using the conventional algorithm of the sphere-filled method. When the mesentery and the vessels behind it were grasped, these were caused the deformation with the anisotropic property which was specified from the direction of the vessel structure. Then, the detected spheres moved to the direction of composition of two vectors: a vector from the centre of the internal sphere to the point where forceps contact the tissue surface and a vector of the anisotropic direction. Finally, the surface polygons were deformed by following the internal spheres' displacement. The vessel structure deformation was also shown by the displacement of the mesentery model's spheres. Laparoscopic instruments were reconstructed as 3D computer aided design data, and these manipulations were emulated by manipulation of two PHANToM devices (SensAble Technologies Inc.).

3. Result

The surgical maneuvers of a right hemicolectomy could be simulated as shown by Figure 1. Figure 1(a) shows the reconstructed organ models for simulation. The sub-windows of Figure 1(a-1) and (a-2) show the internal spheres of each organ. The size of the internal spheres was designated after consideration of the organ's size and its elastic characteristics. By using these models, a surgeon simulated the day before operation as shown by Figure 1(b). Then, the deformation of the reconstructed models such as grasping and cutting was shown by Figure 1(c). As well, by setting the anisotropic characteristics, simulation of real tissue deformations could be performed. Figure 2 shows a comparison of the model deformation and the surgical maneuvers between this simulation system and real surgery. As shown in this figure, we demonstrated tissue deformation that was similar to real deformation.

4. Conclusion

We developed a laparoscopic surgery simulation system specially designed to practice and plan laparoscopic colectomy with patient-specific data. By using this system, the surgical maneuvers such as grasping of the mesentery and vessels were effectively simulated in real-time. As well surgeons could practice dissecting, isolating and dividing vessels with the laparoscopic virtual instruments. We obtained good feedback about the deformation of the models from many skilled surgeons with much experience of laparoscopic colorectal surgery, although the models have to validate their deformations.

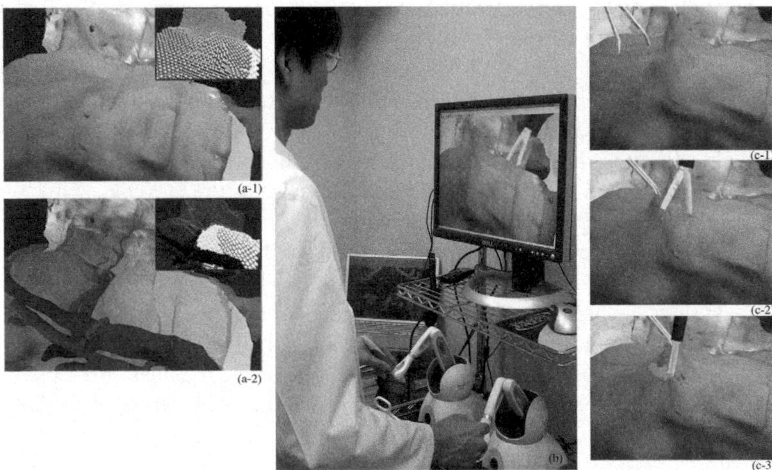

Figure 1. Laparoscopic right hemicolectomy simulation. (a-1) and (a-2) shows the reconstructed organ models for simulation. A surgeon simulated the surgery pre-operatively as shown by (b) while the deformation of the models were shown by (c-1) to (c-3) in time-sequential images.

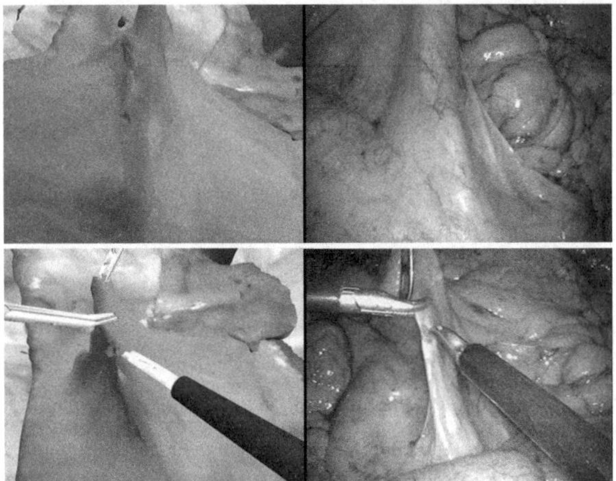

Figure 2. Comparison of model deformation and surgical maneuvers. The upper images show a surgery simulation while the lower show a real surgery.

References

[1] S. Suzuki, N. Suzuki, A. Hattori et al., "Dynamic Deformation of Elastic Organ Model and the VR Cockpit for Virtual Surgery and Tele-surgery," Studies In Health Technology and Informatics 94, Proceedings of Medicine Meets Virtual Reality 11, pp. 354-356, 2003.
[2] S. Suzuki, N. Suzuki, A. Hattori et al., "Sphere-Filled Organ Model for Virtual Surgery System," IEEE Trans. on Medical Imaging, vol. 23, no. 6, pp. 714-722, 2004.
[3] S. Suzuki, N. Suzuki, A. Hattori et al., "Tele-surgery simulation with a patient organ model for robotic surgery training," International Journal of Medical Robotics and Computer Assisted Surgery, vol. 1, no. 4, pp. 80-88, 2005.

Medicine Meets Virtual Reality 15
J.D. Westwood et al. (Eds.)
IOS Press, 2007

467

Development and Evaluation of a Virtual Intensive Therapy Unit - VITU

A THEODOROPOULOS[a], R KNEEBONE[a], B DORNAN[b],
R LEONARD[b] and F BELLO[a,1]
[a]Department of Biosurgery and Surgical Technology, Imperial College London
[b]St Mary's Hospital NHS Trust, London, UK

Abstract. Complex and safety critical healthcare environments like the Intensive Therapy Unit demand highly skilled professionals efficiently interacting with their technologically advanced surroundings and with each other. The ITU environment is daunting to newcomers and contains considerable potential for harm by inexpert treatment. In spite of this, current training is largely workplace based and depends upon observation and supervised practice with real patients. We propose the development of a distributed collaborative environment that recreates key elements of critical care. Centred on a 'virtual bedspace', team members will care for the patient in a way that accurately reflects actual practice and therefore minimises any learning gap. Graded exposure to increasing levels of complexity will ensure that collaborative learning takes place alongside each participant's clinical experience and complements it appropriately.

Keywords. Collaborative environments, virtual intensive therapy unit, team training, patient safety

1. Introduction

The Intensive Care Unit (ITU) is a specialised environment where severely ill patients receive 24 hour individual care. Multi-professional team working is crucial to effective patient management in this setting. Healthcare professionals from medicine, nursing and a range of allied professions work together in a co-ordinated way, combining their expertise for the benefit of each patient. In this high-technology setting, intensive monitoring provides continuous data about cardiac, respiratory, renal and other body systems. Life support systems (such as ventilators and kidney dialysis) are frequently necessary. Invasive procedures are also common, with many patients requiring central venous cannulation, arterial lines, tracheostomy or intercostal drains. High quality patient care in the ITU requires each clinician to gather and interpret complex physiological data, responding immediately to any deterioration. In addition, clinicians must understand and control high-technology equipment, carry out invasive procedures when necessary, and work effectively within a multi-professional team to exercise clinical judgement. The ITU environment is daunting to newcomers and contains considerable potential for harm by inexpert treatment. A report by the Leapfrog Group for Patient Safety [1] mentions that at least one in ten patients who die in ITUs every day would survive if dedicated intensivists – physicians specially trained to care for critically ill patients – were present and managing their care. Current training is largely

---

[1] Corresponding Author: F Bello, Dept. of Biosurgery and Surgical Technology, 10th Floor QEQM Building, St Mary's Hospital, Praed St, London W2 1NY, UK; E-mail: dorothy.F.Bello@imperial.ac.uk

workplace based and depends upon observation and supervised practice with real patients. The aim of this project is to develop a distributed collaborative virtual environment – the Virtual Intensive Therapy Unit or VITU – that recreates key elements of critical care, providing a safe yet realistic adjunct to the clinical workplace with great potential benefit.

2. Related Work

The SimTech project at Stanford University attempts to simulate a virtual 3D environment of an emergency care centre [2]. SimTech focused on the honing of collaborative crisis management skills and perceived the virtual environment as a cost-effective complementary tool to real-life simulation for educational purposes. VPICU stands for Virtual Pediatric Intensive Care Unit and its focus is to improve the quality of care in pediatric intensive care units [3]. The VPICU team argues that intensivists operate in isolation and do not treat enough patients with a particular ailment to determine the optimal medical practice. Furthermore, they do not share their knowledge and experience. They identified the problem as that of communication barriers and addressed it by suggesting the use of real-time patient data acquisition from the bedside. An alternative solution is presented by VISICU [4], a company offering an innovative remote-care strategy designed to improve ITU care processes while leveraging scarce intensivist resources. Its technology combines advanced software systems and telemedicine to create a unique approach for off-site hospital personnel to deliver critical care. The Interactive Trauma Trainer [5] is a human-centred design project to develop a proof-of-concept battlefield surgery decision-making trainer. The project's purpose is to train the user in making appropriate decisions related to the urgent treatment of an incoming casualty with a "Zone 1" neck fragmentation wound. These diverse projects represent efforts to address the lack of alternative simulation-based training in intensive care or trauma situations. Our proposed VITU follows on from these efforts introducing a flexible and powerful scenario scripting and execution framework allowing a range of training possibilities.

3. System Architecture

The VITU is a scenario-based system that follows a client-server architecture in order to support the collaborative interactions taking place in the ITU. The components of the VITU are: Client-side application, Server-side application, Remote administration tool and Scenario database.

The Client-side application is responsible for the rendering of the virtual environment (graphics rendering, sound playback, 3D interactions). The user's avatar interacts with the virtual environment on the client-side at the 3D mesh level. All meaningful user input is captured and forwarded to the server application.

The Server-side application provides the interface to the Scenario database and physiological models, as well as the core logic and data / event handlers. All non-administrative transactions with the Scenario database take place on the server-side. Consequently, any retrieved data that needs to be rendered or reproduced, such as 3D models and sound samples, is dispatched to the respective clients. Events are forwarded to the core logic module where they are processed and appropriate actions scheduled.

The Scenario database holds all information regarding the main entities of the ITU environment, participants and scripted scenarios. It is also used to hold authentication data and any other relevant personal information of the system's registered users. Administration of the database (adding users, scripting new scenarios, etc) is achieved remotely using the Remote administration tool.

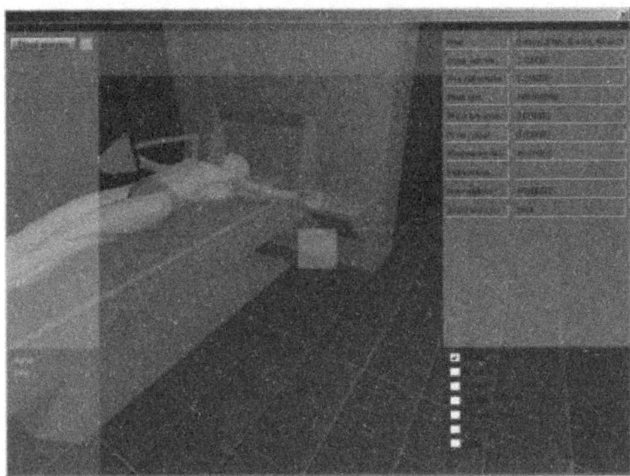

Figure 1. Illustration of the VITU interface during simple scenario execution.

4. Results

By combining scenario scripting capabilities with 3D graphics and physiological modelling, the VITU prototype allows members of the team to conduct the required scenario interactions with the patient and environment. Figure 1 illustrates the initial prototype environment. The VITU has the potential to encourage teaching and learning to take place within a structured educational environment which reflecting the learner's workplace. Graded exposure to increasing levels of complexity ensures that collaborative learning takes place alongside each participant's clinical experience and complements it appropriately.

5. Discussion and Conclusion

The functionality provided by the VITU environment enables the team members to share the same virtual workspace, with the possibility of simultaneous interactions. A powerful scenario scripting and execution framework allows a range of training possibilities from equipment usage to complex clinical care case studies. Specific benefits within this application domain to be investigated are: orientation to the ITU, rehearsal of common / important situations, creation of patient-specific scenarios and consolidation of newly acquired skills.

References

[1]   http://www.leapfroggroup.org/
[2]   http://simtech.stanford.edu/
[3]   http://vpicu.org/
[4]   http://twww.visicu.com/
[5]   http://www.hfidtc.com/public/PDF/ITT.pdf

Medicine Meets Virtual Reality 15
J.D. Westwood et al. (Eds.)
IOS Press, 2007

Low fidelity simulation of temporal bone drilling leads to improved but sub-optimal outcomes

Cory TORGERSON[a] , Ryan BRYDGES[b], Joseph CHEN[a], and Adam DUBROWSKI[b,1]

[a]*Dept. of Otolaryngology,* [b]*Dept. of Surgery, University of Toronto, Toronto, ON, Canada*

Abstract. Novices' learning of temporal bone drilling on a simple (2D) model was compared to learning of the skill on a complex model (3D). Trainees practicing on 2D model required an additional 3D practice to achieve similar final products as those practicing on a 3D model. This implies that during learning fundamental psychomotor adaptations take place, regardless of the exact skill practiced. However to achieve optimal products the depth of drilling must be practiced separately on high fidelity models.

Keywords: Evaluation, otolaryngology, technical skills, training

1. Introduction

While recent attention has focused on the settings where surgical skills can be taught[1], there has been little research on approaches to teaching. The motor learning literature may provide some answers.

In particular, Learning Specificity Theory[2] explains that the greater the resemblance between the practiced task and the task that will be performed in the real world, the more functional the learning. On the contrary, according to the Optimal Challenge Point Framework[3], the difficulty of practice should be adjusted to the

---

[1] Corresponding author: Adam Dubrowski, University of Toronto, Surgical Skills Centre at Mount Sinai Hospital, 600 University Avenue, Level 2-Room 250, Toronto, Ontario, M5G 1X5, Canada. E-mail: adam.dubrowski@gmail.com; phone: (416) 370-4194; fax: (416) 340-3792

trainees' current performance level in order to be most beneficial to the learning process. These two views yield conflicting hypotheses when applied to the acquisition of a precision bone-drilling task by novice surgeons.

This study compared novices' learning of temporal bone drilling skills on a very simple model to their learning of the skill on a more complex model.

2. Methods

Two groups of right-handed medical students practiced precision bone drilling on either high or low fidelity models. The high fidelity model consisted of drilling a 3D shape to fit a cochlear implant in a sawbone block (Figure 1). The low fidelity model consisted of drilling a 2D outline of a square in the same material. At the end of the practice session, both groups performed one additional practice trial on the 3D version of the skill. Practice duration was held constant. Before the practice session and after a 1-hour retention period all participants were tested on the 3D task. In addition a group of otolaryngology fellows was assessed on the 3D version of the task. Outcome variables included expert assessment of final products, and amount of sawbone mass removed during drilling on the pre-test and retention test.

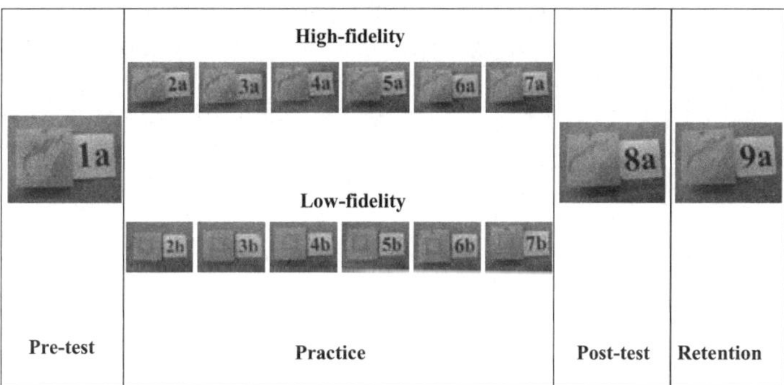

Figure 1. The experimental protocol.

3. Results

Both final product and mass removed dependent measures showed two types of construct validity: they could discern junior from advanced (fellows) performance ($p<.05$), and they could also discern trained and untrained performances within the same novice group of participants ($p<.05$).

The participants in both novice groups showed improvements on the assessment of final products that were retained over the one week period ($p<.01$). However, the group of participants that practiced on the 2D version of the task required an additional 3D practice trial to remove the same amount of bone material as the 3D practice group and the fellows (Figure 2).

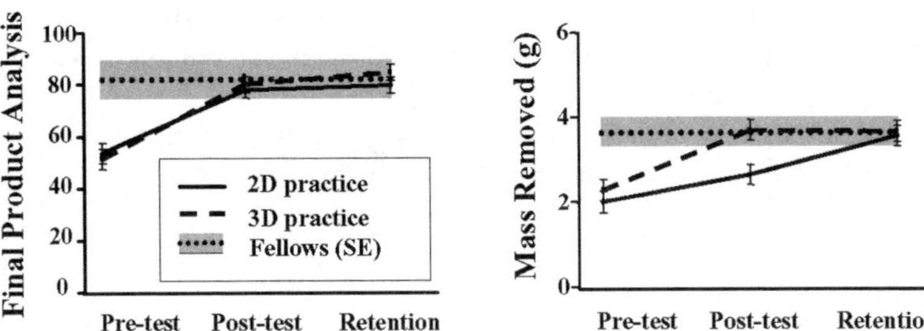

Figure 2.   This figure depicts patterns of results for the two types of outcome variables for both practice groups. The fellows performances are also plotted as a line with shaded area representing the variability.

4. Conclusions

Our results showed that practicing on a high fidelity model (3D) resulted in similar but not identical improvements in outcomes as practicing on a low fidelity model (2D). That is, the group of trainees who practiced on the low fidelity model required an additional 3D practice attempt to remove the same amount of bone mass as the group who practiced on a 3D version of the task and the more advanced group of fellows.

This implies that, during the initial stages of practice, fundamental psychomotor adaptation processes for drilling take place, regardless of the exact skill that is practiced. These processes are most likely related to familiarization with novel instruments and bone material. However specific processes related to the depth of drilling and thus the amount of material removed must be practiced separately on a high fidelity model.

These results support Learning Specificity Theory. Hence, when learning new technical skills in a simulated environment it is pertinent to select models that contain all constructs of the skill. For example, in this study the 2D practice did not adequately train depth of drilling – a construct that is important for optimal performance in the Operating room.

However, our results also imply that the initial familiarization phase may be achieved during a low fidelity practice session. Drilling on low fidelity models contains a high degree of internal feedback, derived from the task itself. Therefore, this form of practice may require less expert resources.

5. References

[1] Hamstra SJ, Dubrowski A, Backstein D. Teaching technical skills to surgical residents: A survey of empirical research. *Clin Orthop Relat Res*. **449**, (2006), 108-15.

[2] Adams JA. A closed-loop theory of motor learning. *J Mot Behav* **3(2)**, (1971), 111-149.

[3] Guadagnoli MA, Lee TD. Challenge point: a framework for conceptualizing the effects of various practice conditions in motor learning. *J Mot Behav* **36(2)**, (2004), 212-224

Medicine Meets Virtual Reality 15
J.D. Westwood et al. (Eds.)
IOS Press, 2007

473

Objective Surgical Performance Assessment for Virtual Hysteroscopy

Stefan TUCHSCHMID [a,1], Michael BAJKA [b], Daniel BACHOFEN [a],
Gábor SZÉKELY [a], Matthias HARDERS [a]

[a] *Virtual Reality in Medicine Group, Computer Vision Lab, ETH Zurich, Switzerland*
[b] *Clinic of Gynecology, Dept OB/GYN, University Hospital Zurich, Switzerland*

Abstract. We present robust methods for objective, structured, and automated assessment of surgical performance in virtual diagnostic hysteroscopy. Surgery specific metrics are based on a hierarchical task decomposition and have been integrated into our simulation setup. Measurements include visible surface quantification, fluid consumption and indicators for safety and economy of movement. Both visual and quantitative results from exemplary interventions of novice and expert surgeons are shown.

Keywords. surgical simulation, performance assessment

1. Introduction

Our research focus is the development of a high-fidelity surgical training simulator for hysteroscopy. The system is designed to allow the acquisition of psychomotor skills as well as training of procedural skills like decision making and problem solving [5]. For the structured learning of surgical skills, objective feedback is crucial. Virtual reality systems may be used for surgical assessment and have been reported to be superior to traditional methods such as direct observation, animal models, videotapes and procedure logs in terms of reliability and validity [10]. However, validated performance assessment on surgery simulators requires objective metrics, which have to be met consistently by a trainee before operating on a patient [4].

Current metrics are usually based on easily obtainable measurements such as the intervention time or surgical tool movements [3]. Darzi et al. [2] pointed out in 1999 that *"a system that can provide unbiased and objective measurement of surgical precision (rather than just speed) could help training, complement knowledge based examinations, and provide a benchmark for certification."* Since then, some effort has been made to develop assessment parameters which relate better to the final objective of the given surgery. Ritter et al. showed that time to completion is a poor metric for the objective assessment of intracorporal knot-tying performance whereas an automated knot quality score can accurately distinguish well-tied knots from poorly tied knots [12]. Rosen et al. used Markov models for the clustering of force/torque signatures in order to reveal the internal structure of a surgical task [14,13]. Moorthy et al. tracked tool motions to

---

[1] Correspondence to: tuchschmid@vision.ee.ethz.ch

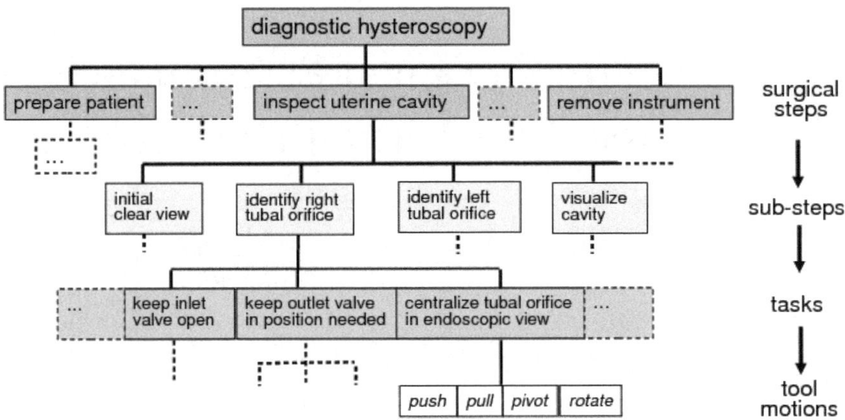

Figure 1. Task decomposition for diagnostic hysteroscopy (extract).

analyze the dexterity of a surgeon to provide performance feedback on the psychomotor skills [9].

A systematic review on the use of medical simulators from 1969 to 2003 identified three key characteristics of a training system to facilitate learning in high-fidelity simulations: feedback possibilities, repetitive practice and curriculum integration [6]. In this paper, we present robust methods for objective, structured, and automated assessment of surgical performance for virtual diagnostic hysteroscopy which provide feedback both during and between repetitions and can be integrated into a teaching curriculum.

2. Objective Surgical Performance Assessment

In order to implement performance assessment for virtual hysteroscopy, the following steps are required: *hierarchical task decomposition* to break down the surgery into its elements, implementation of *surgery specific performance metrics*, and their *integration into the simulation setup* to test reliability and validity of the assessment metrics.

2.1. Hierarchical Task Decomposition

We performed a cognitive task analysis similar to Cao et al. [1] for diagnostic hysteroscopy in order to identify the specific performance metrics. A panel of experienced surgeons split up the diagnostic hysteroscopy procedure into surgical steps (e.g. inspect uterine cavity), sub-steps (e.g. identify right tubal orifice), tasks (centralize tubal orifice in view) and tool motions needed (see Figure 1). In contrast to Moorty et al. we use tool motions and activities merely to evaluate completion of a task or sub-step, while aiming at measuring procedural skills on a higher level.

Table 1. Pseudocode for real-time visualized surface detection.

```
01   enable occlusion query extension;
02   define THRESHOLD;
03   move all triangles to unvisualizedSet;
04   for triangle in unvisualizedSet {
05       reset occlusion query;
06       render triangle;
07       get nrRenderedPixels from occlusion query;
08       visibility[triangle] = nrRenderedPixels / triangleArea[triangle];
09       if (visibility[triangle] > THRESHOLD) {
10           move triangle from unvisualizedSet to visualizedSet;
11       }
12   }
```

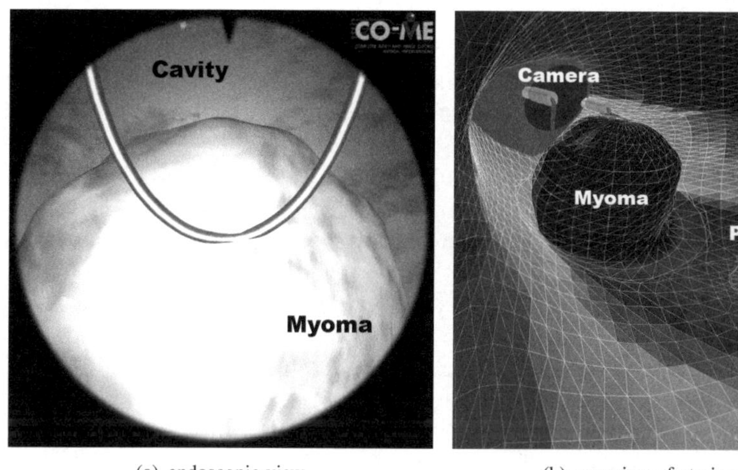

(a) endoscopic view   (b) overview of uterine cavity

Figure 2. Quantification of visualized surface (green: visible, red: invisible from camera viewport).

2.2. Surgery Specific Performance Metrics

The main complications in hysteroscopy are excessive hypotonic fluid absorptions leading to the fluid overload syndrome, intraoperative hemorrhages, and uterine perforations [11,7]. Therefore, we implemented performance metrics that indicate the amount of distension media used, the quality of the endoscopic view, and the safe handling of the hysteroscope. The fluid consumption is computed in real-time by simulating the effects of leakage at the cervix, loss at the continuous flow sheath interface, outflow suction, transtubal loss, and intravasation. We track the movements of the hysteroscope, compute safety and economy of movement parameters such as distance to the uterine wall and the camera path length, and register all collisions.

The most important metric for diagnostic hysteroscopy is the quantification of the properly visualized surface. Part of the uterine surface may be concealed from the endoscopic view due to obstructing pathologies, the shape of the uterus, or heavy bleeding. Such a visibility measurement also allows us to mark critical regions which need to be visualized for a complete diagnostic procedure, e.g. on the tubal ostia. Most current graphics cards provide the OpenGL-Extension `GL_ARB_occlusion_query` to query the number of pixels drawn by a primitive. Normally, this feature is used to implement occlusion culling by rendering a bounding box around every primitive, querying the rendered pixels and checking if one or more are visible. However, occlusion querying can also be used to check all surface triangles for visibility in real-time. Normalizing the rendered pixels with the surface area yields a measure for the visibility of the triangle. If the visibility measure is larger than a threshold value, we mark the surface triangle as visualized and remove it from the test for better performance. Table 1 shows the corresponding pseudo-code. Since the occlusion query counts the actually rendered pixels, it automatically handles the restriction to the viewing frustrum as well as occlusion by surgical tools, pathologies and even floating tissue scraps or bubbles. Figure 2 depicts the actually visualized surface for a typical hysteroscopic scene, where a small polyp is hidden behind a large myoma.

2.3. Integration into the Simulation Setup

To demonstrate reliability and validity of the implemented metrics, we integrated the developed assessment methods into our virtual surgery setup and measured learning curves for both novice residents and expert clinicians. The goal was to perform an optimal diagnostic hysteroscopy as defined in the task decomposition, including but not limited to inserting the hysteroscope, setting in- and outlet valves, and navigating the camera inside the uterine cavity. After properly establishing the hydrometra, the task was to examine the complete uterine cavity while maintaining clear viewing conditions by adjusting the in- and outflow valves.

In general, structured feedback given by a teacher or the simulator is necessary to improve the learning curve of a trainee [8]. During a trial, immediate auditory feedback was provided in case of a collision with the uterine wall. Moreover, concluding feedback was given after a trial by visually comparing the achieved results with expert data. A sample of such an intervention report is shown in Figure 3. A movie replay of the simulation can be shown to further facilitate self-teaching. Each case was repeated several times in order to establish learning curves.

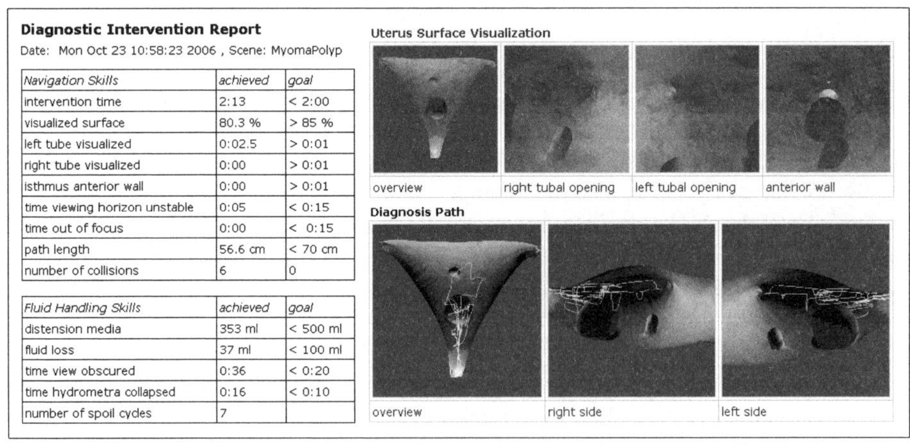

Diagnostic Intervention Report

Date: Mon Oct 23 10:58:23 2006 , Scene: MyomaPolyp

Navigation Skills	achieved	goal
intervention time	2:13	< 2:00
visualized surface	80.3 %	> 85 %
left tube visualized	0:02.5	> 0:01
right tube visualized	0:00	> 0:01
isthmus anterior wall	0:00	> 0:01
time viewing horizon unstable	0:05	< 0:15
time out of focus	0:00	< 0:15
path length	56.6 cm	< 70 cm
number of collisions	6	0

Fluid Handling Skills	achieved	goal
distension media	353 ml	< 500 ml
fluid loss	37 ml	< 100 ml
time view obscured	0:36	< 0:20
time hydrometra collapsed	0:16	< 0:10
number of spoil cycles	7	

Figure 3. Example diagnostic intervention report.

Figure 4 shows a visual summary of three exemplary interventions, obtained from an experienced surgeon (more than 200 hysteroscopies performed), a novice's first trial,

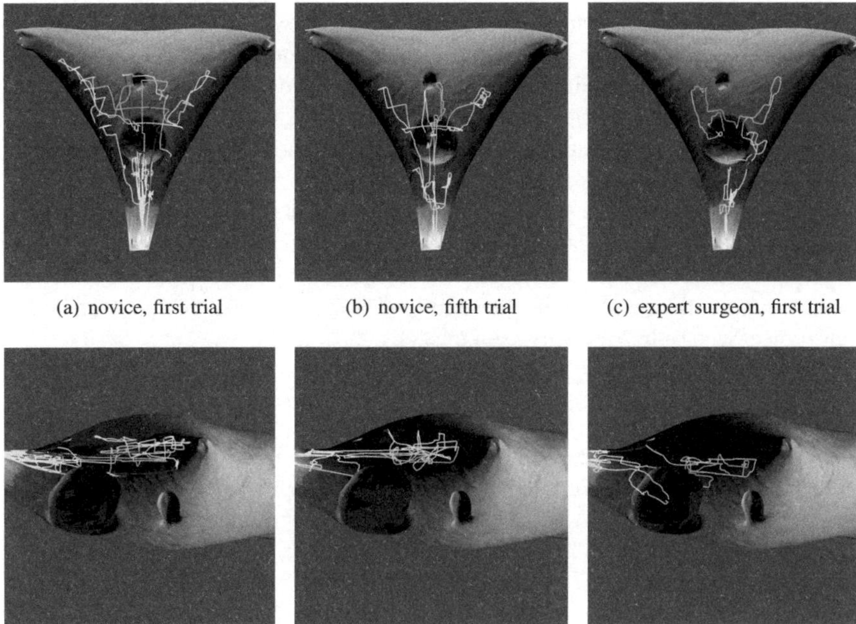

(a) novice, first trial   (b) novice, fifth trial   (c) expert surgeon, first trial

Figure 4. Visualized uterus surface and camera navigation path for novice and expert interventions (top row: view from above, bottom row: view from the left patient side).

and a novice's fifth trial. Uterine surface patches not visualized are marked in red and the navigation path of the endoscopic camera is color-coded with respect to the distance to the uterine surface (red: collision, green: distance more than 10mm). The path of the master surgeon is significantly shorter but still provides optimal surface coverage, while the novice surgeon first exhibits poor economy of movement and insufficient surface coverage, but later on improves performance. The visual impression is confirmed by the quantitative measurements in Table 2.

Table 2. Quantitative performance measurements for novice and expert interventions.

	novice, 1. trial	*novice, 5. trial*	*expert, 1. trial*
surface visualized	87.5%	90.4%	89.4%
distension fluid used	813 ml	538 ml	366 ml
intervention time	3:52 min	2:24 min	1:56 min
time out of focus	2:26 min	1:27 min	0:24 min
path length	120.1 cm	65.5 cm	50.5 cm
number of wall collisions	11	4	1
time colliding	14.9 s	5.9 s	1.8 s
time view obscured	1:18 min	0:20 min	0:37 min

3. Discussion and Conclusions

While the underlying task decomposition achieves a high consensus among experts in terms of task components, the proper setting of threshold parameters has been difficult.

Questions like *"when is the view too obscured/blurred/bright?"* or *"how close does one need to visualize the tubal ostia?"* were settled by finding a trade-off that all experts could agree on. While the preliminary results look promising, further validation is needed before the implemented metrics can be used in an assessment tool. A clinical study is currently carried out to investigate construct and content validity of the implemented performance metrics.

The proposed framework for performance assessment produces reliable and quantitative measurements of surgical performance for diagnostic hysteroscopic interventions. The integration into the clinical curriculum is currently investigated. Screenshots, movies of sample interventions and detailed descriptions of the simulator modules can be found on our project web (http://www.hystsim.ethz.ch).

Acknowledgments

This research has been supported by the NCCR Co-Me of the Swiss National Science Foundation. The authors would like to thank all developers of the hysteroscopy simulator project.

References

[1]   C. G. Cao, C. L. MacKenzie, J. A. Ibbotson, L. J. Turner, N. P. Blair, and A. G. Nagy. Hierarchical decomposition of laparoscopic procedures. *Stud Health Technol Inform*, 62:83–89, 1999.

[2]   A. Darzi, S. Smith, and N. Taffinder. Assessing operative skill. Needs to become more objective. *BMJ*, 318(7188):887–888, Apr 1999.

[3]   A. G. Gallagher and R. M. Satava. Virtual reality as a metric for the assessment of laparoscopic psychomotor skills. Learning curves and reliability measures. *Surg Endosc*, 16(12):1746–1752, Dec 2002.

[4]   A.G. Gallagher, E.M. Ritter, H. Champion, G.Higgins, M. Fried, G. Moses, C. D. Smith, and R. M. Satava. Virtual reality simulation for the operating room: proficiency-based training as a paradigm shift in surgical skills training. *Ann Surg*, 241(2):364–372, Feb 2005.

[5]   M. Harders, M. Bajka, U. Spälter, S. Tuchschmid, H. Bleuler, and G. Székely. Highly-realistic, immersive training environment for hysteroscopy. *Stud Health Technol Inform*, 119:176–181, 2006.

[6]   S. Issenberg, W. McGaghie, E. Petrusa, D. Gordon, and R. Scalese. Features and uses of high-fidelity medical simulations that lead to effective learning: a BEME systematic review. *Med Teach*, 27(1):10–28, Jan 2005.

[7]   M. König, A. Meyer, B. Aydeniz, R. Kurek, and D. Wallwiener. Hysteroscopic surgery–complications and their prevention. *Contrib Gynecol Obstet*, 20:161–170, 2000.

[8]   T. Mahmood and A. Darzi. The learning curve for a colonoscopy simulator in the absence of any feedback: no feedback, no learning. *Surg Endosc*, 18(8):1224–1230, Aug 2004. Clinical Trial.

[9]   K. Moorthy, Y. Munz, A. Dosis, F. Bello, and A. Darzi. Motion analysis in the training and assessment of minimally invasive surgery. *Minim Invasive Ther Allied Technol*, 12(3):137–142, Jul 2003.

[10]   K. Moorthy, Y. Munz, S. Sarker, and A. Darzi. Objective assessment of technical skills in surgery. *BMJ*, 327(7422):1032–1037, Nov 2003.

[11]   A. Pasini and C. Belloni. Intraoperative complications of 697 consecutive operative hysteroscopies. *Minerva Ginecol*, 53(1):13–20, Feb 2001.

[12]   E. M. Ritter, D. A. McClusky, A. G. Gallagher, and C. D. Smith. Real-time objective assessment of knot quality with a portable tensiometer is superior to execution time for assessment of laparoscopic knot-tying performance. *Surg Innov*, 12(3):233–237, Sep 2005.

[13]   J. Rosen, J.D. Brown, L. Chang, M.N. Sinanan, and B. Hannaford. Generalized approach for modeling minimally invasive surgery as a stochastic process using a discrete markov model. *IEEE Trans Biomed Eng*, 53(3):399–413, March 2006.

[14]   J. Rosen, B. Hannaford, C. G. Richards, and M. N. Sinanan. Markov modeling of minimally invasive surgery based on tool/tissue interaction and force/torque signatures for evaluating surgical skills. *IEEE Trans Biomed Eng*, 48(5):579–591, May 2001.

Medicine Meets Virtual Reality 15
J.D. Westwood et al. (Eds.)
IOS Press, 2007

Interactive Physically-based X-ray Simulation: CPU or GPU?

Franck P. VIDAL [a], Nigel W. JOHN [a], Romain M. GUILLEMOT [b]

[a] *School of Computer Science, University of Wales, Bangor, UK*
[b] *CReSTIC / LERI / MADS, Université de Reims Champagne-Ardenne, Reims, France*

Abstract. Interventional Radiology (IR) procedures are minimally invasive, targeted treatments performed using imaging for guidance. Needle puncture using ultrasound, x-ray, or computed tomography (CT) images is a core task in the radiology curriculum, and we are currently developing a training simulator for this. One requirement is to include support for physically-based simulation of x-ray images from CT data sets. In this paper, we demonstrate how to exploit the capability of today's graphics cards to efficiently achieve this on the Graphics Processing Unit (GPU) and compare performance with an efficient software only implementation using the Central Processing Unit (CPU).

Keywords. X-ray simulation, GPU-based volume rendering, Interventional radiology.

Introduction

There is a growing demand for validated virtual environments designed for training Interventional Radiology (IR) procedures. Our research group is actively involved in this task and together with clinical collaborators at the Royal Liverpool Hospital and elsewhere, we are producing a real time simulator for image-guided needle puncture [4]. We exploit the capabilities of modern PC graphics cards to efficiently implement many functions of the simulator. In this paper we demonstrate how to implement one of these functions - physically-based simulation of x-ray images from CT data sets - and compare performance results with an equivalent CPU-based approach.

1. Methods and Tools

Our simulator uses a patient specific data set acquired in DICOM format from a medical CT scanner. Hounsfield values are then converted into linear attenuation coefficients that can be directly used by our determinist simulation algorithm based on the attenuation law (or Beer-Lambert law) that relates the absorption of light to the properties of the material through which the light is travelling. We only consider directly transmitted photons, photon scattering is then ignored. In the case of a monochromatic incident beam, for homogeneous materials, the Beer-Lambert law is: $N_{out} = N_{in} \times e^{-\mu \times x}$, with N_{in} the number of incident photons, x the lenght (in cm) of the x-ray path across the material, μ is the linear attenuation coefficient (in cm^{-1}) of the material, and N_{out} the number of photons after crossed the material. Ray tracing has been shown to be efficient for the fast approximation of x-ray images using triangular meshes [1]. Figure 1 shows that the concept can also be extended to volume data sets, each voxel corresponding to a cube characterized by its linear attenuation coefficient. In this case, a ray is sent through each pixel of the simulated image orthogonal to the viewing direction. Using this approach, the attenuation of the incident x-ray beam is computed for each voxel traversed. Our implementation is optimized by taking into account the fact that the exit-point of the ray into the current voxel is the entry-point of the ray into the next voxel to be processed, which is always within the direct neighborhood of the current voxel. The computation

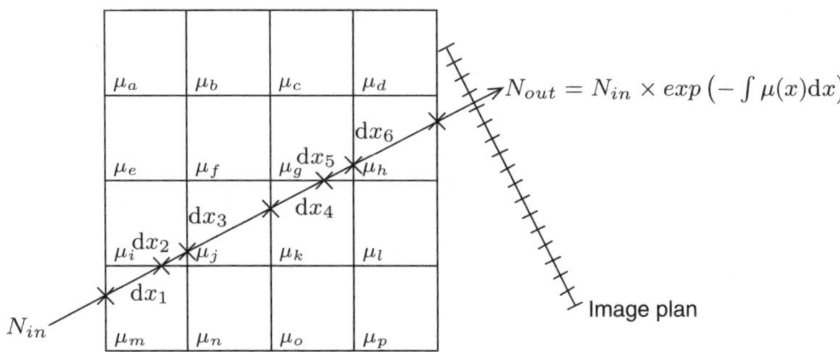

Figure 1. Principle of x-ray simulation in 2D.

time and the image quality will only depend on the number of pixels of that image and the number of voxels of the data set. Two versions of the algorithm have been produced:

CPU-based. The algorithm is well suited for parallel programming. Indeed, each processor available can compute simultaneously a different sub-region of the final image. Thus the algorithm has been implemented using the pthread library to take advantage of parallel computing on multi-processor computers (i.e. with several physical CPUs) or mono-processor computers with hyper-threading (i.e. with only one physical CPU but two logical CPUs).

GPU-based. Ray-casting using 3D textures and ray-tracing have previously been implemented on GPUs (Graphics Processor Units) [2,3] and take advantage of the parallel processing capabilities of this programmable hardware. However, a GPU-based simulation of physically-based x-ray images has not yet been addressed and it is not straightforward to use the GPU to process x-ray attenuation coefficients. We achieve this using OpenGL, the OpenGL Shading Language and 3D texture hardware. Hounsfield values in the body are between -1000 (air) and 1000 (hard bones). The values of the original dataset are clamped between those values, then normalized between 0.0 and 1.0 to be loaded into the texture memory. The fragment program will convert texture values into attenuation coefficients and compute the x-ray attenuation by ray-tracing.

2. Results

Table 1 summarises the performance achieved on different hardware configurations. The time taken (in ms) to perform a predefined animation of 1000 512×512 frames generated from a $512 \times 512 \times 62$ CT data set is recorded. Figure 2 shows examples of the computed images.

Table 1. Performance comparison: average time to compute a 512×512 image (in ms) using a $512 \times 512 \times 62$ CT data set.

	Bi-Xeon 2.4 GHz without hyper-threading	Bi-Xeon 2.4 GHz with hyper-threading	Nvidia GeForce 6400	Nvidia Quadro FX 3400
CPU x-ray attenuation	22421	23661	X	X
GPU x-ray attenuation	X	X	1.876	0.907

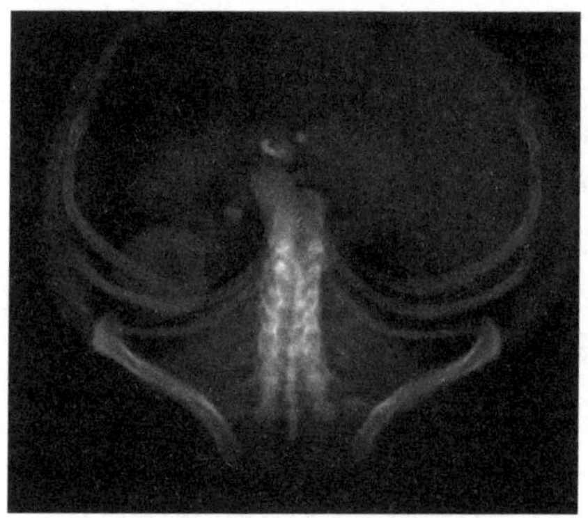

(a) Image computed on the CPU.

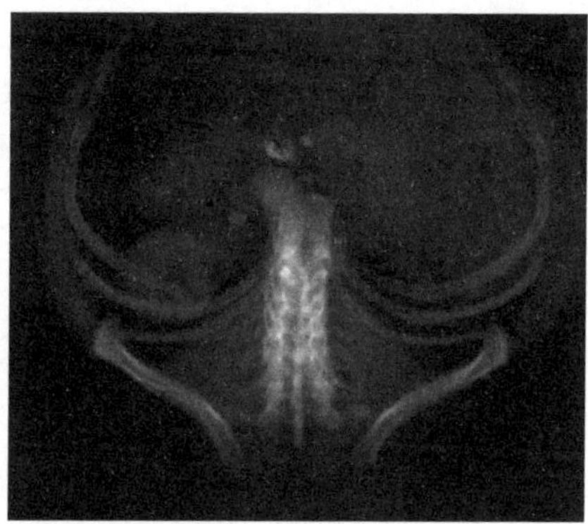

(b) Image computed on a laptop with a Nvidia GeForce 6400 graphics card.

Figure 2. Examples of x-ray simulations.

3. Conclusions/Discussion

The parallised CPU-based simulation of high-resolution images is too slow on bi-processors and prevents real-time interaction. Hyper-threading seems not to improve the performance. However, our GPU-based implementation enables the simulation of x-ray images from volume data in real time, at high resolution, and with the same image quality as software volume rendering on CPUs. The use of the attenuation law also results in more accurate x-ray images than previously reported work.

References

[1] N. Freud, P. Duvauchelle, J. M. Létang, and D. Babot. Fast and robust ray casting algorithms for virtual x-ray imaging. *Nuclear Instruments and Methods in Physics Research Section B: Beam Interactions with Materials and Atoms*, 248(1):175–180, July 2006. DOI: 10.1016/j.nimb.2006.03.009.

[2] J. Krüger and R. Westermann. Acceleration techniques for GPU-based volume rendering. In *Proceedings of IEEE Visualization 2003*, pages 287–292. IEEE Computer Society, Oct. 2003. DOI: 10.1109/VIS.2003.10001.

[3] T. J. Purcell, I. Buck, W. R. Mark, and P. Hanrahan. Ray tracing on programmable graphics hardware. *ACM Transactions on Graphics*, 21(3):703–712, 2002. Proceedings of ACM SIGGRAPH 2002. DOI: 10.1145/566654.566640.

[4] F. P. Vidal, N. Chalmers, D. A. Gould, A. E. Healey, and N. W. John. Developing a needle guidance virtual environment with patient-specific data and force feedback. In H. U. Lemke, K. Inamura, K. Doi, M. W. Vannier, and A. G. Farman, editors, *CARS 2005: Computer Assisted Radiology and Surgery*, volume 1281 of *International Congress Series*, pages 418–423. Elsevier, May 2005. DOI: 10.1016/j.ics.2005.03.200.

Medicine Meets Virtual Reality 15
J.D. Westwood et al. (Eds.)
IOS Press, 2007

Device Connectivity for Image-Guided Medical Applications

Jochen VON SPICZAK[a,b,1], Eigil SAMSET[a,e,f], Simon DIMAIO[a,f], Gerhard
REITMAYR[c], Dieter SCHMALSTIEG[d], Catherina BURGHART[b] and Ron KIKINIS[a,f]

[a]*Brigham and Women's Hospital, Boston, MA, USA*
[b]*Technical University of Karlsruhe, Karlsruhe, Germany*
[c]*Cambridge University, Cambridge, UK*
[d]*Graz University of Technology, Graz, Austria*
[e]*University of Oslo, Rikshospitalet, Oslo, Norway*
[f]*Harvard Medical School, Boston, MA, USA*

Abstract. The integration of medical devices with software applications is crucial
for image-guided medical applications. This work describes a general device interface that has been designed for high-frequency streaming of multi-modal events,
thus providing maximum performance and flexibility for such applications. Several sample applications and performance tests are provided to demonstrate the usability of the concept.

Keywords. General Device Interface, Middleware, Event Streaming, OpenTracker,
Image-Guided Intervention.

Introduction

Tracking and navigation systems, peripheral devices, image acquisition, image visualization, and data logging play an indispensable role in image-guided medical applications. In order to interconnect a wide variety of interventional devices in a flexible and
extensible manner, it is necessary to have a software framework that provides high-
level hardware abstraction, efficient handling of data streams in real time, and transparent network support. The system described in this paper augments a software framework originally developed for high-bandwidth event streaming in VR applications to
meet the extended requirements to interconnect a variety of heterogeneous medical
devices for high-performance image-guided medical applications.

1. Related Work

Many existing solutions for connecting medical hardware devices with surgical planning and navigation interface software do not exploit the full potential for processing

---

[1] Corresponding Author: Jochen von Spiczak, E-Mail: jochen@bwh.harvard.edu
This study was supported in part by the NIH U41-RR019703 and NSF EEC-9731748 grants.

events coming from arbitrary sources, and are not easily generalizable. The extent of such connectivity is illustrated in Figure 1.

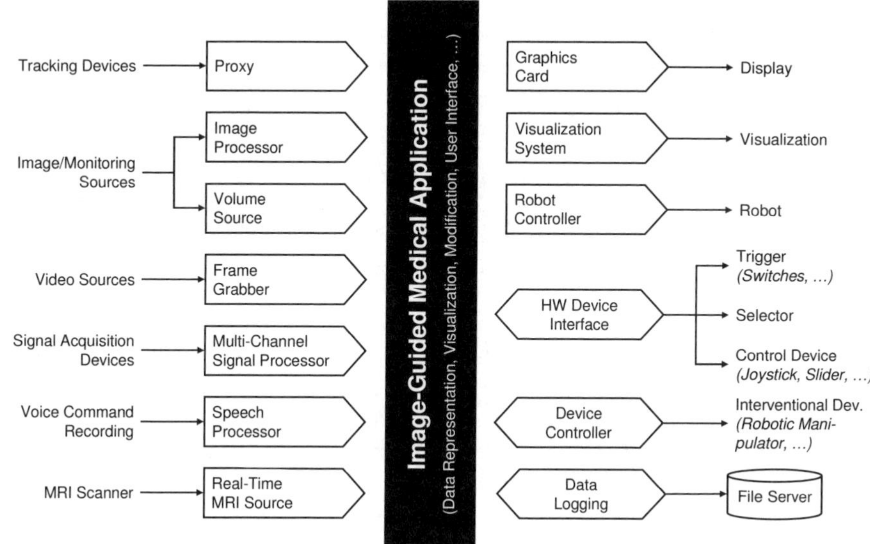

Figure 1. Taxonomy of hardware devices that need to be supported.

Prior work can be divided into two main categories. First, there are systems for high-frequency, real-time streaming of event data using a highly optimized, fixed data structure for the streamed events that can be accessed, copied, and processed with minimum delay. The fixed event structure limits the applicability of such systems to its dedicated field of application [1]. Second, there are systems for asynchronous process-ing of multi-modal events, the content of which can be flexibly defined. Such systems typically achieve lower performance due to the associated overheads [2].

2. Tools and Methods

A general device interface for image-guided medical applications was designed. It in-cludes the definition of a common protocol and facilitates data logging, network trans-mission, and an efficient method for configuring variable hardware setups. In addition, translation components for several different types of devices have been implemented—these can be extended by the user as required.

As the underlying concept, we introduce high-frequency streaming of multi-modal events with generic data types. Events are generated dynamically at runtime—as re-quired by the application—and can contain data of arbitrary types, including composite high-level types defined by the user. The structure of each event can change during its lifetime—information can be added, accessed, modified, and deleted. The present li-brary was developed on the basis of the well established OpenTracker library [1], which provided hardware abstraction for a plurality of tracking systems, but could not support any other devices due to its fixed event data structure. The augmented architec-ture was implemented as a highly extendable C++ library in a strictly object oriented manner. It relies on the concept of generic programming to realize event attributes of generic types. Events can be serialized and distributed in a self-descriptive format for network and file logging support.

3. Results

A number of tests were undertaken to evaluate the overall performance of the system. Performance tests were run on an off-the-shelf computer workstation (Dell Precision™ Workstation 670). A minimal event latency of 50.66 µs could be reached resulting in a throughput of 19.74 kHz. Performance degraded for more complex hardware setups with extensive additional event filtering. Several applications were successfully developed using the proposed approach and thus proving the usability of the framework:

ECG triggered, MRI guided navigation for cardiac interventions: A patient's electrocardiogram (ECG) signal is sampled and encoded in an event. Navigation software for cardiac intervention interprets the heart rate attribute of the incoming event and synchronizes visualization of a set of pre-operatively acquired MRI images of the complete heart cycle with the patient's current heart rate [3].

A dynamic and extensible software framework for Image-Guided Therapy: A software framework called The SIGN[2] was developed, facilitating rapid development of navigation applications for image-guided procedures and therapies that require multi-modal imaging and tracking. For interfacing with a large range of medical devices, OpenTracker was used with an extension library called SPLOT [4].

4. Discussion and Conclusion

The proposed design of multi-modal event streams is suitable for high-performance image-guided medical applications that require both high-bandwidth event streaming and support for multiple heterogeneous devices. The lowest throughput of the system was measured for a setup far more complex than typically required in practice and was still satisfactory for most applications. Dynamic introduction of any number of arbitrarily-typed event attributes with late type-binding during runtime provides significant functional advantages over hard coded, fixed event data-structures, and is more flexible than simpler generic approaches that determine event data types at compile time.

References

[1]   G Reitmayr, D Schmalstieg, *OpenTracker - A Flexible Software Design for Three-Dimensional Interaction.* Virtual Reality, Vol. 9, No. 1, pp. 79-92, Springer, London, Dec. 2005.
[2]   R Carey, G Bell, *The Annotated VRML 2.0 Reference Manual.* Addison-Wesley, 1997.
[3]   E Samset, DF Kacher, P Aksit, GH Reynolds, LM Epstein, FA Jolesz, *ECG Triggered MRI-Guided Navigation for Cardiac Interventions.* In Proc. ISMRM 2006, Seattle, Washington, USA, p. 287.
[4]   E Samset, A Hans, J von Spiczak, SP DiMaio, R Ellis, N Hata, FA Jolesz. *The SIGN: A Dynamic and Extensible Software Framework for Image-Guided Therapy*, MICCAI workshop on Open Source and Data for Medical Image Computing and Computer-Assisted Intervention, Insight-Journal, DSpace Handle http://hdl.handle.net/1926/207.

---

[2] The SIGN and SPLOT are available under the BSD compatible Slicer license (http://www.ncigt.org/sign).

Medicine Meets Virtual Reality 15
J.D. Westwood et al. (Eds.)
IOS Press, 2007

485

Natural Orifice Transluminal Endoscopic Surgery (NOTES): An Opportunity for Augmented Reality Guidance

Kirby G. VOSBURGH[a,b,1] & Raúl SAN JOSÉ ESTÉPAR [b]
[a]CIMIT/ Massachusetts General Hospital
[b]Brigham and Women's Hospital

Abstract. Laparoscopic techniques have gained wide acceptance because they offer a safe and less invasive alternative to open surgery. To further reduce the invasiveness of peritoneal access, the next logical step is to eliminate the incision through the abdominal wall using natural orifices as entry points. This Natural Orifice Transluminal Endoscopic Surgery (NOTES) approach has the potential to replace or augment current techniques. Several research groups have cut through the stomach or colon wall (per-oral transgastric or per-anal transcolonic) to perform organ resections in animal models, and some procedures in humans have been reported anecdotally. Widespread use of these techniques will depend on providing the physician with adequate visual feedback, clear indicators of instrument location and orientation, and support in the recognition of anatomic structures. Compared with laparoscopy, successful endoscopy must accommodate several additional complexities: (1) The flexibility of the endoscope tip complicates the understanding of its distal orientation. Successful navigation inside the stomach and in the abdominal cavity generally requires two years of sub-specialty training. (2) Several surgical targets lie in a retrograde position with respect to an incision in the stomach wall. Efficient and safe access to the pancreas, gall bladder, or the kidneys requires detailed knowledge of the tip placement relative to adjacent anatomic structures. (3) Since there is limited direct access to the abdomen, iatrogenic injuries, such as the accidental cutting of an artery, will be more dangerous and difficult to manage. We present here approaches to resolving these limitations though augmented reality techniques using pre-procedure CT or MRI imaging, real time tracking and reference image registration, and display to the operating physician. As an example, the utility of image registration techniques for orientation for the gastric access puncture is discussed in detail. It is anticipated that such augmentation will make intra-cavitary interventional techniques easier to master and use in practice, and thus more likely to be widely adopted.

Keywords: endoscopy, augmented reality, laparoscopy, image registration, NOTES

1. Introduction

Natural Orifice Transluminal Endoscopic Surgery (NOTES) is a new approach to surgical management of disease in the abdomen. Early stage animal model trials [1.2] and a small number of tests in human patients [3] have provided tantalizing prospects for the performance of surgical resections which leave no visible scars. While the impact of NOTES is being evaluated for many procedures, it may be especially beneficial to obese patients, for whom present techniques may be difficult in practice.

---

[1] kirby@bwh.harvard.edu; #702, 165 Cambridge St., Boston, MA, 02114, USA.

More generally, it will reduce scarring and wound exposure, thereby permitting a faster recovery. However, NOTES presents significant challenges in surgical procedure; it will require new technical approaches through the use of novel instruments to address issues of efficacy, efficiency, and safety. Since the NOTES concept is directed at displacing elective procedures now performed using laparoscopy or laparotomy, the validation of NOTES will be challenging.

A multi-disciplinary, multi-institutional team has identified several barriers to the success of NOTES; here we concentrate on the subset of challenges which may be addressed through advanced navigation and visualization technology; that is, by Augmented Reality techniques.

2. Barriers to the widespread use of NOTES

A group of fourteen leaders in the fields of surgery and endoscopy met in mid-2005 to analyze the barriers to the widespread use of NOTES procedures in the abdomen. [4] They agreed that the significant barriers were:

- Effective access to the peritoneal cavity
- Near-perfect gastric (intestinal) closure
- Prevention of infection
- Development of suturing and anastomotic (non suturing) devices
- **Support for spatial orientation**
- **Development of a multitasking platform to accomplish procedures**
- **Control of intra-peritoneal hemorrhage**
- Management of iatrogenic events
- Identification and management of physiologic untoward events
- Compression syndromes
- Training providers

Of these factors, gastric (or other luminal wall) closure was judged the most important, with the related factor of infection control also being of significant concern. As many as three of these challenges, highlighted in bold type, may be approached through improvements in Augmented Reality (AR) technology.

3. The potential advantages of Image Registered NOTES

Over the past two decades, many investigators have sought to show image and instrument position in 3D models; with several collaborators we have explored the use of real time systems which track instruments and display relevant data in the context of registered 3D models of the patient. This work is based on the recent development of tiny, but very accurate position sensors [5] and very fast interface and software systems [6] which permit complex visualization with no discernible lag. A series of experiments have shown that the presentation of probe position in sparse 3D models and the display of a spatially matched reformatted reference image (Fig. 1) provide valuable support to the operator in positioning intra-corporeal probes and understanding the content of

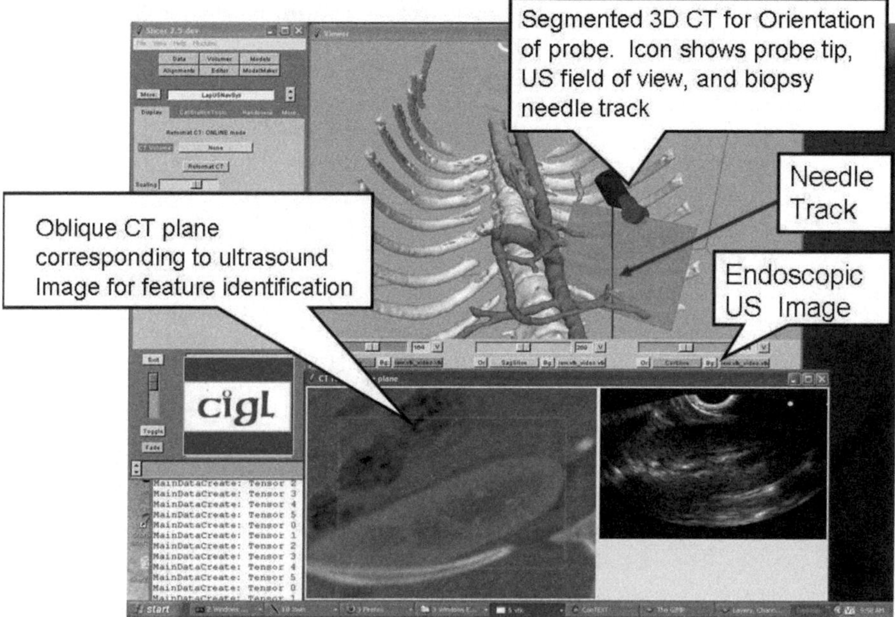

Figure 1. Image Registration System Display

ultrasound images they can provide. These "Image Registration" (IR) techniques have been used to improve task performance in laparoscopy [7] and endoscopy, [8] (Fig 2) and have been explored for guiding transgastric access [9] as a first step in developing image registered NOTES techniques. In these studies, both timed task performance (Fig 3) and analysis of the kinematics data on probe motion were used to quantify the benefits of IR technology.   Our overall conclusion (see the works referenced) is that such augmented reality techniques as Image Registration significantly improve the utility of intra-corporeal ultrasound; this is supported by structured survey analyses of the users, in which they reported much less frustration and need to concentrate when using the IR-augmented systems, while scoring much higher on the task metrics. From a technical perspective, we determined that real time performance was far more

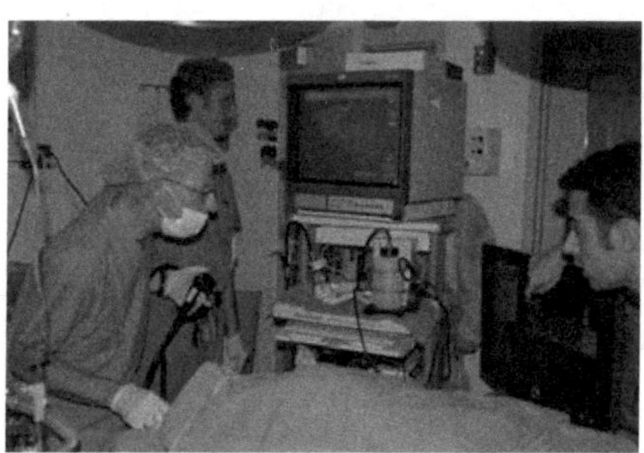

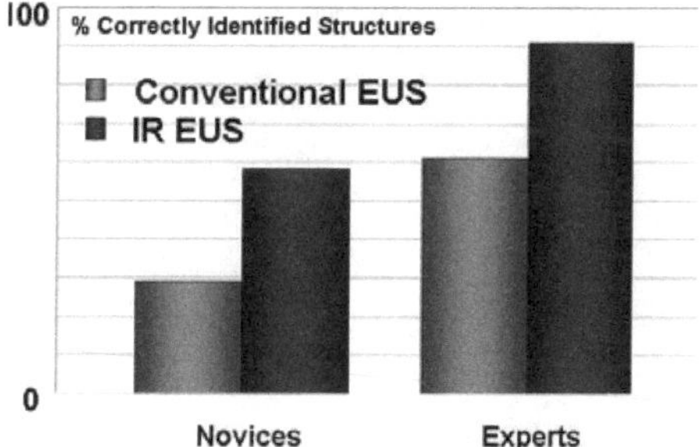

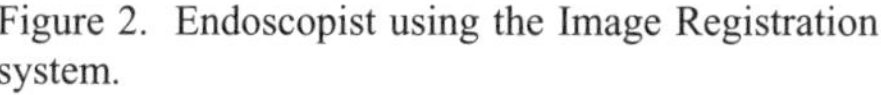

Figure 2. Endoscopist using the Image Registration system.

Figure 3. Percentage of anatomic targets in the abdomen identified in a timed trial using conventional and image registered gastroscopic ultrasound

important than ultra precise registration; an error or a few millimeters was accepted by the physician operators.

Techniques such as Image Registration appear to have many opportunities to support NOTES. These include probe guidance, positioning the probe on a surface in the desired orientation (Fig. 4), showing the anatomic structures distal to the probe (which will be important for puncture sites), and showing the relationship to other instruments.

As an example, consider the challenge of per-oral transgastric access to the abdomen. The operator of the endoscope is above the mouth of the patient, more than 0.5m from the puncture site. Figure 2 shows this relationship in a porcine model test. The operator positions the endoscope probe tip on the stomach wall. Clearly, the probe should not puncture the arteries on the posterior surface or those adjacent to the stomach. Figure 5 shows the arterial structure outside the stomach wall in a surface rendering of a contrast enhanced CT of a

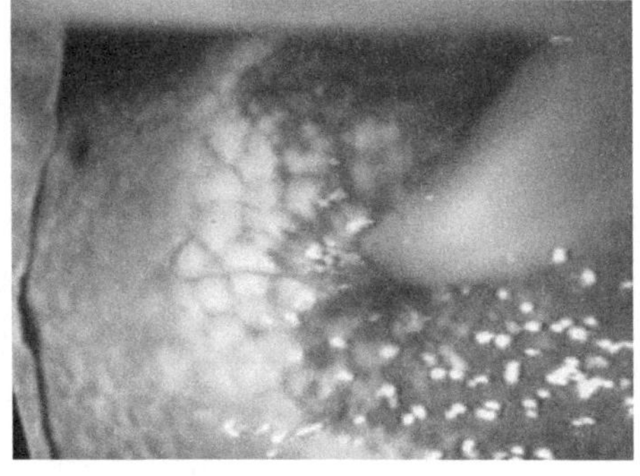

Figure 4. Probe inserted through stomach wall and guided to the boundary of a treated region of the liver. [9]

porcine model in supine position. The endoscopic view shown in Figure 5 (left image) mimics the view that an endoscopist will face; that is, looking down the esophagus toward the anterior stomach wall. While the details of the vascular structure are somewhat different in humans (and among individuals), the principle is that the major vessels distal to the puncture site must not be injured. However, the solution of this is not as simple as just make a pre-procedure CT and then tracking instruments, because the endoscopist will generally inflate the stomach to gain a better working space. This, in turn will press the stomach wall against other vascular structures, and certainly distorts the position of the vessels attached to the

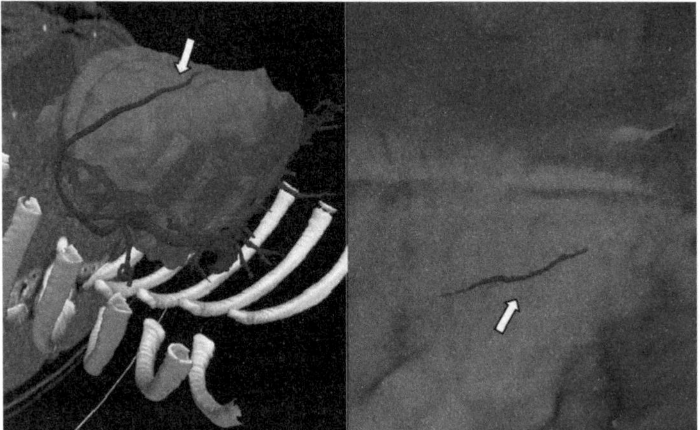

Figure 5. View of the vasculature anatomy of the stomach of a porcine model. The right image is an exterior view of the right part of the specimen. The right gastrodoudenal artery (white arrow) can be seen lying on top of the stomach wall. The left image is an endoscopic view of the same site from the inside of the stomach towards the right-anterior part. The vessel structure has been overlaid with the semi-transparent model of the stomach wall but it will not be visible in a standard endoscopic view.

outer stomach wall. Further evaluation, preferably in human subjects, will be necessary to determine the limitations of the Image Registration technique in this context.

4. Other Augmented Reality Techniques

Path planning in 3D has recently been highly developed by various groups, initially for virtual colonography and then bronchoscopy, notably at Penn State [10] and in the SuperDimension broncoscopic biopsy system. [11] It may also be valuable to compare the expected structure seen thorough the endoscope with that created from a model of the visual field using the CT data, incorporating the visual distortions of the endoscope optics. [12]

Many investigators, notably Aylward and collaborators, [13] have highlighted the details of the vascular structure, which are visible in pre-procedure CT, and intra-procedure optics and ultrasound to provide both orientation and localization of, for example, resection targets. This is particularly appealing in real time, since the blood vessels "move" with the target, which may be displaced form the pro-operative position, subject to respiratory effects, etc.

5. Discussion

From these preliminary results, it is reasonable to expect that Augmented Reality approaches including (but certainly not limited to) Image Registration and similar comparison techniques will be implemented in the clinical practice in NOTES procedures.   The methods developed for the evaluation of existing laparoscopic and endoscopic techniques may also be used to evaluate new NOTES procedures and to compare among various approaches. However, changes in patient posture, as well as respiratory and peristaltic motion will continue to challenge techniques, such as Image Registration, which depend on a reasonable correspondence with pre-procedure images. An eventual solution may be the ability to do real time registration using the details of vascular structure, perhaps acquired by 3D ultrasound.

6. Summary

Augmented Reality approaches may provide the missing links between general surgery, conventional endoscopy, and NOTES by providing contextual information in an intuitive and easily implemented display. The Image Registration technique, which appears (in early tests) to be beneficial for conventional endoscopy and laparoscopic imaging, may be one of many successful approaches to ensuring the practicality and widespread used of NOTES interventions.

7. Acknowledgements

This work was supported by CIMIT® under US Army MRMC Cooperative Agreement DAMD 17-02-2-0006. The information does not necessarily reflect the position of the government, and no official endorsement should be inferred. The authors thank N. Stylopoulos and D. Rattner for helpful comments, and Ascension Technologies and Olympus for equipment donations.

8. References

[1]   Kalloo AN, Singh VK, Jagannath SB, Niiyama H, Hill SL, Vaughn CA, Magee CA, Kantsevoy SV (2004) Flexible transgastric peritonoscopy: a novel approach to diagnostic and therapeutic interventions. *Gastrointest Endosc* 2004:60;114–7.

[2]   Wagh, MS, BF Merrifield, CC Thompson Endoscopic Transgastric Abdominal Exploration and Organ Resection: Initial Experience in a Porcine Model. *Clinical Gastroenterology and Hepatology* 2005:**3**; 892-896

[3]   Rao, et al, Personal communication to ASGE/SAGES Working Group (Ref 4.)

[4]   D. Rattner, A. Kalloo, et al. ASGE/SAGES Working Group on Natural Orifice Transluminal Endoscopic Surgery *Surg Endosc* (2006) 20: 329–333; also published in *Gastrointest Endos* 2006: 63-2.

[5]   MicroBIRD, Ascension Technologies, Burlington, VT, USA

[6]   3D Slicer; www.slicer.org

[7]   Ellsmere J. Stoll J. Wells W 3rd. Kikinis R. Vosburgh K. Kane R. Brooks D. Rattner D. A new visualization technique for laparoscopic ultrasonography. *Surgery. 136(1):84-92, 2004 Jul.* see also Vosburgh, KG, N. Stylopoulos, C. Thompson, R. Ellis, E. Samset, R. San Jose Estepar, Novel real time tracking interface improves the use of laparoscopic and endoscopic ultrasound in the abdomen. Proc. Computer Aided Radiology and Surgery (CARS) 2006, Osaka.

[8]   Vosburgh, KG, N. Stylopoulos, R. San Jose Estepar, RE Ellis, E. Samset, CC Thompson   EUS and CT Improve Efficiency and Structure Identification over Conventional EUS, *Gastrointestinal Endoscopy*, 2006 (in press).

[9]   San Jose Estepar, R, N. Stylopoulos, RE Ellis, E. Samset, C-F Westin, CC Thompson, KG Vosburgh Towards Scarless Surgery: An Endoscopic Ultrasound Navigation System for Transgastric Access Procedures. *MICCAI 2006*;LNCS 4190, I; 445-453 (Springer).

[10] Kiraly, AP, WE Higgins, G. McLennan, EA Hoffman, JM Reinhardt three-dimensional Human Airway Segmentation Methods for Clinical Virtual Bronchoscopy, *Acad. Radiol.* 2002: 9 (10);1553-68.

[11] www.superdimension.com

[12] Helferty, JP. Zhang C. McLennan G. Higgins WE. Videoendoscopic distortion correction and its application to virtual guidance of endoscopy. *IEEE Trans Med Imag.*2001:20(7);605-17.

[13] Aylward SR, J. Jomier, S. Weeks E. Bullitt Registration and Analysis of Vascular Images. *J. Comp. Vision* 2003:55;123-138

Medicine Meets Virtual Reality 15
J.D. Westwood et al. (Eds.)
IOS Press, 2007

491

Immersive Visualization with Automated Collision Detection for Radiotherapy Treatment Planning

J W WARD [a], R PHILLIPS [a,1], T WILLIAMS [b], C SHANG [b], L PAGE [a],
C PREST [a], A W BEAVIS [c]

[a] *Department of Computer Science, University of Hull, Hull, UK*
[b] *Boca Raton Community Hospital, Florida, USA*
[c] *Princess Royal Hospital, Hull and East Yorkshire NHS Trust, Hull, UK*

Abstract. Intensity modulated radiotherapy (IMRT) is a technique for treating cancer tumours using external delivery of radiation. To create a treatment plan the directions of the external radiation beams (typically 5 to 9) need to be specified. Normally the beams are all coplanar due to the added complexity of planning and patient set-up for non-coplanar beams. RTStar provides a virtual environment of a radiotherapy (RT) treatment room that provides a range of views and visualizations that aid a treatment planner to choose non-coplanar beam directions efficiently. RTStar also automatically warns the planner when a collision would occur during patient set-up. A study was conducted on 8 prostate IMRT cancer patients using RTStar to create RT plans using non-coplanar beams. The study demonstrated that these IMRT prostate plans with non-coplanar beams had a dosimetric advantage over their coplanar conterparts.

Keywords. Visualization, radiotherapy planning, collision detection.

1. Introduction

Intensity modulated radiotherapy (IMRT) [1] is a technique for treating cancer using external delivery of radiation. The radiation field is delivered from a number of beam directions (typically 5 to 9) by a linear accelerator. The shape of each radiation beam is matched to the shape of the tumour and the intensity of radiation is modulated across the cross section of the beam via collimation. A challenging task for the treatment planner is choosing the best set of beam directions. Once chosen an inverse planning optimisation algorithm computes the dose intensity across each beam taking into account dose constraints for the tumour and surrounding critical organs (known as organs at risk). Typically, all the beams of the plan are coplanar (i.e. they all lie in the same plane, normally the axial plane of the patient). This coplanar approach guarantees that the rotating gantry of the linear accelerator does

---

[1] Corresponding author: Roger Phillips, Department of Computer Science, University of Hull, Cottingham Road, Hull, East Riding of Yorkshire, UK, HU6 7RX; E-mail: r.phillips@hull.ac.uk

not collide with the patient. Use of non-coplanar beams has been reported [2] but the possibility of a collision and additional set-up complexity reduces their use. We have developed a visualization software, RTStar, that can be used with a commercial radiotherapy planning system to create IMRT plans with non-coplanar beams. RTStar features an interactive immersive environment of a radiotherapy (RT) treatment room. This environment contains the patient and it provides automatic detection of potential collisions between the patient and surrounding equipment. Section 2 describes RTStar's facilities that support RT planning. Sections 3 to 5 present a prostate study where RTStar was used to create IMRT plans with non-coplanar beams. These showed a dosimetric improvement over coplanar plans.

2. Tools and Method

The software application RTStar provides a range of simulations and visualizations based on a virtual RT treatment room. RTStar's initial use was for education and interactive immersive training of RT [3,4]. This paper reports how RTStar was extended to support RT planning and its application to plan non-coplanar beams.

The approach adopted for non-coplanar planning of beams is that the RT treatment is first planned using a set of coplanar beams via a commercial RT treatment plan review system (in our case CMS Focal - see www.cms-stl.com). The treatment plan is then uploaded into RTStar. Using RTStar's flexible visualization and automated collision detection facilities, the RT planner manually adjusts one or more beams to achieve a better position. The objectives in seeking an improved beam direction are typically to obtain a better heterogeneous dose distribution to the planned tumour volume (PTV) or provide better dose sparing to the organs at risk, for example by reducing dose to the dose hot spots.

These revised beam directions are then entered back into the RT planning system and a new treatment plan and its dose is computed.

2.1. Visualization Facilities

The virtual environment created by RTStar contains models of the patient, the RT plan, the treatment couch and linear accelerator, all set within a treatment room. This is known as the *room view* (Figure 1). The elements of the RT plan that can be visualized include the image data sets (typically CT / MRI), segmented volumes for the tumour (CTV, PTV, etc) and surrounding organs at risk (e.g. bladder, rectum), dose distribution for the treatment site, radiation beams and their constituent segments, etc. The models of the couch and linear accelerator are geometrically precise and match the equipment actually used for RT treatment. This as important in order to predict collision between the patient on the couch and the gantry of the linear accelerator. Full interactive articulation of the couch (3 DOFs) and gantry (2 DOFs) is provided to the planner. Dose visualization of the existing plan is provided by the display of various isodose surfaces and a dose colour-wash on the surface of the tumour and organs at risk (Figure 2). This dose visualization enables the planner to locate the hot and cold spots of dose for the current plan and to adjust a beam position to reduce their effect.

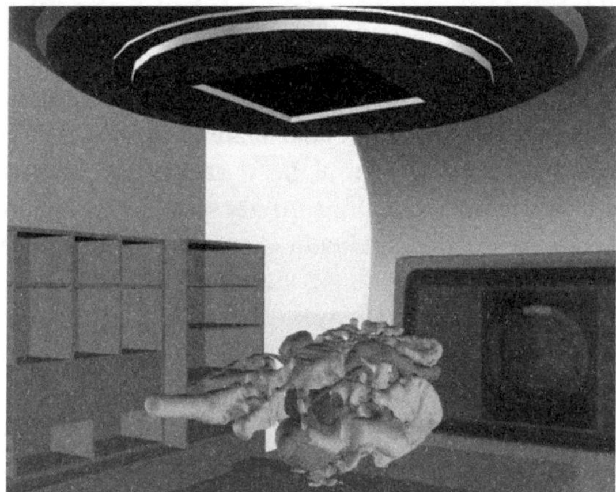

Figure 1. Room view of all segmented anatomy with skin hidden.

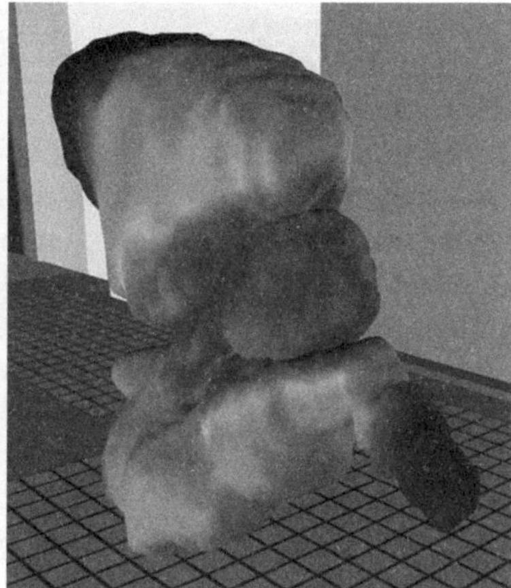

Figure 2. View of bladder (top), tumour (middle) and rectum (bottom) with dose colour-wash on surface of structures.

Visualization controls allow the display of the gantry, couch, image study sets, organs etc to be turned on and off and the transparency and colour of the anatomy and dose can be varied at will.

In addition to the room view, RTStar provides a *beam's eye view* (BEV), i.e. a view formed by looking down the central axis of the beam towards the treatment site. This view is particularly useful in determining the extent of overlap between the tumour and the organs at risk within a beam. This view helps the planner to adjust the beam direction to minimise such overlap.

RTStar uses a dual monitor set-up, with one being a 19" auto-stereo 3D monitor, and the other a conventional 2D monitor. The room view and BEV are divided over these two monitors. The room view can be displayed in stereoscopic 3D, which provides the planner with greater depth perception of the treatment site. The planner is able to navigate around the room view with ease and zoom-in on structures, fly between structures and even view inside structures as required.

Together, the above visualization facilities of RTStar allow the planner to assimilate quickly the juxtaposition between the tumour, surrounding critical organs, the radiation beam and its associated dose distribution and to efficiently and conveniently make adjustments to the beam directions.

2.2. Collision Detection Facilities

Potential collision between the patient, couch and the linear accelerator's gantry is detected automatically by RTStar as the planner adjusts the beam position. This avoids creating RT plans that can not be delivered in the actual treatment room.

Currently RTStar provides a visual warning (i.e. the gantry goes red) when a collision is about to occur between the gantry of the linear accelerator and the couch and patient. This is achieved by creating bounding volumes around the gantry and couch. For prostate and thorax cancer sites a bounding volume for the patient is created from the CT dataset and is extended to cover the whole patient. The bounding volumes include a margin to account for minor variations in actual patient set-up.

3. Prostate Study

The purpose of the study was to investigate the dosimetric advantages of using non-coplanar beams in IMRT plans compared to existing coplanar plans. For the study 8 IMRT prostate cases whose treatment had already been planned at the Boca Raton Community Hospital were randomly selected. Revisions to these existing plans aimed to achieve dosimetric advantage by choosing beam directions that would reduce the radiation dose to the rectum and the bladder.

For these 8 cases the coplanar 7-beam IMRT plans were normalised by setting the prescribed dose constraint that 95% of the tumour volume (D95) be at least 45 Gy. For all cases the 7 gantry angles were evenly spread from 35° to 325°.

Aided by RTStar's visualization facilities the heuristics for selecting better beam positions were established. Using the BEV it became evident that for the two most posterior beams, more than 75% of the rectum intersected the beam targeted on the PTV. Therefore to reduce the rectal dose, these two most posterior beams were rotated anteriorly until the overlap of the PTV on the anterior rectal lumen was reduced to 50% of the visible rectal cross section. This determined the limits of the two most posterior gantry angles for posterior oblique beams. The remaining 5 beams were then evenly arranged between these limits. To reduce the bladder dose, the two anterior beams either side of the AP beam were rotated inferiorly by about 40° to reduce the bladder overlap (Figure 3). Inferiorly tilting the AP beam would further reduce dose to the bladder, however it exposes the penile bulb to radiation which is highly undesirable [5], thus no adjustment was made to the AP beam.

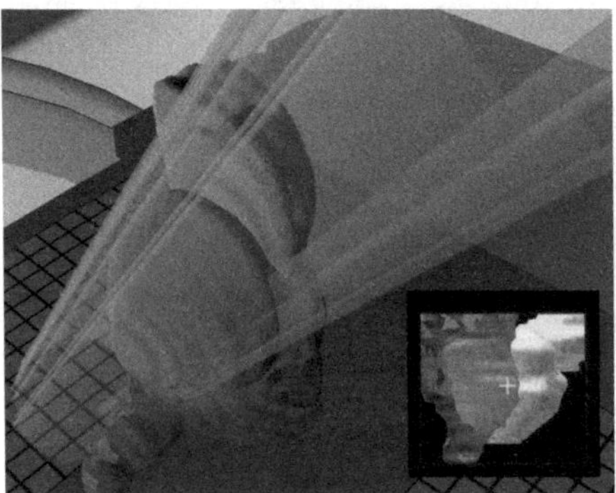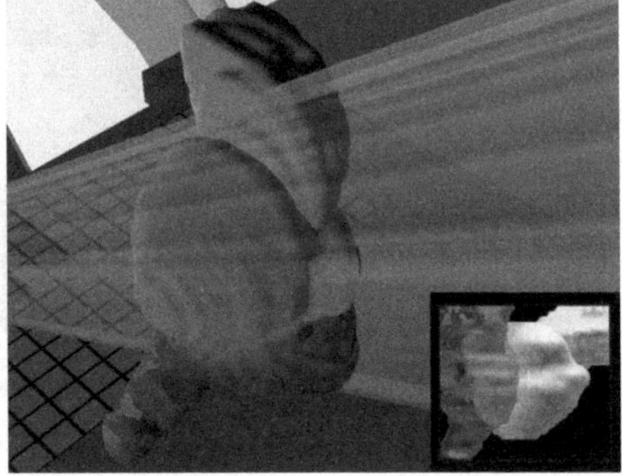

Figure 3. On the left, the view of the original right anterior oblique beam shows that almost the entire bladder overlaps the beam. On the right, a larger portion of the bladder is spared by inferiorly tilting the beam to create a non-coplanar beam. Inset shows the beam eye view (BEV) of the treatment site.

4. Results of Study

Dose homogeneity for the tumour was compared by analysing the global maximal dose (D Global Max) and the average dose of the 5% of the PTV that received the highest dose (D high 5%). A significant reduction in both indicators was observed in the test group as shown in Table 1.

Table 1. Comparison of dose homogeneity for the planned tumour volume (PTV)

	D high 5%			D Global Max		
	Control	Test	Difference	Control	Test	Difference
Max	5115	5025	-140	5416	5373	-191
Min	4828	4780	-5	4960	4864	-23
Mean	4958	4898	-60	5149	5065	-84
SD	108	86	58	146	156	56
t-test (2 sided)	0.022			0.004		

For the organs at risk, i.e. the rectum and the bladder, the mean dose (D mean) was determined. In addition, hot spots of radiation within each organ were analysed. For the rectum, the 10 cc of the rectum that received the highest dose (D 10cc) was determined. Similarly for the bladder the highest dose for 30 cc (D 30cc) was determined. The results for the rectum and bladder are given in Tables 2 and 3.

Table 2. Comparison of dose for the rectum (an organ at risk).

	D mean			D 10cc		
	Control	Test	Difference	Control	Test	Difference
Max	2573	2408	-231	4479	4437	-290
Min	1789	1885	180	3330	3150	20
Mean	2200	2185	-15	4053	3960	-93
SD	234	189	150	421	463	108
t-test (2 sided)	0.708			0.044		

Table 3. Comparison of dose for the bladder (an organ at risk).

	D mean			D 30cc		
	Control	Test	Difference	Control	Test	Difference
Max	4078	3991	-873	4770	4583	-425
Min	1084	838	231	3618	3408	-3
Mean	2767	2412	-356	4329	4159	-169
SD	1084	1037	324	405	409	125
t-test (2 sided)	0.017			0.006		

For the rectum there was no significant difference between the mean dose for the two groups. However, there was a significant reduction for the test group in lowering the mean radiation to the 10 cc hot spot.

For the bladder there was a significant reduction of the mean dose for the test group. Furthermore, there was also a significant reduction for the test group in lowering the mean radiation to the 30 cc hot spot. Together these two statistics indicate that for the bladder there is a significant dosimetric advantage for the test group.

5. Discussion

In the original IMRT plans with their coplanar beam setups, the structures adjacent to the PTV, including a large portion of the rectum and the bladder are exposed to the beams. By tilting two of the anterior oblique beams away from their coplanar positions to provide better dose sparing, a portion of the radiation dose was in fact shifted from the inferior portion of the rectum to its superior section. This contributed to there being no significant change to the mean rectal dose. However the rectal 10 cc high dose region showed a significant improvement due to this dose shifting. Not achieving a significant reduction to the mean rectal dose was rather unexpected as intuitively one would expect a reduction of rectal overlap to give a reduction of mean rectal dose.

However for the bladder, the BEV of these two non-coplanar beams clearly showed that the volume of the bladder in the beam was reduced (Figure 3). Consequently there was both a significant reduction for the test group of both the bladder mean dose and mean dose to the bladder's high 30 cc dose region.

This study also showed an improvement to dose homogeneity within the PTV.

We believe that non-coplanar beam arrangement is the sole factor for these dose improvements. As the two inferiorly tilted beams are further apart from their adjacent beams in terms of entrance point, this creates a more favourable pre-condition for dose intensity modulation.

6. Conclusions

The study reported has demonstrated that non-coplanar beam arrangement for prostate treatment can give better dose sparing to the bladder and reduce the high dose region of the rectum. The virtual simulation facilities of RTStar played a key role in developing and individualising the new set of optimal beam orientations.

The investigators of the reported study found the user-friendly visualization and collision detection facilities very important for IMRT planning with unconventional beam settings, including non-coplanar beam orientation. These facilities provided additional visual information that assisted the evaluation of the spatial relationship between the PTV and adjacent critical structures and helped analyse those organs at risk that intruded into a specific beam. RTStar is now being used to establish heuristics for including non-coplanar beams in plans for other treatment sites.

RTStar is being further developed to allow automatic collision detection for all treatment sites. Ongoing work is investigating creation of a full body model of a patient from PET images, including models of treatment aids, fitting a generic patient model to real patient data, adjustable collision margins, etc.

A software prototype has also been developed where the facilities of RTStar are seamlessly integrated into CMS's Focal RT plan review system.

References

[1]	Webb S, *Intensity-modulated radiation therapy*, Institute of Physics Publishing, Bristol, 2000.

[2]	Price Jr RA, et al, *Advantages of using non-coplanar vs. axial beam arrangements when treating prostate cancer with intensity-modulated radiation therapy and the step-and-shoot delivery method*; Int J Rad Onc Biol Phys 2002, Vol. 53:236-243

[3]	Phillips R, Ward JW, Beavis AW, *Immersive Visualization Training of Radiotherapy Treatment*, Proceedings of Medicine Meets Virtual Reality 13, pp 390-396, Jan 26-29 2005, Long Beach.

[4]	Phillips R, Ward JW, Bridge P, Appleyard RM, Beavis AW, *A Hybrid Virtual Environment for Training of Radiotherapy Treatment of Cancer*, Proc. Electronic Imaging Science & Technology: Stereoscopic Displays & Applications, San Jose, USA, Jan 2006, SPIE Vol 6505, pp 6055008 1-12.

[5]	Steenbakkers RJHM, et al, *Reduction of dose delivered to the rectum and bulb of the penis using MRI delineation for radiotherapy of the prostate*; Int J Rad Onc Biol Phys 2003, Vol. 57:1269-1279.

Medicine Meets Virtual Reality 15
J.D. Westwood et al. (Eds.)
IOS Press, 2007

Obstacle Crossing in a Virtual Environment with the Rehabilitation Gait Robot LOKOMAT

Mathias WELLNER [a,1], Thomas THÜRING [a], Eldin SMAJIC [a],
Joachim VON ZITZEWITZ [a], Alexander DUSCHAU-WICKE [a,b], and
Robert RIENER [a,c]

[a] *Sensory-Motor Systems Group, ETH Zurich*
[b] *Hocoma AG, Volketswil*
[c] *Research Spinal Cord Injury Center, University Hospital Balgrist, Zurich*

Abstract. The rehabilitation robot LOKOMAT has been developed at the Balgrist University Hospital to automate treadmill training of spinal cord injury and stroke patients. A virtual environment setup was implemented to increase patient's motivation and provide biofeedback, consisting of visual, acoustic and haptic modalities. Based on the knee and hip angles of the orthosis, an animated figurine moves through a virtual environment.

This contribution describes the setup of the system and selected technical performance parameters. We focused on delay times caused by the setup, stability of the haptic obstacle rendering and on the level of immersion as judged by four healthy subjects.

Results show that subjects judged the system's performance well (questionnaire scores over 80%). Problems exist though for obstacle rendering (questionnaire scores of 55%).

1. Background, Problem

The rehabilitation robot LOKOMAT (see Figure 1) has been developed at the Balgrist University Hospital to automate treadmill training of spinal cord injury and stroke patients [1].

Virtual environment techniques have the potential to enhance motor rehabilitation [2], especially by creating immersive game-like scenarios [3]. These provide extrinsical motivation cues (rewards and incentives).

The challenge was to combine LOKOMAT and virtual environment techniques to create an immersive, multi-modal obstacle-crossing scenario.

---

[1] Corresponding Author: Mathias Wellner, E-mail: wellner@mavt.ethz.ch

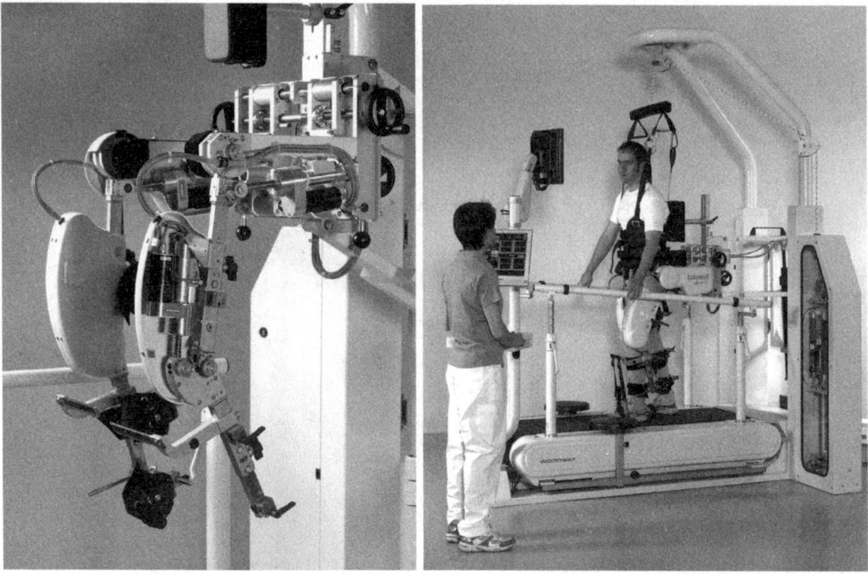

Figure 1. LOKOMAT leg orthosis

2. Tools and Methods

2.1. LOKOMAT *and Haptic Feedback*

The LOKOMAT is driven in a special mode, with the weight and friction of the orthosis being compensated with a model-based controller. The treadmill speed is controlled by the subject, using force sensors to measure the sheer force between feet and treadmill. The resulting force is used to compute the acceleration of the treadmill.

In addition, the LOKOMAT works as a haptic interface. The obstacles are implemented with virtual spring-damper systems. Penetration of the foot tip into the obstacle results in a force driving the foot out of the obstacle. The resulting force in walking direction x can be noted as:

$$F_x = \begin{cases} -K\,\Delta x - B|v_x| \text{ for } \Delta x > 0 \text{ and } v_x > 0 \\ -K\,\Delta x \text{ for } \Delta x > 0 \text{ and } v_x < 0 \\ 0 \text{ for } \Delta x < 0 \end{cases}$$

Δx: penetration depth, K: spring constant, B: damping coefficient, v_x: x-velocity

2.2. *Audio and Visual Feedback*

The audiovisual display consists of a 5.1 Dolby surround sound system and a large projection screen (3×2 m^2). Using polarization technique a 3D image can be seen by the subject. A figurine is visible (see Figure 2), walking over the obstacles in a beach scenario with palm trees and different underground materials (wood, water, grass, gravel).

Sound feedback consists of event-driven sounds (steps, obstacle hits) and background music. To find out signal latencies in the system (due to network latencies and multitasking) we conducted a test by creating a sample sound and measuring the delay

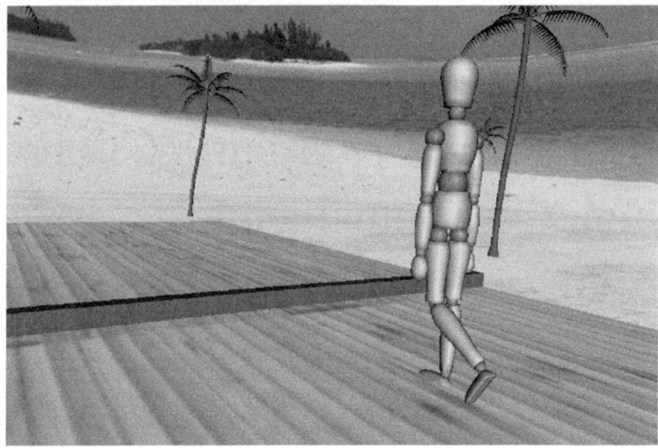

Figure 2. Avatar with beach environment

between triggering signal and speaker output. Due to the measured signal latencies a prediction method was implemented to trigger event-related sounds earlier.

3. Results & Discussion

The results for signal latencies were that the majority of values are between 100 and 150 ms. This is the reason why we needed to implement a prediction method to trigger step sounds earlier.

Tests were conducted with four healthy subjects and a questionnaire was created to evaluate the level of immersion of the scenario. Results indicate that the quality of visual and acoustic feedback are judged well (questionnaire scores are over 80%) and that obstacle force feedback is seen slightly worse (55% for obstacle rendering).

4. Conclusion

The goal of creating an immersive, multi-modal scenario was successfully achieved. Next steps include optimizing the obstacle rendering and conducting experiments to investigate human feedback mechanisms and improve visual and acoustic feedback modalities for obstacle walking.

References

[1]   Robert Riener, Lars Lünenburger, and Gery Colombo. Human-Centered Robotics Applied to Gait Training and Assessment. *Veterans Admin. Journal of Rehabilitation Research and Development*, 2006.
[2]   Dario G. G. Liebermann, Aron S. S. Buchman, and Ian M. M. Franks. Enhancement of motor rehabilitation through the use of information technologies. *Clin Biomech (Bristol, Avon)*, September 2005.
[3]   A. A. Rizzo, I. Cohen, P. L. Weiss, J. G. Kim, S. C. Yeh, B. Zaii, and J. Hwang. Design and development of virtual reality based perceptual-motor rehabilitation scenarios. In *Engineering in Medicine and Biology Society, 2004. EMBC 2004. Conference Proceedings. 26th Annual International Conference of the*, volume 2, pages 4852–4855 Vol.7, 2004.

Medicine Meets Virtual Reality 15
J.D. Westwood et al. (Eds.)
IOS Press, 2007

GPU-Friendly Marching Cubes for Visualizing Translucent Isosurfaces

Yongming XIE, Pheng-Ann HENG, Guangyu WANG, and Tien-Tsin WONG
Department of Computer Science and Engineering
Shun Hing Institute of Advanced Engineering
The Chinese University of Hong Kong

Abstract. Marching cubes has long been employed as a standard indirect volume rendering approach to extract isosurfaces from 3D volumetric data. This paper presents a GPU-friendly MC implementation. Besides the cell indexing, we propose to calculate vertex and normal interpolations by precomputing the expensive equations and looking up these values during runtime. Upon a commodity GPU, our implementation can rapidly extract isosurfaces from a high-resolution volume and render the result. With the proposed parallel marching cubes algorithm, we can naturally generate layer-structured triangles, which facilitate the visualization of multiple-layer translucent isosurfaces without performing computational expensive sorting. The algorithm extracts and draws triangles, in a layer by layer fashion, from back to front.

Keywords. Isosurface extraction, volume rendering, hardware acceleration

Introduction

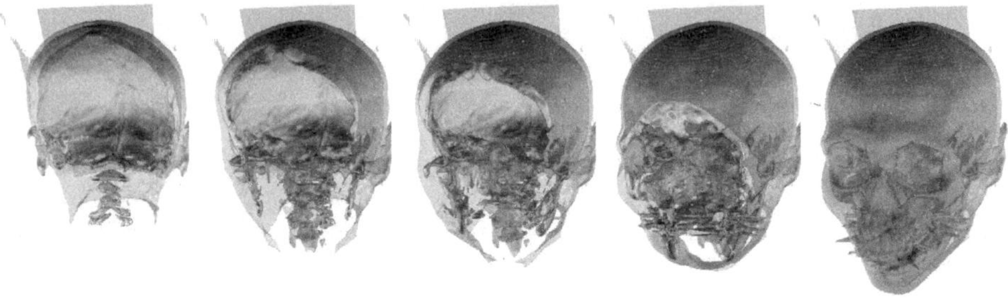

Figure 1. Multiple translucent isosurfaces are visualized, with the proposed GPU-friendly marching cubes algorithm, which draws triangles from back to front. Fine details and the relationship among inner structures are well illustrated.

Isosurfaces have been widely adopted to reveal the complex structures in medical and scientific volume data, due to its fine visual quality. Visualizing multiple layers of translucent isosurfaces (normally represented as triangles) not just generates high-quality rendering results, but also allows viewers to better understand the relationship among internal structures (Figure 1).

This paper proposes a GPU-friendly isosurface extraction method that facilitates the visualization of multiple layers of translucent isosurfaces as demonstrated in Figure 1.

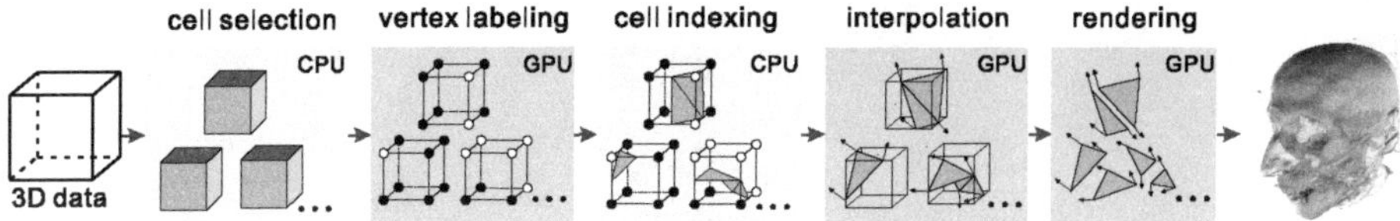

Figure 2. Framework of the proposed method.

Instead of performing visibility sorting, triangles are drawn from the back to front in a layer-by-layer fashion. This approach allows us to visualize the complex translucent isosurfaces in real time. The layer-structured triangles are directly generated by the proposed GPU-based isosurface extractor according to the user-specified isovalues. Our system utilizes the graphics processing unit (GPU) to extract the isosurfaces and achieves an interactive rate even the isosurfaces are on-the-fly generated and rendered.

We employ the classical marching cubes (MC) [4] as our GPU-based isosurface extractor. Most existing GPU-based methods make use of the marching tetrahedra (MT) [2,3,6]. Although MT can resolve the ambiguity, it normally generates excessive number of triangles. Hence, we believe MC is a more cost effective to implement on GPU. By marching the cubes in a layer-by-layer fashion, our method naturally generates triangles in a layer ordering that in turn facilitates our painter style rendering. Moreover, our method explicitly generates triangles within GPU memory. They can be transferred to main memory for further processing. Although we only implement MC algorithm in our framework, it can be trivially modified to most MC variants, such as MC *33* [1], MC* [5].

1. Framework

The framework of the proposed method is shown in Figure 2. There are two parts: extraction and rendering. Extraction is completed by our GPU-friendly MC algorithm. In the rendering part, the extracted geometry is rendered layer by layer, from back to front. Our rendering process facilitated visualization of multiple translucent isosurfaces, without computational expensive sorting. As shown in Figure 2, the proposed algorithm consists of the following main steps:

1. **Cell selection**　In the 3D volume data, active cells are determined.
2. **Vertex labeling**　Each vertex of the active cell is marked, by comparison with the given isovalue.
3. **Cell indexing**　According to the labels, it indexes the active cell in lookup tables, and determines its active edges and how corresponding isosurface vertices must be connected to form triangles.
4. **Normal calculation**　It computes vertex normal by neighboring vertices.
5. **Interpolation**　For each active edges, it computes the position and gradient of the corresponding isosurface vertex by linear interpolation.
6. **Rendering**　Given the extracted geometry, it draws triangles from back to front, with the painter's algorithm.

In the proposed method, cell selection and indexing are executed on CPU. Vertex labeling, normal calculation, interpolation, and rendering are completed by GPU.

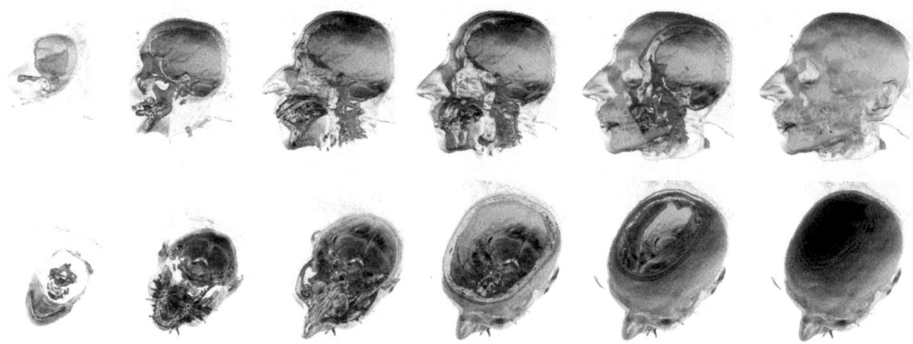

Figure 3. Other rendering results.

2. Results

To evaluate the proposed algorithm, we test it with a variety of 3D medical volume data. Some rendering results are shown in Figure 3. For a high-resolution data set, we can get high-speed interactive isosurfaces extraction and rendering. For low-resolution data, real-time performance can be achieved.

3. Conclusions

In this paper, we present a GPU-friendly MC algorithm. The proposed algorithm can rapidly extract and render isosurfaces from high-resolution 3D volume data. Our framework can be trivially modified to implement a wide range of MC variants. With this framework, we can efficiently visualize multiple layers of translucent isosurfaces, without sorting. The extracted geometry is stored in GPU memory and ready for post-processing. Given the geometry, many other interesting applications can be developed.

Acknowledgement

The work described in this paper was supported by grants from the Research Grant Council of the Hong Kong Special Administrative Region (Project no. CUHK 4223/04E and CUHK 4453/06M) and CUHK Shun Hing Institute of Advanced Engineering.

References

[1] E. V. Chernyaev. Marching cubes 33: Construction of topologically correct isosurfaces. Technical Report CN/95-17, CERN, 1995.

[2] P. Kipfer and R. Westermann. GPU construction and transparent rendering of iso-surfaces. In *Proc. of Vision, Modeling and Visualization 2005*, pages 241–248, 2005.

[3] T. Klein, S. Stegmaier, and T. Ertl. Hardware-accelerated reconstruction of polygonal isosurface representations on unstructured grids. In *Proc. of Pacific Graphics 2004*, pages 186–195, 2004.

[4] W. E. Lorensen and H. E. Cline. Marching cubes: A high resolution 3D surface construction algorithm. *Computer Graphics (Proc. of SIGGRAPH 1987)*, 21:163–169, 1987.

[5] G. M. Nielson. MC*: Star functions for marching cubes. In *Proc. of IEEE Visualization 2003*, pages 59–66, 2003.

[6] F. Reck, C. Dachsbacher, R. Grosso, G. Greiner, and M. Stamminger. Realtime isosurface extraction with graphics hardware. In *EUROGRAPHICS 2004 Short Presentations*, 2004.

Medicine Meets Virtual Reality 15
J.D. Westwood et al. (Eds.)
IOS Press, 2007

503

Can we remember stiffness?

Yasushi YAMAUCHI
*National Institute of Advanced Industrial Science and Technology (AIST), Tsukuba,
Japan*

Abstract. [Aim] This study aims at evaluating how exactly we can understand and remember given force information. [Methods] A forceps is attached to the PHANToM Premium 6DOF's stylus. By manipulating the forceps one can touch virtual objects. Nine subjects participated in this study. First, an object with certain stiffness k_g is presented: the subject can touch and learn its stiffness for 15 seconds. Then, following 15 seconds intermission, 20 objects with gradually different stiffness are presented. The subject touches these objects and chooses one of them, that has the same stiffness as the object presented before the intermission. This test is repeated 16 times for different k_g. [Results] The average 'remembered' stiffness k_r is in close agreement with the given stiffness k_g, but its variation is large ($0.12 < SD/k_g < 0.60$). [Conclusions] We can roughly remember the object's stiffness from force-feedback through a forceps.

Keywords. force-feedback, elasticity, surgical simulator, surgical robot.

Introduction

Several surgical simulators have been developed aiming at surgical education and preoperative rehearsal. Some simulators, such as *VSOne*, arc equipped with force feedback, and others, such as *MIST-VR*, are without force feedback. The surgical robot *da Vinci* has no force feedback, and its operators sometimes feel difference compared with conventional operations.

The force feedback can enhance the visual feedback and augment intuitiveness of the manipulation of surgical devices [1][2]. On the other hand, the force feedback feature requires force sensors and actuators, thus results in more complex and expensive systems.

From an aspect of ergonomics, this study aims at evaluating how exactly we can understand and remember given force information, and how the force feedback is effective for surgical devices.

Method

The task we chose is to touch an object by a forceps and recognize its stiffness. The following two tests are carried out.

1) Difference threshold test

In this test, two objects with different stiffness are presented simultaneously: the minimum difference of stiffness that subjects can distinguish is recorded.

A PHANToM Premium 6DOF is used as a force feedback device. The tip of a forceps is fixed to the stylus of the PHANToM, and is manipulated in an abdominal model (Figure 1). The subjects can 'touch' virtual elastic objects defined in software.

A virtual elastic object is a rectangular plane. When the forceps 'touches' it, a reaction force is generated perpendicular to the plane.

In this test, two virtual elastic objects with different stiffness ($k_0 \pm \Delta k/2$) are presented at once, and the subject answers which object has higher stiffness (Figure 2). The k_0 varies with 0.25, 0.50, 1.00 (N/mm), and the Δk varies with 0.05, 0.10, 0.20 and 0.40 (N/mm).

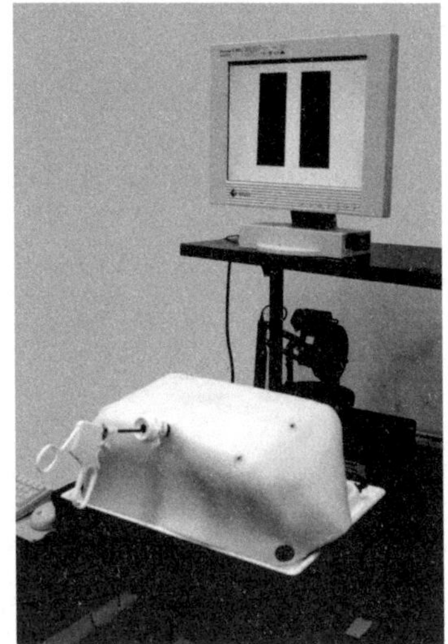

Figure 1 A force-feedback system with a forceps

2) Stiffness recognition test

This test is to reveal how accurate and quantitatively the subjects remember given stiffness information.

The experiment system is as same as the difference threshold test. First, a large virtual elastic object, whose stiffness is randomly selected within 0.15 to 0.90 (N/mm), is presented. The subject touches and learns its stiffness for 15 seconds. After an intermission for 15 seconds, 20 small virtual elastic objects are presented (Figure 3). The stiffness of these objects is gradually different from 0.05 to 1.00 (N/mm). The subject touches them and chooses one that is assumed to have the same stiffness as the large object presented before.

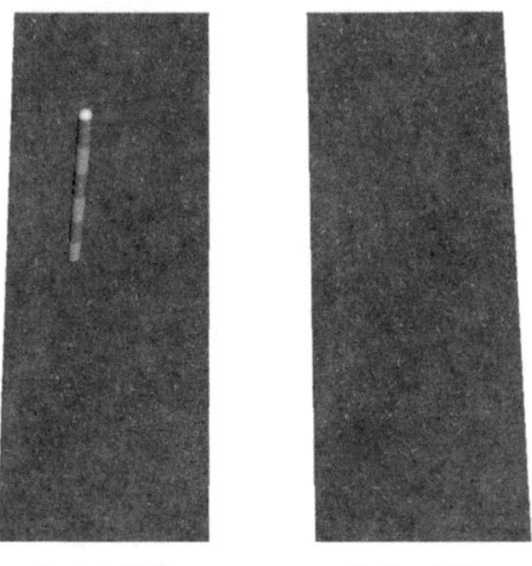

Figuer 2 Touching two objects with different stiffness

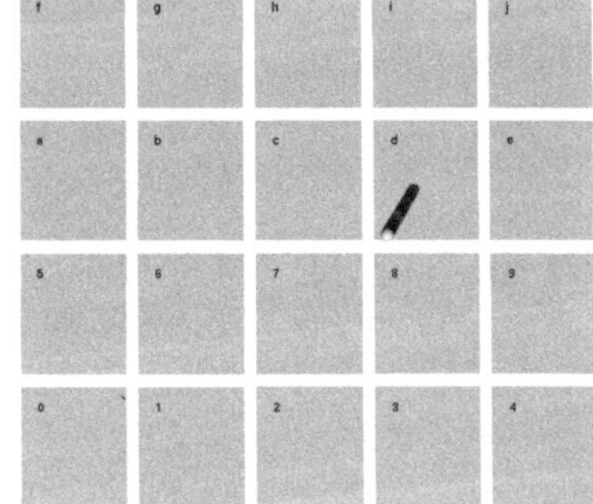

Figure 3 Touching one of the 20 virtual objects with different stiffness

Result

Nine subjects without experience of laparoscopic surgery participated in this study. To eliminate the learning effect, five training tasks are carried out before each test.

Table 1 shows the result of the difference threshold test. k_0 is the mean stiffness of two objects, and Δk is the difference of stiffness. The values are the ratio of the correct answers, and * indicate the combination of the k_0 and Δk where the ratio is statistically high (binominal test, $p < 0.05$).

Figure 4 shows the result of the stiffness recognition test. The horizontal axis k_g indicate the real stiffness of the large virtual elastic object, and vertical axis k_r indicates the average of 'remembered' stiffness, that the subjects chose one of 20 small objects. Error bars indicate standard deviation (SD). The k_g and the average of k_r correspond well, but the variance is large: the ratio of SD to k_g reaches from 0.12 to 0.60.

Discussion

In the difference threshold test, larger Δk and bigger k_0 resulted in higher ratio of correct answers. This result implies that this test follows Weber's Law, and its Weber's ratio is approximately 20%. This ratio is far high compared with that of the vision (about 2%). In the stiffness recognition test, the variance of remembered stiffness is much larger than Weber's ratio.

In conclusion, we can remember the difference of stiffness, but roughly.

Table 1 Ratio of correct answer for each combinations of stiffness (k_0) and difference of stiffness (Δk) *: $p < 0.05$

		Δk (N/mm)			
		0.05	0.10	0.20	0.40
	0.25	0.78*	0.94*	1.00*	1.00*
k_0 (N/mm)	0.50	0.67	0.83*	1.00*	1.00*
	1.00	0.44	0.56	0.22	0.39

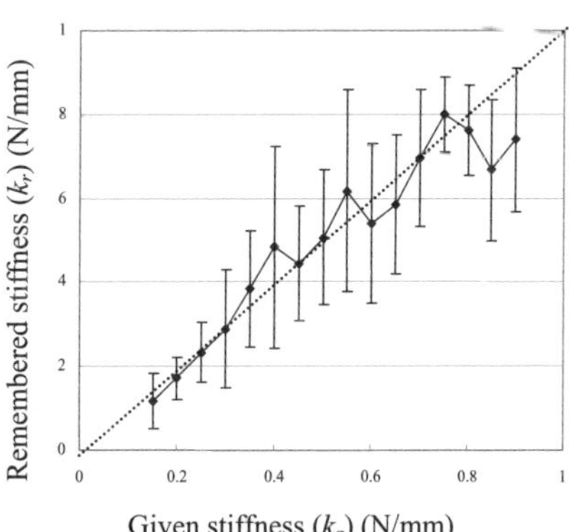

Figure 4 The result of the stiffness recognition test. The given stiffness (k_g) of the large virtual elastic object vs. the 'remembered' stiffness (k_r).

References

[1] Gerovich O, Marayong P, Okamura AM. The effect of visual and haptic feedback on computer-assisted needle insertion. Comput Aided Surg 2004;9(6):243-9.

[2] den Boer KT, et al. Sensitivity of laparoscopic dissectors. What can you feel? Surg Endosc 1999;13(9):869-73.

Weber's Law:
A just-noticeable difference in a stimulus is proportional to the magnitude of the original stimulus.

Medicine Meets Virtual Reality 15
J.D. Westwood et al. (Eds.)
IOS Press, 2007

VR Enhanced Upper Extremity Motor Training for Post-Stroke Rehabilitation: Task Design, Clinical Experiment and Visualization on Performance and Progress

Shih-Ching Yeh[1], Albert Rizzo[2], Margaret McLaughlin[1], Thomas Parsons[2]
[1]Integrated Multimedia Systems Center, [2] Institute for Creative Technologies
University of Southern California
shihchiy@usc.edu , arizzo@usc.edu, mmclaugh@usc.edu, TParsons@ict.usc.edu

1. Background &Overview

Stroke is the leading cause of serious, long-term disability among American adults. Each year over 700,000 people suffer a new or recurrent stroke, and nearly 500,000 (71%) survive with some form of enduring neurological disability. Upper extremity (UE) motor impairment is a common consequence of stroke and often produces significant challenges for patients as they engage in everyday instrumental activities of daily living [1][2]. Fortunately, research has shown that such lost UE function can be recovered or improved via systematic, repetitive and task-oriented motor training. However, motor-training tasks used for conventional therapy are questionable due to limited capacity to systematically control stimulus presentations and to precisely capture motor response performance in real time. Virtual reality (VR) enhanced motor training is an emerging therapeutic modality that can serve to deliver UE motor training tasks within consistent, yet modifiable simulated functional environments that mimic real world challenges [3][4]. Further, with the use of advanced sensing systems in VR, a large quantity and wide variety of high quality data can be captured to serve the rehabilitation process. As well, game features can be integrated into the VR training to enhance motivation and promote therapeutic focus and adherence.

We build a VR interactive task: Static Reaching Task. It is designed to have patients reach multiple virtual targets in 3D space with synchronized forearm and hand movement on their paretic side, shown in Fig. 1. The challenges in developing and applying such a system to stroke rehabilitation are addressed below. 1) What strategies we can conduct the precise translated between real world and virtual movements so as to actively drive the patient's behavior? 2) What general forms of kinematic measures can be defined or derived via collected data so as to suitably represent the patient's behavior? 3) How can we quantitatively detect the patient's current status or evaluate the patient's progression via the use of such a VR interactive system?

In this paper, we first describe the system architecture with respect to each division's design and implementation so that it can meet the challenges 1) mentioned above. Then we introduce a variety of interaction measures with regard to their definition, derivation and representation so as to meet the challenge 2). Next we describe a clinical pilot test on stroke patients. And we propose a methodology to detect and visualize the patient's current status and progression via the collected data, in response to challenge 3).

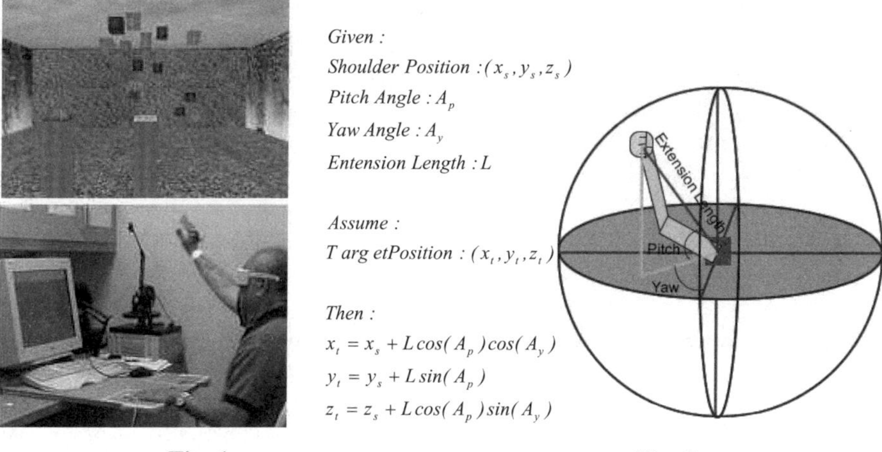

Fig. 1   **Fig. 2**

2. Design of VR System

To construct such an interactive virtual environment, shutter glasses are used to perceive the 3D world of virtual environment and the tracking device, Flock of Birds, is used to interact with virtual environment. Within the virtual environment, multiple cube-shaped targets are distributed simultaneously in 3D space. The subject, with trackers attached to his hands, has to extend the forearm to reach any one of the targets as desired without order requirement. The subject's hand has to move back to a start position between each reaching task.

The target position is a crucial factor in detecting the patient's ability to reach a specific zone in 3D space. It is positioned in a semi-spherical zone that is calibrated to each patient's current range of motion. A certain location within the semi-spherical zone requires a specific combination of pitch, yaw and extension of arm length. Thus, difficulty level can be distinguished according to various settings of the target's position via pitch, yaw and extension of arm length. The algorithm to set the position of the target is given in Fig. 2.

A mapping mechanism is carefully designed to convert measures from the physical world to the virtual environment. An accurate mapping can ensure that the system will drive the patient's activity such that he/she will behave in a way dictated by the therapist's rehabilitation design. First, target position in virtual world has to be allocated accurately with respect to the shoulder joint in real world. Thus, the tracker is put on the patient's shoulder joint upon the activation of program so as to set the initial position, shown in Fig. 3. And the arm length is measured. Second, the hand must have a fixed starting position in the physical world for each trial so that performance can be compared among trials. Thus, the start position in the virtual environment has to map with the start position in the physical world. Visual signs are given in both virtual environment and real world, shown in Fig. 4.

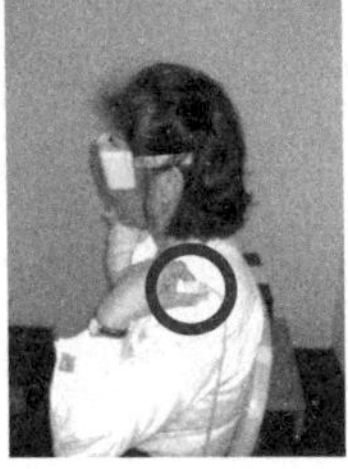

Fig. 3

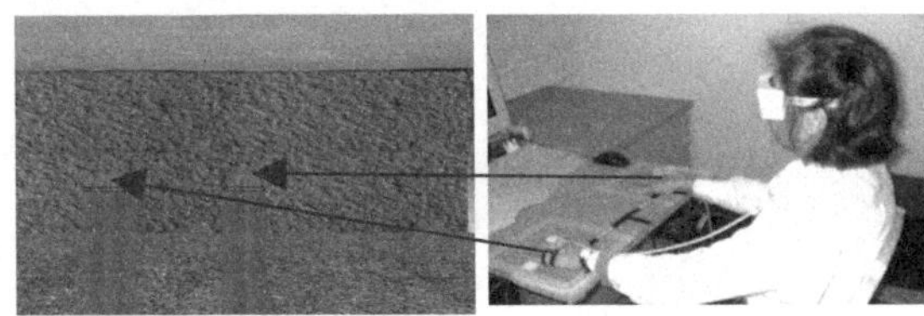

Fig. 4

3. Kinematic Measures

Kinematic measures are designed to evaluate the patient's behavior quantitatively. Status or progression can be visualized from these kinematic measures. Three types of kinematic measures are defined and used: performance time, movement efficiency and moving speed. They are derived from the position and orientation data of the hand tracker, recorded through the whole operation period at a data acquisition rate 60Hz.

Performance time (PT) is defined as the period between the time when the virtual hand started to move from the start position and the time the virtual hand reaches a target in 3D space. It is an index to indicate the moving speed without regard to the moving path. A lower value reveals a higher speed.

Movement efficiency (ME) is defined as the ratio of the actual moving path over the shortest moving path. The shortest moving path is the linear distance between the start position and the position of the virtual target. The actual moving path is the accumulation of linear distance for each time interval through the process of reaching. ME is an index of the patient's moving stability. A lower value of ME indicates a better moving stability.

Moving speed (MS) is defined as the ratio of the actual moving path over performance time. It is an index to indicate moving speed with respect to the moving path. Further, it is in direct proportion to ME while it is in inverse proportion to PT. Thus, it can also represent the integration of speed and stability. A higher value implies a greater degree of integrated speed and stability.

The equations to calculate ME and MS are given in Fig. 5.

4. Clinical Pilot Test

A three-month clinical experiment using this VR task (along with 3 others) was conducted from the USC Keck School of Medicine. Time since the stroke and severity of impairment are the two crucial factors that determine the extent to which patients can hope to improve motor function through the therapeutic process. Thus, the patient who volunteers to be a subject must first be screened. We first screened patient volunteers to see if they could meet the inclusion criteria: 1) stroke at least one month prior to the pilot trial; 2) over the age of 18 years; 3) able to attend 12 training sessions. Subjects were also examined to see if they had a Mini-Mental Status Exam score below 24, significant limitations in passive range of motion, or no active movement in the hemiparetic UE. Five subjects passed the screening and participated in the test. On the first day of participation, the subject was introduced to the VR task, the dynamic reaching test, and tried it out. After the learning session, the subject attended 12 training sessions. Assistance was provided by a physical therapist to avoid any improper movement that might cause pain or injury. Simultaneously, behavioral assessments were applied at three points: pre-training, mid-training (between the 6th and 7th visits) and post-training. Motor performance was evaluated via a standard arm function test: TEMPA. Severity of motor deficit was determined with the UE portion of the Fugl_Meyer [5], a measure of motor function.

5. Case Study: Visualization of Status &Progression

To visualize the current status in regard with each kinematic measure, we map each target's 3D position onto one zone in a pitch-yaw 2D chart that is then coordinated with each kinematic measure to generate a 3D performance map, shown in Fig. 6. Performance of each practice session, containing twenty targets in 3D space, can be visualized via a single performance map. And progression can be visualized from a set of performance maps across different time points. Moreover, all values are classified into three levels and labeled with different colors where red, blue and green stand for "Excellent", "Good" and "Fair" respectively. Further, the trend line across different time points can be derived via the average value of each practice session for each kinematic measure.

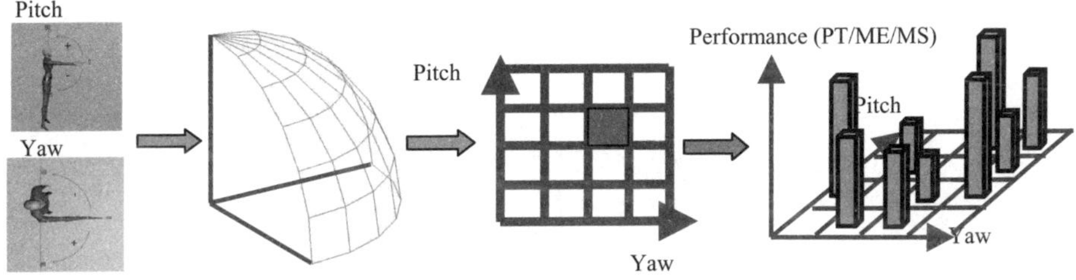

Fig. 6

Since a huge amount of data is collected, subject 103 with one single test case with reaching range 45%~60% (expected extension of arm-length ratio) is selected for case study and representing test results. The information of this selected test case (twenty targets) is presented in Fig. 7. This selected test case is practiced five times as listed in Fig. 8.

The performance maps of kinematic measure MS, for all practice sessions, are displayed in Fig. 9. It shows that most zones turn into "Excellent" level after five practice sessions while half of them are at "Good" level and the other half are at "Fair" level at the first practice session. The trend line, shown in Fig. 10, also shows that average performance of PT is in a positive trend toward better performance from first practice session to fifth practice session. Namely, performance PT is improved after five practice sessions.

```
Trial  size   pit    yaw    % of arm length
1      3      15     45     45
2      3      15     -15    60
3      3      0      60     50
4      3      45     75     45
5      3      30     45     50
6      3      15     90     60
7      3      75     60     60
8      3      0      75     60
9      3      0      45     45
10     3      75     45     50
11     3      15     60     45
12     3      60     30     50
13     3      0      15     45
14     3      0      30     60
15     3      15     30     50
16     3      90     15     50
17     3      30     30     45
18     3      60     60     60
19     3      45     15     45
20     3      0      -15    50
```

Fig. 7

$$ME = \frac{Actual\ Moving\ Path}{Shortest\ Path} \qquad MS = \frac{Actual\ Moving\ Path}{Performance\ Time}$$

Fig. 5

Session ID	Date
PS1	02-21-06
PS2	02-22-06
PS3	02-28-06
PS4	03-01-06
PS5	03-03-06

Fig. 8

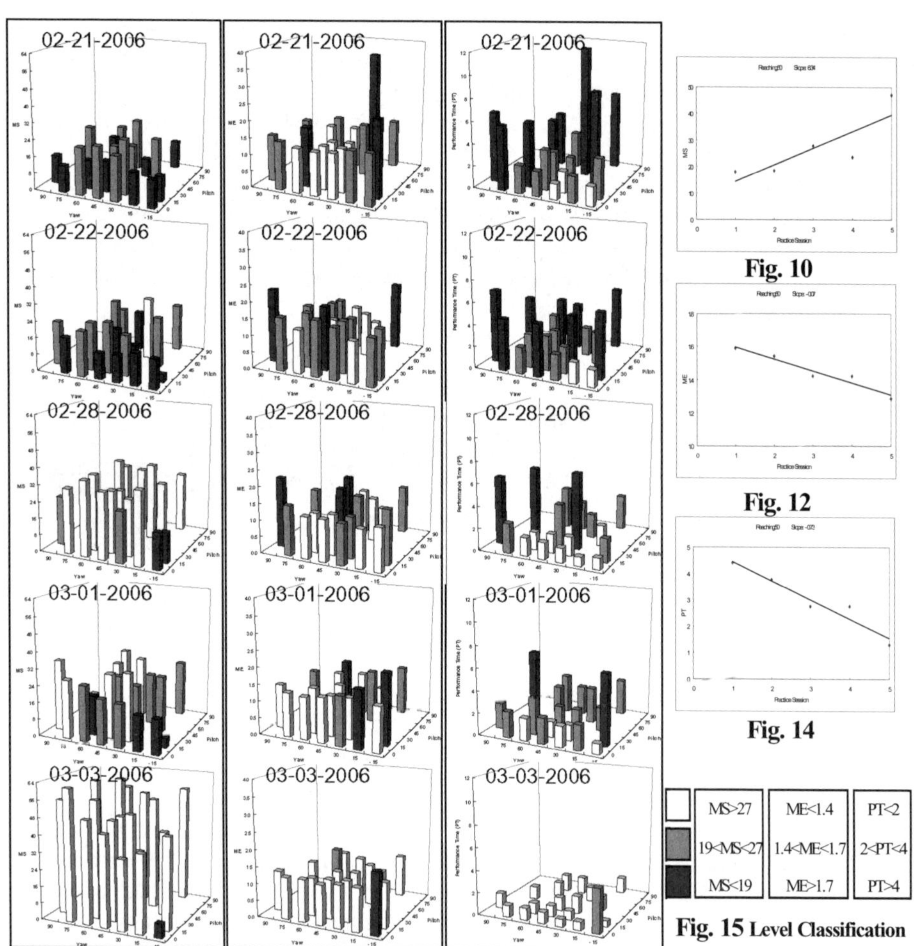

Fig. 15 Level Classification

Fig. 9 MS   **Fig.11 ME**   **Fig. 13 PT**

The performance maps of kinematic measure ME, for all practice sessions, are displayed in Fig. 11. It shows that the percentage of "Excellent" level is increased after five practice sessions. The trend line, shown in Fig. 12, also shows that average performance of ME is in a negative trend toward better performance from first practice session to fifth practice session. Namely, performance ME is progressed after five practice sessions.

The performance maps of kinematic measure PT, for all practice sessions, are displayed in Fig. 13. It shows that most zones turn into "Excellent" level at fifth practice sessions. The trend line, shown in Fig. 14, also shows that average performance of PT is in a negative trend toward better performance from first practice session to fifth practice session. Namely, performance PT is advanced after five practice sessions.

Further, they are classified into three levels and labeled with different textures in each Fig., shown in Fig. 15.

6. Conclusion &Future work

A VR enhanced upper extremity motor training task is designed well both in patient-specific need and in therapy perspective. The system equippes with an important feature which is the capability to actively drive human kinematic behavior via a combination setting of environmental parameters. Further, it is successfully applied to a clinical pilot test on five stroke patients.

Representative kinematics measures: Performance Time, Movement Efficiency and Moving Speed are defined suitably to represent kinematic features. Methodology is proposed to visualize the status and progression on a base of kinematics measures. The case study clearly revcales the patient's current status of hand arm movement with respect to his/her motion range composed of pitch, yaw and arm length. Further, progression is found and visualized quantitatively over a series of practice sessions on all three kinematic measures.

In regard with the future work, new technology advances need to be investigated such that system interfaces, such as 3D displays or tracking devices, can be replaced with more portable and cheaper devices. Such efforts can pragmatically evolve this interactive system into a home based rehabilitation tool. A larger scale clinical test on a larger sample of patients and with healthy controls is underway so that the functionality of the system can be verified and/or improved. Further, automatic diagnostic tools that measure current status and progression are being developed in our lab for future clinical use.

Reference

1. Mayo NE, Wood-Dauphinee S, Cote R, Durcan L, Carlton J. Activity, participation, and quality of life 6 months poststroke. Arch Phys Med Rehabil. 2002;83:1035-1042.
2. Jonsson AC, Lindgren I, Hallstrom B, Norrving B, Lindgren A. Determinants of quality of life in stroke survivors and their informal caregivers. Stroke. 2005;36:803-808.
3. Holden MK. Virtual environments for motor rehabilitation: review. Cyberpsychol Behav. 2005:8 (3):187-211.
4. Weiss PL, Katz N. The potential of virtual reality for rehabilitation. J Rehabil Res Dev. 2004;41 (5):vii-x.
5. Fugl-Meyer AR, Jaasko L, Leyman, I, Olsson S, Steglind S (1975). The post-stroke hemiplegic patient. 1. A method for evaluation of physical performance. Scand J Rehab Med, 7, 13-31.

Medicine Meets Virtual Reality 15
J.D. Westwood et al. (Eds.)
IOS Press, 2007
© 2007 The authors. All rights reserved.

Clinical Evaluation of the KAIST-Ewha Colonoscopy Simulator II

Sun Young Yi[a], Hyun Soo Woo[b], Woojin Ahn[b], Woo Seok Kim[b], and
Doo Yong Lee[b]

[a]*Department of Internal Medicine, Ewha Womans University, Seoul, Republic of Korea*
[b]*School of Mechanical, Aerospace and Systems Engineering, KAIST
Daejeon, Republic of Korea*

Abstract. This paper presents clinical evaluation of the KAIST-Ewha Colonoscopy Simulator II that is extended from the previous version jointly developed by KAIST and Ewha Womans University. Realism validation was carried out twice before the clinical evaluation. Nine fellows and six residents participated in this part of clinical evaluation study, and they were divided into two groups, simulation-trained and control groups. The control group was assessed through five colonoscopies to actual patients under supervision before starting the traditional patient-based training. They will be assessed again after the regular training is over. The simulation-trained group is being trained with two specially designed training scenarios. The subjects in this group will be also assessed through five colonoscopies to actual patients after completing the training. The study is in progress, and this paper reports preliminary results of the study.

Keywords. Colonoscopy Simulator, Clinical Validation

Introduction

Rigorous clinical evaluation involving physicians is integral to success of medical simulators. Clinical studies have been reported recently to asses realism, complexity and usefulness of the commercialized colonoscopy simulators, Simbionix GI-Mentor and AccuTouch [1-4]. It is shown that these simulators are particularly useful in the early part of the learning curve of the colonoscopy training [5,6]. This paper presents preliminary results of clinical evaluation in progress for the KAIST-Ewha Colonoscopy Simulator II [7].

1. Method

Realism of the simulation was first studied using questionnaire survey. Three colonoscopy experts and two fellows performed simulation using the developed simulator. The subjects were asked to express agreement or disagreement to a set of questions on the five-point scale. The result of the first survey was used to improve and modified the simulator. The second survey was, then, carried out in similar fashion.

Next, training efficacy of the simulator is being studied. Two training scenarios are used for the simulation-based training, which have different colon flexures and degrees of difficulty. The training scenario A is designed to teach practical skills to navigate the colon using combination of torque and up-down angulations. The scenario B is designed to teach skills to manage a loop formed in the sigmoid colon. The subjects should vigorously move and twist the colonoscope to straighten the loop and shorten the bowel. The simulator has a scoring system which is developed based on the performance criteria established by analyzing the experts' recorded simulation profiles including motion, force and torque.

Validation of training efficacy is in progress with participation of fifteen subjects including nine fellows and six residents. The subjects are divided into two groups, simulation-trained (n=9) and control (n=6). Before the control group began the traditional patient-based training, they had been assessed through five colonoscopies to actual patients under close supervision by experts.

Final assessment of the control group will be carried out after completion of the patient-based training. The subjects in the simulation-trained group will be also assessed through five colonoscopies to actual patients after completion of the simulation-based training.

2. Preliminary Results and Discussion

Figure 1 shows the results of the realism validation. In the first survey, the subjects agreed that visual graphics; force and haptic feel; and colonoscope control were satisfactory. Graphics rendering for air control and loop management was improved and satisfactory in the second survey. We can see that realism of the simulation is satisfactory in the all five categories in the second survey. Figure 2 shows the learning curves of three of the subjects in the simulation-trained group until they finished the training scenario A. The shaded region in each graph indicates the requirement to pass the particular criteria. These results show that the targeted colonoscopy skills are being acquired through the simulation-based training. The study is in progress, and consists of two phases. In the first phase, performance of the colonoscopies to actual patients by the group with no-training will be compared with the simulation-trained group. In the second phase of the study, the performance of the actual colonoscopies by the patient-trained group will be compared with the simulation-trained group to asses the training efficacy and efficiency of the developed colonoscopy simulator.

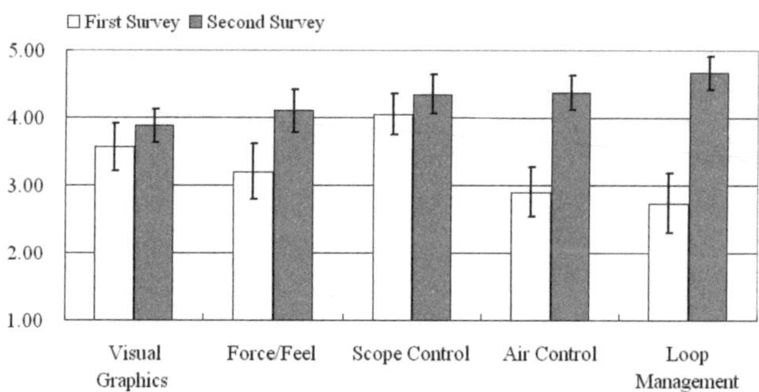

Figure 1. Result of the realism validation

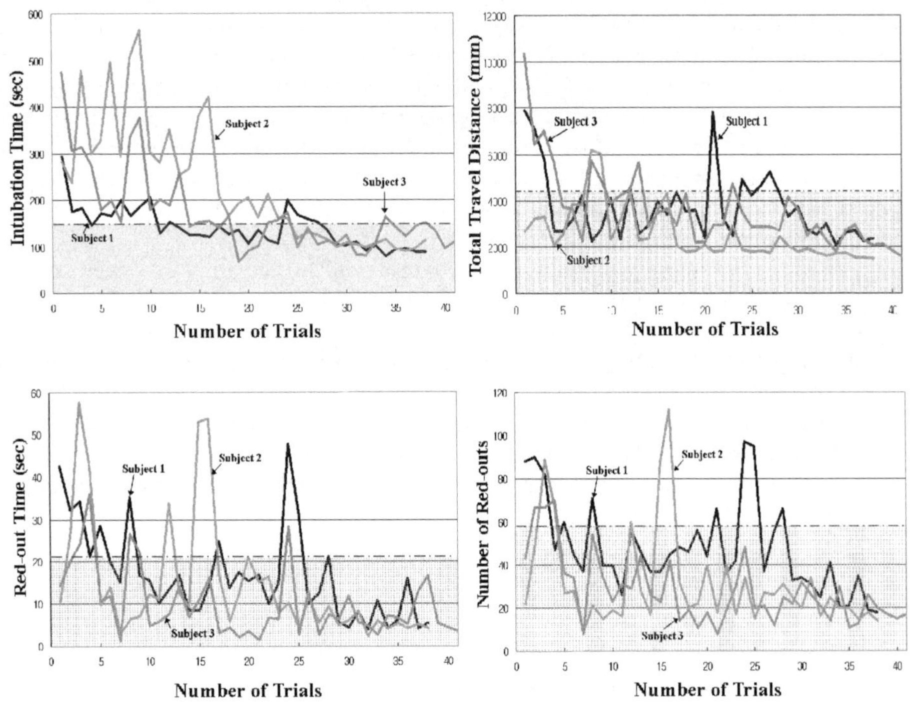

Figure 2. Learning curves of three of the subjects in the simulation-trained group

References

[1]   L. Aabakken, S. Adamsen, and A. Kruse, "Performance of a colonoscopy simulator: experience from a hands-on endoscopy course," Endoscopy, vol. 32, pp. 911-913, 2000.

[2]   Simbionix, Ltd., http://www.simbionix.com.

[3]   R.E. Sedlack and J.C. Kolars, "Validation of a computer-based colonoscopy simulator," Gastrointestinal Endoscopy, vol. 57, no. 2, pp. 214-218, 2003.

[4]   Immersion, Co., http://www.immersion.com.

[5]   G. Ahlberg, R. Hultcrantz, E. Jaramillo, A. Lindblom, and D. Arvidsson, "Virutal reality colonoscopy simulation: a compulsory practice for the future colonoscopist?" Endoscopy, vol. 37, pp. 1198-1204, 2005.

[6]   J. Cohen, S.A. Cohen, K.C. Vora et al., "Multicenter, randomized, controlled trial of virtual-reality simulator training in acquisition of competency in colonoscopy," Gastrointestinal Endoscopy, vol. 64, no. 3, pp. 361-368, 2006.

[7]   S.Y. Yi, H.S. Woo, W.J. Ahn, J.Y. Kwon, and D.Y. Lee, "New colonoscopy simulator with improved haptic fidelity," Advanced Robotics, vol. 20, no. 3, pp. 349-365, 2006.

Medicine Meets Virtual Reality 15
J.D. Westwood et al. (Eds.)
IOS Press, 2007

Virtual Worlds for Teaching the New CPR to High School Students

Patricia YOUNGBLOOD, PhD[a,1], Leif HEDMAN, PhD[b, c], Johan CREUTZFELD,MD[c], Li FELLANDER-TSAI, MD, PhD[c], Karl STENGARD,PhD[d], Kim HANSEN[a], Parvati DEV,PhD[a], Sakti SRIVASTAVA, MD[a], Laura KUSUMOTO, MS[e], Arnold HENDRICK[e] and Wm. LeRoy HEINRICHS, MD, PhD[a]

[a]SUMMIT (Stanford University Medical Media and Information Technologies), [b]Umea University, [c]Karolinska Institutet , [d]Huddinge SHS, and [e]Forterra Systems, Inc.

Abstract: In this study we created a virtual 3D world for learning to manage medical emergencies and evaluated it with 24 high school students in the USA and Sweden. We found that students in both groups felt immersed and found the online simulation easy to use. Scores for flow and self-assessed flow were significantly higher for the RHS group as compared to the HG group (p=.001 and .023 respectively; Mann Whitney U test). Self-efficacy scores for the HG group were significantly higher after training (p=.016 Mann Whitney U test). Males in the RHS group scored significantly higher on flow and self assessed flow than females (p=.006 and p=.023 respectively; Mann Whitney U test). This study demonstrates the potential value of using MMOS for learning to respond to medical emergencies.

Keywords: CPR training, flow, high school students, MMOS, self-efficacy, serious games, simulation, virtual worlds

Introduction

Two major studies have demonstrated the ineffectiveness of standard Cardio-Pulmonary Resuscitation (CPR) training of healthcare professionals [1],[2]. Despite the prevailing belief that using resuscitation manikins along with didactic instruction is an effective training methodology, about 25% of those trained immediately before testing on manikins failed correct performance. The purpose of our project was to create, evaluate, and assess learning outcomes when using virtual 3D worlds for training high school students to respond appropriately to a medical emergency requiring CPR.

1. Methods

In this project, the research teams designed, developed and evaluated a new approach to training laypersons to conduct CPR, using Forterra Systems, Inc.'s OLIVE (On-Line, Interactive, Virtual Environment) game development platform. In Massively, Multi-player, Online Simulation (MMOS), also called "virtual worlds", students/trainees play the role of a character ("avatar") in a scenario. Students interact with other characters ("avatars") in the virtual world by using the keyboard and mouse to control their avatar's actions/movements and headsets with voice over IP to communicate in real time with the other players. After the role-play, trainees participate in an instructor-led discussion of their performance in the scenario.

Researchers at Stanford University in CA along with teams from Karolinska Institutet and Umea University in Sweden and game developers at Forterra Systems Inc. worked collaboratively to design and implement studies at two sites—one with students at Redwood High School (RHS) in San Mateo County, CA and one with students at Huddinge Gymnasium (HG) in Stockholm, Sweden. The collaborators jointly designed the CPR scenarios, which were developed by the Forterra group, and implemented by the research teams, including the students' biology teachers, following the same research protocol. Figure 1 shows the virtual 3D world where high school students are conducting CPR on their teacher, who has suffered a cardiac arrest.

During the spring semester of 2006, evaluation studies were conducted with 24 high school students in the USA and Sweden. All students participated in the training scenarios and completed scales and questionnaires immediately following the role-plays. Ease of use, realism, total flow experience and self-efficacy were assessed. Both groups had been trained in how to conduct CPR, using the traditional manikin-based method. In the RHS group there were 8 females and 4 males; 10 were completing their fourth year in high school, one was completing the third year, and one was completing the first year. In the HG group, there were 5 females and 7 males, whose ages ranged from 16 to 20. For each scenario, four students interacted with each other in the same "virtual world" to practice the steps they would take to rescue the victim, who has had a cardiac arrest. After each role-play, the teacher conducted a debriefing session with the students to review their actions and identify the best ways to respond to the situation.

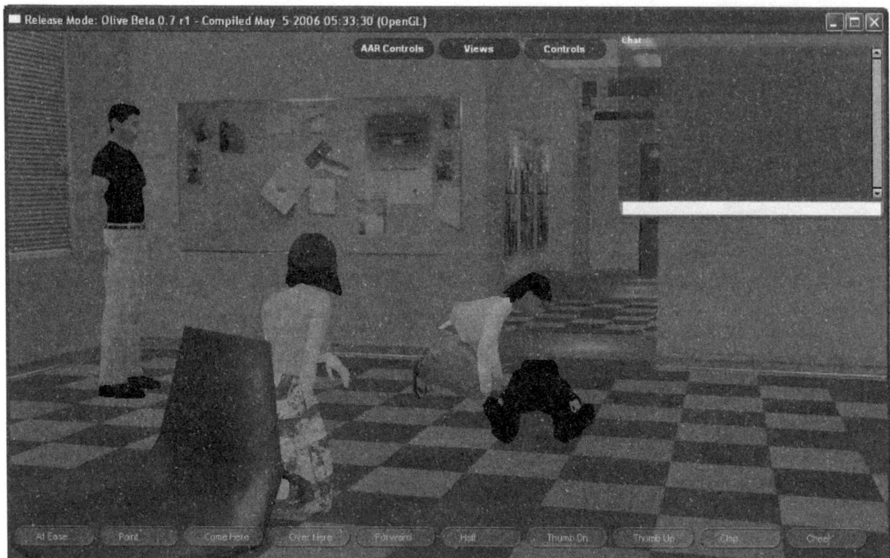

Figure 1: High school students conducting CPR on their teacher.

We performed both parametric (T-test) and non-parametric (Mann-Whitney U) tests using Statistica 7.0. The two analyses gave very similar results.

2. Results

2.1. Background variables

When asked about frequency of videogame play, the mean for the RWH group was 2.88 on a scale of 1-5 (where 3= once a month). Similarly, the mean for the HG group was 2.50 (where 3=once a week). No significant differences between the two groups were found for the background variables of immersion, computer experience and technical difficulty.

2.2. Ease of Use

Results indicate that on a scale of 1-5 (1=low and 5=high), the mean scores for RHS students and HG students respectively were 3.83 and 4.00 for "Extent of Immersion" and 3.97 and 4.00 for "Ease of Use" questions. In addition, RHS students indicated an increase in their confidence in reacting to a medical emergency before and after the training from a mean score of 3.97 to 4.46. When asked how useful they felt the new training system would be for learning to react to a medical emergency, the RHS students' mean score was 4.68. When asked if this type of simulated training would have a part in the education of tomorrow, the HG students' mean score was 4.60.

2.3. Flow experience and Self-efficacy

In addition to ease of use, the researchers sought data on two affective learning outcome variables: students' total flow experience [3] and self-efficacy before, during and after training [4],[5],[6]. These process variables are especially important to better understand the user's experience when engaging in simulation exercises.

There were no significant differences for the two groups –on the two indices of total flow experience used in this study: flow in scenario number 2 (assessed with 8 questions just after the scenario) and self-assessed flow (assessed by one "direct" question on their experience of flow). Hence, the measurements of total flow were stable.

The scores for flow were moderate to high for both groups (above 50), and very high for the RHS group (mean score of 81 of a maximum score of 100). T-tests showed that both total flow and self-assessed flow were significantly higher for the RHS group as compared to the HG group (p= .0003 and .0078, respectively). Non-parametric (Mann-Whitney U) tests revealed the same pattern; flow as well as self-assessed flow was significantly higher for the RHS group as compared to the HG group (p= .0009 and .0232, respectively).

Self-efficacy was relatively high (above the mean of 3.5) for both groups. However, no significant difference in self-efficacy was found between the two groups. Since self-efficacy was measured both before and after the training scenarios for the HG group, it was possible to evaluate whether self-efficacy changed with training for this group. Self-efficacy was significantly higher (p= .0158 Mann-Whitney) after training for this group.

2.4. Gender differences

With regard to the HG group, both the T-test and Mann-Whitney U test showed no significant differences between males and females regarding immersion and the affective learning outcome variable self-efficacy. However, females had less experience with computers (P=.04, T-test). For the RHS group, there were significant gender differences regarding the affective variable flow as measured by our two indices: total flow and self-assessed flow. Females had significantly lower scores for total flow and self-assessed flow than males (P=.0083 T-test; P=.0063 Mann-Whitney U test) and (P=.0061 T-test; P=.0232 Mann-Whitney U test) respectively. As mentioned before no such differences were found for the HG group.

3. Discussion

The data from these two studies support the use of MMOSs for teaching students to respond appropriately to a medical emergency requiring CPR. Both groups of students indicated they like the new interactive method of learning with Serious Games, and they would like more of the curriculum presented in this way. Our findings clearly indicate that both student groups' practice was associated with positive experiences of flow; their scores were generally high (above 50) on the Karolinska Flow Instrument. Students in the RHS group rated Total flow especially high, indeed higher than the ratings of the HG students. A reasonable explanation could be that the two groups of students may have coped differently with some of the technical difficulties using the prototype educational game.

For the second affective learning outcome variable - self-efficacy [5],[6] – the data showed no difference between the two groups. However, self-efficacy was relatively high (above the mean of 3.5) for both groups. It is believed that when simulation is used as a training method it improves students' confidence in related, real world tasks. Since both groups had equal opportunity to practice the tasks, both would be expected to experience a greater sense of self-efficacy after the training. Self-efficacy for the HG group was significantly higher after training in the scenarios. Consequently, for this group practice seems to have improved their self-efficacy. For practical reasons, the RHS group was not evaluated before training, so we have no before and after scores of self-efficacy for this group.

With regard to the affective learning outcome variable total flow, quite unexpected gender differences were found for the RHS group, but not for the HG group. RHS females had a significantly lower total flow than males; a difference that can be explained by the frequency of computer use. Although there were fewer boys than girls in the RHS group, it may be that the boys spend more time playing video games and therefore they found the virtual world easier to use. The RHS students, especially the boys, were highly immersed in the game. Games could be a diversion that is more appealing to high school boys than girls.

We also considered the cultural differences between the two groups. A major difference between the two groups of students is that the HG group may have been more achievement oriented with a curriculum that is professionally focused. In contrast, the RHS group is comprised of students in a "continuation" high school in which students are focused on the minimum competency necessary for achieving a high school diploma in preparation for employment. In fact, most of the RHS students have had school interruptions of 12-24 months for dealing with issues of pregnancy, family health, or legal detention, all factors that contribute to age and life-experience differences.

4. Conclusions

While manikin-based training continues to be the most appropriate method for learning the basic psychomotor skills of CPR [7], this study demonstrates the potential added value of MMOS for situated learning in which laypersons are able to practice the sequence of actions necessary to respond appropriately to different medical emergencies.

Acknowledgements

This study was supported by a research grant from the Wallenberg Global Learning Network (WGLN).

References

[1]   Wik L, Kramer-Johansen J, Myklebust H, et al. Quality of cardiopulmonary resuscitation during out-of-hospital cardiac arrest. JAMA. 2005;293:299-304.

[2]   Abella BS, Alvarado JP, Myklebust H, et al. Quality of cardiopulmonary resuscitation during in-hospital cardiac arrest. JAMA. 2005;293:305-310.

[3]   Hedman L, Sharafi P. Early use of Internet-based educational resources: effects on students' engagement modes and flow experience. Behaviour & Information Technology 2004, 23, 2:137-146.

[4]   Pintrich PR, Smith DA, Garcia T, McKeachie WJ. Reliability and predictive validity of the motivated strategies for Learning Questionnaire (MSLQ), Educational and Psychological Measurement, 1993,53:801-813.

[5]   Bandura A. Self-Efficacy: The Exercise of Control, 1997, New York: Freeman.

[6]   McGaghie W, Issenberg SB, Petrusa ER, Scalese RJ. Effect of pracice on standardized learning outcomes in simulation-based medical education. Medical Education 2006; 40: 792-797.

[7]   Wallin CJ, Meurlin L, Hedegård J, Hedman L and Felländer-Tsai L. Target-focused medical emergency team training using a human patient simulator: effects on behaviour and attitude. In Press 2006; Medical Education.

[1]Corresponding author: Patricia Youngblood, PhD, SUMMIT, 251 Campus Dr. MSOB x232, Stanford University School of Medicine, Stanford, CA 94305-5466 and E-mail address: <u>youngblo@stanford.edu</u>

Medicine Meets Virtual Reality 15
J.D. Westwood et al. (Eds.)
IOS Press, 2007

Towards an understanding of conventional surgical haptics for use in MIS[1]

John S. ZELEK [a,2], and Hao XIN [a]

[a] *Systems Design Eng., Univ. of Waterloo, Canada*

Abstract. In order to define what haptics to provide to surgeons during MIS (minimally invasive surgery), it is important to determine what a surgeon experiences via the tactile modality during conventional and laparoscopic surgery. We performed a set of experiments towards this goal using a laparoscopic tool during a push and gasp task, using an Omni haptic device to simulate the elastic properties of biological tissue. We found attenuation during both tasks, more so for passive (pushing) than active (gasping) activities.

Keywords. MIS, wearable haptics, tactile, kinesthetic

Introduction

The sense of touch (haptics) is a complex experience, arising from sensory receptors in the skin of the fingers pads, together with information arising in the joint and muscle receptors. This rich sensory information is crucial to many aspects of our daily lives: it is how we explore our world, how we communicate, work and play. Typically, we are not aware of how this sensory information is utilized, until it is lost or degraded. Vision is inherently subject to illusions which arise from distance-size subjectivity and depth being only implictly encoded in the 2D image. Alternatively, touch provides direct assessment of size and volume and provides object perceptual properties such as hardness, compliance, texture, temperature, weight, etc. Many robot-like devices currently exist which provide force feedback resolved to a single point. We are interested in producing wearable haptics for application in MIS using technology we have developed based on being able to produce forces using stacked miniature pager motors driven such that mechanically they are out of phase. In order to know what haptic experience to provide for MIS, we first need to quantify what the haptic experience is in conventional surgery. Minimally invasive surgery (MIS) can take 2 forms: (1) free-form: user holds probe-equipped with sensors (i.e., laparoscopic surgery); and (2) controlled: programmed robotic arms uses a probe. Some haptic feedback is experienced during laparoscopic surgery. In both cases of MIS, in varying degrees [1], hand-eye coordination is hindered and direct touching of the tissue is not possible. Because often surgeons rely on the sense of touch to deter-

[1] The authors would like to acknowledge the National Science and Engineering Research Council (NSERC) and PRECARN for their partial support.

[2] Corresponding Author: Systems Design Eng., Univ. of Waterloo, Waterloo, ON, Canada, N2L 3G1; E-mail: jzelek@uwaterloo.ca.

mine nature of the tissues, for instance to distinguish a nerve from a vessel, or healthy from cancerous tissues, the loss of direct contact with the tissues is one of the primary limitations of this new surgical approach. Nonetheless, MIS with smaller incisions and reduced tissue trauma translates into reduced wound complications, patient discomfort and hospital stays.

Currently available force sensing technology [2] includes force sensing resistor and capacitor-based elements and array systems. The alternative technology are strain gauge based sensors (i.e., such as force-torque sensors) and accelerometers, for detecting ridges [3]. Kinesthetic information can be captured via small accelerometers and bend sensors for joint angles. There are 2 types of grips: (i) precision grip is any grip that involves the thumb and one or more fingers with or without the palm serving passively as a prop; and (ii) power grip in which objects are strongly squeezed by the fingers alone or squeezed by the fingers, thumb, and actively by the palm [4]. Human precision grips for retrieval, holding, pinching and handling of objects are further classified in terms of the number of fingers in the grip. Basic categories of surgical instruments include specialized implements for the functions of cutting, grinding, and dissecting; clamping; grasping and holding; probing; dilating or enlarging; retracting; and suctioning.

Experiments

Our initial experiments have evaluated pushing and grasping using a laparoscopic tool to exert a force unto an object with elastic properties, essentially imitating the motion of surgeons when they poke at tissues to determine compliance. The grasping task involves picking up an object a pre-defined distance. The complete haptic information is captured using pressure sensors and an accelerometer to quantify the force and the kinesthetic data, respectively. To simulate the elastic properties of biological tissue but still maintain tight control over force exertion, the PHANToM Omni device from SensAble was used. The laparoscopic tools used is a tapered Maryland grasper with a plastic body. One Memsic dual-axis accelerometer is attached to the body of the graspers to capture the changes in horizontal and vertical tilts. Two Tekscan FlexiForce pressure sensors, mounted at the end-effector and the handle of the laparoscopic graspers, are used to capture the force component of the haptic information. The sensor on the handle is placed at the contact point between the thumb and the handle for both graspers. During the data capture phase, the PHANToM device is configured such that the pushing and grasping tasks moves the haptic arm for a distance of approximately 40mm to ensure comparability across different data streams. Data capture was conducted under four conditions or four spring stiffness: 0, 0.1 N/mm, 0.2 N/mm, and 0.3 N/mm.

We found minor differences in the motion of the grasper between the push and the grasp task, with more fluctuation in the vertical direction. There are more fluctuations in the motion of the grasper during the grasp task. The range of angle change is larger, and the differences between different spring stiffness are also more prominent. At the location of the end-effector, there appears to be more variation in pressure during the pushing task. However, the corresponding pressure data from the handle seems more uniform, suggesting a loss of information from the end-effector to the handle. The same effect is observed, though to a lesser extent, during the grasping task. The data suggests that there could be differences in the application of force depending on the task, and that

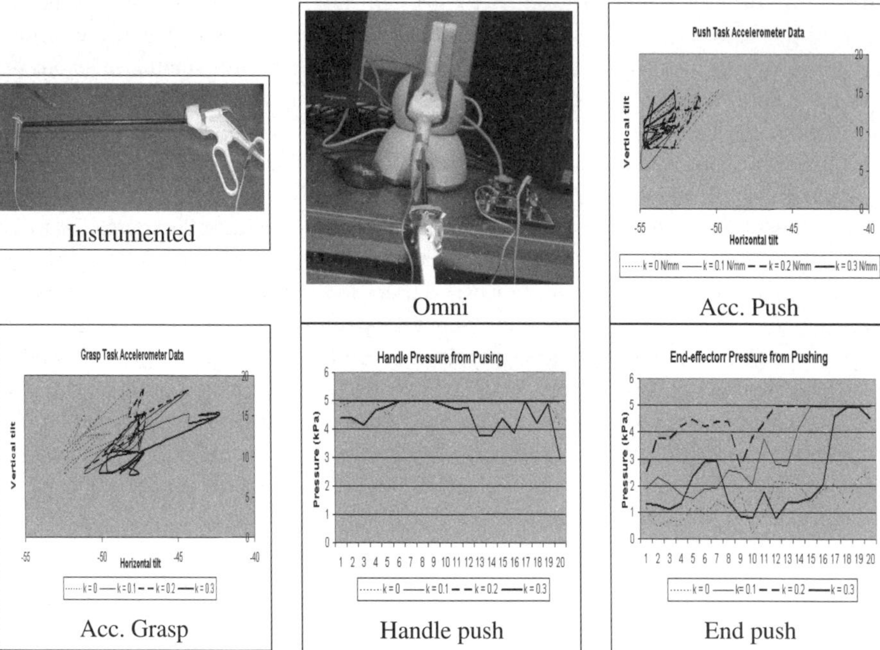

Figure 1. From top left to right and down: (i) instrumented Maryland grasper; (ii) Omni setup; (iii) Accelerometer data for push task; (iv) Accelerometer data for grasp task; (v) Handle pressure from pushing; and (vi) End-effector pressure from pushing.

the laparoscopic tool might be attenuating the force information such that the information availability is reduced.

In Closing

This preliminary experiment suggests that the laparoscopic grasper, and perhaps other laparoscopic tools, could be reducing the amount of haptic information available to the surgeons. We intend to repeat these experiments with other surgical tools so that we can develop models of the haptic experience during various procedures. This will help define what the augmented wearable haptics need to provide so that the MIS haptic experience is similar to conventional surgery.

References

[1]   T. Ortmaier, H. Weiss, and V. Falk, "Design requirements for a new robot for minimally invasive surgery," *Industrial Robot: An international journal*, vol. 31, no. 6, pp. 493–498, 2004.

[2]   J. Tegin and J. Wikander, "Tactile sensing in intelligent robotic manipulation - a review," *Industrial Robot*, vol. 1, 2005.

[3]   H.-Y. Yao, V. Hayward, and R. Ellis, "A tactile enhancement instrument for minimally invasive surgery," *Computer Aided Surgery*, vol. 10, pp. 233–239, July 2005.

[4]   M. Marzke, "Precision grips, hand morphology, and tools," *American Journal of Physical Anthropology*, vol. 102, pp. 91–110, 1997.

Medicine Meets Virtual Reality 15
J.D. Westwood et al. (Eds.)
IOS Press, 2007

Author Index